Pediatric Emergency Medicine

Moses Grossman, MD

Professor and Vice-Chairman, Department of Pediatrics, University of California, San Francisco

Chief, Department of Pediatrics, San Francisco General Hospital, San Francisco, California

Ronald A. Dieckmann, MD, MPH

Associate Clinical Professor, Departments of Pediatrics and Medicine, University of California, San Francisco

Director of Pediatric Emergency Medicine, Department of Emergency Services, San Francisco General Hospital, San Francisco, California

99 Contributors

J. B. Lippincott Company
Philadelphia
New York
St. Louis
London
Sydney
Tokyo

Pediatric Emergency Medicine

A Clinician's Reference

Acquisitions Editor: Charles McCormick, Jr.
Project Editor: Tracy Resnik
Indexer: Sandra King
Art Director: Ellen C. Dawson
Cover and Interior Designer: Arlene Putterman
Production Manager: Helen Ewan
Production Coordinator: Kathryn Rule
Compositor: Tapsco, Inc.
Printer/Binder: R. R. Donnelley & Sons Co.

1 3 5 6 4 2

Library of Congress Cataloging-in-Publication Data

Pediatric emergency medicine : a clinician's reference /
    [edited by] Moses Grossman, Ronald A. Dieckmann; 99
    contributors.
        p.   cm.
    Includes index.
    ISBN 0-397-51017-9
    1. Pediatric emergencies—Handbooks, manuals,
etc.   I. Dieckmann, Ronald A.   II. Grossman, Moses.
    [DNLM: 1. Emergencies—in infancy & childhood—
handbooks, manuals, etc.   WS 39 P371]
    RJ370.P452   1991
    618.92'0025—dc20
    DNLM/DLC
    for Library of Congress   90-6033
                                                    CIP

The authors and publisher have exerted every effort to
ensure that drug selection and dosage set forth in this
text are in accord with current recommendations and
practice at the time of publication. However, in view of
ongoing research, changes in government regulations,
and the constant flow of information relating to drug
therapy and drug reactions, the reader is urged to check
the package insert for each drug for any change in
indications and dosage and for added warnings and
precautions. This is particularly important when the
recommended agent is a new or infrequently employed
drug.

Figures 59-1 to 59-6 © 1987 Robert E. Markison.

To my wife, Verle, for her love and support over forty years,
and to our children and grandchildren.

M.G.

To my wife, Patty Gates,
To my parents,
And to Lauren and Marlowe,
For their love, inspiration, and hope.

R.A.D.

Contributors

Editors ■

MOSES GROSSMAN, MD
Professor and Vice-Chairman, Department of Pediatrics, University of California, San Francisco

Chief, Department of Pediatrics, San Francisco General Hospital, San Francisco, California

RONALD A. DIECKMANN, MD, MPH
Associate Clinical Professor, Departments of Pediatrics and Medicine, University of California, San Francisco

Director of Pediatric Emergency Medicine, Department of Emergency Services, San Francisco General Hospital, San Francisco, California

Associate Editor ■

KENT R. OLSON, MD
Assistant Clinical Professor, Department of Pharmacy, University of California, San Francisco

Medical Director, San Francisco Bay Area Regional Poison Center, San Francisco General Hospital, San Francisco, California

Contributing Authors ■

ALAN ADLER, MD
Chief Resident, Department of Pediatrics, San Francisco General Hospital, University of California, San Francisco, San Francisco, California

NICK G. ANAS, MD
Director, Pediatric Intensive Care, Children's Hospital of Orange County, Orange, California

BYRON Y. AOKI, MD
Associate Professor of Pediatrics, School of Medicine, University of Hawaii

Director, Pediatric Intensive Care, Kapiolani Medical Center, Honolulu, Hawaii

PAUL S. AUERBACH, MD
Associate Professor, Departments of Medicine and Surgery, Vanderbilt University

Director, Division of Emergency Medicine, Vanderbilt University Hospital, Nashville, Tennessee

STUART A. BAIR, MD
Assistant Clinical Professor, Departments of Pediatrics and Psychiatry, University of California, San Francisco, San Francisco, California

WILLIAM BANNER, Jr., MD, PhD
Associate Professor, Department of Pediatrics, University of Utah

Attending Physician, Division of Critical Care, Primary Children's Hospital, Salt Lake City, Utah

HENRY M. BARTKOWSKI, MD
Assistant Clinical Professor, Department of Neurosurgery, Ohio State University

Assistant Chief of Neurosurgery, Columbus Children's Hospital, Columbus, Ohio

CAROL D. BERKOWITZ, MD
Associate Professor, Department of Pediatrics, University of California, Los Angeles

Director, Pediatric Clinic, Harbor-UCLA Medical Center, Los Angeles, California

JAMES BETTS, MD
Director, Trauma Services, Children's Hospital and Medical Center, Oakland, California

RAYMOND L. BRAHAM, BDS, LDS RSC, MScB
Clinical Professor (Pediatric Dentistry), Department of Growth and Development, School of Dentistry, University of California, San Francisco

Clinical Professor (Dentistry), Department of Pediatrics, University of California, San Francisco, San Francisco, California

RICHARD H. CALES, MD
Associate Professor, Departments of Medicine and Surgery, University of California, San Francisco, California

MICHAEL L. CALLAHAM, MD
Professor, Department of Medicine, University of California, San Francisco

Chief, Division of Emergency Medicine, Moffitt-Long Hospital, San Francisco, California

STEVEN C. CASSIDY, MD
Fellow, Division of Pediatric Cardiology, Department of Pediatrics, University of California, San Francisco, San Francisco, California

SAMUEL F. CIRICILLO, MD
Resident, Department of Neurosurgery, University of California, San Francisco, San Francisco, California

PHILIP H. COGEN, MD, PhD
Assistant Professor, Division of Pediatric Neurosurgery, Departments of Surgery and Pediatrics, University of California, San Francisco

FELIX A. CONTE, MD
Professor, Department of Pediatrics, University of California, San Francisco

Co-Director, Pediatric Endocrinology Unit, University of California, San Francisco, San Francisco, California

MARY ANN COOPER, MD
Assistant Professor, Division of Emergency Medicine, Department of Surgery, University of Illinois

Director of Research, Division of Emergency Medicine, Department of Surgery, University of Illinois, Chicago, Illinois

KEVIN P. COULTER, MD
Assistant Clinical Professor, Department of Pediatrics, University of California, San Francisco

Assistant Director, Pediatrics Clinic, San Francisco General Hospital, San Francisco, California

KENNETH DRASNER, MD
Assistant Professor, Department of Anesthesiology, University of California, San Francisco, San Francisco, California

MICHAEL S. EDWARDS, MD
Associate Professor, Department of Neurosurgery, University of California, San Francisco

Director, Department of Pediatric Neurosurgery, University of California, San Francisco, San Francisco, California

MARTIN R. EICHELBERGER, MD
Associate Professor, Department of Pediatrics and Surgery, George Washington University, School of Medicine and Health Sciences, Washington, D.C.

Chief, Trauma Services, Children's Hospital National Medical Center, Washington, D.C.

DONNA M. FERRIERO, MD
Assistant Professor in Residence, Departments of Neurology and Pediatrics, University of California, San Francisco, San Francisco, California

JEFFREY R. FINEMAN, MD
Fellow, Division of Pediatric Critical Care, Department of Pediatrics, University of California, San Francisco, San Francisco, California

ILONA J. FRIEDEN, MD
Assistant Clinical Professor, Departments of Pediatrics and Dermatology, University of California, San Francisco, San Francisco, California

PIERRE GAUDREAULT, MD
Clinical Assistant Professor, Department of Pediatrics, University of Montreal

Director, Pharmacology and Toxicology Section, Saint Justine Hospital, Montreal, Quebec, Canada

EDWARD C. GEEHR, MD
Associate Professor, Departments of Medicine and Surgery, Albany College of Medicine

Chief, Division of Emergency Medicine, Albany College of Medicine, Albany, New York

ALAN M. GELB, MD
Associate Clinical Professor, Department of Medicine, University of California, San Francisco

Chief, Department of Emergency Services, San Francisco General Hospital, San Francisco, California

M. J. GOLDENHERSH, MD
Clinical Instructor, Department of Pediatrics, University of California, Los Angeles

WILLIAM V. GOOD, MD
Assistant Professor in Residence, Department of Ophthalmology, University of California, San Francisco

AIDAN R. GOUGH, JD
Professor of Law, Santa Clara University, Santa Clara, California

CHANDRA G. GORDEN, MD
Fellow, Division of Pediatric Infectious Diseases, SFGH, Department of Pediatrics, University of California, San Francisco, San Francisco, California

DAVID W. GRIFFIN, MD
Clinical Instructor, Department of Pediatrics, University of Minnesota, Minneapolis, Minnesota

JONATHAN GRISHAM, MD
Attending Physician, Emergency Department, Children's Hospital and Medical Center, Oakland, California

MELVIN M. GRUMBACH, MD
Professor, Department of Pediatrics, University of California, San Francisco, San Francisco, California

ANTHONY J. HAFTEL, MD
Director, Department of Pediatric Emergency Medicine, Los Angeles Children's Hospital, Los Angeles, California

SANDRA JO HAMMER, RN, MSN
Nurse Manager, Department of Emergency Medicine, Children's Hospital and Medical Center, Oakland, California

GRAEME HANSON, MD
Assistant Clinical Professor, Departments of Pediatrics and Psychiatry, University of California, San Francisco, San Francisco, California

JAMES HANSON, MD
Attending Physician, Intensive Care Unit, Children's Hospital and Medical Center, Oakland, California

DEE HODGE, III, MD
Director, Division of Pediatric Emergency Medicine, LAC-USC Medical Center, Los Angeles, California

JULIAN T. HOFF, MD
Professor and Chairman, Division of Neurosurgery, University of Michigan, Ann Arbor, Michigan

JULIEN I. E. HOFFMAN, MD
Professor, Departments of Pediatrics and Physiology, University of California, San Francisco

Senior Staff Member, Cardiovascular Research Institute, University of California, San Francisco, San Francisco, California

NICOLETTE S. HORBACH, MD
Assistant Professor, Department of Obstetrics, Gynecology and Reproductive Science, University of California, San Francisco, San Francisco, California

LEONARD B. KABAN, MD
Chief, Department of Oral and Maxillofacial Surgery, University of California, San Francisco, San Francisco, California

MICHAEL T. KELLEY, MD
Assistant Professor, Departments of Emergency Medicine and Toxicology, Ohio State School of Medicine, Columbus, Ohio

KENNETH W. KIZER, MD
Associate Clinical Professor, Department of Medicine and Community Health, University of California, Davis

Director, California Department of Health Services, Sacramento, California

THOMAS K. KOCH, MD
Assistant Professor, Departments of Neurology and Pediatrics, University of California, San Francisco, San Francisco, California

MARION A. KOERPER, MD
Associate Clinical Professor, Department of Pediatrics, University of California, San Francisco

Director, Hemophilia Treatment Center, University of California, San Francisco, San Francisco, California

DANIEL V. LANDERS, MD
Assistant Clinical Professor, Department of Obstetrics, Gynecology and Reproductive Science, University of California, San Francisco, San Francisco, California

ROBERT H. LEVIN, PharmD
Clinical Professor, Departments of Clinical Pharmacy and Family/Community Medicine, University of California, San Francisco, San Francisco, California

FRANK R. LEWIS, Jr, MD
Professor, Department of Surgery, University of California, San Francisco

Chief, Department of Surgery, San Francisco General Hospital, San Francisco, California

JACK W. McANINCH, MD
Professor, Department of Urology, University of California, San Francisco

Chief, Department of Urology, San Francisco General Hospital, San Francisco, California

MICHAEL McGUIGAN, MD
Director, Toronto Poison Control System, Hospital for Sick Children

Associate Professor, Departments of Pediatrics and Clinical Pharmacology, University of Toronto, Toronto, Ontario, Canada

ROBERT E. MARKISON, MD
Assistant Professor, Department of Surgery, University of California, San Francisco

Chief, Division of Hand Surgery, San Francisco General Hospital, San Francisco, California

JAMES D. MARKS, MD
Assistant Clinical Professor, Department of Anesthesiology, University of California, San Francisco, San Francisco, California

KATHERINE K. MATTHAY, MD
Associate Professor in Residence, Departments of Pediatrics and Cancer Research Institute, University of California, San Francisco, San Francisco, California

WILLIAM C. MENTZER, MD
Professor in Residence, Departments of Laboratory Medicine and Pediatrics, University of California, San Francisco

Director, Division of Hematology and Oncology, San Francisco General Hospital

Director, Northern California Sickle Cell Center, San Francisco, California

MERLE E. MORRIS, MD
Clinical Professor (Pediatric Dentistry), Department of Growth and Development, School of Dentistry, University of California, San Francisco

Clinical Professor (Dentistry), Department of Pediatrics, University of California, San Francisco, San Francisco, California

MARY ELLEN MORTENSEN, MD
Assistant Professor, Department of Clinical Pediatrics, Ohio State University

Medical Director, Central Ohio Poison Center, Columbus, Ohio

JOHN A. OGDEN, MD
Professor, Department of Orthopedic Surgery, University of South Florida

Chief of Staff, Shriners Hospital, Tampa, Florida

GARTH S. ORSMOND, MD
Associate Professor, Division of Cardiology, Department of Pediatrics, University of Utah, Salt Lake City, Utah

RUTH ANN PARISH, MD
Assistant Professor, Department of Pediatrics, University of Washington, Seattle, Washington

JOHN COLIN PARTRIDGE, MD
Assistant Clinical Professor, Department of Pediatrics, University of California, San Francisco

Assistant Chief, Newborn Nursery, San Francisco General Hospital, San Francisco, California

DELMER J. PASCOE, MD (deceased)
Clinical Professor, Departments of Pediatrics and Ambulatory and Community Medicine, University of California, San Francisco

Director, Children's Health Center, San Francisco General Hospital, San Francisco, California

RONALD M. PERKIN, MD
Associate Professor, Department of Pediatrics, Loma Linda University Medical Center

Director, Division of Pediatric Intensive Care, Loma Linda University Medical Center, Loma Linda, California

LAWRENCE H. PITTS, MD
Professor, Department of Neurosurgery, University of California, San Francisco

Chief, Department of Neurosurgery, San Francisco General Hospital, San Francisco, California

M. ANTHONY POGREL, MB, ChB, BDS, FDS, RCS, FRCS
Assistant Professor, Department of Oral and Maxillofacial Surgery, University of California, San Francisco, San Francisco, California

ANTHONY A. PORTALE, MD
Assistant Professor in Residence, Department of Medicine and Pediatrics, University of California, San Francisco, San Francisco, California

GARY S. RACHELEFSKY, MD
Clinical Professor, Department of Pediatrics, University of California, Los Angeles

Director, Allergy Research Foundation, Los Angeles, California

MICHAEL D. REED, PharmD
Associate Professor, Department of Pediatrics, University of Virginia, Charlottesville, Virginia

ABRAHAM RUDOLPH, MD
Professor, Departments of Pediatrics and Obstetrics, Gynecology and Reproductive Sciences, University of California, San Francisco

Chairman, Department of Pediatrics, University of California, San Francisco

Senior Staff Member, Cardiovascular Research Institute, University of California, San Francisco, San Francisco, California

COLIN D. RUDOLPH, MD, PhD
Assistant Professor in Residence, Department of Pediatrics, Division of Gastroenterology, University of California, San Francisco, San Francisco, California

MARK A. SCHIFFMAN, MD
Director, Division of Pediatric Emergency Medicine, Oakland Children's Hospital and Medical Center, Oakland, California

JAMES S. SEIDEL, MD, PhD
Professor, Department of Pediatrics, University of California, Los Angeles

Chief, Pediatric Acute Care Clinic and Ambulatory Pediatrics, Harbor-UCLA Medical Center, Torrance, California

VAL SELIVANOV, MD
Attending Physician, Department of Emergency Services, San Francisco General Hospital, San Francisco, California

MICHAEL SHANNON, MD, MPH
Assistant Professor, Department of Pediatrics, Harvard Medical School

Consultant, Massachusetts Poison Control System, Boston, Massachusetts

JOSEPH E. SIMON, MD
Assistant Clinical Professor, Department of Pediatrics, Medical College of Georgia

Medical Director, Pediatric Emergency Department, Scottish Rite Children's Hospital, Atlanta, Georgia

SCOTT J. SOIFER, MD
Assistant Professor in Residence, Departments of Pediatrics and Cardiovascular Research Institute, University of California, San Francisco

Director, Division of Pediatric Intensive Care, University of California, San Francisco, San Francisco, California

RICHARD L. SWEET, MD
Professor and Vice-Chairman, Department of Obstetrics and Gynecology, University of California, San Francisco

Chief, Department of Obstetrics and Gynecology, San Francisco General Hospital, San Francisco, California

ELLEN TALIAFERRO, MD
Associate Clinical Professor, Department of Surgery, University of California, San Francisco

Attending Physician, Department of Emergency Services, San Francisco General Hospital, San Francisco, California

S. ALAN TANI, PharmD
Assistant Clinical Professor, Department of Pharmacy, University of California, San Francisco

Poison Information Specialist, San Francisco Bay Area Regional Poison Center, San Francisco, California

MILTON TENENBEIN, MD
Associate Professor, Department of Pediatrics and Pharmacology, University of Manitoba

Director, Emergency Services, Winnipeg Children's Hospital

Director, Manitoba Poison Control Center, Winnipeg, Manitoba, Canada

PEARL T. TOY, MD
Assistant Professor in Residence, Department of Laboratory Medicine, University of California, San Francisco

Director, Blood Bank, San Francisco General Hospital, San Francisco, California

RONALD R. TOWNSEND, MD
Assistant Professor in Residence, Department of Radiology, University of California, San Francisco, San Francisco, California

JAY H. TUREEN, MD
Assistant Clinical Professor, Department of Pediatrics, University of California, San Francisco, San Francisco, California

GEORGE F. VAN HARE, MD
Assistant Professor of Pediatrics, Department of Pediatric Cardiology, University of California, San Francisco, San Francisco, California

DONALD D. VERNON, MD
Assistant Professor, Department of Pediatrics, University of Utah

Attending Physician, Division of Critical Care, Primary Children's Medical Center, Salt Lake City, Utah

SYLVIA F. VILLARREAL, MD
Assistant Clinical Professor, Department of Pediatrics, University of California, San Francisco, San Francisco, California

SUMAN WASON, MD
Assistant Professor, Department of Pediatrics, University of Cincinnati College of Medicine

Consultant, Cincinnati Drug and Poison Information Center, Cincinnati, Ohio

PEGGY S. WEINTRUB, MD
Assistant Clinical Professor, Department of Pediatrics, University of California, San Francisco, San Francisco, California

MARY L. WILLIAMS, MD
Associate Professor in Residence, Departments of Dermatology and Pediatrics, University of California, San Francisco, San Francisco, California

OLGA F. WOO, PharmD
Assistant Clinical Professor, Department of Pharmacy, University of California, San Francisco

Poison Information Specialist, San Francisco Bay Area Regional Poison Center, San Francisco, California

TIMOTHY S. YEH, MD
Assistant Clinical Professor, Department of Pediatrics, University of California, San Francisco

Director, Pediatric Intensive Care, Children's Hospital and Medical Center, Oakland, California

GRACE YOUNG, MD
Assistant Professor, Department of Pediatrics, George Washington University, School of Medicine and Health Sciences

Assistant Medical Director, Emergency Medical Trauma Center, Children's Hospital National Medical Center, Washington, D.C.

MICHAEL YOUNG, MD
Assistant Clinical Professor, Department of Medicine, University of California, San Francisco

Attending Physician, Department of Emergency Services, San Francisco General Hospital, San Francisco, California

TERRANCE J. ZUERLEIN, MD
Attending Physician, Department of Pediatrics, The Children's Mercy Hospital, Kansas City, Missouri

D. DEMETRIOS ZUKIN, MD
Attending Physician, Department of Emergency Medicine, Children's Hospital and Medical Center, Oakland, California

Foreword

Emergency medical services generally have not been organized to consider the special needs of infants and children. Some 15 years ago, Drs. Grossman and Pascoe directed attention to the special considerations in recognizing and managing emergencies in pediatric practice in their publication, *Quick Reference to Pediatric Emergencies*. This new volume, *Pediatric Emergency Medicine: A Clinician's Reference,* is a logical sequence to the earlier publication. The unique talents of Drs. Grossman and Dieckmann have been combined in this venture.

For the past 30 years, in his position of Chief of Pediatric Services at San Francisco General Hospital, Dr. Moses Grossman has been confronted with the pediatric problems encountered in the inner city. He is truly the *complete pediatrician:* a superb clinician, compassionate physician, and masterful teacher. Dr. Ronald Dieckmann, as Director of Pediatric Emergency Medicine at San Francisco General Hospital, has been actively involved in organization of emergency services for children and in teaching pediatric emergency medicine.

In recent years, societal and economic pressures have brought about a dramatic change in the practice of medicine. As costs of health care, and particularly inpatient care, have exploded in the United States, we are no longer afforded the luxury of hospitalization to observe the injured and sick child without well-documented justification. This has placed increasing responsibility on those who care for children in ambulatory settings or in the Emergency Department to make appropriate diagnoses and decisions.

Drs. Dieckmann and Grossman have provided a comprehensive but succinct review of the numerous clinical problems encountered by the pediatrician, emergency physician, or family physician, including acute illness, trauma, poisonings, and psychological and social issues.

Pediatric Emergency Medicine: A Clinician's Reference is an outstanding aid in the assessment of emergencies in pediatrics and will be greatly appreciated by pediatricians, emergency physicians, family physicians, residents, nurses, and students. It should be in every office and Emergency Department that provides services to children.

Abraham Rudolph, MD
San Francisco
1990

Preface

Publication of the first pediatric emergencies textbook, *Quick Reference to Pediatric Emergencies,* by Delmer Pascoe, Moses Grossman, and their colleagues at San Francisco General Hospital in 1973 laid the cornerstone for a new subspecialty. The landmark first edition of *Quick Reference to Pediatric Emergencies,* and its subsequent two editions in 1978 and 1984, developed from a universal desire to improve the standards of emergency care for children. The series of editions enjoyed worldwide popularity and helped shape the early development of pediatric emergency medicine as a sovereign medical subspecialty.

Since the last edition of *Quick Reference to Pediatric Emergencies,* Delmer Pascoe died, and Ronald A. Dieckmann assumed the co-editorship of the textbook. In addition, over the last several years, major changes have occurred in the clinical practice of emergency pediatrics: important scientific advances have redefined standards for diagnosis and treatment, and interest in emergency pediatrics has magnified throughout the country. Moreover, comprehensive management *systems* have been recently implemented in several areas to coordinate the entire continuum of emergency services now available for children—including injury and illness prevention, home and prehospital care, emergency department and in-hospital care, as well as interfacility patient transfer.

Pediatric Emergency Medicine: A Clinician's Reference, while in direct lineage from *Quick Reference to Pediatric Emergencies,* embodies the metamorphosis which has occurred since the last edition of the old series. *Pediatric Emergency Medicine: A Clinician's Reference* is truly a hybrid of its two parent disciplines: pediatrics and emergency medicine. While pediatric emergency medicine was originally the product of pediatrics in the 1970s, the field gained its second parent in the 1980s, during the period of robust scientific inquiry and clinical research that accompanied maturation of emergency medicine as a primary specialty. *Pediatric Emergency Medicine: A Clinician's Reference* has adopted an orientation to clinical assessment and treatment that joins the principles of emergency practice with the tenets of ambulatory pediatrics.

Pediatric Emergency Medicine: A Clinician's Reference distills a vast body of new scientific knowledge for application to clinical practice. Cardiopulmonary resuscitation, pulmonary disease, pain syndromes, trauma, toxicology, environmental medicine, antibiotic treatment, immunodeficiency states, and emergency procedures, for example, are key subject areas in the book that have undergone substantial revisions in recent years. A new section in the present volume addresses clinical and organizational issues in pediatric emergency medical services (EMS) systems—concepts currently receiving much national attention in conferences, publications, and state and Congressional legislation.

Another prominent feature of *Pediatric Emergency Medicine: A Clinician's Reference* is its broad, national authorship. Ninety-nine contributors from many institutions throughout the United States collaborated in the first edition. This reflects the editors' desire for an eclectic presentation of the subject areas by recognized authorities in pediatrics, emergency medicine, pediatric emergency medicine, trauma, and toxicology. Statements in the chapters are the authors' own, and bibliographies are provided for further reading.

Pediatric Emergency Medicine: A Clinician's Reference is written for the clinician: pediatrician, emergency physician, pediatric emergency specialist, family practitioner, nurse, and other health professional involved in the emergency care of children. It is especially directed at the new generation of students and residents-in-training, who are constantly seeking to understand and apply the cutting edge of medical knowledge to sick and injured children, and to teach the state-of-the-art to their immediate successors.

The format for *Pediatric Emergency Medicine: A Clinician's Reference* is concise and problem-oriented. The departure from the diagnosis-oriented style of *Quick Reference to Pediatric Emergencies* reflects the editors' attempt to achieve greater consistency with the practical sequence of diagnosis and care in the Emergency Department or acute clinic setting. Every chapter follows the same organization, so that the reader can readily elicit information on pathophysiology, clinical findings, ancillary data, treatment, and disposition. Numerous tables and illustrations are intended to improve access to key information.

There are fourteen sections. The first section examines the organization of emergency medical services; the next eleven sections address various problems seen in the emergency setting—presented by the nature of the complaint or by organ system; and the last two sections, "Quick Reference" and "Emergency Drugs," are a potpourri of useful data for the fingertips of the busy practitioner, including a complete list of important drugs, with doses and special considerations in clinical practice.

Pediatric Emergency Medicine: A Clinician's Reference is written for use in the clinical area, and not as a library reference. It will be most useful when immediately available at the physician's desk and even at the bedside of the patient. When combined with basic knowledge, compassion, and finesse, this volume will have its best value in the care of our young patients and their families.

Moses Grossman, M.D.
Ronald A. Dieckmann, M.D.

Acknowledgments

We would like to thank all of our contributors for their informative, organized and updated chapters; these form the skeleton and muscle of this volume. We are also greatly indebted to Ms. Hana Ono, Nancy Ward, Patricia Green, Carol Shea, and the department staffs in Emergency Services and Pediatrics, San Francisco General Hospital. Finally, we are most grateful for the devoted efforts of our publisher, Mr. Charles McCormick, Jr., and our manuscript editor, as well as the many individuals at JB Lippincott Company who transformed the manuscript into a useful and usable book.

Contents

IV ■ Emergent Complaints

V ■ Nonemergent Complaints

VI ■ Pain Syndromes

VII ■ Trauma

VIII ■ Toxicology *Associate Editor: Kent R. Olson*

IX ■ Environmental Emergencies

X ■ Organ System Disorders

XI ■ Infectious Diseases

XII ■ Psychosocial Emergencies

XIII ■ Quick Reference

XIV ■ Emergency Drugs

Index

Pediatric Emergency Medicine

I

Emergency Medical Services for Children

1 Organization of Emergency Medical Services for Children

Ronald A. Dieckmann

A wide spectrum of medical and traumatic conditions occurs in childhood. The range in severity is vast, from minor annoyances such as bee stings, colds, and splinters to life-threatening conditions such as anaphylaxis, meningococcemia, and multiple-system trauma. Pediatric emergencies are managed in many different settings—the home, the ambulance, the physician's office, and the hospital. This chapter examines the formal systems of emergency care that have evolved for treating childhood diseases and misadventures. Increasingly, the individual service components of pediatric emergency care systems are being combined into a coordinated, interdependent continuum of care called *emergency medical services for children (EMSC).*

EMSC ■

A total system of emergency care must provide comprehensive services—prevention, prehospital care, in-hospital care, and rehabilitation. In the United States, general emergency medical service (EMS) organizations oversee emergency care within a countywide or, occasionally, multicounty area. Over the last two decades, EMS systems have rapidly improved their capacity to deliver timely, competent service to sick and injured patients of all ages. The challenge of the 1990s is to bring the benefits of general EMS systems more fully to the pediatric population, by further emphasizing the EMSC subset of EMS. EMSC includes evaluation and treatment of emergencies in children, from birth to about 14 years of age. Further development of EMSC will decrease morbidity and mortality from childhood emergencies.

ORGANIZATIONAL MODEL FOR EMSC

EMSC has three major phases: the entry phase, the response phase, and the hospital phase. Figure 1-1 shows the usual sequence of field communications,

personnel mobilization, ambulance triage, and hospital care that constitutes the EMSC continuum. This organizational model must function completely within the overall EMS system, although children are managed with special treatment algorithms and by field triage guidelines that ensure transport to receiving departments qualified to manage pediatric emergencies.

The *entry phase* begins when the patient is identified (1) and the emergency care system activated, usually through the 911 telephone access (2). The medical dispatch center (3) receives the request for help and determines the mode of response. Several options for emergency response are possible (4): The dispatcher can immediately dispatch an emergency medical technician (EMT) ambulance on a highest priority basis (code 3 response) or on second priority basis (code 2). In serious emergencies, the dispatch center may ask the fire department to co-respond to the scene to assist EMTs. When the emergency is an ingestion or toxic exposure, the dispatcher first consults the regional poison center to determine the urgency of ambulance response.

The *response phase* may involve fire-department personnel, EMTs on basic life support (BLS) ambulances, or EMTs on advanced life support (ALS) ambulances (paramedics), according to medical dispatch protocols. EMTs assess the scene (5), then establish base hospital or communication center contact (6). At the base hospital or communication center, nurses or doctors with prehospital training direct field treatment by radio and determine appropriate patient triage (7). EMTs transport the patient to an emergency department approved for children (EDAP) (8) or a hospital with equipment and personnel capable of stabilizing pediatric emergency patients.

The *hospital phase* of the EMSC model includes primary EDAP stabilization (9), in-hospital care when appropriate (10), and secondary transport (11) to a pediatric critical care center (PCCC) or pediatric

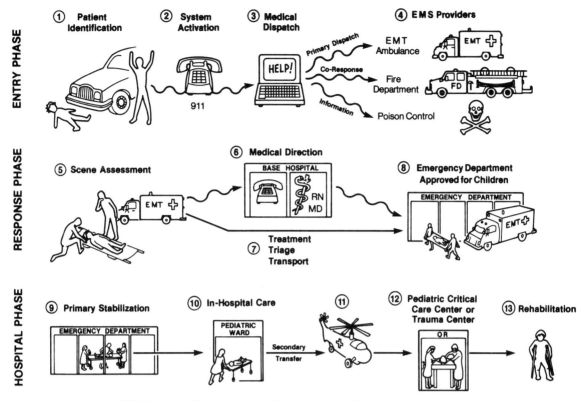

ENTRY PHASE

RESPONSE PHASE

HOSPITAL PHASE

FIGURE 1–1. The continuum of emergency medical services for children.

trauma center (PTC) (12) in selected cases. The continuum ends with rehabilitation (13) of the child and family. Performance throughout the entire spectrum of EMSC is monitored and modified through data collection and quality assurance (QA) (see Chapter 4).

Few EMS systems have developed EMSC to this performance level. Such EMSC design is possible only in cities with superior resources in pediatrics, critical care, and trauma. Rural systems and less-endowed urban EMS systems must evaluate the community's capabilities and modify this EMSC model for local conditions. In many systems, transfer guidelines and agreements with tertiary hospitals for pediatric critical care and trauma care are fundamental.

History of EMS and EMSC ■

EMS *prehospital* systems were originally designed for adults, either for trauma or for cardiac disease. The Emergency Medical Services Act (Cranston Act) of 1973 established the first national framework for EMS.

This landmark legislation arose from the experiences in several regions, particularly Miami and Los Angeles, where systematic organization of prehospital services led to better outcomes for emergency patients. The act established the foundation for EMS administration, training, communications, and transportation and research in emergency care.

Personnel training and equipment, treatment standards, and QA for prehospital pediatric emergencies were not addressed in initial EMS development. However, as measurable improvements in hospital outcomes for adults treated within organized prehospital systems became widely documented, attention was directed at an apparent discrepancy in prehospital care for children.

Table 1-1 summarizes the findings and conclusions of recent major studies of pediatric emergency medical services in the United States. These authors provide a cogent argument that children suffer higher unnecessary morbidity and mortality from a broad range of medical and traumatic conditions. The most egregious problems include:

TABLE 1–1. *Major Studies in Pediatric Emergency Medical Services*

Author	Year	Location	Findings/Conclusions
Haller	1983	Baltimore	Introduction of trauma center reduced morbidity and mortality in adults, but not in children.
Ramenofsky	1983	Mobile	1. Ambulance "false alarms" for children common. 2. 56% of prehospital calls for children were trauma. 3. ALS used less in children than adults (47% vs. 82%). 4. Public education in children's emergencies needed.
Eisenberg	1983	Seattle	1. Out-of-hospital pediatric arrests have 7% survival vs. 20% in adults. 2. Asystole is first rhythm in 77% of cases. 3. Ventricular fibrillation has highest survival in children.
Ramenofsky	1984	Mobile	1. 53% of field pediatric trauma deaths were possibly preventable. 2. Most common problems in unnecessary deaths were delay in recognition (77%), field care (36%), transport (23%), vs. definitive care problems in only 17%.
Fifield	1984	Minneapolis	1. Low ambulance transport rate (5.4%) for children. 2. Low acuity level in transported cases. 3. Personnel training must emphasize medical problems in 0–5 year group, and trauma in adolescents. 4. Current EMS data collection not suitable for children.
Seidel	1984	Los Angeles	1. Field trauma death rates higher for children than adults. 2. Death rates highest where no pediatric center. 3. Ambulances need pediatric equipment standards and treatment guidelines.
Applebaum	1985	Jerusalem	1. Most common prehospital pediatric emergencies: seizures, trauma, cardiac arrests. 2. Ambulance providers had poor ALS skills for children. 3. No arrest victims survived.
Seidel	1986	Los Angeles	1. 40% of paramedic programs have <10 hrs. of pediatric training. 2. Ambulance equipment for children is severely deficient. 3. More training of paramedics and better equipping of ambulances will improve outcome for children.
Tsai	1987	Fresno	1. CNS events, trauma, and ingestions were most frequent problems in field. 2. ALS is rarely used in children, and attempts are often unsuccessful. 3. Alternative methods for ALS delivery are needed. 4. Better medical control of pediatric cases is necessary.
Losek	1987	Milwaukee	1. Of 114 pediatric arrests, out-of-hospital survival occurred in 8%. 2. Endotracheal intubation was successful in 67%, IVs in 32%. 3. Survival was related to endotracheal intubation (in <18 mos) witnessed arrests, and ventricular fibrillation.

1. Long delays by parents and medical dispatchers in identifying significant illness and injury
2. Dangerous underuse of ambulances for serious illness and overuse for minor trauma
3. Inadequate pediatric training for paramedics, and rapid decay in technical competence with pediatric field ALS maneuvers
4. Poor success rates by paramedics, compared to rates for adults, in performing field endotracheal intubation
5. Inadequate equipping of ambulances for childhood emergencies
6. Mistriage of patients to emergency departments incapable of pediatric care
7. Inappropriate delays in secondary transport of patients requiring specialized care in the operating room or pediatric intensive care unit.

Development of Regional EMSC Systems ■

In 1980, Los Angeles implemented the first voluntary EMSC that established two levels of receiving facil-

TABLE 1–2. *System Development Model, Emergency Medical Services for Children*

EMS Component	Function of Component	Areas for Component Development
Entry Phase		
1. Patient identification	Prevention of morbid event	Public/parent education in injury prevention
	Early recognition of distress	Public, parent, EMT, and physician education in early recognition of serious illness/injury in children
2. System activation	Rapid access to medical response system	911 capability in all counties
		Parent/public education in 911 access
3. Medical dispatch	Processing raw field information	Dispatcher training in recognition of pediatric emergencies
	Appropriate dispatching of response personnel	Strict dispatch protocols, with pediatric considerations
		Pre-arrival instructions to initiate field care before EMT arrival
		Priority dispatch guidelines to ensure timely response and appropriate skill level of personnel
4. EMS Providers		
a. Poison control center	Provide assistance in toxicologic emergencies	Formal integration of poison control centers in EMS
		Direct communication from medical dispatch to poison center to assist scene care and guide transport and priority dispatch
b. Fire department	Co-response to scene	Training in pediatric emergencies and basic life support (BLS) techniques for children
c. Ambulance	Trained field response	Training in pediatric emergencies
Response Phase		
5. Field assessment	Recognition of illness and injury	EMT training in advanced life support (ALS)
	Field stabilization	Proper pediatric equipment in ambulances
6. Base hospital	Monitoring of field assessment	Special training of base hospital radio personnel (MICNS and/or MDs) in pediatric emergencies
	Specific radio direction for ALS interventions	Strict field criteria for paramedic radio contact to base hospital
7. Field treatment	Field treatment	Field clinical protocols for pediatric receiving facility
8. Transport to pediatric receiving facility	Delivery of patient to ED with pediatric capability	Designation of emergency department approved for pediatrics (EDAPs)
		Designation of pediatric critical care centers (PCCC)
		Designation of pediatric trauma centers (PTCs)
Hospital Phase		
9. Primary EDAP stabilization	Resuscitation	Emergency department (EDAP) protocols for pediatric care
	Stabilization	Immediate pediatric specialist back-up
		Coordinated group paging system plan for multispecialty care
10. In-hospital care	Pediatric ward care	In-hospital pediatric ward with pediatric capability
11. Secondary transport	Transfer of critical cases to definitive care	Secondary transfer guidelines
		Criteria for patient selection
		Written transfer agreements
12. PCCC or PTC	Definitive care	Tertiary care capability
13. Rehabilitation	Rehabilitation care	Last portion of continuum of care for child and family

ities for children within the EMS: EDAPs and PCCCs. The criteria for EDAP and PCCC designation encompassed standards for staffing, consultation, training, equipment, and ancillary services appropriate for the pediatric patient.

Los Angeles's worthy effort to organize pediatric emergency services focused national attention on EMSC, resulting in a 1986 federal grant to support EMSC. By 1990, twelve states have received funds for research and development of emergency care systems for children.

The EMSC Planning Process ■

Effective regional EMSC planning requires broad-based committee participation: physicians, nurses, paramedics, hospital administrators, and EMS authorities must be represented. Key physician groups include pediatricians, emergency medicine specialists, pediatric emergency specialists, pediatric surgeons, and pediatric intensivists.

A comprehensive EMSC plan addresses the following elements:

1. Assessing regional needs and problems
2. Coordinating appropriate public and private agencies
3. Developing system goals
4. Implementing the EMSC design
5. Reviewing ongoing QA activities
6. Establishing a reliable information system
7. Modifying EMSC based on mandatory, periodic review of system performance.

TABLE 1–3. *Modified Los Angeles Criteria for an Emergency Department Approved for Children (EDAP) and Pediatric Critical Care Center (PCCC)*

EDAP Criteria
  A. Professional staff
    1. All emergency department physicians and one RN per shift certified in ACLS.
    2. 50% of emergency department physicians board-eligible or certified in pediatrics or emergency medicine.
    3. Designated board-certified pediatric consultant immediately available 24 hours a day.
    4. Designated pediatric quality assurance consultant.
    5. Designated pediatric liaison nurse.
    6. Pediatric representative on hospital emergency care committee.
  B. Equipment, supplies, and drugs suitable for children
  C. Treatment protocols for children
  D. Policies and procedures for transfer of critically ill and injured children to pediatric critical care centers
  E. Policies and procedures for child abuse identification, evaluation, and referral

PCCC Criteria
  Meets EDAP criteria, plus
    1. General pediatric intensive care unit
    2. Pediatric ward
    3. Level I or II trauma center
  A. Personnel
    1. In-house specialists 24 hours per day: emergency medicine, pediatrics, general surgery, anesthesia
    2. Available subspecialists within 30 minutes
    3. Child protection team to manage child abuse, neglect, and sexual abuse
  B. Ancillary services
    1. Clinical laboratory with microtechnique, blood bank, and comprehensive other pediatric lab capability
    2. Pediatric radiology
    3. Inhalation therapy
    4. Rehabilitation
    5. Pharmacy
  C. Organization
    1. Transport reviews
    2. Morbidity and mortality reviews
  D. Policies
    1. Resuscitation
    2. No resuscitation
    3. Child abuse
    4. Organ donation
    5. Transfers
    6. Rehabilitation referral

(* Modified from Committee on Pediatric Emergency Medicine of the American Academy of Pediatrics, California Chapter 2, and the Los Angeles Pediatric Society, Standards of Care for Pediatric Patients, 1988.)

Table 1-2 summarizes areas of EMSC that deserve special attention in the overall design. These are based on the EMSC model illustrated in Figure 1-1.

EMSC PERFORMANCE GUIDELINES

Guidelines for EMSC operation should include the following:

1. Criteria for EDAP and PCCC designation (Table 1-3) (rural systems require less stringent standards)
2. Field policies for establishing radio contact with the base hospital or communications center for medical direction in pediatric emergencies
3. Field triage guidelines to identify specific patients for either EDAP or PCCC or PTC field destination
4. Field treatment protocols for children (see Chap. 2).

Epidemiology of Pediatric Prehospital Emergencies ■

Characteristics of children transported by ambulance are different than those brought directly to the emergency department. While about 25–35% of all ED patients are less than 18 years old, only 10% of ambulance patients are children. The acuity level of the prehospital patient is typically low (80% have "minor" emergencies not requiring ALS).

The age ranges of prehospital cases is bimodal: patients are either *very young (0–5 years)* with seizures, trauma, respiratory difficulty, or accidental ingestion as their presenting complaint, or *adolescent,* usually with trauma or altered mental status from intentional ingestions. By contrast, the most common diagnoses of pediatric patients arriving directly in the ED are lacerations, otitis media, pharyngitis, or a simple contusion.

Most transported patients arrive during the summer, on weekends, and between 1–9 p.m. They are unlikely to require ALS, such as intravenous cannulation or endotracheal intubation. However, when ALS is required, success rates in the field are low, especially in children under 18 months. When prehospital cardiopulmonary arrest occurs, it is usually a bradyasystolic arrest, and survival is unlikely (5–10% vs. adult survival of 20%). Medications are infrequently administered in the prehospital setting; most common are oxygen, diazepam, or epinephrine.

Bibliography ■

Applebaum D: Advanced prehospital care for pediatric emergencies. *Ann Emerg Med* 1985; 14:656–659.

Eisenberg M, Bergner L, Hallstrom A: Epidemiology of cardiac arrest and resuscitation in children. *Ann Emerg Med* 1983; 12:672–674.

Fifield GC, Magnuson C, Carr WP, Deinard AS: Pediatric emergency care in a metropolitan area. *J Emerg Med* 1984; 1:495–507.

Haller JA, Shorter N, Miller D, et al: Organization and function of a regional pediatric trauma center: Does a system of management improve outcome? *J Trauma* 1983; 23(8):691–696.

Losek JD, Heunes H, Glaeser P, et al: Prehospital care of the pulseless, nonbreathing pediatric patient. *Am J Emerg Med* 1987; 5(5):370–374.

Ramenofsky ML, Luterman A, Curreri PW, et al: EMS for pediatrics: Optimum treatment or unnecessary delay. *J Pediatr Surg* 1983; 18(4):498.

Ramenofsky ML, Luterman A, Quindlen E, et al: Maximum survival in pediatric trauma: The ideal system. *J Trauma* 1984; 24(9):818–823.

Seidel JS, Hornbein M, Yoshiyama K, et al: Emergency medical services and the pediatric patient: Are the needs being met? *Pediatrics* 1984; 73(6):769–772.

Seidel JS: Emergency medical services and the pediatric patient: Are the needs being met? II. Training and equipping emergency medical services providers for pediatric emergencies. *Pediatrics* 1986; 78(5):808–812.

Tsai A, Kallsen G: Epidemiology of pediatric prehospital care. *Ann Emerg Med* 1987; 16:284–292.

2 Prehospital Care of Medical and Traumatic Emergencies

Ronald A. Dieckmann

While organized prehospital systems clearly have improved hospital outcomes for adult patients with cardiac and traumatic conditions, the history of prehospital care for children is still too short to evaluate the benefits of field intervention. Published reports on prehospital care in pediatric emergencies have pointed out multiple deficiencies in the treatment of children within adult-oriented models of emergency medical services (EMS). Problems in personnel training, ambulance equipment, medical direction, field triage, and emergency department (ED) preparedness appear to account for widespread errors in pediatric prehospital care and may be responsible for significant unnecessary disability and death (see Chapter 1).

The benefits of any field intervention in children must be weighed against the costs of subsequent delay in transport to definitive care and the risk (and possible pain) of the intervention itself. Proximity to a properly equipped and staffed ED, especially an emergency department approved for children (EDAP), pediatric critical care center (PCCC), or pediatric trauma center (see Chapter 1), renders on-scene advanced life support (ALS) justifiable for only a few serious clinical conditions (e.g., apnea, airway obstruction, hypoglycemia, status epilepticus, unstable cardiac dysrhythmias, or full arrest). Immediate transport to an ED, with ALS en route, is appropriate for many childhood emergencies in which field care is unlikely to improve the outcome. A clinical scenario in which field ALS may delay transport and in fact worsen outcome is the severely traumatized child who needs immediate surgical management in the ED or operating room.

Clinical Spectrum of Prehospital Pediatrics ■

Most children evaluated in the field have one of five conditions: trauma, respiratory illness, seizures, al-
tered mental status, or ingestion of a potentially dangerous substance. These conditions prompt early activation of the EMS by parents or caretakers. Yet because the acuity level among transported children (especially those with minor trauma or ingestions) is typically low, field ALS is needed in only about 25% of total pediatric cases. However, for several uncommon but serious clinical problems, the timeliness and quality of prehospital ALS may profoundly influence outcome.

Table 2-1 presents the five most common prehospital clinical problems in pediatrics, and the uncommon but important problem of shock/cardiac arrest. Major clinical issues for each problem are noted, as well as areas for emphasis in prehospital system planning and administration.

Aeromedical Transportation and Treatment ■

Enhanced aeromedical capabilities in EMS provide an excellent means for transferring children from primary receiving hospitals to definitive-care tertiary facilities. Typically, aeromedical personnel are highly skilled nurses and/or physicians from critical-care areas. Treatment guidelines appropriate to the advanced training levels among aeromedical providers usually differ from those for ground ambulance providers with emergency medical technician (EMT) backgrounds. Aeromedical transport of the critically ill or injured child is addressed in Chapter 5.

Field Procedures ■

Most field care for pediatric emergencies consists of simple first aid and basic life support (BLS). In some systems, EMTs are trained only to a BLS level. In other systems, a major discrepancy exists between personnel capabilities in pediatric and adult emer-

8

TABLE 2–1. *Important Clinical Problems in Prehospital Pediatric Care*

Condition	Clinical Issues	Areas for Emphasis
Trauma	Recommended "platinum half-hour" total time from injury to operating room limits appropriateness of all field ALS.	Field guidelines and medical direction must enforce "scoop-and-run" philosophy.
	Head injury usually determines outcome.	Manage airway/breathing/spine in field.
		Attempt IVs en route to hospital.
	Multiple-injury child may appear stable.	Trauma and critical care triage policies.
		Direct transport to pediatric trauma centers and pediatric critical care centers.
	Minor trauma may not require ambulance transport.	Public, parents, and physicians need better education on prudent use of ambulances.
Respiratory Illness	Early recognition of distress key to survival.	Public, parents, and physicians need better education on early identification of distressed child.
		Provider training will improve recognition skills in field.
	Acute bronchospasm is a common, serious field emergency.	Inhaled sympathomimetics are best first-line agents in asthma.
	Airway patency and adequate breathing are first priorities.	Endotracheal intubation training and re-training for paramedics is essential.
Seizures	Diagnosis of "febrile seizure" cannot be determined in field.	All children with seizures require hospital transport.
	Status epilepticus is dangerous and may be difficult to manage in field.	Rectal diazepam is a rapid alternative to parenteral administration.
Altered Mental Status	Hypoglycemic coma requires immediate field treatment to avert brain injury.	Administer $D_{25}W$ or $D_{50}W$ in all suspected hypoglycemic children.
	Beware of complications from recreational drugs, especially cocaine and its derivatives.	All children with impaired sensorium need ED evaluation.
Ingestions	Sympathomimetics and alcohol are common agents in adolescents.	Develop close liaison between poison centers, medical dispatch, and base hospitals.
	Accidental ingestions are common in toddlers.	Activated charcoal is best agent for field use, instead of ipecac.
Shock/cardiac	Vital signs are poor indicators of perfusion.	Provider training must accent assessment skills.
	Vascular access is difficult in <18 mos.	Intraosseous drugs and fluids may be life-saving in the field.
	Survivors from arrest are usually in ventricular fibrillation.	Personnel training in early defibrillation of children is necessary.
		Endotracheal drugs are excellent to begin resuscitation.
	Sudden infant death syndrome (SIDS) and blunt trauma arrests cannot be resuscitated.	Field guidelines must emphasize interaction with "injured family," not ALS interventions.

gencies: EMTs provide BLS to children but ALS to adults.

BLS includes immobilizing the spine, opening the airway, administering oxygen, giving mouth-to-mouth or mouth-to-nose-and-mouth ventilation, administering chest compression, stopping external hemorrhage, and splinting extremities. ALS includes endotracheal intubation, electrical defibrillation, cardiac monitoring, intravenous cannulation, and administration of parenteral medications. Only paramedic EMTs are trained and certified to perform major ALS interventions in the field, under the radio direction of nurses and physicians at the base hospital or paramedic communication center.

Successful application of ALS skills to serious childhood emergencies is hindered by:

1. Inadequate training of prehospital personnel in recognition and treatment
2. Decay of skills
3. Technical difficulties posed by smaller and less familiar anatomy
4. Restrictive regional policies controlling the scope of paramedic practice.

The ALS interventions likely to provide the greatest benefit in the field are *endotracheal intubation, defibrillation,* and *alternative vascular access techniques* to facilitate rapid drug and fluid administration.

ENDOTRACHEAL INTUBATION

Endotracheal intubation establishes a definitive airway, reverses most respiratory insufficiency, and provides a conduit for delivery of key resuscitative medications (epinephrine, atropine, diazepam, lidocaine, and naloxone). See Chapter 139 for the procedure. Direct laryngoscopy also permits effective removal of a foreign body with Magill forceps.

Endotracheal intubation may be the only field procedure of unequivocal value to the critically ill or injured child even in a rapid urban ambulance transportation system. Bag-valve-mask-assisted breathing in children is notoriously ineffective on scene and en route to the hospital. Endotracheal intubation can be well executed in the field by trained paramedics, with documented success rates of over 75% in children over 18 months.

On the other hand, prolonged field intubation attempts are dangerous, and traumatic or esophageal intubations are potentially life-threatening. Therefore, pediatric field intubation must occur within a controlled prehospital system that ensures adequate training and skills retention, capable on-line medical

---

TABLE 2–2. *Supplies and Equipment for Pediatric Prehospital Basic and Advanced Life Support*

Supplies		Equipment	
1. Endotracheal tubes	*Uncuffed sizes:* 2.5, 3, 3.5, 4.0, 4.5, 5.0, 5.5, 6.0	1. Bag-valve-mask resuscitator	*Child and adult*
	Cuffed sizes: 6.0, 6.5, 7.0, 7.5, 8.0	2. Clear masks	Standard and non-rebreathing:
2. Oral airways	Sizes 0, 1, 2, 3, 4, 5		*Neonatal,*
3. Needles	*Butterfly:* 21, 23, 25		*infant, child,*
	Over-the-needle: 14, 16, 18, 20, 22, 24		*adult*
	Intraosseous: 16	3. Nasal cannulae	*Child and adult*
4. 3-Way stopcock (for intraosseous infusions)		4. Laryngoscope handle	
5. Infusion sets	*Minidrip:* 60 gtts/min	5. Laryngoscope blades	*Curved:* 0, 1, 2
	Standard: 15 gtts/min		*Straight:* 0, 1, 2
6. IV solutions, normal saline	100 ml, 250 ml, 500 ml, 1000 ml	6. Stylets for endotracheal tubes	6f, 14f
7. Suction catheters	6f, 8f, 10f, 14f		
8. Feeding tubes (for endotracheal drugs)	5f, 8f	7. Blood pressure cuffs	*Neonatal,*
9. Arm boards	*Neonatal, infant, child*		*Infant, Child*
10. Bulb syringe	1, 2, 3 oz		*Adult:* arm,
11. Diapers	*Small, medium, large*		thigh
		8. Spine board	*Child and adult*
		9. Femur splint	*Child and adult*
		10. Rigid neck collar	*Child and adult*
		11. Cardiac monitor-defibrillator	4.5 and 8 cm paddles
		12. Magill forceps	*Child and adult*

direction, and a strict field intubation policy. In most settings, paramedics should be limited to two intubation attempts of no more than 30 seconds' duration each. The very young child has extremely limited tolerance to the hypoxia induced by intubation maneuvers, even with adequate (usually 3 minutes) preoxygenation with 100% oxygen.

DEFIBRILLATION

Early defibrillation is imperative for ventricular fibrillation and ventricular tachycardia arrests and must precede all other forms of ALS. See Chapter 6 for the procedure. While ventricular dysrhythmias are unusual in children (<10% of all arrests), meaningful survival from pediatric cardiac arrest is rare except when ventricular fibrillation is the treated rhythm. Routine defibrillation of asystolic arrests will probably not affect outcome. However, apparent asystole on the cardiac monitor may, in fact, be fine ventricular fibrillation. Therefore, a prudent clinical approach to the child with ostensible asystole might involve either an early trial of electricity or review of a second electrocardiographic plane to confirm true asystole.

VASCULAR ACCESS

Failure to establish vascular access is a frequent prehospital problem in pediatric care and is especially common in children under 18 months old, the group most likely to experience serious medical illnesses and cardiopulmonary arrest. Alternative techniques

TABLE 2–3. *Pediatric Prehospital Care Drug List*

Drug	Dose	How Supplied
Atropine	0.02 mg/kg IV, IO, ET minimum dose = 0.1 mg maximum dose = 1 mg, 2×	1 mg/10 ml prefilled syringe
Bretylium tosylate	5 mg/kg IV, IO maximum dose = 30 mg	500 mg/10 ml
Activated charcoal	1 g/year of age PO or by NG tube	15 g or 50 g bottles
Dextrose 50% ($D_{50}W$) (dilute 1:1 with water or NS for $D_{25}W$ solution for <2 years)	less than 2 yrs: 1–2 ml/kg IV of $D_{25}W$ older than 2 yrs: 0.5–1 ml/kg IV of $D_{50}W$	25 g/50 ml prefilled syringes
Diazepam	0.1–0.3 mg/kg slow IV, IO, ET, PR	10 mg/2 ml prefilled syringes
Diphenhydramine	1 mg/kg slow IV, IO, IM	50 mg/ml ampule
Epinephrine 1:1,000 1:10,000	0.01 mg/kg SQ 0.01–0.2 mg/kg IV	1 mg/ml ampule (1:1,000) 1 mg/10 ml (1:10,000)
Ipecac	15 ml/dose PO Repeat once	15 ml unit dose
Lidocaine 2%	1 mg/kg IV, IO, ET	100 mg/5 ml prefilled syringe
Mannitol 25%	1 mg/kg IV	25 g/100 ml
Metaproterenol (Dilute to 3 ml with NS)	0.1–0.3 ml/dose by hand-held nebulizer or mask	0.3 ml vials
Morphine sulfate	0.1–0.2 mg/kg slow IV	10 mg/ml prefilled syringe
Naloxone	less than 2 yrs: 0.4 mg/IV, IO, IM, ET older than 2 yrs: 2 mg/IV, IO, IM, ET	0.4 mg/ml or 2 mg/ml ampule
Sodium bicarbonate	0.5–1 mEq/kg IV, IO with adequate ventilation	5 mg/2 ml prefilled syringes

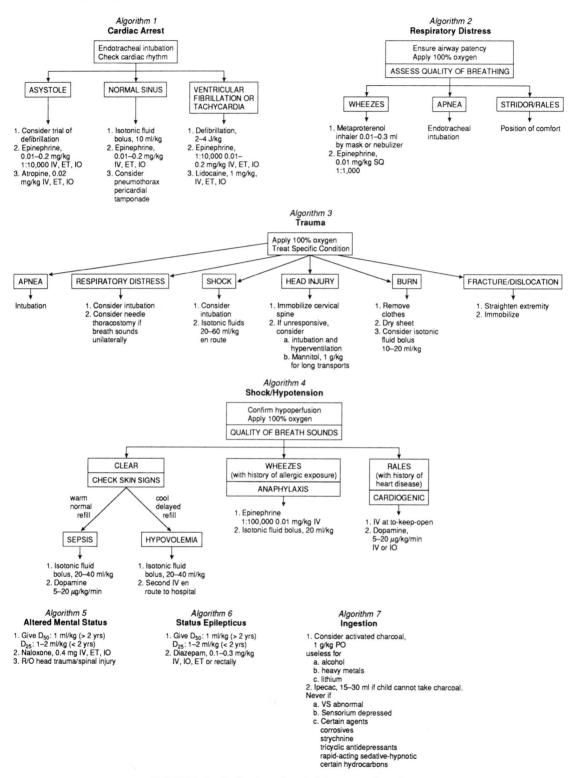

Algorithm 1
Cardiac Arrest

Endotracheal intubation
Check cardiac rhythm

ASYSTOLE

1. Consider trial of defibrillation
2. Epinephrine, 0.01–0.2 mg/kg 1:10,000 IV, ET, IO
3. Atropine, 0.02 mg/kg IV, ET, IO

NORMAL SINUS

1. Isotonic fluid bolus, 10 ml/kg
2. Epinephrine, 0.01–0.2 mg/kg IV, ET, IO
3. Consider pneumothorax pericardial tamponade

VENTRICULAR FIBRILLATION OR TACHYCARDIA

1. Defibrillation, 2–4 J/kg
2. Epinephrine, 1:10,000 0.01– 0.2 mg/kg IV, ET, IO
3. Lidocaine, 1 mg/kg, IV, ET, IO

Algorithm 2
Respiratory Distress

Ensure airway patency
Apply 100% oxygen
ASSESS QUALITY OF BREATHING

WHEEZES

1. Metaproterenol inhaler 0.01–0.3 ml by mask or nebulizer
2. Epinephrine, 0.01 mg/kg SQ 1:1,000

APNEA

Endotracheal intubation

STRIDOR/RALES

Position of comfort

Algorithm 3
Trauma

Apply 100% oxygen
Treat Specific Condition

APNEA

Intubation

RESPIRATORY DISTRESS

1. Consider intubation
2. Consider needle thoracostomy if breath sounds unilaterally

SHOCK

1. Consider intubation
2. Isotonic fluids 20–60 ml/kg en route

HEAD INJURY

1. Immobilize cervical spine
2. If unresponsive, consider
   a. intubation and hyperventilation
   b. Mannitol, 1 g/kg for long transports

BURN

1. Remove clothes
2. Dry sheet
3. Consider isotonic fluid bolus 10–20 ml/kg

FRACTURE/DISLOCATION

1. Straighten extremity
2. Immobilize

Algorithm 4
Shock/Hypotension

Confirm hypoperfusion
Apply 100% oxygen
QUALITY OF BREATH SOUNDS

CLEAR
CHECK SKIN SIGNS

warm normal refill

cool delayed refill

SEPSIS

1. Isotonic fluid bolus, 20–40 ml/kg
2. Dopamine 5–20 µg/kg/min

HYPOVOLEMIA

1. Isotonic fluid bolus, 20–40 ml/kg
2. Second IV en route to hospital

WHEEZES
(with history of allergic exposure)
ANAPHYLAXIS

1. Epinephrine 1:100,000 0.01 mg/kg IV
2. Isotonic fluid bolus, 20 ml/kg

RALES
(with history of heart disease)
CARDIOGENIC

1. IV at to-keep-open
2. Dopamine, 5–20 µg/kg/min IV or IO

Algorithm 5
Altered Mental Status

1. Give D_{50}: 1 ml/kg (> 2 yrs) D_{25}: 1–2 ml/kg (< 2 yrs)
2. Naloxone, 0.4 mg IV, ET, IO
3. R/O head trauma/spinal injury

Algorithm 6
Status Epilepticus

1. Give D_{50}: 1 ml/kg (> 2 yrs) D_{25}: 1–2 ml/kg (< 2 yrs)
2. Diazepam, 0.1–0.3 mg/kg IV, IO, ET or rectally

Algorithm 7
Ingestion

1. Consider activated charcoal, 1 g/kg PO
useless for
   a. alcohol
   b. heavy metals
   c. lithium
2. Ipecac, 15–30 ml if child cannot take charcoal.
Never if
   a. VS abnormal
   b. Sensorium depressed
   c. Certain agents
      corrosives
      strychnine
      tricyclic antidepressants
      rapid-acting sedative-hypnotic
      certain hydrocarbons

FIGURE 2–1. Pediatric prehospital treatment algorithms.

for vascular access include not only endotracheal drugs, but also intraosseous (IO) and rectal drugs. When properly used and controlled, these routes are safe, effective, and simple.

Extending these modalities to the prehospital environment is key to optimal field care. The IO method is useful for a wide range of drugs and fluids, including epinephrine, atropine, anticonvulsants, and isotonic solutions. It is most appropriate for children under 3 years old. (The procedure is described in Chapter 139.)

Another important alternative to intravenous treatment is rectal diazepam, which is rapidly effective for the young child in status epilepticus.

In every field situation where vascular access is attempted by traditional or alternative methods, the time needed to complete the intervention and the accompanying transport delay must be carefully weighed against expected benefit.

Pediatric Prehospital Equipment, Supplies, and Drugs ■

Successful evaluation and treatment of pediatric prehospital emergencies requires proper equipment, supplies, and drugs. Table 2-2 lists appropriate ambulance equipment and supplies and Table 2-3 lists recommended prehospital pediatric drugs.

Pediatric Prehospital Treatment Guidelines ■

Algorithms for prehospital treatment of specific conditions are illustrated in Figure 2-1. These recommendations must be adapted by community clinical advisory committees. Field application of these algorithms is determined by radio direction from the base hospital or paramedic communication center. Sometimes physicians may request that field care deviate from written guidelines; for example, often no treatment is the most appropriate field approach.

An accurate history and physical exam at the scene require an age-appropriate assessment and careful observation of the child with the parent (see Chapter 3). A calm, reassuring approach to the ill or injured "family" will ameliorate treatment and transport; whenever possible, *keep the parent with the child during the prehospital experience*. All pediatric patients assessed by prehospital personnel require transport to the hospital, unless the radio control center authorizes specific release of the patient.

3 The Child in the Emergency Department

Sandra Jo Hammer

Ill and injured children form a disparate population whose emergency care requires skillful, knowledgeable practitioners and specialized, rapidly available equipment and resources. The quality of children's medical care has been profoundly influenced by progress in diagnosing and treating childhood illness and injury, recent sociologic trends, and national fiscal policies.

Characteristics of Population ■

Pediatric patients account for about 25–35% of the total emergency department (ED) population. The percentage of critically ill and injured children is small compared to adult ED populations, perhaps 5–10%.

Common ED diagnoses are otitis media, upper respiratory infections, gastroenteritis, conjunctivitis, and minor trauma. Complex and life-threatening medical and surgical emergencies also affect children, especially those under 2 years old. Previously healthy infants develop sepsis or meningitis; school-age children suffer acute exacerbations of their medically controlled conditions. Children live longer with serious chronic illness.

Injury continues to be the leading cause of pediatric mortality between age 1 year and early adulthood. Sources include vehicular injuries, drownings, burns, toxic ingestions, and falls. Nonaccidental trauma, including homicide, suicide, and child abuse, may be on the rise, and this trend may have significant implications for EDs.

UTILIZATION PATTERNS

Generally, parents use EDs for minor illnesses rather than for well-child care, reflecting the primary-care provider's lack of availability for nonurgent and advice services, especially on weekends and evenings. Because parents or caregivers in the most vulnerable populations (poor, migrant, homeless, minority) appear to greatly overestimate the child's illness and overutilize ED services, they comprise a disproportionate share of the ED population. Pediatric ED patients are often referred by private physicians and primary-care providers after regular office hours. Moreover, children are often not covered by private or public health insurance or this insurance is inadequate, leading to delays in seeking care and preventable mortality and morbidity. Table 3-1 summarizes the changing characteristics of the overall pediatric ED population.

TABLE 3–1. *Changing Characteristics of Pediatric ED Populations*

Larger number of children with chronic illness.

Growing number of children with sequelae from complex chronic illness.

Increasing numbers of "vulnerable" children, overusing services for minor problems.

Earlier recognition of child physical/sexual abuse by health care providers.

Increasing rates of NAT (non-accidental trauma).

Greater primary-care ED referral after hours and weekends.

Enhanced recognition of potentially life-threatening illness by pediatricians, with earlier ED referral.

Low rate of ambulance use for major emergencies.

Regionalization of pediatric tertiary (e.g., burns, psychological, critical care) and trauma care with concentration of specialty patients in individual institutions.

Less federal financial support for routine health care and for preventive care in the community, with resultant ED use as a "last resort."

TABLE 3–2. *Developmental Approaches for Pediatric Physical Assessment*

Age Group	Developmental Characteristics	Nursing Actions
Infants	Often experience separation anxiety after 6 months of age	Have parent hold baby for most of examination.
		Distract infant with brightly colored toys or by talking. Small stuffed animals that clip onto stethoscopes are effective for distracting infants and toddlers while assessing breath sounds.
Toddlers	Eager to please	Explain what pleases you (for example: "Holding still will make it easier for me to listen to you.").
		Show pleasure when child cooperates.
	Need to feel autonomous	Have child help to unbutton shirt.
	Fantasies are prevalent	Use child's fantasies to elicit cooperation (for example: "I'm going to listen to you with my stethoscope to hear if you have any ducks quacking inside.").
	Fear separation from parents	Have parent hold child while you listen to child's chest.
	Learn through sensorimotor experiences	Explain what you will do with child in short sentences using sensory terms.
		Allow child to play with equipment; (for example, have him "blow out the light" from otoscope, listen to his own heartbeat with stethoscope).
Preschoolers	Ask lots of questions	Give child opportunity to ask questions.
		Answer with simple, short, responses.
		Answer only what is asked.
	Attempt to cope with new situations	Encourage play to help child relate to ED experience.
	Have prominent fears of castration	Tell child which part of body you will examine.
School-aged children	Are absorbed with concrete aspects of situations	Supply child with technical explanations about what occurs
		Use simple drawings such as an upside-down tree to explain pulmonary anatomy.
	Understand body mechanics	Use examination time as an opportunity to teach about health.
	May need privacy	Ensure privacy while listening to child's chest; parents may need to leave room momentarily.
	Feel peers are important	Emphasize ED experience as a unique event to share with friends.
Adolescents	Definitely need privacy	Decide who will be present during physical examination before examination.
	Think logically and concretely	Be straightforward in your approach; do not be condescending.
	Have concerns about results of their treatment	Advise adolescents of their response to aerosols and other treatments.
		Keep them informed of expected outcomes of treatment.
		Report evidence of normal physical examination findings as well as abnormal ones.

(From Wabschall J: Nursing management of children during a mild to moderate asthma attack. *J Emerg Nursing* 1986;12:137.)

Evaluation ■

Rapid, comprehensive assessment of the child in the ED requires an age-specific orientation. Table 3-2 outlines such a developmental approach. Because children range from tiny infants to adolescents of more than 80 kg, it is most important to appreciate the child's physical ability to respond to injury and illness, as well as his or her psychosocial and cognitive capabilities to cooperate, communicate, and understand. In the pre-school and early school age child not in physical distress, play therapy with draw-

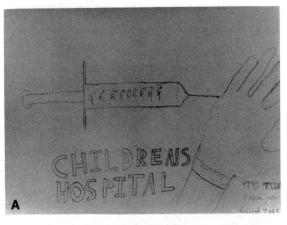

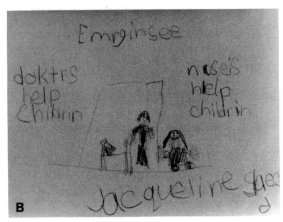

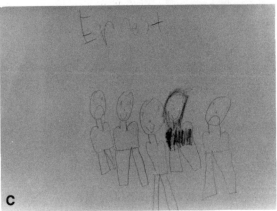

FIGURE 3–1. Children's artwork: How they view the ED. (*A*) Nine-year-old trauma victim resuscitated in the ED. (*B*) Six-year-old child who has never been to an ED. (*C*) Six-year-old asthmatic with many previous visits to the ED.

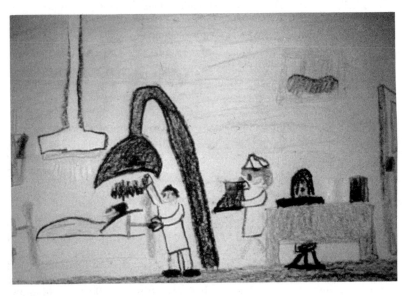

FIGURE 3–2. A child's view of the inside of the ED.

TABLE 3–3. *Predictive Model: Six Observation Items and Their Scales*

Observation Item	1 Normal	2 Moderate Impairment	3 Severe Impairment
Quality of cry	Strong with normal tone or content and not crying	Whimpering or sobbing	Weak or moaning or high pitched
Reaction to parent stimulation	Cries briefly then stops or content and not crying	Cries off and on	Continual cry or hardly responds
State variation	If awake, stays awake or if asleep and stimulated, wakes up quickly	Eyes close briefly, awake or wakes with prolonged stimulation	Falls to sleep or will not rouse
Color	Pink	Pale extremities or acrocyanosis	Pale or cyanotic or mottled or ashen
Hydration	Skin normal, eyes normal and mucous membranes moist	Skin, eyes are normal and mouth slightly dry	Skin doughy or tented and dry mucous membranes and/or sunken eyes
Response (talk, smile) to social overtures	Smiles or alerts (≤2 mo)	Brief smile or alerts briefly (≤2 mo)	No smile, face anxious, dull, expressionless or no alerting (≤2 mo)

Score: <10 only 2.7% had a serious illness.
11–15 26.2% had a serious illness.
>16 92.3% had a serious illness.
(From McCarthy PL, et al: Observation scales for febrile children. *Pediatrics* 1982; 70:806. Copyright American Academy of Pediatrics, 1982, reprinted with permission)

ing may be effective to allay anxiety (See Figure 3-1).

Acute pediatric illness is often difficult to detect and qualitate. Unlike the directed anatomic exam that underlies adult physical diagnosis, the overall condition of the ill child is best derived from an observational model (Table 3-3). Such simple observations of physical state such as color, hydration, quality of

TABLE 3–4. *Triage Categories*

Category	Definition	Access to ED	Examples of Patient Complaint
I Emergent	Life and/or limb threatening Unstable	Immediate (seconds)	Cardiac arrest, seizures, obvious respiratory distress. Fractures with vascular compromise.
II Urgent	Stable, potentially unstable	As soon as possible (minutes)	Sickle-cell crisis, displaced extremity fractures without vascular compromise. Moderate dehydration <10%. Wheezing with accessory muscle use.
	Should be reassessed every 15 minutes until treated.		
III Nonurgent	Stable, no obvious distress	As soon as space becomes available	Simple lacerations with controlled bleeding, mild dehydration <5% Fevers <38.5°C in children >6 mo.
	Should be reassessed every 30 minutes until treated.		
IV Stable	Stable, no distress	When space and personnel available	Impetigo, abrasions, colds without fever.
	Should be reassessed every hour.		

(Adapted from Thompson J, Dains J: Comprehensive triage. Reston, Va.: Reston Publishing Co., 1982)

TABLE 3–5. *Characteristics of a Dedicated Pediatric Area*

A. Adjacent but separate from adult ED.
B. Muted wall colors, cool shades, cartoon or familiar character murals on walls.
C. Separate waiting area for parents and siblings.
D. Separate desk and telephone extension.
E. Rooms that provide privacy yet allow easy visibility, suction, and oxygen in all rooms.
F. Comfortable chairs, including rockers for parents.
G. Controlled, heated environment.
H. Gurneys with side rails, basinettes and cribs available.
I. Activities for children and parents.
   1. Waiting area—closed-circuit cable TV with child-care information. Permanent, easily washable play scapes, carpeting.
   2. Pediatric ED—diversional materials, books, coloring books with crayons, washable toys, magazines, and child-care information available to parents.
   3. Informational/educational area—pamphlets, books on injury and illness prevention and common pediatric problems.
J. Small kitchen area with premade formulas, juice, bottles, crackers, baby foods; coffee available to parents.
K. Separate treatment room for painful procedures (IV starts, LPs, bladder taps).

cry, and social response may be more sensitive and predictive of serious illness than a physical exam. *Approaching the child in a kind, gentle, reassuring manner is key.* A warm, private environment and gentle instrumentation is likewise valuable.

The Injured Family ■

EDs are chaotic and frightening to patients and families. Acute injury and illness affect not only the child but also his or her nuclear and extended families and community. Parents are abruptly faced with supporting the child while coping with their own concerns, anxieties, and responsibilities, especially to other siblings. Ordinarily, the ED staff should limit access to children in the ED, even from concerned, well-meaning (or hostile) relatives and visitors. Separating the parent and child, however, is unnecessary and unwise except during periods of intensive resuscitation or when parental anxiety has a negative effect on the child's coping. Usually, with adequate explanation, the parent is an ally and assistant.

Siblings of ED patients are confronted with their own fears and anger about perceived illness, pain, and causality. Sibling guilt may be overwhelming, especially when the child, during the course of normal sibling rivalry resolution, had secretly wished harm upon the other child. The ED provider must anticipate sibling reactions and appropriately prepare parents for adverse reactions and regressive behaviors (see Chapter 127). Therefore, every injured or ill child is best viewed as an "injured family." Every family must be sustained and supported by active staff participation, frequent discussion, and honest, frank communication about ED procedures and the child's status. Very often, social services and clergy are helpful.

Triage ■

ED nursing triage identifies and prioritizes the level of need for emergency services. With growing demands for emergency services, triage serves an ever-increasing role in quality ED care.

A basic knowledge of normal pediatric growth and development, both physiologic and psychosocial, provides a framework to detect variations and deviations. Familiarity with age-adjusted physiologic parameters such as heart and respiratory rates, temperature, and blood pressure is essential. A triage setting with minimal distractions allows for the rapid collection of subjective and objective nursing data, comforts the ill and uncomfortable child and family, and facilitates appropriate management of acute pediatric illness. Communicating with the parent and child clearly, honestly, and concisely are hallmarks of effective triage.

Assignment of a triage classification reflects not only data collection about disease severity, but also the ED's ability to treat the child expeditiously. Table 3-4 give examples of triage categories. A triage system is most effective and efficient when it is customized for each facility, ED capability, and predicted volume. This allows flexibility and reallocation of personnel to meet the sudden volume increases inherent in ED populations.

The following data should be recorded at triage:

1. *General appearance:* Use observational model.
2. *Temperature:* Collected in centigrade scale by the most accurate route: rectally, orally, axillary, tympanic membrane. Antipyretics may be administered based on standing departmental order.
3. *Pulse:* Apical, noting rate and rhythm. Document pulses distal to suspected fractures.
4. *Respirations:* At-rest respiratory rate; note quality (grunting, flaring, retracting).
5. *Blood pressure:* Use proper cuff size (two-thirds distance from elbow to shoulder).

Pediatric ED ■

Ideally, facilities that treat children should have a dedicated pediatric area and staff. In a general ED, the nurse assigned to pediatrics is often viewed as expendable and is reassigned to the adult area, causing long waits for pediatric patients and families and markedly decreasing nursing interventions. This is dangerous and alienating. Moreover, noisy environments may harm the child and parents. Child-sensitive environments and activities in the ED may make waiting more bearable and may greatly decrease psychological distress. Table 3-5 describes the characteristics of a dedicated pediatric area.

Each child is best managed in the ED by a designated primary physician-nurse team. The essential components in providing effective ED care are communication, teamwork, planning, practice, and education. Role expectations must be established for the combined team effort and goals must be set for patient care in the department.

ED Disposition ■

Discharge from the ED, usually the final phase of care, should be preceded by home instructions, both verbal and written (see Chapter 143), prescriptions, and arrangements for follow-up care. If the child has no source of primary health care, arrange for this before the child leaves the ED. Preventive education is an essential responsibility of nurses and physicians during patient discharge. After a morbid event, the injured family is especially receptive to such education. Pamphlets and referral information may reinforce verbal instruction.

If admission is indicated, provide a careful explanation to the child and parent, including the reason for admission and the anticipated course. Ensure that the patient is admitted to the clinical unit or intensive care unit (ICU) as soon as possible after the admission decision. The ED is an inappropriate environment for extended treatment or monitoring of an unstable patient.

When admission to the ICU is indicated, the parents should accompany the child to the unit and be introduced to the ICU care providers, thereby preserving continuity.

If transfer to another facility is necessary, tell the parents as soon as the decision is made. Indicate the time of transfer and the planned transfer method (transport team, aeromedical, family). Also explain how to find the receiving facility, the unit the child is being admitted to, and the receiving physician's name.

Bibliography ■

Christoffel K, Garside D, Tokich T: Pediatric emergency department utilization in the 1970s. *Am J Emerg Med* 1985; May:177–181.

Kelley S: Pediatric emergency nursing. Norwalk, Conn.: Appleton and Lange, 1988.

Liptak G, Super D, Baker N, et al: An analysis of waiting times in a pediatric emergency department. *Clin Pediatr* 1985; 24(4):202–209.

Smith R, McNamara J: Why not your pediatrician's office? A study of weekday pediatric emergency department use for minor illness care in a community hospital. *Pediatr Emerg Care* 1988; 4(2):107–111.

Thompson J, Dains J: Comprehensive triage. Reston, Va.: Reston Publishing Co., 1982.

Wabschall J: Nursing management of children during a mild to moderate asthma attack. *J Emerg Nursing* 1986; 12(3): 134–141.

4 Medical Direction and Quality Assurance

Richard H. Cales

Emergency medical services for children (EMSC), a subset of the overall emergency medical services (EMS) system, accounts for about 10% of prehospital care (Figure 4-1) and 25–35% of emergency department (ED) care. Medical direction and quality assurance for both the individual patient and the EMS system are essential components.

Models ■

Medical direction entails supervision of all medical aspects of EMSC, including planning, implementation, and evaluation of medical care by specially qualified physicians. *Quality assurance* safeguards clinical care and provides public accountability for EMSC operation. Together, they provide the foundation for medical practice in EMSC.

MEDICAL DIRECTION

Medical direction—either on-line or off-line—has *prospective, concurrent,* and *retrospective* aspects. On-line and off-line refer to the direct or indirect relationship, respectively, between the responsible physician and the telecommunications radio network that orchestrates prehospital care from the paramedic base hospital or communication center. Paramedics are permitted to give advanced life support (ALS) to children in the field only under strict radio direction by physicians or physician extenders.

On-line medical direction refers to *concurrent* medical supervision of prehospital care (that is, at the time care is actually rendered), through scene management of field care or through radio supervision. Physicians or, in some states, mobile intensive care nurses (MICNs) functioning as physician extenders provide on-line medical direction for overall EMS. Centralizing on-line medical direction of all field care for children into one source facilitates quality care because it concentrates patient-care re-sponsibilities among a small group of trained physician specialists who clearly understand the procedures, capabilities, and triage process of the entire prehospital sector as well as the special problems and needs of children with emergency conditions. Centralized medical direction is particularly important in pediatric emergencies because of their infrequency, high acuity, and unfamiliarity.

Off-line medical direction, in contrast, involves *prospective* responsibility for developing pediatric standards, such as base hospital call-in criteria and treatment protocols for emergency medical technicians (EMTs) and paramedics (EMTs-P). Off-line physicians also hold *retrospective* responsibility for evaluating patient care and system performance.

Off-line medical direction of pediatric prehospital care is optimally provided by a pediatric emergency physician with special expertise in EMS or an emergency physician with appropriate pediatric training. EMS medical directors not fully versed in pediatric emergency care must obtain additional input from qualified pediatric specialists. Unfortunately, many communities continue to provide medical direction via committee, resulting in ineffective medical leadership and accountability.

QUALITY ASSURANCE

Quality assurance (QA) for EMSC, as for other medical care, encompasses three basic approaches—*input, process,* and *outcome.* Comprehensive QA programs also incorporate *risk management,* which attempts to reduce legal exposure by anticipating and, ideally, minimizing medical misadventures (see Chapter 132 on medicolegal issues).

Input

Input measures for EMS are inventories of system resources, especially standards that precisely define

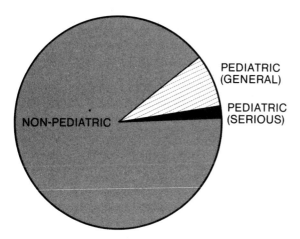

FIGURE 4–1. EMS system for prehospital emergencies.

performance expectations. Such measures may be based on face validity (expert opinion) or, less commonly, on scientific validity (research).

EMSC standards address all aspects of care, including prevention, system access, prehospital care, inhospital care, and, when necessary, rehabilitation and follow-up. Prehospital care standards include "the five T's": training, treatment, triage, transport, and transfer. Standards for pediatric receiving facilities apply to either of two general types of facilities: emergency departments appropriate for pediatrics (EDAPs) or highly specialized hospitals equipped to manage specific pediatric conditions (i.e., trauma and critical care) (see Chapter 1). EDAPs are qualified to provide care for most pediatric emergencies and usually serve as general EDs as well.

EMS transfer standards or protocols provide particular benefit for pediatric patients, who often present to hospitals unequipped to provide definitive care, especially in rural areas, and who need expeditious transfer to more appropriate pediatric hospitals.

Process

Process measures assess the quality of care by evaluating compliance with input measures. Examples are review of prehospital medical records for compliance with pediatric field treatment protocols and designation of pediatric hospitals. Prehospital records, hospital charts, and, when available, specialized databases such as trauma and toxicology registers are key to such efforts. Additionally, verification of the ongoing capability of qualified pediatric receiving hospitals ensures continuing system performance for pediatric cases.

Incident reports, vital to effective risk management, document departures from normal operating procedures. Although not part of the medical record, they provide insurers with confidential information regarding episodes that might result in litigation.

Outcome

Outcome measures, which evaluate the results of resources and care, provide the most definitive single QA indicator. Endpoints include mortality and, more difficult to quantify, morbidity.

Risk Management

Risk management, properly implemented, not only reduces legal exposure but also improves medical quality. With dwindling fiscal resources for medical care, increasing expectations of EMS systems, and more frequent EMS litigation, risk management has become essential for system survival.

QA Overview ■

Optimal QA combines the strengths of input, process, and outcome to detect individual problems and, more importantly, trends that require additional attention. Oversight should be provided by a multidisciplinary group that includes emergency physicians, pediatricians, nurses, hospital administrators, and prehospital providers.

Patients appropriate for review can be identified by *random sampling* or *focused selection*. *Random sampling* of patients without high-risk features, whether transported by ambulance or presenting to the ED, typically includes a statistically insignificant sample such as 5% of all patients, yet provides important QA data. Review of a larger proportion of such low-yield patients is neither necessary nor cost-effective. *Focused selection* provides significant cost savings by focusing review on patients with high-risk conditions, identified through generic screens such as Code 3 ambulance runs and high-acuity ED presentations. Combining both methods increases yield while maintaining an efficient QA process.

Particular attention should be paid to patients who stand to benefit most from EMS system intervention. By correlating severity with outcome, reviewers can identify unexpected survivors and deaths, thereby identifying patients meriting additional review while quantifying the overall quality of care.

However, QA efforts are for naught if they do not result in changes that improve quality. Achieving this goal requires four steps:

1. Identifying problems
2. Updating standards
3. Re-evaluating compliance
4. Reassessing the effect of changes.

Using this approach, the EMS system assumes a pro-active role in detecting and resolving problems with the quality of care before they reach crisis proportions.

Bibliography ■

Donabedian A: The quality of medical care: Methods for assessing and monitoring the quality of care for research and for quality assurance programs. *Science* 1978; 200: 856–864.

Holroyd BR, Knopp R, Kallsen G: Medical control: Quality assurance in prehospital care. *JAMA* 1986; 256:1027–1031.

Tsai A, Kallsen G: Epidemiology of pediatric prehospital care. *Ann Emerg Med* 1987; 16:284–292.

Williamson JW, Aronovitch S, Simonson L, et al: Health accounting: An outcome-based system of quality assurance: Illustrative application of hypertension. *Bull NY Acad Med* 1975; 51:727–738.

5 Interfacility Transport of the Critically Ill and Injured Child

Timothy S. Yeh and Byron Y. Aoki

In the last decade, major advances have occurred in the care of critically ill and injured children treated within the emergency medical services (EMS) system. These advances have led to the development of a comprehensive pediatric critical care system with prehospital, emergency department (ED), and in-hospital phases. The in-hospital phase also includes the component of *interfacility transport* (Figure 5-1). Chapters 1, 2, and 3 have presented the appropriate design for prehospital and ED management of critical pediatric patients. This chapter focuses on stabilization and subsequent interfacility transport of the severely ill or injured child to a pediatric intensive care unit (PICU) or a pediatric critical care center (PCCC).

The development of critical care centers for children has also brought the implementation of transport systems to deliver these patients safely to specialized facilities. Outcomes are improved when severely ill or injured children are treated in tertiary-care centers. Therefore, EMS training and triage must emphasize early identification of such patients to enhance transport to appropriate receiving centers. Whenever possible, patients should be transported directly from the field to a PCCC, as outlined in Chapter 1. Strict field triage criteria and capable on-line radio direction of paramedic ambulances are essential to this process. Often, however, critical-care transports occur secondarily as interfacility transports between the primary receiving facility, either an ED or an inpatient unit, to a PICU.

The number of patients requiring critical care is small, about 2–5% of all children transported in the EMS system. But the problems encountered in these patients are diverse, and their definitive treatment requires the resources of facilities with trained staff, a wide range of pediatric in-house subspecialists, and equipment appropriate for the care of critically ill children. Since few facilities have PICUs, especially in rural areas, interfacility transport is an important means of providing equal access for all children requiring pediatric intensive care.

Components of Interfacility Transport System ■

All pediatric critical care transport systems have the same basic components: *the communications system, the transport team, and the equipment.* Each referring facility and region should have specific standards for their transport systems. Ideally, general agreements for interfacility transfers should be carefully discussed and negotiated prospectively to expedite individual case management. Tertiary-care centers that provide critical-care services for children must evaluate regional critical-care needs, in concert with other hospitals and tertiary centers, medical professionals, and EMS representatives, to develop the systems best suited for their areas.

Transport Responsibilities ■

Interfacility transport of critically ill and injured children requires good communication, cooperation, and an understanding of the capabilities and limitations of all parties involved. The interfacility transport is a joint effort and a shared responsibility between the referring and receiving institutions. The care providers may be separated into *the referring facility staff, the receiving facility staff,* and *the transport team.*

RESPONSIBILITIES OF THE REFERRING FACILITY STAFF

The referring physician's role begins with the initial resuscitation and stabilization. After this, a decision must be made as to whether the patient will require

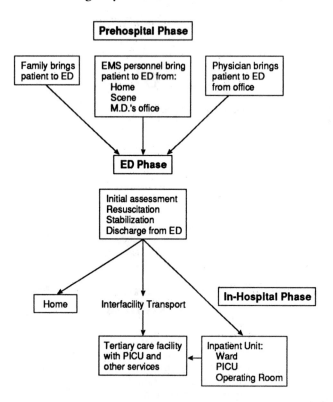

FIGURE 5-1. Pediatric critical care system.

transport to another facility. Pre-established transfer guidelines may aid this determination. In the initial call to the tertiary center, sufficient information must be exchanged to determine the patient's current status, the appropriate mode of transport, the need for further stabilizing measures, and the approximate time the transport team will arrive. Information from the referring physician should be documented on a standardized checklist, such as Table 5-1. Because time is very precious, the information transmitted must be pertinent, concise, and easily understood.

In the time between PICU contact and the arrival of the transport team, the referring physician should maintain contact with the tertiary center to assess and treat changes in the patient's condition appropriately. Limited ED staff and equipment may dictate what can actually be done for the patient before transfer. Admission to the pediatric ward, general ward, or general ICU may provide a better environment for monitoring and ongoing care, especially when the time before transfer is long. All practitioners who care for critically ill or injured children must develop not only skills for initial assessment and stabilization of critical conditions, but also a familiarity with the pediatric critical-care resources available in their own facility and region.

RESPONSIBILITIES OF THE RECEIVING FACILITY STAFF

The PICU or tertiary receiving facility must activate the transport team as soon as possible. The receiving facility decides on the mode of transport. Staffing limitations in either the PICU or the transport team, as well as traffic and weather conditions, may delay dispatch of the transport team. If such a delay occurs, it is the tertiary center's responsibility to decide on the best course of action. Referral to another PICU may be necessary, and the tertiary center should facilitate this by contacting other critical-care units for the referring physician. Meanwhile, the PICU physician staff continues to assist the referring physician in stabilizing the patient and preparing for transfer.

RESPONSIBILITIES OF THE TRANSPORT TEAM

Once the transport team arrives at the referring facility, it may assume full responsibility for the patient or it may work with the referring physician until departure. The transport team contacts the PICU before leaving to discuss further therapeutic interventions and the patient's current status. If any sudden or unexpected changes occur, the transport team may need to contact the PICU during transport.

TABLE 5–1. *Transport Information*

Patient Name
Age/Date of birth
Weight

Referring physician's name
Referring hospital name
City, phone number
Patient location (ER, OR, ICU)

Brief history of present illness

Vital signs including HR, RR, BP, Temp

Brief description of physical exam with pertinent findings
  including
    Color
    Character of respirations
    Pulses/perfusion
    Neurologic function (level of consciousness, tone,
      posture, pupils, Glasgow Coma Score)
    Hydration
    Urine output

Laboratory studies (relevant studies)
X-rays and other diagnostic studies

Current therapy

Need for isolation (e.g. Varicella)

Summary of patient status
  General assessment
  Significant problems by organ system

Questions/Discussion of on-going therapy

Communications ■

The communications system must provide a mechanism for initiating the transport and for ongoing consultation. Many tertiary-care centers provide toll-free telephone numbers for easy access. Once the transport team arrives, appropriate interaction and exchange of information must take place between the transport team and the referring facility personnel to ensure a smooth transition in patient care. Finally, the communications system must be able to maintain continued contact between the transport team and the receiving hospital during the actual transport.

The Transport Team ■

The transport team must be able to provide the level of care required for the patient. Team personnel may consist of any of the following: physician (attending, PICU or equivalent fellow, pediatric resident), PICU nurse, mobile intensive care nurse (MICN), respiratory therapist, paramedic or emergency medical technician (EMT), as well as a pilot for air transports. The actual composition of the team is best determined by the medical director of the PICU transport service, who is in the best position to know the skills and capabilities of the transport team personnel and to match them with the patient's needs. Although most pediatric transport teams include a physician, there are many excellent interfacility transport services that use critical-care nurses or paramedics. Personnel must be skilled in pediatric critical-care assessment and technical skills, such as intravascular access and endotracheal intubation. The referring physician familiar with the type of transport team used by the regional tertiary center is best able to help the tertiary center assign the necessary personnel.

Equipment and Vehicles ■

The mode of transport must be based upon the patient's best interests and not the convenience of either the referring or receiving facility. Geographic constraints such as distance (greater than 150–200 miles) and terrain (mountain ranges and large bodies of water) may dictate the use of fixed-wing air transport. Helicopter transport may be ideal in situations in which ground transportation times would be unreasonable due to distance or traffic problems. In some instances, however, ground transport is preferable, such as when inclement weather makes air transport impossible or when no suitable landing site is available. Regardless of the mode of transport selected, the vehicle must be able to provide the transport team with a mobile intensive care unit, including a portable ventilator, compressed gases, suction capabilities, and electric power for monitors and other equipment. Some transport vehicles have gurneys and isolettes designed specifically for different ages. The small pediatric patient with a relatively large body surface area is particularly susceptible to excessive heat loss, necessitating warming lights or temperature-controlled isolettes.

Most transport teams carry their own pediatric supplies, in addition to the equipment supplied in the vehicle. These include intubation and ventilation equipment (laryngoscopes, endotracheal tubes, suction catheters), intravenous catheters, intravenous fluids, monitoring equipment (stethoscope, blood pressure cuffs, thermometer, ECG monitor, pulse oximeter), and drugs. All equipment is sized appropriately to accommodate the anatomic differences in the growing infant and child.

Which Patients Should Be Transferred? ■

Criteria have been recently promulgated for primary field triage of severely ill and injured children to a receiving hospital capable of providing pediatric critical-care services. Such standards have the greatest application in the urban EMS system with many hospitals that have variable capabilities for providing pediatric care within a relatively limited geographical area. On the other hand, guidelines for interfacility transport depend on many variables that are specific to institutions, regions, and patients. Therefore, only broad guidelines are appropriate; individual case management should be based on the relative capabilities of the referring and receiving facilities. Table 5-2 provides a example of recently proposed criteria for pediatric interfacility transfers in northern and central California.

In practice, most children transferred to PICUs have either neurologic emergencies (particularly head trauma) or respiratory problems, often requiring therapeutic interventions such as intubation and mechanical ventilation. When the characteristics of the overall group of children in critical-care units are analyzed, differences are significant depending on where the child is hospitalized. Pediatric patients receiving intensive care in community hospitals tend to be older (10–18 years) and are often trauma or ingestion victims, while the patients in PICUs are younger (70% <5 years) and have respiratory disease, cardiovascular problems, or trauma. The referring physician must understand the capabilities of his or her hospital to decide whether the patient can receive optimal care there. Many hospitals can provide excellent care to critically ill adult patients but cannot offer the same services to children. Generally speaking, *younger patients requiring mechanical ventilation, aggressive cardiovascular support, extensive or complex surgical procedures, or management of*

TABLE 5–2. *Pediatric Interfacility Transfer Guidelines*

The following patients presenting to centers without pediatric critical care capability may benefit from immediate transfer to a pediatric critical care center or trauma center:

I. Physiologic Features
1. Glasgow Coma Scale of 8 or less
2. Respiratory failure or need for mechanical ventilation
3. Shock refractory to volume therapy
4. Blood transfusion requirements exceeding 40 ml/kg
5. Unstable cardiac dysrhythmias
6. Heart failure
7. Cardiopulmonary arrest
8. Severe hypothermia or hyperthermia
9. Hepatic failure
10. Renal failure
II. Anatomic Features
1. Fractures with neurovascular or compartment injury
2. Fractures of the axial skeleton
3. Suspected or actual spinal injuries
4. Traumatic amputations with potential for replantation
5. Head injury with
    Cerebrospinal fluid leak
    Significant depressed skull fracture
    Need for intracranial pressure monitoring
6. Penetrating wounds requiring complex operative repair
7. Flail chest
8. Electrocution
9. Major burns or inhalation injury
III. Etiologic Features
1. Near drowning
2. Refractory status epilepticus
3. Significant envenomation
4. Potentially life-threatening ingestions

(Modified from recommendations from the Pediatric Intensive Care Network of Northern and Central California, 1988–1989)

intracranial hypertension should be cared for in an ICU that is staffed by personnel experienced in the care of critically ill children. These centers can also provide the equipment and subspecialty consultants most appropriate for pediatric patients.

Preparing the Patient for Transport ▪

The number of critically ill and injured children is small. Most transported patients are young; one study found that 85% of the children were less than 6 years of age. Their problems are usually complex and involve multiple organ systems. Nearly two-thirds of these patients have neurologic or respiratory problems. The physician must therefore be prepared to rapidly treat children of all ages and sizes with a wide variety of disorders.

A practical approach to emergency evaluation and therapy is most useful for both the initial intervention and subsequent transport. A transport checklist (Fig. 5-2) may be helpful. The following are important stabilization guidelines:

Respiratory System
☐ Maintain adequate to high paO2 or oxygen saturation; the primary concern is to avoid hypoxemia—use FiO2 1.0 throughout stabilization and transport.
☐ Achieve normal to moderately alkalotic pH.
☐ *Intubate and ventilate* patient in respiratory failure or patient at risk for developing failure in transit.
☐ Obtain chest x-ray: check endotracheal tube position, barotrauma.
☐ Insert nasogastric tube in all intubated patients.
Cardiovascular System
☐ Maintain adequate/good heart rate, blood pressure.
☐ *Administer fluids, inotropes* as needed to restore blood pressure.
☐ Correct pathologic *dysrhythmias.*
Neurologic System
☐ *Control seizures.*
☐ Aim for *adequate cerebral perfusion pressure* in the patient with a central nervous system insult (estimate if intracranial pressure is unknown).
☐ Use medical *intracranial pressure (ICP) control measures* when ICP elevation is suspected.
Metabolic Problems
☐ Check and correct life-threatening *abnormal electrolytes.*
☐ Address specific pediatric concerns: *glucose, calcium.*
Fluids
☐ Establish *reliable intravenous or intraosseous access.*
☐ Use *appropriate intravenous fluids and rates.* Avoid D5W!
Renal
☐ Establish and *follow urine output.*
Hematologic
☐ Check *hemoglobin, hematocrit:* establish minimum level for adequate oxygen content.
☐ Check for *bleeding:* platelet count, coagulation studies.
Infectious Disease
☐ *Administer antibiotics* for presumed infection.
Temperature
☐ Aim for *euthermia:*
　☐ *Antipyretics* for fever.
　☐ Provide warmth for *hypothermia,* take measures to prevent hypothermia especially in small infants and children
Injury
☐ Apply cervical collar, splints, hemorrhage control, pain control as needed.
Transport Preparation
☐ *Secure* endotracheal tube, intravascular line, tubes and catheters.
☐ *Restrain, sedate* patient as needed.
☐ Have anticipated equipment, medications and supplies readily available.
☐ Take copies of medical record chart, x-rays and specimens.
Air Transport Considerations
☐ *Oxygen:* anticipate drop in partial pressure during ascent; use FiO2 1.0.
☐ Air transport may be contraindicated in patient with *borderline or inadequate oxygen delivery*-severe hypoxemia, anemia.
☐ *Air-filled body cavities:* expand at lower atmospheric pressure.
　☐ Place nasogastric tube—evacuate air from stomach.
　☐ Place chest tube for pneumothorax (even for small ones since they may expand).
　☐ Air in other body cavities—treat as needed.
Call Receiving PICU
☐ Specific suggestions for individual situations.

FIGURE 5–2. Transport preparation checklist.

1. Address patient problems by organ system and by pathophysiology, not by diagnosis. Since multisystem failure may be present and a definitive diagnosis may not be established, identify and treat specific pathophysiologic findings. Examples: hypoxemia, wheezing, hypoglycemia.
2. Focus initial therapy on life-threatening problems; address other problems later. Restore and maintain oxygen delivery first, since the first priority is stabilization of the respiratory and cardiovascular systems. Next, identify and treat other important organ systems, such as the neurologic and skeletal systems.
3. Treat the likely etiologies of the identified problems, since an exact diagnosis is often not known. Therapy may also be provided for presumed life-threatening problems in the absence of definitive diagnosis. Example: presumed intracranial pressure elevation in the comatose head injury patient.
4. Treat the patient without performing the usual diagnostic tests when such procedures may delay urgently needed therapy (e.g., prolonged attempts to obtain blood cultures in a patient with probable septic shock) or further compromise the patient (e.g., a lumbar puncture in a febrile patient with meningismus and hypoventilation).
5. Stabilize the patient before departure to minimize the chances of deterioration en route that would necessitate complex interventions in a poorly controlled environment.
6. Provide early interventions for anticipated problems that would not necessarily be required in the non-transport situation. Example: before departure, intubate the child in respiratory distress who is not in full respiratory failure but may require intervention during transport.
7. Limit therapy and monitoring in transit to essential patient needs. Be as efficient and uncomplicated as possible.

A checklist for preparing a child for transport (Figure 5-2) can be useful to both the referring facility staff and the transport team and should be reviewed in detail before departure.

Bibliography ■

Britten AG, Rogers MC: Transportation of critically ill children. In Roger MC, ed.: *Textbook of Pediatric Intensive Care*. Baltimore: Williams & Wilkins, 1987, p. 1386.

Kissoon N, Frewen TC, Kronick JB, et al: The child requiring transport: Lessons and implications for the pediatric emergency physician. *Pediatr Emerg Care* 1988;4:1.

Pettigrew AH, Singer JM, Falade E, et al: The report of the Pediatric Intensive Care Network of Northern and Central California. US Dept. of Health and Human Services Grant #MCJ-063336, 1986.

Pollack MM, Alexander SR, Clarke N, et al: The superiority of tertiary care pediatric intensive care. *Crit Care Med* 1988, 16(4), p. 376.

II

Cardiovascular Emergencies

6 Cardiopulmonary Arrest and Resuscitation

Ronald A. Dieckmann

Cardiopulmonary arrest in childhood is rare. It typically occurs as a secondary, terminal event, in a process of progressive system failure, precipitated by any of a diverse group of conditions. The actual cascade of pathophysiologic events leading to arrest almost always follows one of two final common pathways: either respiratory insufficiency or hemodynamic collapse. Respiratory insufficiency is the more common pathway and usually involves the infant.

Resuscitation from cardiac arrest in children is successful in only about 5–10% of cases. Several important problems account for poor outcome. First, there is a critical gap in scientific knowledge of the complex pathophysiology of cardiopulmonary arrest and of the effectiveness of current methods of treatment. Current standards for resuscitation are derived from animal models, adult experience, and anecdotal cases in childhood. Second, delayed response to serious childhood illness and injury frequently precludes early institution of potentially life-saving interventions. Such failures in response include problems in recognition of distress by parents and health-care providers, and slow mobilization of available community emergency medical services (EMS). Last, technical difficulties in airway management and vascular access and inadequate preparedness for major pediatric emergencies often limit the timeliness and quality of care in the prehospital setting and in the early emergency department (ED) phase of resuscitation.

Etiology ■

Table 6-1 presents the common causes of cardiac arrest in children. Of all etiologies, the most frequent is *sudden infant death syndrome (SIDS)*, a still poorly understood disorder of autonomic regulation of cardiopulmonary function in infants. SIDS is responsible for up to 40% of all nontraumatic deaths in childhood. There is no known treatment for this condition. *Respiratory insufficiency*—usually secondary to infectious conditions, bronchospasm, near-drowning, or airway obstruction—is the most likely treatable cause of cardiac arrest. When treatment is effectively instituted at this stage, salvage is possible in 75–90% of cases.

Primary cardiac arrest occasionally occurs in children, usually in a child with known congenital heart disease or acquired cardiomyopathy who suffers a sudden lethal dysrhythmia or pump failure. The post-open heart operative period is a common setting for such an event.

Trauma deserves special emphasis, since injuries are by far the most likely reason for field emergency care in pediatrics (see Chapter 2) and the most common cause of deaths in children over 1 year of age. Serious childhood trauma is usually blunt and multisystem (head, chest, abdomen), with motor-vehicle accidents or falls as the mechanism of injury. Life-threatening pathophysiology in traumatized children may develop from respiratory insufficiency, hemodynamic collapse, or central nervous system (CNS) insult. Identifying and managing the pre-arrest state of childhood trauma is especially important because of high salvageability of such victims within well-organized systems for prehospital and ED trauma care.

PROFILES OF THE CARDIAC ARREST VICTIM

Three distinct clinical profiles of the pediatric arrest victim predominate:

1. The very young child, about 3–6 months old, suffering from respiratory infection and insufficiency, or SIDS
2. The toddler with severe underlying disease of the cardiopulmonary system or CNS, who is admitted to the hospital and has an in-hospital arrest
3. The older child, 7 or 8 years old, who arrests from closed head and multiple systems injuries after a traumatic event.

TABLE 6–1. *Common Etiologies of Pediatric Cardiopulmonary Arrest*

Sudden Infant Death Syndrome (SIDS)	***Trauma***
	Motor vehicle accident
Respiratory Insufficiency	Fire—smoke inhalation
Lower airway	Falls
infections	Electrocution
Upper airway	
infections	***Central Nervous System Disorders***
Bronchospasm	
Drowning	***Seizures***
Aspiration/airway	Meningitis
obstruction	Hydrocephalus
	Tumors
Shock	Head trauma
Congenital heart	
disease	***Poisoning/Metabolic Disorders***
Cardiomyopathy	Reye's syndrome
Dehydration	Hypoglycemia
Sepsis	Hyperkalemia
Anaphylaxis	

Prognostic Variables ■

Outcome from true cardiac arrest in children is poor. Those who do survive are likely to have experienced witnessed arrests, with ventricular fibrillation as their presenting rhythm. They will have usually received early advanced life support (ALS), particularly electrical countershock; epinephrine; and field endotracheal intubation (positive predictive value for children under 18 months). The association of survival with witnessed arrest is well demonstrated for all patient populations and reflects the higher survivability when time from the precipitating event to definitive ALS is brief. Delays of more than 10 minutes have been uniformly related to poor outcome. When downtime is long enough that more than two epinephrine doses do not return spontaneous cardiac activity, mortality is almost certain; there have been no survivors among 70 such cases in three published studies.

Of all variables, presenting rhythm has the highest predictive value for survival from arrest. The most common rhythm of childhood arrest is bradyasystole, a terminal spectrum of electrical degeneration associated with hypoxia, that probably begins with bradycardia and ends with asystole. This rhythm is the first rhythm in about 95% of out-of-hospital arrests and about 90% of in-hospital arrests. Survival is less than 5%.

Ventricular dysrhythmias, primarily ventricular fibrillation and ventricular tachycardia, make up most

of the remaining patients. Children predisposed to these rhythms are older, usually with such associated conditions as congenital heart disease, metabolic disorders, traumatic myocardial contusion, electrocution, or viral myocarditis. When electrical countershock is applied early in this population, survival is probably 30–50%. Among all reported cases, where outcome from out-of-hospital arrest is linked to rhythm, about half of the successfully resuscitated children had ventricular fibrillation or ventricular tachycardia.

Finally, direct laryngoscopy for foreign body removal, and reversal of respiratory arrest by intubation and mechanical ventilation are key variables in overall survival. Successful prehospital intubation is correlated with resuscitation from full arrest in the patient under 18 months. Unfortunately, intubation success rates by field responders are less than 50% for this age group. Training, continuing re-training, and medical direction for field pediatric intubation must be well organized and carefully monitored to achieve consistent success.

Treatment ■

PREPAREDNESS

Preparedness, the principal ingredient for optimal resuscitation, includes prospective organization of drugs and equipment, rehearsals, and ongoing personnel training. Legible wall charts or pocket "code cards" help avoid common errors in memorization of age-adjusted weights, blood pressures, heart and respiratory rates, endotracheal tube sizes, and per-kilogram drug doses (See Chapter 133). During the resuscitation, all ALS interventions must be orchestrated by a single code team captain, a physician who assigns specific tasks to team members, ensures timely administration of drugs, and orders appropriate procedures. The captain's responsibilities also include setting prudent limits for the duration of the resuscitation attempt, critiquing the resuscitation with team members retrospectively, and communicating directly with the family. The captain's duties are summarized in Table 6-2.

Anticipation of arrest—especially with certain high-risk patients—is also part of proper preparedness. Table 6-3 lists major high-risk patients and circumstances.

PROCEDURAL CONSIDERATIONS

Securing reliable intravascular access is often the rate-limiting step in pediatric resuscitation. Both percutaneous and open cutdown cannulations of peripheral

TABLE 6–2. *Responsibilities of the Resuscitation Team Captain*

Assigns specific tasks to team members, prospectively if possible.
Ensures successful endotracheal intubation and effective ventilation.
Gives exact drug orders in a timely manner on a per-kilogram basis.
Orders all procedures (e.g., defibrillation, endotracheal drugs, vascular or intraosseous access, thoracostomy, pericardiocentesis).
Orders appropriate ancillary tests (e.g., laboratory analyses, radiographs, ECGs).
Determines therapeutic endpoint.
Determines patient disposition (e.g., intensive care unit admission, immediate transfer to tertiary facility).
Ensures accurate documentation of resuscitation.
Communicates directly with family.
Conducts retrospective critique with team members.
Contacts medical examiner (coroner) and primary physician as needed.

TABLE 6–3. *High-Risk Patients and High-Risk Situations for Cardiopulmonary Arrest*

High-Risk Patients
    Unstable neurologic status
    Shock
    Respiratory insufficiency
    Patient with underlying cardiopulmonary or CNS disease
    Neonates
High-Risk Situations
    Diagnostic Procedures
        Lumbar puncture
        Thoracocentesis
        Parenteral administration of cardiopulmonary depressant medications
    Therapeutic Maneuvers
        Intubation
        Extubation
        Thoracostomy
        Change of FiO_2
        Deep venous line placement
        Vagal stimulation
            Suctioning
            Tube feeding
            Nasogastric tube insertion

veins are associated with poor success rates, long delays, and frequent complications. Because of these difficulties in conventional techniques, both *endotracheal and intraosseous drug administration need to be considered early in resuscitation.*

ENDOTRACHEAL DRUGS

The four resuscitative drugs currently acceptable for endotracheal administration are epinephrine, atropine, lidocaine, and naloxone. Pharmacokinetic studies in children are not available, but overall efficacy is probably equal to intravenous administration, although several reports suggest higher doses for the endotracheal route. The most efficacious method for endotracheal drug administration is first to dilute the desired agent to 3–5 ml with normal saline, then to instill the solution directly into the trachea through a feeding tube inserted past the tip of the endotracheal tube. Table 6-4 lists the specific sequence for this procedure.

INTRAOSSEOUS INFUSIONS

The intraosseous (IO) or intramedullary infusion technique is now recognized as *effective* for all resuscitative drugs and fluids, *safe* to growing bones, and *simple* to teach and execute. (See Chapter 139.) This technique is best used in tandem with the endotracheal route, to allow early drug delivery while conventional intravenous access is sought.

The procedure is appropriate for prehospital field use in an adequately controlled EMS system. Either

the distal femur or the proximal tibia are suitable sites for needle insertion.

ELECTRICAL COUNTERSHOCK

Electrical countershock is a life-saving procedure in ventricular fibrillation, ventricular tachycardia, and unstable supraventricular tachycardia. *Reperfusion is directly correlated with speed of delivery of electrical current.* For infants, 4.5-cm paddles are appropriate; for children over 10 kg, use 8-cm paddles. Paddles can be applied in standard sterno-apical locations; if only adult paddles are available, they can be used anterior-posterior. A good conductive agent is nec-

TABLE 6–4. *Technique for Endotracheal Drug Administration*

Draw calculated drug dose into 10-ml syringe.
Dilute drug with normal saline to total volume of either 5 ml or 1 ml/kg if patient < 5 kg.
Insert tip of umbilical artery catheter or pediatric feeding tube past distal tip of endotracheal tube.
Instill solution directly into trachea.
Follow with injected air to clear tubing.
Ventilate three times with bag to disperse solution into distal tracheobronchial tree.

essary, together with firm application of paddles to the chest wall. Exact paddle size and the location and dose of electricity may be less important than a careful technique that ensures tight contact and timely repeat administrations. Table 6-5 presents specific steps in pediatric countershock.

The Resuscitation Sequence ■

The team captain delegates procedural tasks whenever possible and ensures that the following interventions are accomplished in a controlled, sequential fashion:

1. *Establish unresponsiveness and quality of cardiopulmonary effort.* Carefully look, listen, and feel to determine that an arrest has actually occurred.
2. *Open the airway.* Use the head-tilt/chin-lift maneuver, avoiding hyperextension of the neck. Too vigorous head-tilt may occlude the trachea or compromise the cervical spine in an injured patient. Therefore, use a jaw-thrust, instead of a head-tilt, when spinal injury is suspected. Suction

---

TABLE 6–5.   *Technique for Delivering Electrical Countershock*

Ensure indication is present, usually shock or full arrest with tachydysrhythmia or ventricular fibrillation.
When patient is conscious, consider light anesthesia with intravenous diazepam, 0.1–0.2 mg/kg.
Apply electrode jelly to lower left sternal border and at left posterior axillary line at level of cardiac apex. When adult paddles are used, select locations on the anterior and posterior left chest.
Use 4.5-cm paddles for infants; 8-cm paddles for children over 10 kg.
Rub jelly into chest wall to lower skin impedance.
Record the ECG.
Select appropriate electrical dose, based on rhythm and mass of patient.
Attempt *synchronized* cardioversion first if rhythm is tachydysrhythmia. Use *asynchronized* cardioversion (defibrillation) if rhythm is ventricular fibrillation or if synchronized cardioversion fails twice to convert tachydysrhythmia.
Apply paddles firmly to chest wall.
Ensure there is no contact between team personnel and patient or bed.
Discharge electrical current.
If sinus rhythm does not return, repeat the procedure with double the current.

---

may be needed to clean the airway of secretions, blood, foreign bodies, etc.
3. *If the airway remains obstructed* despite initial attempts to establish patency, implement the following maneuvers to evacuate a possible aspirated foreign body. For the older child, deliver 6–10 rapid subdiaphragmatic abdominal thrusts using the heel of the hand (modified Heimlich maneuver), with the patient supine. In the infant, give four sharp back blows with the heel of the hand between the securely held shoulder blades, then deliver four chest thrusts (instead of abdominal thrusts) to the mid-sternum.

   Repeat the sequence. If several series of maneuvers fail to establish patency, do immediate direct laryngoscopy to visualize the area of obstruction, and remove an obvious foreign body with Magill forceps. If this procedure does not relieve obstruction, perform endotracheal intubation. (See Chapter 139.) Very rarely, even endotracheal intubation fails to establish an effective airway. In such cases, do a needle cricothyroidotomy to bypass the obstruction. (See Chapter 139.)
4. *Secure the airway.* Insert an oropharyngeal or nasopharyngeal airway device when intubation equipment is not immediately available. (A conscious child will not tolerate the oropharyngeal device.) Otherwise, do immediate endotracheal intubation. The size of the tube can be approximated from the diameter of the patient's fifth digit, by age $\left(\dfrac{\text{Age in years} + 16}{4}\right)$, or taken from the wall chart for pediatric sizes. (See Chapter 133.)
5. *Ensure adequate breathing.* If breathing is absent or ineffective and endotracheal intubation is delayed, do assisted breathing with a properly-fitted bag-valve-mask apparatus. When bag-valve-mask ventilation is used, the technique is facilitated when one rescuer holds the mask firmly and the second rescuer does inflations. Slower, controlled inflations of the chest will provide optimal ventilation. (Refer to Table 6-6 for appropriate rate of ventilation for age.) Watch the chest rise to confirm successful ventilation. Next, insert a nasogastric tube and evacuate the stomach contents.

   Rarely, equipment for bag-valve-mask ventilation and endotracheal intubation is either unavailable or unsuccessful. In such cases, either mouth-to-mouth or mouth-to-nose-and-mouth ventilation may be considered. Use body substance precautions, if possible, to prevent disease transmission from victim to rescuer. When these methods are used, nasal oxygen per cannula applied to the resuscitator may enhance oxygen delivery.

TABLE 6-6. *Parameters for Cardiopulmonary Resuscitation in Children*

| Age | Breathing Rate | Compressions | | Hand Placement for Compression |
		Rate	Depth	
Less than 1 year	20 per minute	100–120	0.5–1 inch	2 or 3 fingers at midsternum, one finger below nipple line, or 2 thumbs at midsternum with hands encircling chest
1–7 years	15 per minute	80–100	1–1.5 inches	Three fingers or heel of one hand, 2 fingers above xyphoid
Over 7 years	12 per minute	80–100	1.5–2 inches	Heel of both hands with body pressure, 2 fingers above xyphoid

6. *Examine for a pulse.* If none is palpable, begin chest compressions at the appropriate rate while supporting the back with the opposite hand or with a pediatric backboard. Use proper hand placement on the sternum (See Figure 6-1 and Table 6-6). Assess the effectiveness of chest compressions by palpating the brachial or femoral pulse.

7. *Attach "quick look" paddles or cardiac monitor* for rapid read-out of electrical rhythm. If ventricular fibrillation, ventricular tachycardia, or supraventricular tachycardia is present, deliver electrical countershock as outlined on treatment algorithm Figure 6-2. If asystole is present, obtain a second electrocardiographic plane to ensure that rhythm is indeed flatline, rather than fine ventricular fibrillation, or proceed with two "trial" defibrillations at 2 and 4 joules/kg.

8. *Establish intravascular access.* Either a percutaneous peripheral venous approach, preferably in the upper extremity or external jugular vein, or the intraosseous approach is acceptable. Femoral vein cannulation using a standard percutaneous approach, an open cutdown technique, or Seldinger guide-wire technique, is an effective alternative method for rapid access. In the individual with difficult access, drug therapy may be initiated with epinephrine administered through the endotracheal tube into the trachea, or sublingually in non-intubated patients.

9. *Initiate pharmacologic therapy.* Treatment algorithm Figure 6-2 indicates the order of drug administration. Drug delivery requires both careful titration on a per-kilogram bases and timely repeat doses, where appropriate. Table 6-7 lists drugs by dose, unit form, and route.

10. *If reperfusion occurs, continue cardiac monitoring and consider the need for inotropic support with dopamine, dobutamine, or epinephrine infusions* (see Chapter 8). Document the patient's

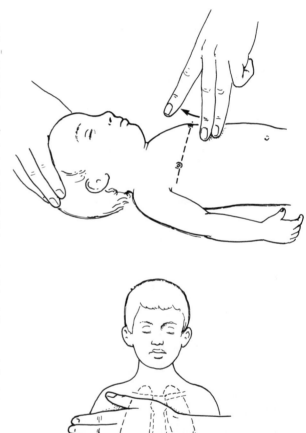

FIGURE 6-1. Chest compression technique for the infant (above) and child (below).

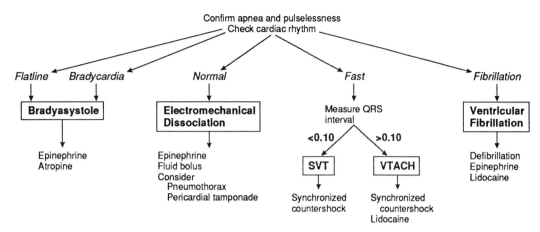

FIGURE 6–2. Algorithm for drug therapy in cardiopulmonary resuscitation.

neurologic status. Titrate the fluid infusion at the minimal rate possible, to avoid overhydration. Admit the child to the intensive care unit or arrange for immediate transfer to a pediatric critical care center.

11. *Ensure proper documentation.* An identified recorder, usually a nurse, must precisely list the time, dose, and exact name of every drug and procedure during the resuscitation. Data on the patient's response to therapy (e.g. rhythm, pulse, blood pressure, neurologic status) are essential in the resuscitation record. The captain must review and sign the document.

12. *Communicate the results of resuscitation to parents immediately.* Follow the guidelines in Chapter 127 if death occurs.

13. *Conduct a retrospective critique,* including any decision to terminate resuscitation. Staff questions and concerns must be handled and grief reactions acknowledged and validated.

Pharmacology of Resuscitation ■

The role of drugs in resuscitation has recently been revised. Only a few pharmacologic agents are proven to enhance survival; many drugs that were previously administered routinely in resuscitation are probably either ineffective or overtly dangerous. Further, drugs known to be efficacious in *low-flow* states (e.g., atropine, naloxone) may not be efficacious in *no-flow* states.

DRUGS KNOWN TO BE EFFECTIVE

The *alpha agonists* are our best drugs in cardiac resuscitation. They activate alpha receptors in the aorta and trigger intense vasoconstriction, thereby increasing aortic diastolic pressure and coronary artery perfusion. Animal studies have isolated two types of alpha receptors in the aorta: α_1 and α_2. Since epinephrine holds both α_1 and α_2 agonistic properties, it appears to be a better drug than pure α_1 agonists, such as methoxamine or phenylephrine.

A persuasive body of experimental data and anecdotal reports suggest that *the current recommended dose of epinephrine (0.01 mg/kg or 10 μg/kg) may be too low, especially in asystolic arrests.* Indeed, doses of 10–20 times current American Heart Association recommendations (i.e., up to 100–200 μg/kg) may be necessary to achieve adequate coronary and cerebral blood flow during arrest. These higher dose forms have not been well evaluated in children for either safety or effectiveness.

The *antidysrhythmics* (lidocaine and bretylium) are secondary agents for use in either post-defibrillation ventricular fibrillation or ventricular tachycardia or in perfusing ventricular tachycardia. No agent is known to have an advantage over another for these indications. One acceptable regimen is three boluses of lidocaine (to 3 mg/kg total) before giving bretylium.

DRUGS PROBABLY INEFFECTIVE IN FULL ARREST

The anticholinergic drug *atropine* is quite effective in the hemodynamically unstable child with bradycardia and secondary hypoperfusion. When used in true cardiac standstill, however, it has no proven benefit. In adults, clinical trials have failed to show any advantage of atropine over normal saline in full arrest, but such studies have not yet been extended to the young arrest victim.

TABLE 6-7. *Drug Doses in Pediatric Resuscitation*

Interventions	Dose	Route	Comment
Epinephrine USP 1:10,000	0.01–0.2 mg/kg	ET, IV, IO, SL	Repeat every 5 minutes
0.1 mg/ml			Higher dose range is more effective.
10-ml syringe = 1 mg			
Atropine sulfate	0.02 mg/kg	ET, IV, IO	Repeat every 5 minutes
0.1 mg/ml			Minimum dose = 0.1 mg
10 ml = 1 mg			Maximum dose = 1 mg twice
$NaHCO_3$ 8.4% solution	0.5–1 Eq/kg	IV, IO	Use with caution, *only with intubated patient*
1 mgEq/ml			
50-ml syringe = 50 mEq			
Lidocaine HCl	1 mg/kg	ET, IV, IO	Repeat 1 mg/kg ×3, every 8 minutes then follow bolus with infusion, at 20–50 μg/kg/min
10 mg/ml			
25 ml syringe = 25 mg			
Bretylium tosylate	5 mg/kg	IV, IO	Maximum dose = 30 mg/kg
50 mg/ml			Use after lidocaine fails
10 ml = 500 mg			
$D_{25}W$ and D_{50}	1–2 ml/kg: <2 yrs of $D_{25}W$	IV, IO	Check Chemstix, give for value ≤100 mg%
Mix D_{50}, 1:1 with water or NS to get $D_{25}W$ or $D_{25}NS$	0.5–1 ml/kg: >2 yrs of $D_{50}W$		Avoid IO administration
Naloxone	0.4–2 mg (children)	ET, IV, IO	Pure opiate antagonist
0.4 mg/ml	0.4 mg (neonates)		
1 ml ampule = 0.4 mg			

Electrical countershock: 2 watt-sec/kg asynchronized for ventricular fibrillation, 1 watt-sec/kg synchronized for ventricular tachycardia (use asynchronized mode if synchronized fails), 0.5 watt-sec/kg asynchronized for supraventricular tachycardia.

Similarly, the opiate antagonist *naloxone* will reliably reverse pulmonary, CNS, and possibly cardiovascular depression in the opiate-overdosed patient, but probably exerts no important action in the setting of cardiac standstill. Nor does *routine dextrose administration* have any established value. Rapid bedside chemstrips for serum glucose determination will identify those few hypoglycemic patients who actually need dextrose. The chemstrip technique avoids unnecessary administration in the normoglycemic or hyperglycemic patient, where the safety of concentrated dextrose solutions is unknown.

DRUGS POSSIBLY DANGEROUS

Sodium bicarbonate has been used widely in cardiac arrest to treat metabolic acidosis, a condition purported to lower fibrillation threshold, attenuate pressor response to catecholamines, and compromise cardiovascular performance. Newer investigations have demonstrated instead myriad adverse metabolic reactions to bicarbonate administration, including hyperosmolality, hypernatremia, hypokalemia, metabolic alkalosis, and tissue hypoxia from leftward shift of the hemoglobin-oxygen dissociation curve. Bicarbonate may also directly depress myocardial and CNS function.

Bicarbonate administration immediately increases serum carbon dioxide tension, which may induce paradoxical intracellular acidosis by rapid diffusion across lipid membranes. Organ dysfunction ensues. *A child in arrest should not receive bicarbonate unless he or she is intubated and adequately ventilated.* Indications for bicarbonate use are poorly defined, since outcome studies have not yet confirmed benefit from use of this agent in true arrest.

Long downtimes or persistent metabolic acidosis may be relative indications. Use of bicarbonate may be life-saving in perfusing, unstable patients in the pre-arrest state with tricyclic antidepressant overdoses, or hyperkalemia.

Calcium is indicated only for patients with certain known, specific metabolic disturbances: hypocalcemia, hyperkalemia, hypermagnesemia, and calcium channel blocker overdose. Except for this extreme minority of arrest patients, calcium will be ineffective and possibly harmful. Calcium is an established endogenous chemical mediator of brain cell injury and death after reperfusion. Administration of calcium may cause neuronal as well as cardiac injury in patients who experience return of spontaneous circulation.

Isoproterenol is contraindicated in full arrest because of its beta-adrenergic-mediated reduction in aortic diastolic pressure and resultant decrease in coronary artery perfusion.

Terminating the Resuscitation ■

When initial resuscitative efforts fail to restore spontaneous perfusion, the captain is faced with a decision to discontinue ALS. The following questions will help establish a therapeutic endpoint:

1. Was the arrest witnessed or unwitnessed?
2. What was the presenting rhythm?
3. Are extenuating factors present, especially hypothermia or barbiturate overdose?
4. Did the child respond to critical ALS interventions (endotracheal intubation, electrical countershocks, or epinephrine)?
5. What is the total downtime?

An unwitnessed, asystolic arrest is unlikely to respond to any therapy. *If the child is warm and no extenuating factor is present, resuscitation should continue through intubation and reversal of hypoxia and respiratory acidosis, electrical countershock when appropriate, and three epinephrine doses.* If hypothermia is suspected, efforts to revive the child are indicated until the heart is warm, since hypothermia (and barbiturates) confer a powerful protective effect on brain and organ survivability (see Chapter 95).

If the arrest rhythm is VF, VT, or SVT, resuscitation should usually continue until either reperfusion or asystole. Multiple countershocks may be necessary. Protracted resuscitative efforts are indicated for the patient with intermittent periods of spontaneous circulation. However, in the child with no response and no extenuating factors, mortality is likely.

Sometimes, reperfusion develops but the child has suffered overwhelming brain injury. As our technologies for cardiopulmonary resuscitation continue to evolve, this scenario may become more common, until better strategies for cerebral resuscitation become available. The brain-dead child warrants consideration for organ donation. This possibility requires a most sensitive approach with the bereaved family. Key elements in communicating with the family about the death of a child in the ED are presented in detail in Chapter 127.

Bibliography ■

American Heart Association: Standards and guidelines for cardiopulmonary resuscitation and emergency cardiac care. *JAMA* 1986; 255:2961–2969.

Dieckmann R: Pediatric advanced life support: A critical analysis. In Barkin R: *The emergently ill child.* Rockville, Md., Aspen Publications, 1987, pp. 345–355.

Eisenberg M, Bergner L, Hallstrom A: Epidemiology of cardiac arrest and resuscitation in children. *Ann Emerg Med* 1983; 12:672–674.

Zaritsky A: Advanced pediatric life support: State of the art. *Circulation* 1986; 74:124–128.

Zaritsky A, Nadkarni V, Getson P, et al: CPR in children. *Ann Emerg Med* 1987; 16:1107–1111.

7 Neonatal Resuscitation

John Colin Partridge

Six to ten percent of full-term newborn infants and up to 80% of premature infants require resuscitation in the immediate postnatal period. Respiratory support is more commonly needed than cardiac support, since respiratory insufficiency and hypoxia usually precede cardiac arrest.

The perinatal brain is relatively resistant to asphyxic damage, yet infants requiring resuscitation are at risk for death or severe sequelae. An Apgar score of 0–3 after 10 minutes is associated with a 69% mortality during the first year; 20% of survivors have a major handicap. Adequate preparation, identification of high-risk circumstances for intrapartum asphyxia, and prompt and skillful neonatal resuscitation may minimize sequelae or prevent death.

Etiology and Pathophysiology ∎

Normal labor and delivery is associated with fetal hypoxemia, hypercarbia, and metabolic acidosis. The normal neonate responds with hyperpnea and tachycardia. The newborn who cannot establish adequate ventilation develops progressive hypoxemia and mixed acidosis. Irreversible shock and death follow if resuscitation is not immediately instituted. These cardiopulmonary events during asphyxia are accompanied by severe metabolic derangements of glucose, calcium, and potassium metabolism.

Ninety percent of infants suffering perinatal asphyxia have had intrapartum complications resulting from altered placental gas exchange, altered maternal perfusion of the placenta, or maternal hypoxemia. (See Table 7-1.)

Clinical Findings ∎

Apgar scoring: Clinical assessment of the degree of depression and of the need for resuscitation usually are based on Apgar scores. Each of five signs is scored 0, 1, or 2 at one and five minutes after birth. (See Table 7-2.) With increasing severity or duration of asphyxia, the Apgar deteriorates in a predictable manner: first color, then respiration, then tone, then reflex, and finally heart rate. The profoundly bradycardic or gasping infant necessitates *immediate* aggressive resuscitation without awaiting Apgar scoring. Apgar scores should not be used in the emergency setting to predict short- or long-term morbidity or mortality.

Vital signs: Accurate assessment of the vital signs in the neonate requires familiarity with normal values. (See Table 7-3.)

Physical examination: Assess the maturity of the infant and perform a directed physical examination of the infant once resuscitation is underway or the infant is stable. Evaluate the character of respiratory activity, quality and symmetry of breath sounds, heart sounds, and murmurs. Observe for pallor, cyanosis, peripheral capillary refill, and meconium staining. Assess neuromuscular tone, level of alertness, and amount of spontaneous activity. Evaluate for choanal atresia, palatal defects, copious oropharyngeal secretions (tracheoesophageal fistula), or scaphoid abdomen (diaphragmatic hernia). Observe for birth trauma.

Treatment ∎

See Figure 7-1.

GENERAL PRINCIPLES

The ABCDs of neonatal resuscitation are *A*irway, *B*reathing, *C*irculatory support, and *D*rug resuscitation. Resuscitation for neonates differs from older children because of the neonate's unique physiology. The most important distinguishing features are:

1. Smaller collapsible airways
2. Fluid-filled lungs, which may be immature and lacking in surfactant

TABLE 7-1. Perinatal Factors Associated With a Need for Resuscitation

Maternal
Preterm labor, postdates pregnancy
Infection (chorioamnionitis)
Hypertension, hypotension
Diabetes mellitus
Cardiac disease
Respiratory disease
Acute or chronic drug intoxication
Anemia, hemoglobinopathy
Anomalies or genetic abnormalities

Uteroplacental
Uterine anomalies
Multiple gestation
Placenta previa
Abruptio placentae
Uteroplacental insufficiency
Abnormal labor pattern

Umbilical Vascular
Cord compression, prolapsed cord
Cord avulsion

Fetal
Cephalopelvic disproportion
Abnormal presentation
Erythroblastosis fetalis

Neonatal
Prematurity, postmaturity
Meconium aspiration
Respiratory distress syndrome
Congenital infection, pneumonia, sepsis
Birth trauma
Anomalies
Hypothermia

3. Patency of ductus arteriosus, foramen ovale, and ductus venosus
4. Immature CNS regulation of respiration
5. Labile and responsive pulmonary vascular resistance

6. Thermal instability
7. A dive reflex
8. Pulmonary and cardiac right-to-left shunting
9. Predilection for hypothermia and hypoglycemia.

ORGANIZATION

Team approach: Resuscitation is best performed by an organized team with a designated leader, with each person assigned prospectively and prepared for specific tasks. The leader should be responsible for managing the airway and directing the team. A "code card" with normal values, equipment sizes, and drug doses will help prevent errors. (See Tables 7-4 and 7-5.) Administer drugs only after adequate ventilation and circulation is established. Drugs must be given in the proper order, for the proper indication, and in precise doses by safe routes.

Preparation: Whenever possible, anticipate the high-risk delivery so that the team is ready and assembled. Notify obstetrics, the nursery staff, and ancillary services (e.g., respiratory therapy, radiology, or a transport team). If time and equipment permit, monitor the fetus by stethoscope or, preferably, by continuous electronic fetal monitoring. Scalp sampling is rarely feasible in the emergency department setting. Evaluate amniotic fluid for meconium staining, bleeding, and purulence.

Set-up: Increase the room temperature to 27°C. Turn on the overhead radiant warmer. Heating lamps or warm blankets are acceptable if no radiant heat source is available. Turn on the oxygen source, check the anesthesia bag, and attach an appropriate-sized face mask. Ensure that proper equipment is available and functioning. (See Tables 7-4 and 7-6.) Prepare an endotracheal tube and suction apparatus. In situations of anticipated profound fetal distress, open an umbilical catheterization tray and draw up drugs for a chemical resuscitation.

TABLE 7-2. Apgar Scoring Method

Sign	Score		
	0	1	2
Color (**A**ppearance)	Blue, pale	Pink body, blue extremities	All pink
Heart rate (**P**ulse)	Absent	<100	>100
Reflex irritability (**G**rimace)	Absent	Grimace to stimulation	Cough or sneeze to stimulation
Muscle tone (**A**ctivity)	Limp	Some flexion of extremities	Active motion, full flexion
Respiratory effort (**R**espiration)	Absent	Slow, irregular	Lusty cry

TABLE 7–3. *Normal Ranges for Neonatal Values*

Heart Rate		*Hematocrit*	
100–160 beats/min		45–65%	
Respiratory Rate		*Blood Glucose*	
40–60 breaths/min		45–130 mg/dl	
Temperature			
36.0–37.3°C (axillary)			

	Mean	Systolic	Diastolic (mm Hg)
Blood Pressure			
Birth weight			
1 kg	25–44	39–59	16–36
2 kg	32–51	42–65	22–42
3 kg	38–57	50–74	26–46
4 kg	42–62	58–80	32–42

	pH	P_aCO_2 (torr)	P_aO_2 (torr)
Arterial Blood Gases			
Time			
Birth (cord. art.)	7.23–7.25	49–56	13–22
10 min	7.20–7.22	39–55	40–69
30–60 min	7.31–7.33	35–41	70–83
Several hours	7.34	35	74

ROUTINE MANAGEMENT AT BIRTH

For all infants, including those in distress:

1. Hold the infant at the level of the placenta with the head slightly dependent until the cord is clamped and cut.
2. Quickly clamp and cut the cord; do not strip blood from the cord.
3. Hand the infant off to the resuscitating team.
4. Place the infant supine in slight Trendelenburg position under the radiant warmer, with the infant's head toward the resuscitation leader.
5. Immediately assess status (a several-second Apgar scoring) to decide the need for intervention. Monitor the heart rate by auscultation with a stethoscope or by palpation of the umbilical arterial pulse.
6. Clear the oropharynx by gentle *brief* suction.
7. Gently stimulate the infant by rubbing the back or lightly slapping the soles of the feet. Vigorous or prolonged stimulation is not efficacious and may be detrimental.
8. Towel-dry the face and then the body.
9. Assign the Apgar scores at one and five minutes.

10. If the infant is bradycardic, apneic, or moderately or severely depressed, begin resuscitation efforts immediately. (See Figure 7-1.)

RESUSCITATION

Begin management based on initial assessment and the one-minute Apgar score. *Vigorous infants* (Apgar scores of 7–10) should need only gentle stimulation, temperature maintenance, and suction to clear the oropharynx. Evacuate gastric contents only after the infant is stable for 5 minutes. The *moderately asphyxiated infant* (Apgar score 4–6) is apneic, cyanotic, and slightly bradycardic (heart rate 90–100 bpm), with a normal or elevated blood pressure. The infant responds promptly to stimulation or blow-by oxygen and usually gasps before cyanosis resolves. A delayed response requires positive-pressure ventilation. The *severely asphyxiated infant* (Apgar score 0–3) is apneic, pallid or ashen, profoundly bradycardic (heart rate 0–50 bpm), hypotonic, and poorly responsive. Blood pressure is low, capillary refill delayed. The infant responds slowly to aggressive resuscitation; color often improves before gasping occurs.

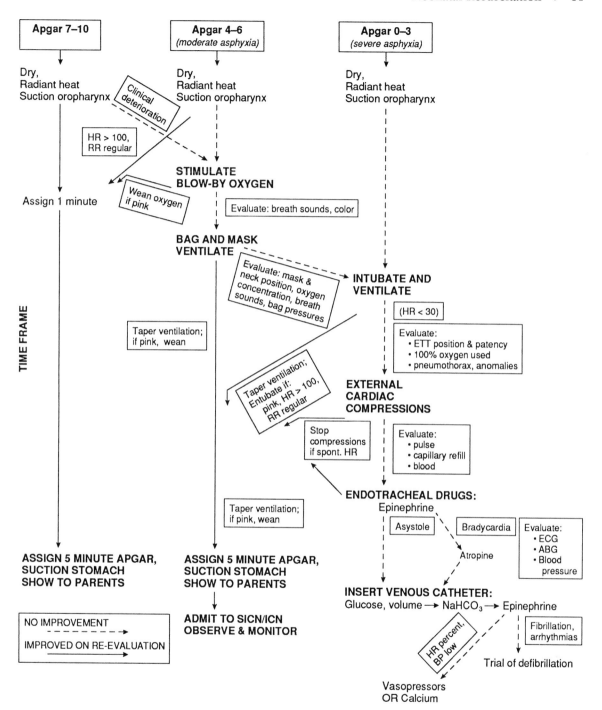

FIGURE 7–1. Guide to neonatal resuscitation.

TABLE 7–4. *Resuscitation Equipment: Guidelines by Birth Weight*

Birth Weight (g)	Oral Airway*	Endotracheal Tube†		Suction Catheter Size (Fr)	Umbilical Artery Catheter‡	
		Size (mm)	Depth (cm)		Size (mm)	Depth (cm)
<1,000	000	2.5	7	5	3.5	7
1,000–1,500	000	2.5–3.0	7–8	5–6	5	7–8
1,500–2,500	00	3.0	8–9	6	5	8–9
2,500–3,000	0	3.0–3.5	9–10	6–8	5	9–10
>3,000	0	3.5	10–11	8	5	10–11
>4,000	0	4.0	11–12	8	5	11

* Oral airways rarely necessary since jaw lift is usually successful in maintaining airway patency
† Endotracheal tubes—general guidelines
    1. Size of fifth digit = approximate ETT size
    2. Use largest tube that fits with small air leak
    3. Place circumferential line at vocal cords
‡ Umbilical catheters—general guidelines
    1. Use 5 Fr whenever possible
    2. Insert to depth = (umbilicus to inguinal crease) × 2 + length of umbilical stump

DRUG RESUSCITATION

The severely depressed infant needing cardiac massage is likely to require drug resuscitation to restore heart rate, cardiac output, respiration, and metabolic homeostasis (see Figure 7-1). See Table 7-5 for appropriate drugs and doses.

Endotracheal instillation of epinephrine, atropine, or naloxone allows rapid administration and rapid absorption in the immediate phase of resuscitation when vascular access is not yet established. Double intravenous doses, inject the drug into the endotracheal tube (or preferably directly into the trachea with a feeding tube or umbilical artery catheter), and follow with positive-pressure ventilation and cardiac massage. Use umbilical venous cannulation for other emergency drug administration or volume expansion during resuscitation. Umbilical arterial catheterization is indicated for continuous blood pressure monitoring and arterial blood gas analysis after the immediate stabilization. (See Chapter 139 for the technique of umbilical vessel catheterization.) Peripheral venous access may be difficult and time-consuming. Intraosseous or intracardiac administration are rarely necessary in the newborn.

EVALUATION ■

1. *Evaluate the response to each component of resuscitation.* Continue Apgar scoring at five-minute intervals during the resuscitation to determine the need for continued efforts and to adjust the level and the intensity of the intervention. Match the continuing intervention to the level required by the infant's current status.

2. *Evaluate environmental effects on resuscitation.* Prevent hypothermia by radiant heat and humidification and by heating the oxygen source.

3. *Obtain ancillary data* (Table 7-7) once the infant's condition stabilizes.

4. When expected improvement does not follow resuscitative intervention, *investigate for problems with the equipment, asphyxiating complications* such as pneumothoraces, or *congenital anomalies.*

5. *Taper the resuscitative efforts as Apgar scores improve.* Overly aggressive resuscitation may cause laryngospasm, pneumothorax, or bradycardia or may increase risks for intraventricular hemorrhage, chronic lung disease, or retinopathy in the premature infant. Abrupt cessation of resuscitation may cause clinical deterioration.

6. *Evaluate the advisability of transport and admission.* Transport the infant to the nursery or ward once Apgar scores are over 6 and the infant is stabilized. Admit or transfer all infants needing resuscitation or pharmacologic intervention after birth to a neonatal intensive care unit. A semi-intensive care nursery or transitional-care nursery is adequate for moderately asphyxiated child, or an intensive care nursery for a severely asphyxiated child. Monitor all resuscitated infants for signs of asphyxic organ damage.

7. *Establish criteria for continuing resuscitative efforts.* Risks of asphyxic neurologic sequelae are

TABLE 7–5. *Neonatal Resuscitation Drugs*

Drug (Stock Concentration)	Indication	Dose	Route
Epinephrine (10-ml ampules of 0.1 mg/ml sol [1:10,000 dolution])	Asystole, bradycardia, flat ECG	*Bolus* 0.01–0.03 mg/kg (=0.1–0.3 ml/kg)	IV, ET, UVC
		Infusion 0.05–1.5 μg/kg/min	IV, UVC
Atropine (10-ml ampules of 0.1 mg/ml sol)	Bradycardia	0.01–0.03 mg/kg (0.1–0.3 ml/kg)	IV, ET, UVC
Glucose (D$_{10}$W)	Blood glucose < 40	*Bolus* 2–3 ml/kg	IV, UVC
		Infusion 6 mg/kg/min (=100 ml/kg/day)	IV, UVC
Volume Expanders (whole blood, saline Lactated Ringer's 5% albumin sol)	Hypovolemia, hypotension	10–20 ml/kg	IV, UVC
Sodium Bicarbonate (10-ml ampules of 1 mEq/ml solution)	Severe metabolic acidosis (pH < 7.1), hyperkalemia	1–2 mEq/kg (2–4 ml/kg) [dilute 1:1 with sterile water)	IV, UVC
Calcium	Decreased cardiac output, 2° hypocalcemia, hyperkalemia		IV, UVC (emergency)
Chloride (10-ml ampules, 100 mg/ml, of 10% solution)		20 mg/kg (0.2 ml/kg)	
Gluconate (10-ml ampules, 100 mg/ml, of 10% solution)		100 mg/kg (1 ml/kg)	IV
Naloxone (Neonatal) (2-ml ampules of 0.02 mg/ml solution)	Acute narcosis	0.01 mg/kg (1 ml in preterm, 2 ml in term infant)	IM, IV, UVC
Dopamine (5-ml ampules of 40 mg/ml)	Hypotension	*Infusion* 5–20 μg/kg/min	IV
Isoproterenol (5-ml ampules of 0.2 mg/ml sol [1:5,000 dilution])	Hypotension, bradycardia, decreased cardiac output	*Infusion* 0.05–1.0 μg/kg/min	IV
Lidocaine (5-ml ampules of 20 mg/ml solution)	Ventricular tachycardia	*Bolus* 1 mg/kg	IV
		Infusion 10–50 μg/kg/min	IV
Defibrillation	Ventricular tachycardia, paroxysmal atrial tachycardia, ventricular fibrillation	0.5–2 watt-sec/kg	

TABLE 7–6. *Neonatal Resuscitation Equipment Checklist*

	Prehospital/ Field	Emergency Department
Warm blankets	+	
Heat lamp or radiant warmer		+
Thermometer, temp. probe	±	+
Oxygen source (warm, humid)	+	+
Lighting	+	+
Infant stethoscope	+	+
Suction catheter with syringe	+	
Suction catheter with machine	±	+
Face masks (preterm, term)	+	+
Self-inflating bag, pop-off	+	
Anesthesia bag, manometer		+
Endotracheal tubes (2.5–4.0)	+	+
Stylet	±	±
Sterile needles, syringes, stopcocks	+	+
Oral airways (000–0)	±	±
Laryngoscope (0 and 1 Miller blades)		+
Spare bulbs and batteries		+
Cord tie, clamps	+	+
Hemostat, forceps, scissors, scalpel	+	+
Umbilical catheters (3.5 and 5 Fr)		+
Resuscitation drugs	+	+
Sterile attire, drapes		+
ECG monitor		+
Blood pressure monitor		+
Blood gas machine		+
Glucose reagent sticks	+	+
Defibrillator	±	+
Umbilical catheter tray		+
Thoracostomy tray		+

+ = Essential
± = Desirable

generally minimal until more than 15 minutes of resuscitation, even with Apgars of 0–3. Severe acidosis (pH <7.0) is not a reason to withhold or withdraw resuscitative efforts. Thus, a delay in initiating intervention must not deter attempts at cardiopulmonary resuscitation.

8. *Document the resuscitation and the response to intervention.*

Special situations may necessitate changes in the routine sequence of resuscitation. Table 7-8 describes

TABLE 7–7. *Ancillary Data During Neonatal Resuscitation*

Complete blood count, hematocrit, differential
Blood glucose, calcium, magnesium, electrolytes
Arterial blood gases
Blood culture
Chest x-ray
ECG monitoring
Transcutaneous oxygen and saturation monitoring
Blood pressure monitoring

TABLE 7–8. *Conditions Requiring Alterations in Resuscitation Technique*

Condition	Signs	Intervention
Meconium Aspiration	Staining of skin or amniotic fluid, fetal distress	Suction oropharynx before delivery of shoulders
		Laryngoscope, ETT suction before breathing starts
Respiratory Distress Syndrome	Premature infant with tachypnea, cyanosis, retractions, flaring, grunting	Judicious use of oxygen
		Marked distress → intubate
		Ventilate at rapid rates, low pressures, and with end-expiratory pressures
		Avoid trauma
		Maintain temperature and metabolic homeostasis
		Treat with antibiotics
Shock	Intrapartum bleeding, cord accidents, trauma, twins, sepsis; pallor, slow capillary refill, hypotension, bradycardia	Insert umbilical catheter
		Volume expansion. Consider inotropes.
		Culture; treat with antibiotics if infection suspected
Maternal Drugs		
Opiate addiction	Apnea, bradycardia	Intubate and resuscitate
		Avoid naloxone
		Severe → diazepam or paregoric
Cocaine	Hypertonia, irritability, hyperreflexia, seizures	Support ventilation
		Seizures → phenobarbital
		Examine for anomalies
Alcohol	Hypoglycemia, hypotonia, inadequate ventilation	Support ventilation
		Monitor blood glucose
		Examine for anomalies
Pneumothorax*	Sudden-onset cyanosis, respiratory distress, unequal breath sounds, chest transilluminates	Increase oxygen Needle aspiration, then tube thoracostomy
Anomalies		
Choanal atresia*	Pink crying, blue quiet	Position prone Maintain oral airway
Diaphragmatic hernia*	Scaphoid abdomen, decreased breath sounds, cyanosis	Gastric decompression
		Endotracheal intubation
		Oxygenate and ventilate
		Observe for pneumothorax
Tracheo-esophageal fistula*	Excess oral secretions, distended abdomen, respiratory distress, aspiration	Elevate head
		Keep NPO
		Oropharyngeal suction

* Requires surgical evaluation and treatment.

selected conditions that may require emergent interventions.

Bibliography ∎

Apgar V: A proposal for a new method of evaluation of the newborn infant. *Current Res Anesth Analg* 1953; 32:260–267.

Benitz WE, Frankel LR, Stevenson DK: The pharmacology of neonatal resuscitation and cardiopulmonary intensive care. Part I: Immediate resuscitation. *West J Med* 1986; 144:704–709.

Brown KJ, Purvis RJ, Forfar JO, et al: Neurologic aspects of perinatal asphyxia. *Dev Med Child Neurol* 1974; 16:567–580.

Cunningham MD, TePas KE: Newborn care in the delivery room. In: Knuppel RA, Drukker JE (eds.): *High-risk pregnancy: a team approach.* Philadelphia: WB Saunders, 1986, pp. 495–516.

Mulligan JC, Painter MJ, O'Donoghue PNP, et al: Neonatal asphyxia. II. Neonatal mortality and long-term sequelae. *J Pediatr* 1980; 96:903–907.

Nelson KB, Ellenberg JH: Apgar scores as predictors of chronic neurologic disability. *Pediatrics* 1981; 68:36–44.

Neonatal advanced life support. Standards and guidelines for cardiopulmonary resuscitation (CPR) and emergency cardiac care (ECC). *JAMA* 1986; 255:2933–2951.

Ostheimer GW: Resuscitation of the newborn infant. *Clin Perinatol* 1982; 9:177–190.

Versmold HT, Kitterman JA, Phibbs RH, et al: Aortic blood pressure during the first 12 hours of life in infants with birth weight 610 to 4,220 grams. *Pediatrics* 1981; 67:607–613.

8 Shock

Ronald A. Dieckmann and Anthony J. Haftel

Shock has been called "the rude unhinging of the machinery of life"—an apt description of the profound system failure associated with the shock state. A more scientific definition is oxygen starvation; if shock is untreated, profound hypoxia and death ensue. Shock is progressive: it proceeds from a compensated to an uncompensated phase and ultimately to an irreversible phase. Shock is not hypotension; in fact, the compensated phase is usually normotensive. Successful treatment is premised on early recognition and aggressive management.

Pathophysiology ■

Shock is inadequate delivery of oxygen to tissues. This pathophysiologic state can be created by a breakdown of any of the separate components in the delivery process. Table 8-1 presents these key components and their relationships. There are two major determinants of oxygen delivery: oxygen content and cardiac output. Oxygen content is determined by oxygen saturation and red blood cell mass. Cardiac output is determined by heart rate and stroke volume. Stroke volume is the product of preload, contractility, and afterload. Every clinical entity causing shock represents the failure of one or more of these vital components.

In most of the conditions that produce shock in children, decreased stroke volume is the primary problem, usually from volume loss. The incremental phases of organ response to hypovolemia are well described and have reproducible clinical correlates. Table 8-2 indicates the features of the compensated, uncompensated, and irreversible phases of hypovolemic shock, with the clinical characteristics of each phase.

The pathophysiology of septic shock differs somewhat from other forms of shock. Powerful endotoxins and chemical mediators orchestrate the complex hemodynamic response to host-pathogen interaction. A *hyperdynamic phase* occurs early, marked by diffuse cellular dysfunction and decreased systemic vascular resistance. A decompensated *cardiogenic phase* follows, as cardiopulmonary function deteriorates and vascular resistance increases. Table 8-3 depicts the clinical characteristics associated with pathophysiologic stages of septic shock.

Etiologies ■

There are many clinical causes of shock. A clinically useful classification defines three major categories: *hypovolemic, cardiogenic,* and *distributive* shock. Table 8-4 lists common clinical entities associated with each major shock category. Clinical findings in the different shock states often overlap, because pathophysiologic changes share common pathways; therefore, immediate bedside differentiation may be impossible. Late phases of shock from any etiology are clinically indistinguishable.

Clinical Findings ■

Survival from shock requires early identification. Once decompensation and significant hypotension develop, the probability of mortality is high. Recognition of shock in children is complicated by several special problems in rapid assessment:

1. Perfusion may be mistakenly equated with blood pressure, and early signs of hypovolemic compensated shock (cool skin with delayed capillary refill, tachycardia) are missed.
2. Blood pressure may be obtained incorrectly or with improper equipment; findings are often not adjusted for age. *Normal systolic blood pressure is 60 mm Hg in infants and 80 + 2 × age (in years) for children over 2 years. Normal diastolic pressure is two-thirds systolic pressure* (see Figure 11-1).
3. The child cannot provide key history or cooperate with the examination.
4. Diagnosis is delayed or obscured by overemphasis on insensitive ancillary tests, sometimes in the face of persuasive clinical signs of shock.

TABLE 8–1. *Six Determinants of Tissue Oxygen Delivery*

Physiologic Equation:

Tissue Oxygen = Oxygen Content[a] × Cardiac Output[b]

Specific Components:

[a]*Oxygen content = (1) Red Cell Mass × (2) Oxygen Saturation*

[b]*Cardiac Output = (3) Heart Rate × Stroke Volume*

Stroke Volume = (4) Preload × (5) Contractility × (6) Afterload

5. The child is inadequately monitored during ancillary testing (laboratory procedures, radiographs, or computerized axial tomography) and decompensation develops suddenly and unexpectedly.
6. Sequential examinations are not performed in ambiguous cases.

When frank hypotension is present, the diagnosis of shock is easy, but effective treatment depends on basic differentiation between hypovolemic, cardiogenic, and distributive shock. Table 8-5 summarizes several key clinical signs that will rapidly distinguish these entities. Usually, historical features will facilitate early etiologic classification and direct treatment (e.g., the parents' report of gastrointestinal losses through persistent diarrhea suggests hypovolemia; high fever at home, lethargy, and poor color indicate

TABLE 8–2. *Phases of Hypovolemic Shock: Clinical Characteristics*

Phase	Characteristics
Compensated	Normal blood pressure
	Peripheral vasoconstriction
	Increased heart rate
	Normal CNS
	Normal cardiac output
	Reduced urine output
	Reduced CVP
	Reduced stroke volume
	Increased myocardial contractility
Uncompensated	Decreased blood pressure
	Decreased CNS
	Anuria
	Acidosis
	Decreased cardiac output
Irreversible	Major organ failure
	Cellular death imminent

TABLE 8–3. *Phases of Septic Shock: Clinical Characteristics*

Early Phase (Hyperdynamic)	Late Phase (Cardiogenic)
Febrile	Hypothermic
Warm extremities	Cold, mottled extremities
Bounding pulse	Weak, thready pulse
Normo/hypertensive	Hypotensive
Tachycardic	Tachycardic
Tachypnea	Bradypnea
Decreased SVR	Increased SVR
Increased cardiac output	Decreased cardiac output
Polyuria	Oligo/anuria
Normal capillary refill	Prolonged capillary refill
Hypoxia	Hypoxia
Normal CNS	Obtunded, comatose
Respiratory alkalosis	Metabolic acidosis
Normal coagulation	DIC
Hyperglycemia	Hypoglycemia

possible sepsis; difficulty breathing and poor feeding in a child with congenital heart disease suggest heart failure). *Whenever presented with an infant or child who appears seriously ill, the physician must consider whether the patient is in shock.*

Any history of underlying medical problems must be elicited. The physical exam requires special attention to perfusion status. *In children, the most sensitive measures of perfusion are skin signs, once the patient is warm.* Be certain to expose the child adequately for examination, but be careful not to induce hypothermia, as this will rapidly exacerbate hypoperfusion and will cloud assessment. Delayed capillary refill (>2 seconds) with pale, cool, clammy, or mottled skin is a sensitive and specific sign of hypovolemia. Since vasoconstriction occurs first in the lower extremities, check the skin at the kneecaps. In a patient with distributive shock, skin signs are different, as noted in Table 8-5.

After skin signs, the next important measures of perfusion are *heart rate and respiratory rate.* While sensitive, these signs are nonspecific, since a variety of factors—including anxiety, fever or drugs—may be present. *Pulse pressure* is better than systolic pressure, but often the diastolic pressure in children is difficult to obtain accurately without a Doppler device. Palpated central pulses may also be diminished. In the stable, cooperative patient the "tilt test" is a useful indicator of perfusion: Record heart rate and blood pressure two times with the child supine, then twice again after the child has been sitting up for two minutes. Heart rate increases of 20 per minute or blood pressure drops of more than 10 mm Hg are good evidence for moderate to severe hypovolemia.

TABLE 8–4. *Shock Categories and Common Etiologies*

Hypovolemic	Cardiogenic	Distributive
Hemorrhagic Trauma GI bleeding DIC Coagulopathy Neonatal CNS bleed *Fluid and Electrolyte Loss* Diarrhea DKA Gastroenteritis Polyuric states Hyperthermia Mineralocorticoid deficiency Cystic fibrosis *Plasma/Protein Loss* Burns Nephrosis Peritonitis and third space losses	*Cardiogenic* Hypoplastic left heart Aortic coarctation Aortic stenosis Anomalous coronary artery Postoperative cardiomyopathy *Dysrhythmia* Bradycardia Supraventricular tachycardia Ventricular tachycardia AV Block *Infectious* Myocarditis Pericarditis Endocarditis *Obstructive* Tamponade Pulmonary embolus Pneumothorax	*Sepsis* Gram-negative sepsis Meningococcemia *Neurogenic* *Drug* Antihypertensives Barbiturates *Anaphylaxis*

Blood pressure is poorly correlated with hypovolemia during the compensated phase and is difficult to obtain and interpret; when low, however, it usually accurately indicates hypoperfusion. *Mental status abnormalities,* confusion, agitation, or lethargy, may also indicate advanced hypoperfusion. Since hypoxia, drugs, and head trauma may also be present, this parameter is nonspecific. *Elevated jugular venous pressure,* when detected in the setting of hypoperfusion, may be quite useful. This finding occurs with increased right heart pressures—specifically, cardiogenic shock or obstructive conditions such as pericardial tamponade and tension pneumothorax.

A careful, *complete* physical examination may reveal other key differential findings. Rales in the chest with a cardiac gallop and hepatosplenomegaly are cardinal signs of cardiogenic shock, an etiologic category that must be excluded at the onset, since treatment of this condition depends on augmenting pump function and not on volume administration. Indeed, fluid administration may cause rapid deterioration in such patients.

Other clues in physical assessment should identify non-cardiogenic shock so that fluid therapy can be initiated immediately. Certain findings may also assist specific diagnosis. Fever and petechial rash signal

TABLE 8–5. *Differentiating Shock States*

	Hypovolemic	Cardiogenic	Distributive
HR	Rapid (postural deterioration)	Rapid (postural improvement)	Rapid (slow with neurogenic)
Gallop	—	+	—
S1	Loud	Soft	Loud
Ext Jug	Low	High	Low
Capillary Fill	Poor	Poor	Normal
Lungs	Clear	Wet	Clear
Heart	Small	Large	Small

sepsis. Blunt trauma necessitates a highly expectant approach to occult abdominal injury, especially to the liver and spleen.

Ancillary Tests ■

Shock is a clinical diagnosis. Ancillary tests may augment clinical findings but are secondary. Ancillary tests have their greatest utility for specific diagnosis and focused treatment after successful stabilization.

Important laboratory data for any child in shock include arterial blood gases, complete blood count, electrolytes, creatinine, BUN, CO_2, platelet count, coagulation studies, and urinalysis. *Ensure that blood is immediately sent for type and crossmatch.* A chest radiograph is often extremely helpful in borderline cases, but must be obtained in a closely monitored setting. This simple film readily differentiates cardiogenic from non-cardiogenic shock and provides a valuable guide to initial volume administration. The presence of a large heart with pulmonary vascular congestion dictates a therapeutic plan using aggressive inotropic support and minimal volume, whereas a small heart silhouette with decreased pulmonary vascular markings establishes a non-cardiogenic etiology that requires vigorous volume resuscitation.

Perform an ECG in all unstable patients. Other studies, including blood and urine cultures, erythrocyte sedimentation rate, and spinal fluid analysis, may be helpful, depending on the suspected condition. CT scanning may significantly improve diagnostic accuracy in some conditions, especially trauma, where internal abdominal hemorrhage is suspected.

Treatment ■

Once shock is recognized, an aggressive management approach will greatly improve survival (see Figure 8-1). The goal of emergency department care is to reverse pathophysiology. Specific treatment of precipitating conditions often follows resuscitation and stabilization.

1. First, *intubate the unstable, hypotensive patient early.* Reversal of hypoxia and acidosis in uncompensated phases of shock is absolutely imperative. Even if the patient is breathing spontaneously, endotracheal intubation will secure the airway and ensure optimal ventilation and oxygenation. Apply 100% oxygen initially in all cases.
2. *Follow respiratory status with pulse oximetry or serial arterial blood gases* to ensure adequate breathing.
3. *Apply a cardiac monitor.* Closely observe heart rate and rhythm to assess pump function, to detect worsening of cardiopulmonary status, and to gauge the adequacy of therapy. Bradycardia suggests hypoxia or neurogenic shock. Treat specific dysrhythmias.
4. *Secure intravenous access* using two large-bore IV catheters in non-cardiogenic forms of shock or one secure IV line for cardiogenic shock. When IV access is impossible or delayed, establish one or multiple intraosseous lines.

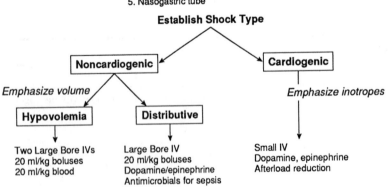

FIGURE 8-1. Management of decompensated shock.

5. *If non-cardiogenic shock is present,* immediately infuse 20 ml/kg of isotonic saline or crystalloid. If the patient remains hypotensive or hypoperfused, follow with a second 20 ml/kg bolus. Begin increased maintenance infusion rate to replace calculated volume losses and ongoing losses.

   If additional volume is needed to maintain perfusion after 40 ml/kg, use type O negative, type specific, or crossmatched blood at 20 ml/kg, depending on perfusion status. Packed cells mixed with normal saline or fresh whole blood are acceptable. Consider fresh frozen plasma, if packed cells are given, especially if a bleeding diathesis is suspected.

   Continue to push volume until either perfusion is restored or clinical signs of volume overload develop (increased jugular venous pressure, rales, cardiac gallop, hepatosplenomegaly). If shock continues, begin dopamine. A CXR may help guide therapy at this point if assessment is ambiguous. *Do not begin inotropic support until volume restoration is complete.*

   If trauma is the underlying problem, control external hemorrhage. Whenever penetrating injury of the chest or contiguous anatomic regions is present, consider tension pneumothorax or pericardial tamponade. Immediate needle or tube thoracostomy or pericardiocentesis may be indicated (see Chapter 139 for procedures).

6. *If distributive shock is diagnosed* and the patient is still hypotensive after volume challenge, proceed to immediate epinephrine or dopamine infusion. Start dopamine at 5–10 µg/kg/min and increase drip rate quickly to restore perfusion. The pneumatic antishock garment may have value in refractory cases.

7. Sepsis is the most likely cause of distributive shock in children. If sepsis is suspected, expect that high dopamine infusion rates may be necessary. *Titrate the dopamine infusion at the bedside every two minutes until perfusion is restored.* Rates over 30 µg/kg/min may be necessary. Occasionally, a second or third inotropic agent is needed; epinephrine (0.05–1.0 µg/kg/min) and/or dobutamine (5–20 µg/kg/min) are excellent additive agents. Multiple infusions can be piggybacked into one line. Begin systemic antimicrobials immediately.

8. *If cardiogenic shock is present,* establish an IV line with 5% dextrose in water at a to-keep-open rate. Initiate a continuous infusion of dopamine, starting at 5–10 µg/kg/min, and titrate the dopamine infusion. Use epinephrine and/or dobutamine in addition to dopamine if necessary.

   Afterload reduction with nitroprusside (0.5–7.0 µg/kg/min) is indicated if inotropic supports fails.

9. *Insert Foley catheter.* Urine output is a sensitive measure of perfusion status and adequacy of therapy. Ensure at least 1 ml/kg/hr output, measuring every 15–30 minutes.

10. *Insert nasogastric tube* to decompress stomach

11. Ensure that all six components of tissue oxygen delivery are optimized (see Table 8-1).

12. Restore homeostasis by reversing associated metabolic abnormalities, such as hypoglycemia or hypocalcemia

Once initial stabilization is accomplished, further diagnostic interventions are indicated. Specific treatment recommendations for individual conditions are described in detail elsewhere:

Complications ■

The sequelae of shock are diverse and reflect the universal systemic derangements that accompany tissue oxygen starvation. Table 8-6 lists the most common serious complications.

Disposition ■

All children with suspected shock require inpatient care. Patients with compensated forms of hypovolemic shock who respond readily to oxygen and IV

TABLE 8–6. *Complications of Shock*

Brain injury or death
Acute renal failure
"Shock lung"
Disseminated intravascular coagulation (DIC)
Hepatic dysfunction
Pancreatic ischemia
Gastrointestinal hemorrhage

fluids ordinarily can be managed on the pediatric ward. However, all children with cardiac failure or decompensated non-cardiogenic shock require admission to a critical care unit capable of treating children or immediate transfer to a pediatric critical care center.

Bibliography ■

Crone RK: Acute circulatory failure in children. *Pediatr Clin North Am* 1980; 27:525–538.

King EG, Chin WD: Shock: an overview of pathophysiology and general treatment goals. *Crit Care Med* 1985; 1(3): 547–561.

Levin DI, Perkin RM: Shock in the pediatric patient (Part I). *J Pediatr* 1982; 101:163–169.

Pollock MM, Ring JC, Fields AT: Shock in infants and children. *Emerg Med Clin North Am* 1986; 4(4):841–857.

Rimar JM: Shock in infants and children: assessment and treatment. *MCN* 1988; 13(2):98–105.

Williams TM: Shock in the pediatric patient. *Indiana Med* 1988; 81(1):18–20.

Witte MK, Hill JH, Blumer JL: Shock in the pediatric patient. *Adv Pediatr* 1987; 34:139–173.

9 Congestive Heart Failure

Julien I. E. Hoffman

Congestive heart failure (CHF) is a syndrome in which either the heart cannot maintain adequate circulation to tissues, or it accomplishes perfusion through compensatory mechanisms that themselves produce organ dysfunction. CHF in childhood usually presents in the first year of life in patients with congenital heart disease.

Etiology ■

Table 9-1 lists the multiple etiologies for CHF in childhood. Heart failure can occur from excessive pressure, excessive volume, or defects in myocardial function due to either pump failure or dysrhythmias. Different congenital lesions tend to precipitate CHF at different times during infancy, as noted in Table 9-2. Older children with acute CHF often have an acquired cardiac defect such as myocarditis or cardiomyopathy.

Pathophysiology ■

Increased volume or pressure and/or myocardial dysfunction results in:

1. Dilatation and hypertrophy of the involved chambers, with resulting *cardiomegaly.*
2. Increased sympathetic tone due to stretching of atrial receptors, with accompanying *tachycardia, pallor,* and *sweating.*
3. Retention of salt and water, with resulting *edema* and *oliguria.*

EFFECT ON VENTRICLES

Most lesions causing CHF affect the left ventricle predominantly, so that most children have left heart failure alone or combined with right heart failure. Pure right heart failure does occur, but it is relatively uncommon.

Nonspecific signs of CHF include:
1. Irritability, difficulty in feeding
2. Excess sweating, especially in young children
3. Poor arterial pulses, low blood pressure, pallor due to vasoconstriction, and low urine output due to low cardiac output
4. Gallop rhythm.

Left heart failure
1. End-diastolic pressure rises because of dilatation, and perhaps because of reduced compliance.

    Congestive heart failure may predispose the patient to pulmonary infection. If cold sweating of the extremities is evident, the diagnosis of heart failure is probable, even if there is also pulmonary infection.
2. Hepatomegaly is absent in pure left heart failure.
3. Pulsus alternans is the only direct evidence of left heart failure.

Right heart failure
Hepatomegaly, peripheral edema, and raised jugular venous pressure indicate *right heart failure.*

1. The liver edge may be pushed down by lung hyperinflation.
2. Peripheral edema is often absent, especially in infants.
3. Raised jugular venous pressure is often difficult to detect in infants, who can have CHF with minimal elevation of systemic venous pressure.

Treatment ■

Provide specific therapy when appropriate:
1. Give glucose, calcium, or magnesium if these are deficient.
2. Remove excess blood volume in hypervolemia.
3. Give packed red cells for anemia.
4. Pace ventricles with slow heart rates.
5. Return tachycardias to sinus rhythm by drugs or electrical countershock.

53

TABLE 9–1. *Causes of Congestive Heart Failure*

Excessive Pressure Load	*Excessive Volume Load*	*Defects in Myocardial Function*

Left-Sided Lesions
Coarctation of the aorta, especially in infancy
Aortic stenosis, especially in infancy
Systemic hypertension, especially due to acute glomerulonephritis
Cor triatriatum or mitral stenosis
 	
Right-Sided Lesions
High pulmonary vascular resistance
Pulmonic stenosis
Obstructed pulmonary veins
Premature closure of the foramen ovale
	Large Left-to-Right Intracardiac Shunts
	Common causes:
	  Ventricular septal defects
	  Patent ductus arteriosus
	  Endocardial cushion defects
	  Complex heart disease
	Uncommon causes:
	  Total anomalous pulmonary venous connection without obstruction
	  Large left to right shunts in secundum atrial septal defects
	
	Regurgitation through any of the Heart Valves
	
	Arteriovenous Fistulae
	
	Anemia
	
	Hypervolemia, often Iatrogenic
		Myocarditis
		
		Other Cardiomyopathies
		
		Anomalous Origin of the Left Coronary Artery
		
		Coronary Artery Disease (e.g., mucocutaneous lymph node syndrome)
		
		Severe Anemia
		
		In Neonates
		Hypocalcemia
		Hypomagnesemia
		Hypoglycemia
		Severe acidemia
		Post-asphyxia
		
		Severe Tachycardia or Bradycardia

Increase oxygen supply with cold humidified supplementary oxygen, especially if there is cyanosis or pulmonary edema.

TABLE 9–2. *Congenital Conditions Causing CHF at Different Times During Infancy*

Newborn Period
Hypoplastic left heart
Arteriovenous fistula
Large placental–fetal transfusion
Regurgitation of the pulmonic or tricuspid valves
Third-degree AV block
Paroxysmal atrial tachycardia (PAT)

First Month
Aortic coarctation with patent ductus arteriosus
Ventricular septal defect
Total anomalous pulmonary venous return
Tricuspid atresia
Truncus arteriosus

First Six Months
Transposition of the great vessels
Ventricular septal defect
Patent ductus arteriosus
Truncus arteriosus with large left-to-right shunt

Six to 12 Months
Ventricular septal defect
Endocardial fibroelastosis
Total anomalous pulmonary venous return

Decrease oxygen consumption by:
1. Bed rest; the most comfortable position is the semi-Fowler. Infants may be placed in a special seat.
2. Lower body temperature, if high. Keep neonates at neutral thermal temperature (abdominal skin temperature of 36–37°C).
3. Sedation; morphine 0.1 mg/kg intramuscularly may be given for marked restlessness.
4. Paralysis with a neuromuscular blocker, intubation, and mechanical ventilation may be life-saving in the sickest patients.

Control salt, water, and calorie intake:
1. Withhold oral feedings if the child is very ill.
2. In infants, empty the stomach to prevent regurgitation and aspiration. The stomach is often atonic and dilated in these very ill infants.
3. Restrict fluid intake initially to 750 ml/m² of body surface area or 65 ml/kg/day if there is severe failure. Be less restrictive in less severe failure. Keep sodium intake low by avoiding added salt and foods high in sodium; if necessary, use salt substitutes.

Establish diuresis:
For severe failure, especially with marked pulmonary edema, give intravenous furosemide (1 mg/kg). Usually, oral agents are adequate: furosemide (1–3 mg/kg, 1–4 times daily); chlorothiazide (25–50 mg/kg/day); hydrochlorothiazide (1–2 mg/kg/day); or metolazone (0.2–0.4 mg/kg once daily) if the other agents are ineffective. These diuretics all cause po-

tassium loss, which can be treated with oral potassium (2 mEq/kg/day).

Digitalize:

1. The digitalizing dose is the theoretical total amount needed to achieve a good effect. This is at first an approximation and may have to be increased or decreased.
2. The dosages for digitalization and maintenance are given in Table 9-3.
3. If any digitalis preparation has been given within the preceding week, obtain a full ECG and consult a cardiologist, or else start on maintenance dosage. *Check serum potassium and creatinine before starting to digitalize.* If potassium is low, reduce digitalizing dose. If creatinine is high, reduce maintenance dose after consultation.
4. The digitalizing dose should be given in three portions: either ½, ¼, ¼ or ⅓, ⅓, ⅓; the latter is easier to calculate and less likely to cause dosage errors. These doses should be given six to eight hours apart. *Always check the dose and be careful of the decimal point.*
5. A rhythm strip that shows good P waves should be obtained two hours after each dose (that is, at the most likely time for digoxin-induced arrhythmias to occur). If arrhythmia occurs, treat for digitalis toxicity as outlined below.
6. Additional loading doses may be needed if the congestive failure does not improve, after cardiologist consultation.
7. If digitalization is stopped because of toxicity before the planned digitalizing dose is complete, base the maintenance dose on the actual digitalizing dose given.
8. Give the first maintenance dose 8 to 12 hours after the last digitalizing dose.
9. If patient vomits a dose, do not repeat.

Employ vasodilator therapy in severe presentations:

1. Use an IV infusion of sodium nitroprusside for severe cardiac failure after cardiac surgery or when other therapies are ineffective. Start at 0.5 μg/kg/ min, and regulate by response of blood pressure and blood flow. Raise head of bed to obtain maximal venous pooling. Do not exceed 10 μg/kg/ min, and check frequently for metabolic acidosis.
2. For chronic ambulatory use, give oral hydralazine (0.5 mg/kg 2–4 times daily, to a maximum of 5 mg/kg/day), prazosin (25 μg/kg 2–3 times daily, to a maximum of 250 μg/kg/day), or captopril (0.1 mg/kg 2–4 times daily, to a maximum of 6 mg/ kg/day). Assess effectiveness by clinical response and widened pulse pressure with a normal mean blood pressure.

Treatment of Severe Pulmonary Edema ∎

This condition constitutes a grave pediatric emergency and necessitates an aggressive approach in the emergency department to reverse pathophysiology and restore pump function.

1. Provide 100% oxygen, by positive-pressure through an endotracheal tube if hypotension or respiratory insufficiency is present. If the child is not in severe distress, oxygen by mask or by bag-valve-mask ventilation may be adequate.
2. Morphine sulfate, 0.1 mg/kg IV, or subcutaneously in less severe cases.
3. Place tourniquets proximally on three limbs. Every 15 minutes, remove one tourniquet and place it on the free limb so that no limb has a tourniquet for more than 45 minutes.
4. Administer furosemide (Lasix), 1 mg/kg, IV.
5. Begin to digitalize (see above).
6. If there is no rapid improvement, give aminophylline, 5 mg/kg, IV, over three to five minutes. Monitor for bradycardia during infusion.
7. For pulmonary edema and severe congestive heart failure unresponsive to usual therapy, either dopamine or isoproterenol is effective, as long as there are no obstructive lesions.

TABLE 9–3. *Doses for Digitalization and Maintenance*

Age	Digitalization*	Maintenance Dose†
Premature	30 μg/kg	10 μg/kg/day
Full term to 2 years	45 μg/kg	15 μg/kg/day
Over 2 years	30 μg/kg	10 μg/kg/day

* Total digitalizing dose of digoxin (Lanoxin) IM or IV, divided into 3 portions.
† Daily maintenance dose of oral digoxin, divided into 2 doses per day.

8. If the child is unresponsive to above treatment, proceed to endotracheal intubation and ventilation, after full pre-oxygenation with 100% oxygen and rapid sequence induction.

Digitalis Toxicity as a Complication of Management ■

DIAGNOSIS

The following are signs of digitalis toxicity:
1. Very long PR interval (50% greater than control interval)
2. Second- or third-degree atrioventricular block
3. Marked sinus bradycardia
4. Appearance of ventricular ectopic beats (especially a bigeminal rhythm), paroxysmal atrial tachycardia (especially with 2:1 AV block), ventricular tachycardia, or even ventricular fibrillation. The appearance of ventricular bigeminal rhythm or paroxysmal supraventricular tachycardia with 2:1 AV block in a patient on digoxin should always be regarded as evidence of digitalis toxicity.
5. Neonates and young infants usually have atrioventricular conduction anomalies; older children usually have ectopic rhythms.

Caveats in diagnosis and treatment of suspected toxicity:
1. Slight lengthening of the PR interval and sagging of the ST segment are not evidence of toxicity.
2. Vomiting in the absence of other evidence of toxicity is not an indication to stop digoxin.
3. Toxicity can occur even when the serum digoxin concentration is normal.

TREATMENT

1. Stop digoxin.
2. If there is a dangerous arrhythmia (ventricular tachycardia, paroxysmal atrial tachycardia with block), give IV potassium, provided there is evidence of good renal function and a normal or low serum potassium level. Dilute potassium salt until the concentration is under 80 mEq/liter and give no faster than 0.3 mEq/kg/hour. Monitor the ECG during infusion. *Do not give if there is a second- or third-degree atrioventricular block.*
3. If there is marked bradycardia, try atropine, 0.01–0.02 mg/kg/dose, IV or IM.
4. If toxicity persists, remember that digoxin has a short half-life in the body of about 36 hours. Therefore, careful observation and potassium administration are usually all that is needed. If a longer-lasting agent is used (digitalis leaf, digitoxin) or if the toxicity seems life-threatening, consult a cardiologist at once. If this is not possible, consider the following:
   a. Phenytoin (Dilantin), 1 mg/kg, IV in normal saline, over one to two minutes and repeated every five minutes until improvement occurs or 10 doses have been given. Monitor arterial pressure every one to three minutes and stop if there is marked hypotension.
   b. Propranolol (Inderal), 0.1 mg/kg, IV. (*Caution:* Avoid propranolol in asthmatics.) It may intensify atrioventricular block, so avoid if there is first- or second-degree atrioventricular block. Propranolol may cause CHF to return or worsen.
   c. Calcium disodium versenate (EDTA). Give 30 mg/kg, IV, over two hours. Monitor the ECG continuously and titrate dosage. Stop when signs of toxicity decrease; restart if they reappear. (*Caution:* EDTA may counter the therapeutic action of digoxin and cause the return of congestive heart failure. It may cause hypocalcemic tetany, bronchospasm, or seizures; do not treat by giving calcium because calcium may cause severe arrhythmias. Prevent this complication by giving EDTA slowly and with careful monitoring.)
   d. Digoxin-specific Fab antibodies have been used successfully. Use for life-threatening arrhythmias that do not respond to any other therapy (see chapter 146).
5. For specific arrhythmias, other drugs may be indicated (see Chapter 12.)

Bibliography ■

Artman, M, Graham TP Jr: Guidelines for vasodilator therapy of congestive heart failure in infants and children. *Am Heart J* 1987; 113:994–1005.

Elkins BR, Watanabe AS: Acute digoxin poisonings: Review of therapy. *Am J Hosp Pharm* 1978; 35:268–277.

Hoffman JIE, Stanger P: Congestive heart failure. In Rudolph A (ed) *Pediatrics*, 18th ed. New York: Appleton-Century-Crofts, 1987, pp. 1336–1342.

Parmley WP, Chatterjee K: Vasodilator therapy. *Curr Prob Cardiol* 1978; 2,12:1–75.

Smith TW, Butler VP Jr, Haber E, et al: Treatment of life-threatening digitalis intoxication with digoxin-specific Fab antibody fragments. *New Eng J Med* 1982; 307:1357–1362.

Talner NS: Congestive heart failure in the infant: A functional approach. *Pediatr Clin North Am* 1971; 18:1011–1029.

Zucker AR, Lacina SJ, DasGupta DS, et al: Fab fragments of digoxin-specific antibodies used to reverse ventricular fibrillation induced by digoxin ingestion in a child. *Pediatrics* 1982; 70:468–471.

10 Pericardial Disorders

Julien I.E. Hoffman

Pericardial diseases are uncommon in childhood. However, severe presentations such as suppurative pericarditis and pericardial tamponade require immediate therapy to avert major morbidity or mortality. *Pericarditis* is inflammation of the pericardium. Typically, both the parietal and epicardial layers and the surface myocardium are involved. *Pericardial effusion* is an abnormal collection of fluid in the pericardial cavity. The fluid may be serous, purulent, or bloody. *Pericardial tamponade* is dangerously high intrapericardial pressure from pericardial effusion, with critical obstruction to inflow and outflow of blood.

Etiology ■

Table 10-1 presents the many causes of pericarditis in childhood. The most common etiology is idiopathic or presumed viral infection.

Pathophysiology ■

Pericarditis causes roughening of the opposing pericardial surfaces, irritation of the phrenic nerves, superficial myocardial cell injury, and sometimes inflammation of the adjacent pleura. If the pericardium is lax, a large effusion without tamponade is possible. On the other hand, a small effusion can cause tamponade if the pericardium is thick from prior inflammation or if the effusion forms very rapidly. *Intrapericardial effusion* distends the pericardium, which then separates from the heart. The fluid muffles heart sounds and reduces QRS voltage. *Tamponade* causes a rise in intrapericardial pressure and impairs cardiac relaxation and filling.

In the setting of tamponade, end-diastolic and atrial and venous pressures are raised on both sides of the heart by approximately equal amounts. Jugular venous pressure is raised, and there is hepatomegaly. Stroke volume is low, with tachycardia, low blood pressure, a narrow pulse pressure, and peripheral vasoconstriction. With inspiration, the intrathoracic pressure becomes more negative and the abdominal pressure becomes more positive. Systemic venous return cannot be accommodated in the heart because of limited expansion. Therefore, the jugular venous pressure may rise with inspiration. Moreover, with inspiration, left ventricular output decreases, and blood pressure falls.

Clinical Findings ■

PERICARDITIS

This condition typically presents with the following key findings in history, physical assessment, and ancillary data collection:

1. A history of precordial pain, often relieved by sitting up and leaning forward. Occasionally, pain may be referred to the left shoulder.
2. Auscultation may reveal a pericardial friction rub.
3. The electrocardiogram may show ST and T changes. Early in the disease, the ST segments are elevated in many leads; later, the ST segments return to normal and the T waves invert.
4. Occasionally, the QT segment is shorter than normal for the rate.
5. Nonspecific signs and symptoms of systemic infection, usually a viral syndrome, are often present.

PERICARDIAL EFFUSION

When the effusion is significant, assessment usually reveals:

1. The area of cardiac dullness is widened to percussion, and the left cardiac border of dullness extends beyond the apex beat.
2. The heart sounds are soft all over, and previous murmurs are softer.
3. Low voltage or electrical alternans of QRS complexes may be seen on the electrocardiogram.
4. The cardiac silhouette is widened on chest radio-

TABLE 10–1. *Causes of Pericarditis in Childhood*

Physical Causes:
  Hemopericardium and pericarditis after chest trauma or cardiac surgery
  Serous or serosanguineous effusions after cardiac trauma, cardiac surgery, or myocardial infarction (usually due to autoimmune mechanisms)
  Perforation of right atrium by indwelling lines, even soft silastic catheters.
  Chest wall radiation

Acute Infections:
  Viral—cocksackie A and B, echovirus, mumps virus, adenovirus
  Bacterial—Staphylococcus, Pneumococcus, H. influenzae, Meningococcus
  Mycoplasma, amebae, toxoplasmosis.

Chronic infections:
  Tuberculosis, actinomycosis, nocardiasis
  Fungi
  Hydatid disease
  Anasarca in congestive heart failure, nephrosis, or cirrhosis of the liver
  Collagen vascular disease, especially systemic lupus erythematosus, rheumatoid arthritis, and rheumatic fever
  Metabolic disorders—uremia, myxedema, gout
  Hemodialysis
  Congenital heart disease, cardiomyopathy
  Benign and malignant tumors
  Foreign bodies in the pericardial cavity
Drugs—hydralazine, procainamide, phenytoin, isoniazid, phenylbutazone, methysergide, penicillin, anticoagulants

Common causes in **bold** print.

graph. The shape of the silhouette is not a good guide for establishing the presence or absence of effusion or for differentiating effusion from cardiomegaly; fluoroscopy is of no additional help. Differentiation from cardiomegaly is made best by echocardiography.
5. A diagnostic tap is confirmatory (see Chapter 139 for procedure).

PERICARDIAL TAMPONADE

This is diagnosed entirely by findings on physical examination and independently of the diagnosis of pericardial effusion or pericarditis.

1. Hepatomegaly and a raised jugular venous pressure are present, which may become more pronounced with inspiration.
2. Tachycardia is frequent, often with low blood pressure and low pulse pressure, and sometimes peripheral vasoconstriction manifested by cold, sweating extremities, and peripheral cyanosis.
3. The mainstay of diagnosis is the *pulsus paradoxus,* the fall of blood pressure with inspiration. This is best detected by placing a sphygmomanometer cuff around the arm and measuring blood pressure in the normal way. The cuff is then inflated to just above systolic pressure and deflated slowly until the first Korotkoff's sounds are heard. If the sounds disappear with each inspiration, lower the pressure slowly, in steps of 2 mm Hg at a time, and note when the sounds first persist throughout the respiratory cycle. The difference between the two levels is the amount of pulsus paradoxus. Normally the maximal difference with a very deep breath is under 8 mm Hg. A greater difference can occur with severe respiratory distress in asthma or bronchiolitis. If these conditions are excluded, elevated pulsus paradoxus over 8 mm Hg suggests pericardial tamponade.
4. *The size of the effusion is no guide to establishing the presence or absence of tamponade.*
5. Patients with large hearts or heart failure (e.g., with renal failure or sickle-cell anemia) can develop

effusions and tamponade that may be mistaken for intensification of the heart failure. *Pulsus paradoxus is the key to diagnosing tamponade.* Suspect an effusion with or without tamponade whenever there is sudden or unexpected cardiomegaly, an increase in heart size, or increasing congestive heart failure.

Ancillary Tests ∎

The diagnosis of pericarditis, pericardial effusion, and pericardial tamponade is usually clinical, often with helpful ECG findings. A chest radiograph helps exclude pulmonary processes but is insensitive for evaluating pericardial effusion. *Echocardiography is the best rapid method for diagnosing and quantifying pericardial effusion.* Other ancillary testing is directed at investigation of systemic causes.

Treatment ∎

PERICARDITIS

Pericarditis is not an emergency, but may lead to one. Advise bed rest. Treat the underlying cause specifically if possible. Watch for endocarditis, myocarditis, effusion, and tamponade. Oral anti-inflammatory agents are helpful.

PERICARDIAL EFFUSION

Pericardial effusion signals important associated disease and possible impending tamponade. Institute appropriate diagnostic measures to determine the specific etiology and obtain an immediate cardiologic consultation. When treatment and disposition are not emergent and the patient is being monitored in the emergency department (ED), measure vital signs, venous pressure, and blood pressure frequently, as well as the pulsus paradoxus. Tamponade may develop rapidly when the pericardium reaches its limit of distensibility.

Drainage of the effusion is required if fluid is needed for diagnosis, if suppurative pericarditis is suspected, or if pericardial tamponade occurs. A suppurative effusion must be drained early; consult a surgeon about the need for pericardiectomy.

PERICARDIAL TAMPONADE

This is a major, life-threatening emergency. In early tamponade without hemodynamic instability, the consulting cardiologist may elect conservative treatment with bed rest, diuretics, and acetylsalicylic acid (aspirin). In the ED, apply a cardiac monitor and record vital signs and pulsus paradoxus every half-hour. If the tamponade is severe or increasing, remove fluid emergently with an angiocath or a 20-gauge needle and syringe (see Chapter 139). If the fluid is thick or potentially loculated, consult a surgeon to remove the fluid through a small opening in the pericardium. This can be done even under local anesthesia, allows safe removal of thick fluid, permits manual breakdown of adhesions, and obtains a portion of the pericardium for histologic study.

Disposition ∎

Many patients with acute pericarditis require hospital admission for full evaluation, observation, and treatment. Inpatient treatment may be only symptomatic or it may be specific for the underlying diagnosis. *Admit any child with an acute pericardial effusion that is clinically detectable by physical examination and/or significant pulsus paradoxus.* If evidence of compromised heart filling or hemodynamic instability is present, after resuscitation and stabilization the child requires further management in the intensive care unit or transfer to a pediatric critical care center.

In children with the painful syndrome of acute pericarditis, but without evidence of instability or significant effusion, outpatient management with aspirin and bed rest is appropriate if parental compliance with treatment and follow-up is ensured. Ordinarily, refer patients to their primary physician or, in some cases, to a pediatric cardiologist for follow-up care.

Bibliography ∎

Fowler NO: Diseases of the pericardium. *Curr Probl Cardiol* 1978; 2,10:1–38.

Høier-Madsdenk K, Saunamäki KI, Wulff J, et al: Purulent pericarditis in children. *Scand J Thorac Cardiovasc Surg* 1985; 19:185–188.

Permanyer-Miralda G, Sagrista-Sauleda J, Soler-Soler J: Primary acute pericardial disease: a prospective study of 231 consecutive patients. *Am J Cardiol* 1985; 56:623–630.

Reddy PS, Leon DF, Shaver JA: *Pericardial diseases.* New York: Raven Press, 1982.

Shabetai R: *The pericardium.* New York: Grune & Stratton, 1981.

Spodick DH: The normal and diseased pericardium: current concepts of pericardial physiology, diagnosis and treatment. *J Am Coll Cardiol* 1983; 1:240–251.

11 Systemic Hypertension

Julien I. E. Hoffman

Hypertension refers to systolic, diastolic, or mean arterial blood pressure above the upper limit of normal for the patient's age. Emergency treatment is needed if the patient is symptomatic or if the pressures are high enough to produce systemic complications. Severe hypertension is unusual in childhood; when it occurs, it is usually secondary to pathology in another organ system, often the kidneys.

Normal Standards ■

Normal values for systolic and diastolic blood pressure (Figure 11-1) are based on sphygmomanometer measurements taken with the subject at rest and with minimal anxiety. The figures approximate the 50th and 95th percentiles for each age group. Blood pressures tend to be higher for those excessively tall or heavy for their age, and may be 5–10 mm Hg higher when supine than when sitting up. Differences between pressures in boys and girls are negligible before puberty, and then are related to body size rather than to sex; by 18 years of age systolic pressures are about 8–10 mm Hg higher and diastolic pressures are about 4–5 mm Hg higher in boys than in girls.

Sphygmomanometer measurements are difficult to take in newborn infants and are more accurately taken with oscillometric (Dynamap) or Doppler devices. Arterial pressures are sometimes taken through umbilical arterial catheters or by the flush method, the latter approximating mean pressure. Table 11-1 lists normal mean pressures in newborns.

Table 11-2 describes the procedure for obtaining accurate blood pressures in children. Careful measurement is key to appropriate assessment, treatment, and disposition.

Etiology and Pathophysiology ■

See Table 11-3 for conditions of childhood that are associated with severe hypertension.

Clinical Findings ■

SIGNS AND SYMPTOMS

The important etiologies for severe hypertension in childhood require specific diagnosis. A good history, thorough physical examination, and appropriate ancillary tests will often reveal the underlying problem. Clinical findings in the child with severe hypertension may reflect the primary etiology, or the secondary, systemic effects of elevated blood pressure itself. The following systemic manifestations are cardinal features of *severe* hypertension:

Blood pressure: Exceeds 95th percentile for the patient's age (Figure 11-1) or is increasing rapidly.

Cardiac: Left ventricular hypertrophy, congestive heart failure, pulmonary edema.

Abdominal: Abdominal pain and ileus (e.g., after operative resection of aortic coarctation); flank pain.

Renal: Sudden decrease in renal function; hematuria.

Neurologic: Severe headache, focal or general seizures, focal signs, isolated facial nerve palsy.

Retinal: Visual blurring, retinal hemorrhages and exudates, papilledema, narrowing of arteries, arteriovenous nicking.

Ancillary Data ■

Only a complete blood count and urinalysis are appropriate for initial evaluation in the asymptomatic child with blood pressure elevation alone. Electrolytes, blood urea nitrogen, creatinine, and skull radiographs are also helpful when blood pressure is extremely high or if any systemic manifestations are present. If these tests are inconclusive, obtain a cardiologist consultation before proceeding to more complex tests.

If *major* systemic manifestations are present with hypertension, further evaluation includes an electrocardiogram, chest radiograph, and other specific laboratory tests depending on the clinical findings. *These*

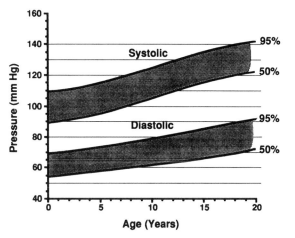

FIGURE 11–1. Normal blood pressures. Averaged, smoothed data for both boys and girls. One week after birth the systolic pressures are about 20 mm Hg lower than is indicated by the left hand sections of the curves, and 1 month after birth they are about 10 mm Hg lower than shown on the graph. Diastolic pressures on the curves are accurate for all ages. The pressures are measured while the children are sitting at rest, and diastolic pressure is taken as the sudden muffling (K4) of the Korotkoff sounds. (Adapted from *Pediatrics* 1987; 79:1–25.)

patients must be admitted to the intensive care unit expeditiously and treated immediately with agents to lower the blood pressure; definitive work-up is then continued on an inpatient basis.

Treatment ■

GENERAL MEASURES

For patients with any systemic manifestations:

1. Bed rest, sedation, low sodium intake.
2. An effective diuretic (metolazone, 0.02 mg/kg IV, or furosemide, 1 mg/kg IV or IM) will cause marked diuresis and will lower blood volume slightly, thus lowering blood pressure. If there is renal failure, *do not* give without consultation.

SPECIFIC MEASURES

Severe Hypertension

Immediate blood-pressure reduction is required within a few minutes in patients with elevated blood pressure and major end-organ abnormalities, such as papilledema, altered mental status, pulmonary edema, or seizures. Any of the following agents is effective, and while therapy may be st₂ emergency department, ongoing treatme place in a properly equipped intensive

1. *Diazoxide (Hyperstat)*, 2 mg/kg, by ₁₄₊₊ jection, without diluting the contents of the vial. A rapid fall in blood pressure may occur in minutes and persist for hours; in this dose severe hypotension is unlikely. The drug can be repeated in 1 mg/kg boluses every 10 minutes until blood pressure is controlled.
2. *Trimethaphan camsylate (Arfonad)* by continuous IV infusion, with careful minute-to-minute monitoring of blood pressure. This agent is seldom used unless all facilities for close observation are present. Dilute the drug to 1 mg/ml and infuse at about 50 to 150 μg/kg/minute; judge the exact dose by frequent blood-pressure measurement. The drug can be very dangerous if blood pressure is not watched continuously. Further, because it is a ganglion-blocking agent, there is some risk of paralytic ileus and urine retention. The drug is very effective at first but loses its effect after 48 hours.
3. *Sodium nitroprusside (Nipride)* by continuous IV infusion, starting with 1 μg/kg/minute and titrated to desired blood pressure. Careful vascular monitoring is imperative, usually with an intra-arterial pressure line. Keep patient at an angle of about 20 degrees to horizontal plane and beware of severe postural hypotension. With long infusions, keep blood level below 12 mg/dl to avoid thiocyanate toxicity. Above a total dose of *3 mg/kg*, the risk of metabolic acidemia is high. Obtain cardiologist consultation in patients with renal disease, since special precautions are necessary.

Moderately Severe Hypertension

Slower hypotensive action, over 10 to 60 minutes, is indicated for patients with increased blood pressure and serious but not life-threatening manifestations

TABLE 11–1. *Normal Mean Pressures in Newborns (mm Hg)*

Birth Weight (kg)	3rd Percentile	97th Percentile
1	28	48
2	29	49
3	34	54
4	43	63

TABLE 11–2. *Technique for Accurate Blood Pressure Measurement*

Apply the cuff firmly to the arm or leg. The inner inflatable bladder must be wide enough to cover 75% of the length of the upper arm or thigh and must extend completely around the circumference of the limb.

Raise the pressure about 20 mm Hg above the level at which the distal arterial pulse disappears, and then lower at a rate of 2–3 mm Hg per second.

The systolic level is the pressure at which the sounds are first heard. The diastolic level is the pressure at which the sounds suddenly muffle. Do not consider disappearance of the sounds to be the diastolic pressure.

For flush pressures, dilate the vessels of the hand or foot by friction or by placing the extremity in warm water. Apply the cuff to the wrist or ankle, elevate the limb above heart level, and squeeze the hand or foot to empty the contained blood; then raise the cuff pressure above the expected systolic pressure. Lower the pressure slowly—about 5 mm Hg per second—and take the pressure at which the hand or foot suddenly flushes. One person watches the extremity and another person watches the mercury column.

(e.g., headache or abdominal pain). The following drugs are usually efficacious:

1. *Hydralazine (Apresoline),* 0.15 mg/kg IM, acts within 20 minutes, and even more quickly when given IV. Give additional doses as needed according to the effectiveness of the first dose; often four to six doses IM per day are effective. The dosage may be increased to 0.6 mg/kg every four to six hours if this is the only drug being used. If hydralazine is not effective in lowering blood pressure, add *reserpine*. If there is no urgency, give reserpine 0.02 mg/kg IM and repeat at four- to six-hour intervals. If the response is inadequate, increase the dose of reserpine to 0.05 mg/kg, and then to 0.07 mg/kg IM.

2. *Reserpine (Serpasil)* may be used as the only drug, especially if hypertension is not very severe and if there is no risk of delaying the fall in blood pressure. Giving hydralazine and reserpine together may diminish the side effects of both drugs.

3. *Alpha-methyldopa (Aldomet)* is an alternative to hydralazine or reserpine. For rapid effect, give 10 mg/kg IV; this lowers pressure in one to two hours. At the same time, begin oral therapy with 5 to 10 mg/kg twice daily.

4. *Nifedipine* 0.15 mg/kg orally is also rapidly effective. Capsules contain 10 or 20 mg. If whole capsule is used, chew and swallow, or break capsule and give solution sublingually. For smaller doses, aspirate the required amount with a tuberculin syringe. Do not expose to light.

5. *Labetalol* blocks both α and β adrenergic receptors and has some direct β adrenergic stimulation that causes vasodilatation; it can be given intravenously in boluses of 0.3 mg/kg every 20 minutes until an acceptable blood pressure is reached. It is not always successful, and should be avoided in asthmatics.

Complications and Caveats ■

1. Be careful to avoid inducing severe hypotension, especially when intravenous drugs are administered.

2. Some of the above drugs, given by any route, may cause severe postural hypotension. Therefore, measure blood pressure supine, sitting, and standing.

3. Be cautious with reserpine if the patient is in heart failure or has asthma. Avoid it in the neonate because it may cause severe nasal obstruction and difficulty in breathing.

4. If the patient has renal failure and alpha-methyldopa is used, give lower doses than suggested above. Also, be cautious in lowering blood pressure, and check renal function frequently. If it is essential to lower the blood pressure but renal function deteriorates, dialysis may be needed.

5. Do not attempt to reduce pressures to normal immediately, especially in chronic hypertension or hypertension due to renal disease. Instead, lower pressures about halfway between initial and ideal pressures.

6. Consult a cardiologist if the cause of hypertension is not easily diagnosed, if there is no response to the recommended drugs in average doses, if severe systemic manifestations are present, or if there are significant side effects of treatment.

7. Maintenance therapy may also be complicated and warrants consultation and mandatory follow-up with the primary physician or consultant.

8. Do not overinvestigate or overtreat mild hypertension. Follow-up alone may be sufficient.

Disposition ■

If pressures are above the 90th percentile, or only slightly above the 95th percentile and the patient is

TABLE 11-3. *Conditions Associated with Hypertension*

I. Measuring errors: "Erroneous" hypertension is sometimes due to use of a too-small blood pressure cuff.
II. Physiologic changes:
    (A) Anxiety and tachycardia.
    (B) Large stroke volume.
        (1) Patent ducts arteriosus, aortic incompetence, arteriovenous fistula, or thyrotoxicosis.
        (2) Bradycardia, including complete heart block.
III. Acute hypertension.
    (A) Central nervous system disorders. Encephalitis, raised intracranial pressure, and diencephalic lesions. Hypertension may occur after intracranial surgery.
    (B) Hypervolemia and hypernatremia. Excessive intravenous fluids and blood, or rarely mineralocorticoid excess.
    (C) Catecholamines:
        (1) Reserpine or rapid intravenous injection of alpha-methyldopa.
        (2) Supersensitivity to added amines. This may be caused by taking sympathomimetic amines as a decongestant, particularly while being treated for hypertension with reserpine or alpha-methyldopa; or by ingesting foods with tyramine (aged cheeses, pickled herring, some wines or beers) while on monoamine oxidase inhibitors.
    (D) Miscellaneous causes:
        (1) Drug abuse (cocaine, amphetamines, phencyclidine).
        (2) Neurologic disorders (familial dysautonomia, Guillain-Barré syndrome, poliomyacute glomerulonephritis).
        (3) Acute renal disease (hemolytic-uremic syndrome, Henoch-Schönlein purpura, acute glomerulonephritis).
        (4) Metabolic disorders (gonadal dysgenesis, acute intermittent porphyria, hypercalcemia).
        (5) Other conditions, especially mercury poisoning, burns, pre-eclampsia, Stevens-Johnson syndrome, leukemia, prolonged bed rest and traction, and bronchopulmonary dysplasia.
IV. Sustained hypertension:
    (A) Coarctation of the aorta.
    (B) Lead poisoning.
    (C) Renal hypertension.
        (1) Acute post-streptococcal glomerulonephritis
        (2) Pyelonephritis
        (3) Renal ischemia due to thrombosis, fibromuscular narrowing, or congenital anomaly
        (4) Congenital renal lesions.
    (D) Endocrine disorders
        (1) Neuroblastomas or pheochromocytomas
        (2) Excessive mineralocorticoids:
        Aldosterone-secreting tumor or hyperplasia of adrenals
        Adrenogenital syndrome due to 11β or 17α hydroxylase deficiency
        Excessive ingestion of licorice
        (3) Excessive glucorticoids:
        Cushing's syndrome
        High-dose glucocorticoid therapy
        (4) Oral contraceptives, testosterone, some other anabolic steroids. (The hypertension may persist for several weeks after stopping the medication.)
        (5) Pre-eclampsia
    (E) Essential hypertension.

---

asymptomatic, all that is needed is an outpatient evaluation consisting of family history, physical examination, and urinalysis and complete blood count. Repeat blood-pressure measurements are imperative on subsequent visits to the primary physician. Advise weight reduction if indicated. If hypertension persists on follow-up, obtain serum electrolytes, creatinine, uric acid, and urea.

For significant (but not severe) sustained hypertension, order additional tests as outlined in ancillary data section above, as well as an electrocardiogram and echocardiogram to evaluate left ventricular hypertrophy. Urine cultures (especially in girls) and appropriate renal and endocrine tests may also be helpful, but selection of these is best done in consultation with a pediatric cardiologist. If the patient is symptomatic from the hypertension, or if there is evidence of any significant end-organ effects, admit the child and obtain specialist consultation.

For severe hypertension with major manifestations, initiate treatment, obtain consultation, and admit the patient to the intensive care unit or arrange immediate transfer to a pediatric critical care center for safe and monitored reduction of blood pressure and for systematic investigations of etiology.

Bibliography ∎

Bauer JH, Reams GP: The role of calcium entry blockers in hypertensive emergencies. *Circulation* 1987; 75 (Suppl V):174–180.

De Quattro V: Treating hypertensive crises: Which drugs for which patient? *J Crit Illness* 1987; 2:24–35.

Garcia JY, Vidt DG: Current management of hypertensive emergencies. *Drugs* 1987; 34:263–278.

Lieberman E: Essential hypertension in children and youth: A pediatric perspective. *J Pediatr* 1974; 85:1–11.

Loggie JH: Hypertension in children and adolescents. I. Causes and diagnostic studies. *J Pediatr* 1966; 74:331–355.

Report of the Second Task Force on Blood Pressure Control in Children, 1987. *Pediatrics* 1987; 79:1–25.

12 Dysrhythmias

George F. Van Hare

Dysrhythmias in childhood are rare. They usually occur in patients with known congenital or acquired heart disease or as a complication of another disorder. Often, reversal of pathophysiology from an underlying systemic process will obviate the need for dysrhythmia therapy.

Occasionally, the dysrhythmia itself is the primary problem; in these cases, rapid identification of the category of dysrhythmia and individualized treatment are imperative. Dysrhythmias associated with hemodynamic instability require emergency therapy. Dysrhythmias in stable patients are less urgent; perform a history, physical examination, and analysis of the electrocardiogram in these patients before treatment.

Classification ■

In the Emergency Department (ED), dysrhythmias are readily categorized into *fast, slow,* or *irregular.* If the rhythm is abnormally fast, inspection of the QRS interval further divides this category of dysrhythmias into *narrow* or *wide complex tachycardias.* Fast or slow rhythms are most likely to require treatment.

Clinical Findings ■

Children with dysrhythmias can be assigned to one of the following severity levels based on history and physical examination: *asymptomatic, mildly symptomatic, seriously ill,* or *critically ill.* The severity level determines the nature and urgency of treatment.

Asymptomatic: The child is completely unaware of the existence of the dysrhythmia.

Mildly symptomatic: Patients may have increased "cardiac awareness" and may report sensations of palpitations, extra beats, "skipped" beats, or "pounding in the chest." Occasionally, dizziness occurs with either bradycardia or tachycardia. Syncope (complete loss of consciousness), secondary to a dysrhythmia, is unusual in children. Asymptomatic and mildly symptomatic patients do not need emergency treatment.

Seriously ill: The seriously symptomatic infant may have congestive heart failure, with a history of fretfulness, irritability, and poor feeding. Diaphoresis, tachypnea, and perioral cyanosis are often present on examination. Blood pressure may be normal with a narrow pulse pressure, thready peripheral pulses, and an enlarged liver. Chest auscultation is often normal, since rales are not usually heard even in the presence of pulmonary edema. Cardiac examination can disclose an abnormally fast or slow heart rate, often with a gallop rhythm.

Older children may complain of shortness of breath, exercise intolerance, a heavy feeling in the chest, and frequently tachycardia. Rales are more common than in infants.

Critically ill: Heart rates sufficiently fast or slow may result in critically low or absent blood pressure, nonpalpable pulses, altered sensorium, or complete loss of consciousness. Preventing cardiopulmonary arrest in critically ill patients requires definitive treatment within two or three minutes of the onset of the dysrhythmia or arrival in the ED.

ECG Data ■

Careful interpretation of the electrocardiogram (ECG) is essential to diagnosis and therapy of dysrhythmias. The essential components include rate, rhythm, axis, P wave, PR interval, QRS complex, ST segment, QT segment, and T wave. *The most important ECG features in childhood are the rate and the QRS complex.* These components must be evaluated against age-specific normals, as illustrated in Figures 12-1, 12-2, and 12-3. Because the QRS complex may be isoelectric in some leads, analyze several leads before considering the dysrhythmia a wide or narrow QRS tachycardia. Table 12-1 summarizes ECG characteristics of the common dysrhythmias.

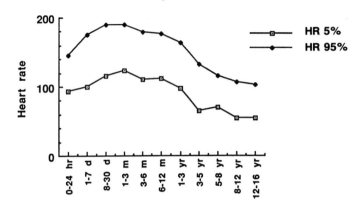

FIGURE 12–1. Electrocardiogram normal standards. Fifth and 95th percentiles for heart rate at various ages. (Adapted from Liebman J, Plonsey R, Gillette PC: Pediatric Electrocardiography. Baltimore: Williams & Wilkins, 1982, pp 82–85. Used by permission.)

Tachycardias: Wide vs. Narrow QRS Complex ■

When a child presents with tachycardia, first evaluate hemodynamic status. Next, check normal heart rate for age (see Figure 12-1) to ascertain that a true tachycardia is present (i.e., rate is greater than the 95th percentile for age). Then, classify the rhythm as a wide or narrow QRS tachycardia by measuring the duration of the QRS complex and comparing it to age norms (see Figure 12-3). While nearly all narrow QRS tachycardias are supraventricular in origin, not all wide QRS tachycardias are ventricular in origin. *Distinguishing between ventricular and supraventricular origin of a wide QRS tachycardia in the ED is usually impossible.* Therefore, hemodynamic status and QRS width alone are the guideposts for treatment.

Narrow QRS tachycardias: The QRS duration is similar to normal sinus rhythm, or less than the 95th percentile for age (usually < 0.10 sec), if a baseline ECG is not available.

Wide QRS tachycardias: The QRS duration is significantly longer than the duration in normal sinus rhythm, or longer than the 95th percentile for age (usually >0.1 sec).

NARROW QRS TACHYCARDIAS

Causes

1. *Sinus tachycardia* (Figure 12-4): There is a normal P wave axis, gradual onset and termination, and rates below 250 beats per minute. Rates above 250 bpm are never sinus tachycardia. Narrow complex tachycardias below 250 bpm are often sinus tachycardia, so this rhythm must be excluded before instituting antidysrhythmic therapy. Causes of sinus tachycardia include fever, pain, dehydration, anxiety, and sepsis.
2. *Atrial tachycardias* (Figure 12-5): P waves precede QRS complexes, and the P wave axis is variable, depending on the site of atrial impulse formation. Short episodes of atrioventricular block (induced by Valsalva or other vagal maneuvers or medica-

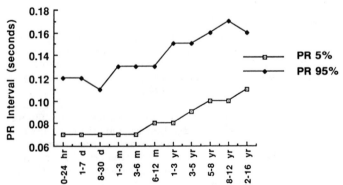

FIGURE 12–2. Electrocardiogram normal standards. Fifth and 95th percentiles for PR interval at various ages.

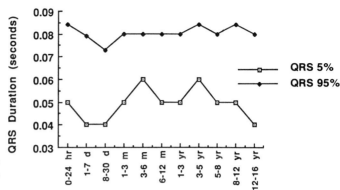

FIGURE 12–3. Electrocardiogram normal standards. Fifth and 95th percentiles for QRS duration at various ages.

tion) do not terminate the tachycardia. There is very little (<10 msec) variation in R-R intervals. Episodes start suddenly, stop suddenly, and end with a QRS complex rather than a P wave. When it is seen in association with significant (grade 2 or higher) atrioventricular block in a patient who has been taking digoxin, digoxin toxicity is the most likely diagnosis (Figure 12-6).

3. *Atrial flutter* (Figure 12-7): The atrial rates are about 300 per minute, or 400–500 in newborns. Atrioventricular conduction may be 1:1 but more often is 2:1 or variable. The characteristic sawtooth appearance of flutter waves may be difficult to appreciate because of superimposition on the QRS and T waves; review lead V1 for clearest P wave configuration. Often, narrow QRS beats are present with frequent wide QRS beats, due to intermittent aberrant conduction.

4. *Atrial fibrillation* (Figure 12-8): Atrial fibrillation represents disorganized activity in the atrium, and there are no discrete regular P waves present. Conduction to the ventricles is quite irregular, and no two R-R intervals are exactly the same, giving an irregularly irregular R-R configuration. While most beats will be conducted with narrow QRS complexes, random aberrantly conducted beats are common, particularly when a short R-R interval follows a longer R-R interval.

5. *Junctional tachycardia:* There are two mechanisms for junctional tachycardia: reentry involving dual pathways in the atrioventricular node, and accelerated junctional focus (junctional ectopic tachycardia) (Figure 12-9).

6. *Accessory pathway reentrant tachycardia* (Wolff-Parkinson-White syndrome) (Figure 12-10): During tachycardia, there is never a delta wave. The P wave follows the preceding QRS complex. There is little or no variation in the R-R interval, and atrioventricular block always terminates the tachy-

cardia, since the atrioventricular node is part of the reentrant circuit. During sinus rhythm, a delta wave is frequently seen.

TREATMENT

Critically ill: Deliver immediate synchronized DC cardioversion at 0.5 watt-seconds or joules/kg (see Table 6-5 for procedure). If unsuccessful, double the dose.

Convert narrow QRS tachycardias in the synchronous mode; wide QRS tachycardias with the synchronous mode; and ventricular fibrillation in the asynchronous mode (defibrillation). In some forms of ventricular tachycardia, the cardioverter-defibrillator may not sense R waves well; if so, use the asynchronous mode. No special precautions are necessary in children on therapeutic doses of digoxin. If there is a concern of high digoxin levels or digoxin toxicity, administer an initial bolus of 1 mg/kg of intravenous lidocaine before cardioversion.

Seriously ill: The patient's hemodynamic status determines the urgency of treatment. If the child is unstable, cardiovert after placement of an intravenous line. More stable patients may be managed in an incremental fashion, as follows:

First, identify and treat underlying exacerbating conditions, such as hypoxia, acidosis, electrolyte abnormalities, drug ingestions and toxicities, and sepsis. Exclude sinus tachycardia, since the treatment of sinus tachycardia is based on correcting the underlying problem.

If sinus tachycardia has been excluded, first attempt a *vagal maneuver* to convert the rhythm back to sinus. Record all maneuvers on an ECG machine. The effect of maneuvers and the mechanism of termination may help in eventually making a diagnosis.

A variety of maneuvers produce a vagal reflex. In many cases, vagal maneuvers terminate tachycardias

TABLE 12–1. *Characteristics of Common Dysrhythmias*

Rhythm	Rate	R–R Intervals	P Wave Axis	P Wave Location	AV Dissociation	Effect of Transient AV Block
Narrow QRS Tachycardias						
Sinus tachycardia	100–250	Regular	Normal	Before QRS	No	Rhythm continues
Atrial flutter	Atrial 300–500	Regular or irregular	—	Flutter waves	No	Rhythm continues
Atrial ectopic tachycardia	120–300	Regular or irregular	Normal or abnormal	Before QRS	No	Rhythm continues
Junctional ectopic tachycardia	120–300	Regular with capture beats	Normal	Dissociated	Usually	Rhythm continues
AV node re-entry tachycardia	120–180	Regular	Superior	Buried on QRS	Rarely	Termination of tachycardia in nearly all
AV reciprocating tachycardia (accessory pathway tachycardia)	120–180	Regular	Superior	After QRS	No	Termination of tachycardia in nearly all
Atrial fibrillation	60–190	Very irregular	—	Fibrillation waves	No	Rhythm continues
Wide QRS Tachycardias						
Ventricular tachycardia	150–260	Regular	Normal or superior	Variable	Frequent	Rhythm continues
Atrial fibrillation with W–P–W	150–300	Very irregular	—	Not well seen	No	Rhythm continues
Antidromic tachycardia with W–P–W	120–180	Regular	Superior	Before QRS	No	Termination of tachycardia in nearly all

AV = atrioventricular, W–P–W = Wolff–Parkinson–White syndrome.

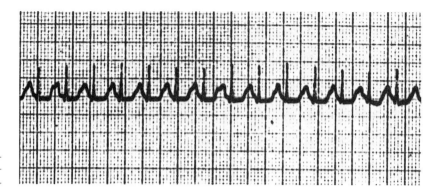

FIGURE 12-4. Sinus tachycardia. P waves are seen superimposed on the preceding T waves.

by inducing transient atrioventricular block, interrupting reentrant circuits. Any of several procedures are acceptable:

1. *Rectal stimulation* by inserting a rectal thermometer or suppository.
2. *Gagging* the infant with a nasogastric tube.
3. *The diving reflex,* elicited by placing a bag of ice with some water over the face large enough to cover the ears, and holding it in that position for 45 seconds.
4. *The Valsalva maneuver* may be elicited by coaching the patient to bear down.
5. *Unilateral carotid massage* is indicated in older patients for 5 seconds. Eyeball pressure should *not* be performed because of the risk of retinal detachment.

If vagal maneuvers fail to terminate the tachycardia, try medical treatment, using any of several different agents (Table 12-2).

1. In children over 12 months of age, try *verapamil* first. Be prepared to manage hypotension with vasopressor drugs or calcium chloride. The drug is contraindicated in children in the first year of life because asystolic arrest has been associated with this drug in this age group. Atropine may be necessary to control bradycardia following conversion of the dysrhythmia.
2. As an alternative to verapamil, or in children under 12 months of age, intravenous *propranolol* is the next choice. Carefully monitor blood pressure and heart rate. Do not give propranolol to children with asthma or congestive heart failure, or to those who have received verapamil.
3. *Digoxin* is effective in most pediatric dysrhythmias. Its disadvantage is that full digitalization takes a long time. Avoid it in patients with Wolff-Parkinson-White syndrome.
4. *Phenylephrine* intravenously evokes a strong vagal reflex, which raises the blood pressure, triggers the baroreceptor reflex, and may terminate the tachycardia.

When vagal maneuvers and medications fail to stop the tachycardia, and the child is seriously symptomatic, proceed to *direct current cardioversion.* Sedate the conscious child with a short-acting barbiturate or

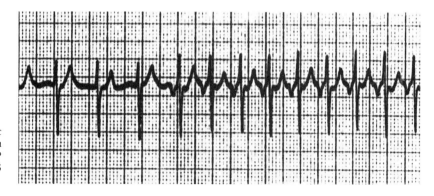

FIGURE 12-5. Atrial ectopic tachycardia. The tachycardia starts suddenly, with inverted P waves seen before the QRS complexes.

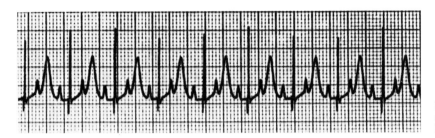

FIGURE 12–6. Atrial tachycardia with 2:1 atrioventricular block, due to digoxin toxicity.

benzodiazepine agent; pretreatment with diazepam or midazolam induces retrograde amnesia (Table 12-3). Some tachycardias do not respond to cardioversion, notably atrial and junctional ectopic tachycardias. In these cases, support blood pressure with vasoactive drugs such as dopamine, consult a cardiologist, and admit the patient to an intensive care unit.

Caveats

When the exact form of narrow complex tachycardia is known, treatment can sometimes be specific, as outlined below. Cardiologist consultation may be warranted.

1. For atrioventricular node reentry and atrioventricular reciprocating tachycardia, *procainamide* may be helpful if initial measures fail.
2. For atrial tachycardias and flutter, procainamide is effective. It may, however, paradoxically increase the ventricular rate, by slowing the atrial rate and shortening the atrioventricular node refractory period, thereby allowing 1:1 conduction of atrial tachycardias. Use only after propranolol or digoxin.
3. If an atrial tachycardia coexists with significant atrioventricular block (e.g., atrial tachycardia with 2:1 conduction, Figure 12-6), digoxin toxicity is likely. Digoxin is contraindicated in this circumstance, as it may precipitate ventricular fibrillation. Stop digoxin and provide hemodynamic support while the effects of digoxin slowly disappear. Carefully control the serum potassium. Consider digoxin antigen binding fragments (Digibind, Burroughs-Wellcome), especially if there has been a recent massive ingestion. Obtain cardiologist consultation and either admit the child to an intensive care unit or arrange a transfer to a pediatric critical care facility.
4. In atrial fibrillation, the goal is to control the ventricular rate. Use verapamil, propranolol, or digoxin, if the child is hemodynamically stable. After the ventricular rate is controlled, procainamide may also convert the dysrhythmia to an organized atrial rhythm (but see Table 12-1 for precautions). However, procainamide may fail and elective electrical cardioversion may be necessary, after consultation with a cardiologist.

WIDE COMPLEX TACHYCARDIAS

Causes

1. *Ventricular tachycardia* (Figure 12-11): Ventricular tachycardia accounts for 95% of wide QRS tachycardias in children. Atrioventricular dissocia-

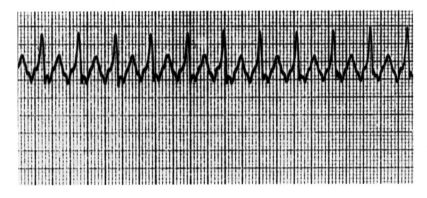

FIGURE 12–7. Atrial flutter. Typical "sawtooth" flutter waves are present with regular 2:1 atrioventricular conduction.

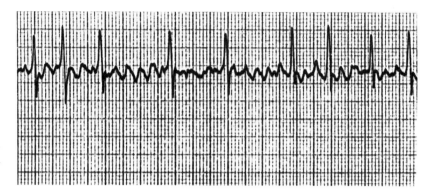

FIGURE 12–8. Atrial fibrillation. There is an "undulating" baseline with no organized atrial activity. The R–R intervals are very irregular, with no two R–R intervals exactly the same duration.

tion is present in about 50% of these. *A hallmark of ventricular tachycardia is the occasional occurrence of fusion beats.* Fusion occurs when the ventricle is depolarized simultaneously by the ventricular focus and a sinus impulse arriving via the atrioventricular node. This results in a QRS complex intermediate in duration and morphology between sinus beats and ventricular beats. Unfortunately, capture and fusion beats are sometimes not recognized. Consider wide QRS tachycardias to be ventricular tachycardia unless another cause has been established. Other possible diagnoses are:

2. *Wide QRS tachycardia in Wolff-Parkinson-White syndrome* (Antidromic atrioventricular reciprocating tachycardia): Accessory pathway-mediated tachycardia, which uses the accessory pathway for antegrade conduction, has wide QRS complexes because the ventricular activation is entirely from the accessory pathway. Atrioventricular dissociation rules out this diagnosis.

3. *Supraventricular tachycardia with aberration:* Any type of narrow QRS tachycardia may occur with wide QRS complexes related to the rapid rate (ab-

erration). This phenomenon is rare in children without pre-existing bundle branch block.

4. *Atrial fibrillation in Wolff-Parkinson-White syndrome:* Some patients with Wolff-Parkinson-White syndrome have accessory pathways that allow conduction with dangerously rapid ventricular rates, due to a short antegrade effective refractory period of the accessory pathway. This life-threatening dysrhythmia is an irregular, fast wide QRS tachycardia. No two R-R intervals are the same.

Treatment

DC CARDIOVERSION: Wide QRS tachycardias are medical emergencies. Direct current cardioversion is the initial treatment of choice in nearly all cases. The procedure is similar to the method for narrow QRS tachycardias (see Table 6-5). However, if the patient is critically ill, sedatives are contraindicated; if the patient is hemodynamically stable with a wide QRS complex, however, employ sedation if at all possible. Unless the rhythm is ventricular fibrillation, synchronize cardioversion to the R wave. If the de-

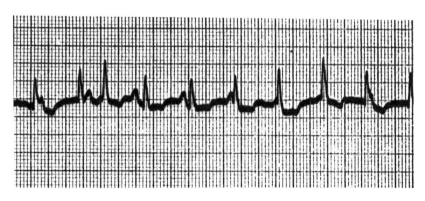

FIGURE 12–9. Junctional ectopic tachycardia. There is atrioventricular dissociation with an atrial rate slower than the ventricular rate. Capture beats occur, which have QRS morphologies nearly identical to the other beats.

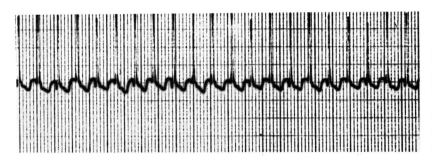

FIGURE 12–10. Reciprocating tachycardia due to an accessory pathway (patient with Wolff–Parkinson–White syndrome). There is no delta wave during tachycardia, and P waves are present, superimposed on the T waves and following the QRS complexes.

fibrillator does not immediately discharge, it may be due to failure of the device to sense the R waves. In this case, switch the device to the asynchronous mode.

MEDICATIONS: If cardioversion fails, especially if the child has atrial fibrillation with an accessory pathway, administer procainamide or lidocaine intravenously. In a patient with ventricular tachycardia who has recurrent sustained or nonsustained ventricular tachycardia or multiform premature ventricular contractions following initial cardioversion, intravenous lidocaine may prevent recurrences of tachycardia.

Bradycardias ■

CAUSES

1. *Sinus bradycardia:* Sinus bradycardia is a regular slow atrial rate with 1:1 conduction. Causes include hypoxia, acidosis, increased intracranial pressure, and hypoglycemia. Drugs such as digoxin and propranolol may also cause significant sinus bradycardia. Mild slowing may be due to increased vagal tone or cardiac conditioning in an athlete.

2. *Atrioventricular block:*
   a. *Third-degree or complete atrioventricular block* (Figure 12-12) may be congenital or surgically induced, or may occur suddenly due to myocarditis. It is recognized as atrioventricular dissociation and regular R-R intervals without capture beats.
   b. *Second-degree atrioventricular block* is classified as Mobitz type 1 (Wenckebach) (Figure 12-13) or Mobitz type 2 (Figure 12-14). Wenckebach conduction is characterized by progressive PR interval prolongation followed by a blocked beat, followed by recovery of conduction). Type 1 generally has a better prognosis than type 2, and responds to medication readily.

TABLE 12–2. *Intravenous Antidysrhythmic Agents*

Agent	Dosage	Comments
Verapamil	0.1–0.2 mg/kg IV 5–10 mg maximum	Beware hypotension; definitely contraindicated under 6 months, probably under 12 months; do *not* give with beta blockers.
Propranolol	0.02 mg/kg IV every 5 minutes, to 0.1 mg/kg	Monitor pulse, blood pressure; contraindicated in asthmatics and in congestive heart failure; do *not* give with verapamil.
Procainamide	15 mg/kg IV over 30 minutes	May cause hypotension; continuous monitoring is essential; cardiology guidance is recommended.
Digoxin	10 μg/kg IV as initial load, 2nd dose in 6 hrs, 3rd at 24 hrs	Do not use in hypokalemia or if digoxin toxicity is suspected (see Table 9-3)
Lidocaine	1–2 mg/kg IV over 15 minutes. Continuous infusion 30–50 μg/kg/minute	
Phenylephrine	0.02 mg/kg IV slowly	Use for raising blood pressure and eliciting a baroreceptor vagal reflex

TABLE 12–3. *Other Agents for Use in Dysrhythmia Management*

Isoproterenol	0.05–0.5 µg/kg/min IV, controlling the infusion to achieve the desired heart rate	Beware insignificant hypertension and tachycardia
Atropine	0.01–0.02 mg/kg IV	Mainly effective when the escape rhythm has narrow QRS complexes
Diazepam	0.10–0.3 mg/kg IV	Monitor respirations
Midazolam	0.035–0.1 mg/kg IV	Monitor respirations

3. *Other causes:* Other causes of bradycardia are: *sinus exit block,* in which sinus P waves intermittently disappear due to block of impulses leaving the region of the node; and frequent *premature atrial contractions,* which occur too early to be conducted to the ventricles and therefore slow the resulting ventricular rate.

TREATMENT

The hemodynamic effect of a slow heart rate depends on how different it is from the patient's usual heart rate. Sudden decreases in rate may be poorly compensated by increases in stroke volume, particularly in those with pre-existing cardiac dysfunction. Moderate bradycardia in normal children will very rarely require treatment. Exceptions include the sudden occurrence of complete atrioventricular block, or pacemaker failure. The urgency of treatment is dictated by the hemodynamic status. Correct underlying causes (e.g., hypoxia) before administering drugs.

1. Medications: Treat bradycardia with atropine first, followed by continuous isoproterenol infusion. This will increase sinus rates and improve atrioventricular conduction, and may increase the rate

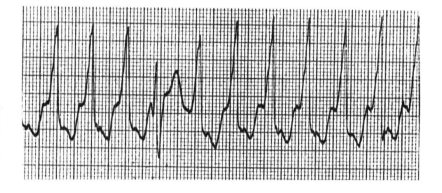

FIGURE 12–11. Ventricular tachycardia. The QRS complexes are wide and bizarre. There is a fusion beat that is intermediate in morphology between the tachycardia beats and sinus beats.

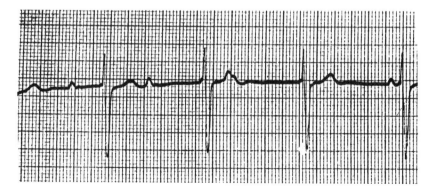

FIGURE 12–12. Third degree (complete) atrioventricular block. Both atrial and ventricular rates are regular but different from one another, with no capture beats.

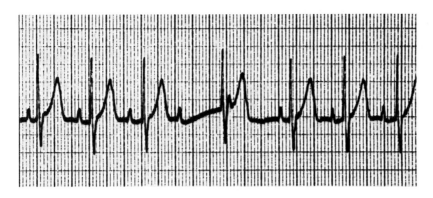

FIGURE 12–13. Wenckebach (Mobitz type 1) second degree atrioventricular block. There is progressive PR interval prolongation followed by a blocked beat. In this patient, there is also a junctional escape beat after the blocked sinus beat.

of subsidiary pacemakers. See Table 12-3 for appropriate doses.

2. Pacing: Following initial stabilization with medications, institute temporary transvenous pacing, particularly in cases with very low ventricular rates (under 30/min) or those with hemodynamic compromise. Transcutaneous pacing may be appropriate for ED resuscitation, pending insertion of transvenous device.

Irregular Rhythms ■

PREMATURE BEATS

Causes

The new onset of frequent premature beats often is the clue to underlying conditions such as digoxin toxicity, other drug ingestions, myocarditis, hypoxia, hypokalemia, hypercarbia, or acidosis.

1. *Supraventricular premature contractions* are recognizable as narrow QRS beats that occur early. They may also have wide QRS complexes due to bundle branch aberration. Those originating in the atrium may be recognized by a premature P wave superimposed on the previous T wave, deforming it.

2. *Ventricular premature complexes* are recognizable as wide, often bizarre early beats, generally without preceding P waves, that produce a compensatory pause before the next QRS complex. The differentiation between ventricular contractions and aberrantly conducted supraventricular contractions is sometimes difficult or impossible from the surface ECG.

Treatment

The physician in the ED will rarely need to treat patients with premature beats of any kind, in the absence of tachycardias. Supraventricular premature contractions virtually never require treatment. Ventricular premature contractions may require treatment if they are:

1. Multiform.
2. Occur in couplets or short runs of ventricular tachycardia.

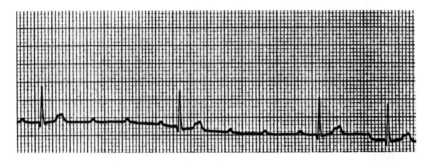

FIGURE 12–14. Mobitz type 2 second degree atrioventricular block. Conduction is 4:1 and an electronic pacemaker is present.

3. Occur in association with a recently converted ventricular tachycardia.
4. Exhibit the "R on T" phenomenon.

Treatment of premature beats is complicated and consultation with a cardiologist may be necessary. Correct inciting factors such as hypoxia and acidosis. If ventricular premature contractions require emergency treatment, the agent of choice is lidocaine, given by a continuous intravenous infusion.

Bibliography ■

Bensen DW: Transesophageal electrocardiography and cardiac pacing: State of the art. *Circulation* 1987; 75(suppl III):III-85.

Flinn CJ, Wolff GS, Dick M, et al: Cardiac rhythm after the Mustard operation for complete transposition of the great arteries. *New Engl J Med* 1984; 310:1635.

Garson A Jr: Medicolegal problems in the management of cardiac arrhythmias in children. *Pediatrics* 1987; 79:84.

Garson A Jr: Atrial flutter in the young: A collaborative study of 380 cases. *J Am Coll Cardiol* 1985; 6:871.

Garson A Jr: Arrhythmias in pediatrics. *Med Clin North Am* 1984; 68:1171.

McNamara DG, Gillette PC: Indications for intracardiac electrophysiologic studies in pediatric patients and the adult with congenital heart disease. *Circulation* 1987; 75(suppl III):III-178.

Mehta AV, Sanchez GR, Sacks EJ, et al: Ectopic automatic atrial tachycardia in children: Clinical characteristics, management and follow-up. *J Am Coll Cardiol* 1988; 11:379.

III
Pulmonary Emergencies

13 Stridor and Airway Obstruction

Ronald A. Dieckmann

Airway obstruction in children causes significant morbidity and mortality, especially in children under 5 years old. Obstruction impedes normal ventilation and oxygenation, and if not recognized and treated in a timely manner, leads to respiratory failure. Respiratory failure leads quickly to respiratory arrest, and ultimately to cardiac arrest. Respiratory dysfunction is the most common etiology for cardiopulmonary arrest in children.

The young child is especially susceptible to severe respiratory dysfunction because of smaller airways and lung volumes, less-developed ventilatory musculature, higher oxygen needs, and easy fatigability. *Stridor*, or noisy breathing, signals partial airway obstruction. Patients presenting with stridor or evidence of airway obstruction require the highest priority for assessment and treatment.

Etiology and Pathophysiology ■

Airway obstruction may occur anywhere in the anatomic pathways of air movement. Etiologies are divided into *upper airway* or *lower airway*. Table 13-1 lists the many causes of airway obstruction in children, based on anatomic distribution. Table 13-2 indicates likely etiologies by age.

The most frequent causes of *upper airway obstruction* are croup, epiglottitis, and foreign bodies. The most frequent causes of *lower airway obstruction* are asthma, bronchiolitis, and foreign bodies. Croup and epiglottitis are discussed in Chapter 115, asthma in Chapter 15, and bronchiolitis in Chapter 116. Evaluation and treatment of foreign bodies in the airway are presented below.

Normal breathing is not audible. *Stridor* is abnormal turbulence of air over obstruction in the airway; the precise quality of the stridor is an important clue to the location of the obstruction. Table 13-3 lists typical sites of obstruction by the quality of stridor. In cases of advanced impedance to air movement, air flow is minimal, so that sounds of breathing or stridorous respirations may be undetectable.

Partial airway obstruction must be considered compromised breathing. Occasionally, congenital conditions such as laryngomalacia or cystic hygroma are stable and well tolerated and rarely produce significant distress. However, if an acute obstruction has occurred, inflammatory or edematous soft tissue swelling may develop rapidly; tiny air passages are occluded in minutes or hours and total obstruction may occur. Hypercarbia and respiratory acidosis, hypoxia, and metabolic acidosis follow.

FOREIGN BODIES IN THE AIRWAY

About 3,000 deaths occur annually in the United States from airway obstruction secondary to aspirated foreign bodies. Children under 5 years old are especially vulnerable; 85% of cases occur in children under 3 years old. Foreign body aspiration at home is the major cause of accidental death in this age group. Often the history is that of a healthy child playing with a small object who suddenly develops sudden coughing, choking, speechlessness, and apnea.

Special hazards in the household include:

Baby aspirin	Coins
Paper clips	Pins and tacks
Plastic wrappers	Peanuts and candy
Eggshells	Pop-tops
Screws and nails	Buttons and beads
Uninflated balloons	Styrofoam
Loose toy parts	Marbles and jacks

Most foreign bodies wind up in the gastrointestinal tract (see Chapter 33); others are placed in the ear, nose, rectum, or vagina. If the object is aspirated into the airway, immediate symptoms are usually present.

TABLE 13–1. *Causes of Stridor and Airway Obstruction*

Upper Airway Obstruction

Nasopharynx
Choanal atresia
Congenital anomalies
Cysts, polyps
Macroglossia (Pierre Robin, hypothyroidism)
Abscess (retropharyngeal, peritonsillar)
Adenotonsillar enlargement
Foreign body
Neoplasm
Poor tongue and pharyngeal control with neuromuscular
   disorder

Larynx and neck
Laryngomalacia
Congenital webs, cysts
Cystic hygroma
Croup
Epiglottitis and tracheitis
Subglottic stenosis
Angioneurotic edema
Laryngeal trauma or laryngospasm
Vocal cord paralysis
Neoplasm
Foreign body

Lower Airway Obstruction
Congenital webs, cysts, vascular anomalies
Subglottic stenosis
Tracheomalacia
Tracheoesophageal fistula
Bronchiolitis
Asthma
Foreign body
Neoplasm

Sometimes, however, there is an asymptomatic interval, then a history of coughing and gagging. Other signs and symptoms depend on where the object is lodged and the degree of obstruction of air flow (see below). In 75% of cases, the inhaled foreign body lodges in the mainstem or lobar bronchus; in 20% of cases, the object is in the upper airway. The laryngeal location is particularly important in children under 1 year.

A special problem is powder aspiration by an infant. In these cases, the asymptomatic period may last hours, then dyspnea, bronchiolitis with pulmonary edema, and atelectasis develop. Mortality is over 20% with significant aspirations. Management involves bronchial washout and general supportive modalities.

Complications from an aspirated foreign body include pneumonia, atelectasis, bronchitis or bronchiectasis, pulmonary abscess, bronchopulmonary fistula, and bronchoconstriction. Delayed presentations occur in about 5% of aspirations; these cases typically present two or more weeks later with pneumonia, hemoptysis, or atelectasis.

Treatment of aspirated foreign bodies requires rigid bronchoscopy under general anesthesia; no other method of removal is safe.

Clinical Findings ■

When stridor is present, determine airway patency. *If air movement is ineffective, postpone all further assessment and immediately open and clear the airway.* The appropriate sequence of techniques for opening the obstructed airway is presented in Table 13-4. If no trauma is present, often a simple jaw thrust will move the mandible and tongue forward and re-establish airway patency.

If foreign body aspiration is suspected in the child who is breathing or coughing spontaneously, the child's natural cough mechanism will usually expel the object. In this situation, do not interfere, since interventions may be dangerous. But if total obstruction is present and the child is neither coughing nor breathing, institute immediate maneuvers to clear the obstruction. For the child under 1 year, employ a series of back blows and chest thrusts. Figures 13-1 and 13-2 (on page 83) illustrate the recommended technique in this age group. The steps are listed in Table 13-5. If the child is over 1 year, apply a series of abdominal thrusts (Heimlich maneuver), as described in Table 13-6.

TABLE 13–2. *Common Causes of Stridor and Airway Obstruction by Age*

Under 1 Year	*1 to 5 Years*	*Over 5 Years*
Congenital anomalies	Foreign body	Adenotonsillar enlargement
Laryngomalacia	Croup	Asthma
Choanal atresia	Epiglottitis	Foreign body
Subglottic stenosis		Neck trauma
Bronchiolitis		

TABLE 13–3. *Quality of Stridor and Site of Obstruction*

Snore
  Nasopharynx

Gurgle
  Tongue
  Tonsils
  Pharynx

High-Pitched Inspiratory Stridor
  Glottis
  Subglottis

Hoarseness
  Larynx

Inspiratory and Expiratory Stridor
  Trachea

Wheeze
  Bronchus
  Bronchioles

If the child is alert, speaking, and breathing independently, keep the patient in a position of comfort—optimally on a parent's lap—and ensure that all diagnostic interventions are gentle, brief, and directed. Vital information can be gleaned from careful observation alone, while obtaining essential history. Rapid assessment of ventilatory adequacy derives from five parameters, as outlined in Table 13-7.

HISTORY

Key elements in the history include:

1. Duration of stridor or respiratory difficulty
2. Quality of stridor (Table 13-3)
3. Exacerbating factors (e.g., crying or feeding worsen laryngomalacia in the infant)
4. Fever
5. Prodromal period of slowly increasing constitutional symptoms (favors viral syndrome)
6. Observed or suspected foreign body aspiration
7. Trauma
8. Drooling (e.g., epiglottitis)
9. Allergic exposures

PHYSICAL EXAMINATION

After rapid assessment of degree of respiratory distress (Table 13-5) and quality of stridor (Table 13-3), further physical evaluation includes special attention to the following features:

1. *Posture.* In upper airway obstruction (e.g., epiglottitis), the child is upright, with neck slightly flexed and head extended; in lower airway obstruction (e.g., foreign bodies), the tripod position is most common.
2. *Depth of breathing.* Obstruction typically decreases depth of breathing and increases rate. In contrast, metabolic acidosis (e.g., diabetic ketoacidosis) will increase depth and rate. Exhaled air on the hand held in front of the child's nose can normally be felt at predictable distances for different ages: under 3 months, 2–3 inches; 4 to 12 months, 4 inches; 12 to 24 months, 5–6 inches.
3. *I/E ratio.* Usually, the ratio of time in inspiration/expiration is 1:1.5. If obstruction is mainly inspiratory (e.g., croup), the ratio may change to 1:1 or 2:1. If obstruction is in the lower airway and primarily expiratory (e.g., asthma), the ratio may become 1:3 or 1:4.
4. *Chest auscultation.* Delay auscultation until last. This part of the physical assessment is least sen-

TABLE 13–4. *Technique for Opening the Airway*

1. Remove obvious foreign bodies (e.g., blood, mucus, vomitus, objects, food) with suction or fingers.
2. Put child in lateral decubitus or prone position to assist drainage; hold infant by feet.
3. If no trauma is present, place child supine, extend neck slightly, and place towel roll under shoulder.
4. For children under 2 years, keep head in *neutral position* without flexion or extension, and place towel roll under occiput.
5. Pull jaw forward by displacing mandible anteriorly with fingers at mandibular angle (jaw thrust).
6. If tongue drops back, pull forward with fingers and wrapped gauze, with hemostat, or with loop of suture through tongue tip.
7. Insert oropharyngeal airway as temporizing measure. Ensure device is sized correctly (distance from edge of mouth to tragus of ear). This will not be tolerated in conscious patient.
8. Use nasopharyngeal airway in older child. In younger child, nasopharyngeal airway may be too traumatic.
9. Begin bag-valve-mask ventilation if breathing inadequate. Use proper mask size; ensure good seal by having second rescuer hold mask on face. Do mouth-to-mouth or mouth-to-nose-and-mouth ventilation, with body substance precautions, if equipment is not available.

TABLE 13–5. *First Aid for Choking Victim Under 1 Year*

1. a. Place the infant face down on the rescuer's forearm in a 60° head-down position with the head and neck stabilized. Rest the forearm firmly against the rescuer's body for additional support.

b. For the choking large infant, an alternate method is to lay the infant face down over the rescuer's lap, with the head firmly supported and held lower than the trunk.

2. Administer four back blows rapidly with the heel of the hand high between shoulder blades.

3. If obstruction is not relieved, turn the infant over to a supine position resting on a firm surface and deliver four rapid chest thrusts (similar to external cardiac compressions) over the sternum using two fingers.

4. If breathing is not resumed, open the victim's mouth by grasping both the tongue and the lower jaw between thumb and finger and lifting (the tongue–jaw lift technique); this draws the tongue away from the back of the throat and may help relieve the obstruction. If the foreign body is visualized, it may be manually extracted by a finger sweep. However, blind sweeps may cause further obstruction and thus should be avoided.

5. If no spontaneous breathing occurs, attempt ventilation with two breaths by mouth-to-mouth or mouth-to-mouth-and-nose technique.

6. Repeat steps 1 to 5 and persist in performing the above techniques as needed while rapidly seeking aid from emergency medical services.

(From Committee on Accident and Poison Prevention, American Academy of Pediatrics: First Aid for the Choking Victim. *Pediatrics* 1988; 81:741)

TABLE 13–6. *First Aid for Choking Victim Over 1 Year*

1. Apply a series of six to ten abdominal thrusts (the Heimlich maneuver) until the foreign body is expelled. The child should be placed on his or her back. The rescuer should kneel at the child's feet if the child is on the floor, or stand at the child's feet if the child is on a table. The astride position is not recommended for small children. The heel of one hand should be placed in the midline between navel and rib cage and the second hand placed on top of the first and pressed into the abdomen with an upward thrust. In small children, the maneuver must be applied gently. It should consist of a rapid inward and upward thrust.

2. If the obstruction is not relieved using the Heimlich maneuver, open the airway using the tongue–jaw lift technique and attempt to visualize the foreign body. No blind finger sweeps should be used.

3. If no spontaneous respirations result, attempt to ventilate the victim. If unsuccessful, repeat a series of six to ten abdominal thrusts.

4. Repeat steps 1 to 3 and persist in performing the above sequence while rapidly seeking aid from emergency medical services.

If the Choking Victim is an Older Child
An older, larger child can be treated as an adult in the standing, sitting, or recumbent (supine) position.

Pediatricians should be familiar with and counsel parents about the dangers and prevention of choking as well as the proper evaluation and first aid measures for treating this emergency.

(From Committee on Accident and Poison Prevention, American Academy of Pediatrics: First Aid for the Choking Victim. *Pediatrics* 1988; 81:741)

sitive. The child may be uncooperative or crying, upper airway sounds may muffle adventitial sounds, or the respiratory rate may be too high to appreciate auscultatory findings at all. Moreover, while rales may be present in patients with associated interstitial or alveolar processes (e.g., bronchiolitis), they are not usually helpful in assessing the degree or level of airway obstruction. The exception is foreign body obstruction of the lower airway, where asymmetry of breath sounds may be useful in localization.

After full assessment of respiratory function, complete a careful physical exam. Associated findings (e.g., septic joint in suspected epiglottitis, penetrating neck injury, or posterior pharyngeal mass in retropharyngeal abscess) will often assist in diagnosis.

Attempts to visualize the airway must be strictly avoided in febrile children with possible epiglottitis, since the swollen epiglottis may clamp down over the larynx during the procedure, precipitating respiratory arrest and making endotracheal intubation difficult or impossible.

Ancillary Data ■

For breathing patients with epiglottitis, airway evaluation and management must take place in the operating room with appropriate personnel and equipment for surgical airway access (see Chapter 115). In all patients with loss of airway patency, if simple maneuvers to relieve obstruction fail (Table 13-4), immediate direct laryngoscopy and endotracheal intubation are imperative.

When airway obstruction is not severe, several radiographic studies are useful. *Posterior-anterior and lateral radiographs of the chest and soft tissues of the neck may reveal the site of obstruction.* Epiglottitis

TABLE 13–7. *Five Parameters for Rapid Assessment of Breathing*

Parameter	Mild	Moderate	Severe
Mental Status	Normal	Agitated	Lethargic
Color	Normal	Pale/mottled	Cyanotic
Air Entry	Normal	Moderately decreased	Markedly decreased
Grunting, Flaring, Retracting	Absent/mild	Moderate	Severe
Respiratory Rate	Normal	Moderately increased	Markedly increased
Newborn	40–45	45–60	60+
6 mos–2 yr	30–40	40–50	50+
2–10 yrs	20–30	30–40	40+
>10 yrs	20	20–30	30+

(Adapted from McGarvey AR: Pediatric respiratory emergencies. *Hosp Phys* 1989; March:24)

and croup have characteristic radiographic findings (see Chapter 115).

When foreign bodies are aspirated into the lower airway, a variety of radiographic abnormalities may be seen: unilateral or bilateral emphysema; mediastinal shift; elevated diaphragm; atelectasis or infiltrates; or the foreign body itself. If the upright chest radiograph is normal (as it is in most cases), obtain expiratory chest radiographs in both right and left lateral decubitus positions; air trapping and hyperinflation of the involved side, with mediastinal shift to the contralateral side, suggest foreign body obstruction. *Fluoroscopy,* which can detect inspiratory mediastinal shifts associated with unilateral bronchial obstruction, further increases the utility of radiography in this condition. Nonetheless, radiography may be completely normal in foreign body aspiration, especially in objects lodged high in the larynx or trachea. Xeroradiography and tomography are rarely helpful and subject the child to high radiation doses.

Flexible fiberoptic bronchoscopy is invaluable in experienced hands. Thorough and speedy evaluation of the upper airway is possible, usually with minimal discomfort to the patient. Minimal sedation and topical airway anesthesia usually obviate general anesthesia. This procedure locates most upper airway foreign bodies and mass lesions, and obtains good visualization of the larynx. Removal of foreign bodies through the flexible bronchoscope, however, is potentially dangerous; general anesthesia and rigid bronchoscopy is often necessary.

Computerized axial tomography (CT) is helpful in selected, stable patients, especially those with mass lesions. *Barium swallow* is indicated in children with suspected tracheoesophageal fistulae, vascular rings, or neuromuscular aspiration syndromes.

Arterial blood gases are useful in evaluation of equivocal cases; alternatively, pulse oximetry will provide sensitive, noninvasive monitoring of oxygen saturation. Other laboratory data is of limited benefit in differentiating causes of airway obstruction, but may offer some value in selected patients.

Treatment ■

ED management of the obstructed airway involves the following approach:

TOTAL OBSTRUCTION

1. Total airway obstruction and apnea requires immediate maneuvers to establish patency (Table 13-4).
2. If simple maneuvers fail, proceed to direct laryngoscopy.
3. If laryngoscopy identifies and alleviates the obstruction (e.g., foreign body removal with Magill forceps), the need for endotracheal intubation is based on the appearance of the airway.
4. If no source of obstruction is identified, or if airway edema or laryngospasm is present, perform endotracheal intubation if possible.
5. If endotracheal intubation is impossible, either because of edema (e.g., airway burns), obstructing masses (hematomas), complicated anatomy, or technical failure, perform needle cricothyrotomy (Chapter 139). A single over-the-needle 14 or 16

gauge catheter, inserted through the cricothyroid membrane, will permit temporary ventilation while arrangements are made for expeditious surgical access to the airway in the operating room.

6. Surgical cricothyrotomy may be possible in older children, but is technically extremely difficult in the younger child. Tracheostomy is contraindicated in the ED.

PARTIAL OBSTRUCTION

Treatment of stridor and partial airway obstruction is premised on protection of the airway. If the child has suspected epiglottitis or impending loss of airway patency, proceed in a speedy controlled manner to protect the airway, as outlined previously.

When immediate airway control is unnecessary in the mild to moderately distressed patient, provide oxygen, establish continuous cardiac monitoring and pulse oximetry, and avoid stressing the child unnecessarily. Place an intravenous cannula for fluid and drug administration, and direct specific therapy at the underlying condition.

Do not leave any child with stridor or respiratory distress unmonitored or unattended during laboratory or radiographic procedures.

Disposition ■

When acute obstruction causes stridor, and definitive airway management is not indicated, admit the child to a monitored inpatient setting. An intensive care unit is imperative if the child is awaiting foreign body removal, has a diagnosis of mild epiglottitis, or has another cause of significant upper airway obstruction. The child with a surgical airway, a nasotracheal intubation, or an endotracheal intubation may require transfer to a pediatric critical care center. Transfer

may be especially warranted if other organ system dysfunction is present or if mechanical ventilation is necessary.

Children with less serious conditions (e.g. moderate croup) can be treated on the pediatric ward or in some cases (e.g., mild croup with no stridor at rest, or laryngomalacia) discharged home with primary physician follow-up.

Prevention plays a major role in reducing the incidence of foreign body aspiration. Educating parents about the dangers of aspiration among preschool-age children given small objects or food items, such as peanuts, seeds, candy, hot dogs, or toys, is key. Additionally, first-aid training of both physicians and parents in treatment of the choking child will avert needless morbidity and mortality from both imprudent overtreatment and ineffectual undertreatment.

Bibliography ■

Abram SH, Fan LL, Cotton EK: Emergency treatment of foreign body obstruction of the upper airway in children. *J Emerg Med* 1984; 2:7–12.

Committee on Accident and Poison Prevention, American Academy of Pediatrics: First aid for the choking victim. *Pediatrics* 1988; 81:740–742.

Gay BB, Atkinson GO, Vanderzalm T: Subglottic foreign bodies in pediatric patients. *Am J Dis Child* 1986; vol 140, pp 165–168.

Hen J: Current management of upper airway obstruction. *Pediatr Ann* 1986; 15:274.

Rothman B, Boeckman CR: Foreign bodies in the larynx and tracheobronchial tree in children. *Ann Otol Rhinol Laryngol* 1980(89):434–436.

Mathew OP: Maintenance of upper airway patency. *J Pediatr* 1985; 106:863.

McGarvey AR: Pediatric respiratory emergencies. *Hospital Physician* 1989; March:24–32.

Mofenson HC, Greensher J: Management of the choking child. *Pediatr Clin North Am* 1985; 32:183–192.

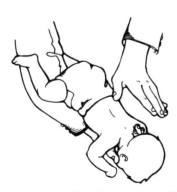

FIGURE 13-1. Technique for administration of back blows in an infant with total airway obstruction

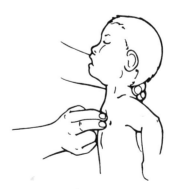

FIGURE 13-2. Technique for administration of chest thrust in an infant with total airway obstruction.

14 Acute Respiratory Failure

Ronald M. Perkin and Nick G. Anas

Respiratory failure is the inability to maintain gas exchange at a rate that matches the body's metabolic demands. The goal in managing the patient with respiratory failure is to ensure adequate gas exchange and oxygen delivery to vital organ systems. Equally important to achieving blood gas homeostasis is providing sufficient blood flow (i.e., cardiac output and distribution) and maximizing the capacity for gas exchange (i.e., hemoglobin content).

Respiratory disorders are common pediatric emergencies. Early recognition of distress and timely treatment is imperative. The unique anatomy of the airways and thoracic cage, as well as special physical and physiologic factors in breathing, make young children more susceptible than older ones to respiratory failure.

Hypercapnic Respiratory Failure (Ventilatory Failure) ■

Ventilatory failure results when alveolar ventilation is inadequate to eliminate the carbon dioxide (CO_2) produced by the body during cellular metabolism. This is reflected in an elevated arterial CO_2 tension ($PaCO_2$).

PATHOPHYSIOLOGY

The carbon dioxide produced by cellular metabolism ($\dot{V}CO_2$) is eliminated almost entirely by the lungs. $PaCO_2$ is directly related to $\dot{V}CO_2$ and inversely related to alveolar ventilation (V_A). V_A is the difference between minute ventilation (V_E) and the physiologic dead space ventilation (V_D) that does not participate in gas exchange. *Minute ventilation (V_E) is the product of tidal volume (V_T) and respiratory rate.* Tidal volume is the amount of gas inspired in a single breath and includes both the anatomic dead space volume and alveolar volume.

ETIOLOGIES

Table 14-1 presents common causes of ventilatory failure.

Increased $\dot{V}CO_2$ rarely causes ventilatory failure by itself because most patients can augment V_E to eliminate the extra CO_2. However, an increased $\dot{V}CO_2$ may precipitate ventilatory failure in patients whose poor neurologic or pulmonary function prevents them from increasing V_E.

An increased $PaCO_2$ results from alveolar hypoventilation in most patients with ventilatory failure.

Increased V_D may occur among patients with obstructive and restrictive diseases, but may be the predominant cause of hypoventilation in patients with pulmonary vascular diseases.

CLINICAL FINDINGS

Respiratory distress is the objective sign of a patient with cardiorespiratory failure; dyspnea is the subjective symptom. Dyspnea describes any state in which the patient becomes conscious of difficulty or effort in breathing or the need for greater respiratory efforts to satisfy air hunger. Dyspnea may be predominantly inspiratory or expiratory.

Signs of hypercapnic respiratory failure are many and varied (Table 14-2). Drowsiness is frequent, unlike the agitation of hypoxemia. If the adequacy of ventilation cannot be clinically evaluated with confidence, obtain an arterial blood gas measurement.

In addition to increased $PaCO_2$, hypercapnic respiratory failure depresses the arterial oxygen tension (PaO_2). The relationship between $PaCO_2$ and PaO_2 is given by the simplified calculation at sea level: $150 - (pO_2 + pCO_2) = (A\text{-}a)O_2$ gradient. An elevated $(A\text{-}a)O_2$ gradient, over 10–20 mm Hg, an important, simply derived marker of ventilation/perfusion abnormalities.

Acute changes in $PaCO_2$ cause a reciprocal change in arterial pH. Sudden respiratory acidosis depresses organ function and may trigger lethal cardiac dysrhythmias. Increases in $PaCO_2$ will also increase cerebral blood flow, which may result in intracranial hypertension in brain-injured patients.

TABLE 14–1. *Etiologies of Ventilatory Failure*

I. Increased carbon dioxide production
  A. Fever, shivering
  B. Exercise (seizures, pain, agitation)
  C. Trauma
  D. Sepsis
  E. Hyperthyroidism
  F. Burns
  G. Excessive glucose administration
II. Decreased alveolar ventilation—normal lungs
  A. Depressed ventilatory drive
    1. Sedation (narcotics, tranquilizers)
    2. Brain injury or illness
    3. Abnormal control of breathing
    4. Alkalosis
    5. Seizures
  B. Neuromuscular disease or weakness
    1. Spinal cord
      a. Tetanus
      b. Trauma
    2. Anterior horn cell
      a. Poliomyelitis
      b. Werdnig Hoffman disease
    3. Peripheral nerve
      a. Acute inflammatory polyneuropathy
      b. Diphtheria
    4. Neuromuscular junction
      a. Myasthenia gravis
      b. Botulism
      c. Organophosphate poisoning
      d. Tick paralysis
      e. Snake bite
      f. Pharmacologic
    5. Muscle
      a. Polymyositis
      b. Hypokalemia, hypophosphatemia
      c. Fatigue
      d. Muscular dystrophies
  C. Upper airway obstruction
    1. Secretions
    2. Head position
    3. Pharyngeal hypotonia
    4. Subglottic edema or mass
    5. Infections—croup and epiglottitis
    6. Tracheomalacia
    7. Foreign body
    8. Laryngospasm
    9. Large tonsils or adenoids
  D. Thorax, pleural, abdomen
    1. Trauma and flail chest
    2. Pneumothorax
    3. Pleural effusion
    4. Chest or abdominal surgery
    5. Abdominal distention
    6. Burn eschar
III. Decreased alveolar ventilation—abnormal lungs
  A. Obstructive diseases
    1. Asthma
    2. Bronchitis
    3. Bronchopulmonary dysplasia
    4. Bronchiolitis
    5. Cystic fibrosis
  B. Alveolar diseases
    1. Pneumonia
    2. Adult respiratory distress syndrome
    3. Congestive heart failure
    4. Pulmonary contusion
IV. Increased dead space ventilation
  A. Reduced pulmonary blood flow
    1. Pulmonary hypertension
    2. Shock
    3. Pulmonary emboli
  B. Alveolar overdistention
    1. Asthma
    2. Bronchiolitis
    3. Foreign body
    4. Positive end expiratory pressure (excessive)

Hypoxemic Respiratory Failure ■

Hypoxemic respiratory failure exists when the PaO_2 is 50 mm Hg or less in the absence of intracardiac right-to-left shunting. In this circumstance, cellular metabolism is jeopardized and abnormal cell function results. Abnormalities in central nervous system and cardiac function are the most frequently observed manifestations of arterial oxygenation failure, because these two organ systems are particularly sensitive to hypoxemia.

PATHOPHYSIOLOGY

The physiologic derangements responsible for a low PaO_2 are:

1. Low inspired oxygen concentration
2. Hypoventilation
3. Ventilation/perfusion mismatching
4. Shunt
5. Diffusion impairment.

ETIOLOGIES

Hypoxemia may occur as a result of changes in the composition of alveolar gas, such as a reduced in-

TABLE 14–2. *Symptoms, Signs, and Warnings of Respiratory Failure*

Hypercapnia	*Hypoxemia*
Headache	Cyanosis
Drowsiness, coma	Confusion, agitation, restlessness
Sweating	Shortness of breath
Tachycardia, hypertension	Sweating
Peripheral vasodilation	Tachycardia, hypertension, dysrhythmias
Apnea	Bradycardia, hypotension (particularly in association with
Excessive work of breathing, shortness of breath	evidence of pulmonary hypertension and/or shock)
Stridor, wheezing	Peripheral vasoconstriction
Paradoxical chest wall–abdominal motion	Rales by auscultation
Reduced air entry by auscultation	Murmur by auscultation
Asymmetric air entry by auscultation	

spired oxygen concentration (e.g., high altitude) or an increased carbon dioxide tension (discussed earlier).

In addition to the composition of alveolar gas, the adequacy of gas exchange is determined by the balance of ventilation and pulmonary perfusion. The relationship of ventilation to perfusion in any given segment of pulmonary tissue is expressed as the $\dot{V}/\dot{Q}$ ratio. The condition of normal distribution of ventilation and perfusion is designated as a $\dot{V}/\dot{Q}$ ratio of 1.0; values above 1.0 represent either an abnormal increase in ventilation or a decrease in perfusion, and values below 1.0 suggest either decreased ventilation or increased perfusion.

Low $\dot{V}/\dot{Q}$ units (less than 1.0) are usually produced when a unit of lung is underventilated because of increased airway resistance (bronchitis, asthma, bronchiolitis, small airway disease) or decreased lung compliance (atelectasis, pulmonary edema, pneumonia). When $\dot{V}/\dot{Q}$ is zero, a shunt is present. Common causes of intrapulmonary shunting include alveolar filling processes (pneumonia, aspiration, pulmonary edema) or closure of airways (atelectasis, foreign body, endobronchial mass). Extrapulmonary shunts occur only in patients with structural defects in the heart or anomalies of the central blood vessels.

High $\dot{V}/\dot{Q}$ units (greater than 1.0) are produced when a unit of lung is underperfused because of vascular occlusion (pulmonary emboli), loss of capillary bed, or obliteration of vascular bed (pulmonary vascular disease).

The final determinant of gas exchange is the ability of oxygen and carbon dioxide to diffuse across the alveolar-capillary membrane. Interstitial edema or fibrosis and a reduction in the cross-sectional area of the pulmonary capillary bed may cause diffusion abnormalities sufficient to result in hypoxemia.

CLINICAL FINDINGS

Signs of hypoxemic respiratory failure are many and varied (Table 14-2). Remember that hypoxemia may be heralded by an altered mental status and restlessness without a sensation of distress.

Ancillary Data ■

The cause of respiratory failure is determined by history, physical examination, interpretation of arterial blood gases and pH and chest roentgenogram.

The signs and symptoms of respiratory failure (Table 14-2) are nonspecific but useful for assessing the severity of the disease, predicting its course, and dictating the urgency of evaluation and therapy. The diagnosis of respiratory failure is assisted by the measurement of arterial blood gases. Acute respiratory failure is present when the pCO_2 is greater than 55 mm Hg (assuming there is no pre-existing lung disease) or the PaO_2 is less than 50 mm Hg (assuming there is no cyanotic congenital heart disease).

Immediate therapy is often dictated by pH, since this value reflects how well $PaCO_2$ and bicarbonate concentration are matched. An elevated $PaCO_2$ associated with a normal pH may not lead to endotracheal intubation and ventilatory support; on the other hand, the same $PaCO_2$, associated with a low pH, might require such interventions. Similarly, hypoxemia with a normal pH does not require the same urgent therapy as hypoxemia with a low pH.

Once the PaO_2 is measured, calculate the $(A-a)O_2$ gradient. Recall that hypoxemia with a normal $(A-a)O_2$ gradient is due to hypoventilation, while that with an increased gradient is usually due to ventilation/perfusion mismatch.

A chest roentgenogram is immediately required to evaluate need for immediate intervention (i.e., pneumothorax, pleural effusion, or malposition of an endotracheal tube in a previously intubated patient). Further diagnostic tests and therapy are guided by findings on the chest roentgenogram. If available, obtain previous films for comparison.

Ensure continuous monitoring of the patient both by physical examination and bedside technology. Physical monitors are level of consciousness, respiratory rate and effort, color, heart rate and rhythm, and perfusion.

Available monitors include continuous pulse oximetry, transcutaneous PaO_2 and $PaCO_2$ electrodes, end-tidal CO_2 samples, and chest wall impedance leads to monitor respiratory rate and assess qualitatively the depth of respiration. Serial assessment of arterial blood gases, pH, and hemoglobin concentration may be indicated.

Treatment ■

The methods for increasing alveolar ventilation, administering oxygen, improving lung volume, and increasing pulmonary blood flow as well as the management of specific disorders are outlined in other chapters. Table 14-3 summarizes treatments for either hypercapnia and/or hypoxemia.

Begin therapy by ensuring airway patency and applying 100% oxygen. Remove or bypass anatomic obstructions to air flow (soft-tissue swelling, secretions, blood, foreign bodies, and aspirated material) whenever they cause ventilatory failure. Intubate the trachea if suctioning, opening the airway, removing foreign bodies, and other noninvasive measures fail to improve ventilation. General indications for endotracheal intubation are:

1. Prevention or reversal of upper airway obstruction in asphyxiating or comatose patients
2. Protection of the airway and lungs against the aspiration of gastric and oropharyngeal contents in patients who lack a gag reflex
3. Facilitation of tracheopulmonary toilet
4. Mechanical ventilation
5. Positive end-expiratory pressure (PEEP).

Administering supplemental oxygen will increase PaO_2 whenever the cause of the hypoxemia is hypoventilation, ventilation/perfusion mismatch, or a diffusion impairment. However, when a shunt, either anatomic or severe physiologic, is the cause of hypoxemia, supplemental oxygen will not be effective.

TABLE 14–3. *Therapeutic Measures to Improve Respiratory Function*

I. Improve ventilatory function
  A. Decrease carbon dioxide production
    1. Reduce fever
    2. Control infection
    3. Seizure control
    4. Careful sedation
    5. Relieve pain
    6. Muscle relaxation if indicated
  B. Increase alveolar ventilation
    1. Airway control
      a. Correct head position
      b. Pulmonary toilet, secretion removal
      c. Racemic epinephrine
      d. Oral or nasal airway placement
      e. Endotracheal tube placement
    2. Remove foreign body
    3. Relieve bronchospasm
      a. Beta-adrenergic agonists
      b. Theophylline
      c. Anticholinergic agents
      d. Corticosteroids
    4. Improve ventilation regulation
      a. Naloxone
      b. Respiratory stimulants
    5. Improve lung compliance and volume
      a. Diuretics
      b. Positive airway pressure
    6. Mechanical ventilation
  C. Decrease physiologic dead space
    1. Improve pulmonary blood flow
    2. Optimize lung volume; reduce hyperinflation
    3. Increase cardiac output
II. Improve arterial oxygenation
  A. Provide supplemental oxygen
    1. Face mask
    2. Nasal cannula
    3. Endotracheal tube
  B. Improve ventilation (see IB)
  C. Decrease intrapulmonary shunt
    1. Patient position
    2. Positive airway pressure
    3. Diuretics
  D. Optimize cardiac output

Disposition ■

Any child with respiratory distress by clinical exam or blood gas determination requires hospital admission. An $(A-a)O_2$ gradient, or $AaDO_2$ greater than 30 mm Hg, even in the absence of significant distress, indicates admission. Recognition of early respiratory insufficiency combined with aggressive treatment will avert unnecessary morbidity and mortality. *Delays in identification and treatment of respiratory distress are the most important preventable features in cardiac arrest in young children,* since most pediatric cardiac arrests are secondary to untreated respiratory arrest.

Often, admission to a pediatric intensive care unit (ICU) or transfer to a properly equipped and staffed pediatric critical care center is necessary. This includes all children with unstable airways, intubated children, or patients with progressive respiratory disease not responding to treatment in the emergency department or clinic. Observation of children with respiratory distress in the emergency department or clinic is often dangerous, due to deficiencies in monitoring capability. Early admission to a more controlled ward or ICU setting is appropriate.

Bibliography ■

Alonzo GG, Dantzker DR: Respiratory failure, mechanisms of abnormal gas exchange, and oxygen delivery. *Med Clin North Am* 1983; 67:557–571.

Dantzker DR: The influence of cardiovascular function on gas exchange. *Clin Chest Med* 1983; 42:149–.

Newith CJL: Recognition and management of respiratory failure. *Pediatr Clin North Am* 1979; 26:617–643.

Redding GJ, Morray JP, Rea C: Respiratory failure in childhood. In: Morray J, ed.: *Pediatric intensive care.* Norwalk, Conn: Appleton & Lange, 1987, pp. 107–.

15 Asthma

M.J. Goldenhersh and Gary S. Rachelefsky

About 10% of all children in the United States suffer from asthma. Asthma accounts for significant illness-related school absenteeism and causes major morbidity, as well as mortality, in childhood. Chronic undertreatment or delay in aggressive care in the distressed child accounts for substantial preventable death and disability. Of all pediatric acute asthma-related Emergency Department (ED) visits, 15–20% require hospitalization.

Asthma is reactive airway disease. *Wheezing is not asthma.* A variety of conditions causing lower airway obstruction (e.g., foreign bodies, bronchiolitis) may present with wheezing (see Chapter 13). Moreover, the severe asthmatic may have an expiratory flow rate too low to produce wheezing.

Etiology and Pathophysiology ■

The asthmatic child has reactive airways. While the precise underlying defect in asthma is unknown, both autonomic dysfunction and sensitizing external irritants are key components in the pathophysiology. Infection, allergic exposures, noxious inhaled substances, or psychological stress may trigger bronchoconstriction. Once airway narrowing begins, if treatment is not instituted in a timely manner, a downward cycle of increasing lower airway obstruction occurs, with release of powerful chemical mediators, increased mucus production, and rapid inflammatory response. The resulting ventilation/perfusion imbalance causes progressive hypoxia, then hypercarbia. Therapy is aimed at interrupting airway constriction and reversing hypoxia and hypercarbia, as well as treating the precipitating condition.

Clinical Findings ■

HISTORY

Physical examination alone is often an unreliable gauge of illness severity. Therefore, past medical history as well as the present history are key to evaluation. Table 15-1 lists important historical features to guide assessment and treatment. Table 15-2 presents major risk factors that signal life-threatening presentations. When major risk factors are present, a heightened sense of urgency is imperative.

PHYSICAL EXAMINATION

Simple inspection of the pediatric patient is extremely informative: note the child's level of alertness, anxiety, and restlessness, as well as rate and depth of respirations, retractions (intercostal, substernal, suprasternal, and sternocleidomastoid muscles), nasal flaring, and ability to speak. Skin color is also helpful. As respiratory insufficiency becomes more marked, the child becomes mottled, then cyanotic. The stoic adolescent, fully dressed, may show subtler signs of respiratory difficulty (pallor, glassy eyes, diaphoresis, nasal flaring, and/or tracheal tug). To evaluate asthmatic children fully, undress and expose them completely for physical assessment.

Tachycardia, which is almost always present, correlates with the level of bronchoconstriction and hypoxia; a heart rate over 150 beats per minute suggests either severe hypoxia or sympathomimetic abuse. Expiratory prolongation, diminished breath sounds, and wheezing are hallmarks of acute asthma. Wheezing is turbulent airflow and progresses from expiratory to expiratory *and* inspiratory with increasing severity of obstruction. Wheezing may be audible, limited to auscultatory findings, or absent. A completely silent chest is an ominous finding and may indicate a grave degree of obstruction. Pulsus paradoxus (a drop in systolic blood pressure ≥ 10 mm Hg with inspiration) indicates severe bronchoconstriction.

Ancillary Data ■

There is little correlation between physician assessment of pulmonary function and objective measures. Expiratory flow rates, if available, are far more sen-

TABLE 15–1. *Pertinent History*

Present Attack
Daily asthma medications prior to attack
Identifiable precipitating factor(s)
Time course of symptom onset and duration
Medications tried (doses, timing, side effects, patient
   response)

Past Exacerbations
Identifiable precipitating factor(s)
Frequency of attacks
Duration of attacks
Previous steroids
Response to past therapy
Hospitalizations
Previous endotracheal intubation

sitive. Peak expiratory flow rate (PEFR) is *extremely* helpful in assessing initial asthma severity and gauging subsequent response to medical therapy. PEFR can usually be elicited in any child 5 years or older. Reference values are readily available and are graphed according to patient height, sex, and race. Many asthmatics who have been educated about peak flow monitoring will have a record of past peak flow rates (including optimal flow during "well" periods), which assists interpretation of ED readings. Spirometry, if available, allows a more detailed evaluation of pulmonary function, but requires more sophisticated equipment and more patient cooperation. In the very young, frightened child suffering from a severe asthmatic event, flow measurements are typically unreliable.

Blood gas measurements, the "gold standard" of acute asthma evaluation, are indicated in any patient who fails to respond to initial therapy. Pulse oximetry provides a noninvasive transcutaneous measurement of pO_2 and an accurate ongoing monitor of oxygen

saturation. Hypoxemia is present in all patients with acute asthma; the degree of hypoxemia correlates well with the degree of acute airway obstruction. Hypercarbia follows hypoxemia. Initially, pCO_2 will be low because of respiratory compensation for hypoxemia; with increasing fatigue and worsening bronchoconstriction, pCO_2 rises. *A $pCO_2 > 40$ mm Hg suggests severe disease, unless the child has chronic CO_2 retention.* In advanced cases, metabolic acidosis may accompany hypoxemia and respiratory acidosis.

Chest radiographs rarely add to the diagnosis or treatment of acute asthma. *Unless symptom history or auscultatory findings suggesting infection, collapse or pneumothorax are present, do not obtain routine chest radiographs.*

Other helpful tests include electrolytes (for vomiting, dehydration, or chronic theophylline overdose with hypokalemia), complete blood count (anemia may aggravate hypoxia), sinus radiographs (a Water's view in younger children rules out suspected sinusitis), and/or sputum gram stain and culture/sensitivity (if complicating bacterial pneumonia or allergic bronchopulmonary aspergillosis is suspected). A theophylline level in patients on maintenance therapy may be helpful. While the "therapeutic range" is usually 10–20 μg/ml, dosing must be individualized to each child's optimal range. Table 15-3 reviews ancillary tests in the evaluation of asthma.

Treatment ■

Severe asthma requires aggressive management to avert ventilatory failure. Figure 15-1 (on page 94) outlines the overall approach in the ED. The following are mainstays of care:

AIRWAY SUPPORT

If airway obstruction is so severe that breathing is totally ineffective or absent, proceed to immediate

TABLE 15–2. *Risk Factors for Life-Threatening Asthma*

Early onset of severe asthma, particularly less than 1 year of age.
Frequent need for hospitalization to control asthma.
History of endotracheal intubation.
Dependence on corticosteroids, either oral or inhaled.
Noncompliance or abuse of medication.
Labile asthma with pronounced "morning dipping".
"Brittle" asthma with unexpected rapid deterioration of pulmonary function.
Teenager with longstanding asthma of early onset.
Depressive symptoms with chronic asthma.

TABLE 15–3. *Ancillary Data*

Pulmonary Function Tests
  Peak Expiratory Flow Rate
  Spirometry
Arterial Blood Gas
Electrolytes
Theophylline Level
Complete Blood Count
Chest Radiographs
Sinus Radiograph
Sputum Gram Stain, Culture, Sensitivity

intubation and positive-pressure ventilation. This is rarely necessary. Almost every child deserves an initial trial of management with oxygen and adrenergic agents, and possibly isoproterenol, before proceeding to intubation.

OXYGEN

Provide continuous moisturized low-flow oxygen by an age-appropriate delivery system (nasal cannula or mask for an older child, hood for infants). Asthmatics are not at risk for hypercarbia induced by oxygen therapy. The very young child (<18 months) may have an initial transient worsening and decreased pO_2 for up to 10 minutes following beta-agonist therapy. Therefore, it is imperative to combine supplemental oxygen with inhalation treatment in small children.

BETA-2 AGONIST AEROSOL THERAPY

Sympathomimetics are the most potent of all bronchodilators and are the first-line medication for acute asthma. Inhaled beta-2 agonist bronchodilators, when compared with injectable epinephrine, have fewer side effects and at least equal efficacy. The inhalation mode of administration offers major advantages: medication is delivered directly to the site of action, with minimal systemic absorption; pharmacokinetics are not impeded by severe obstruction; and acceptability is high in the distressed child. Moreover, painful injections are avoided. These agents are best administered by oxygen-powered nebulizers. Avoid pressurized nebulization (IPPB) because of the theoretical risk of increasing airway obstruction and extrapleural air. Older children can hold the mouthpiece to inspire the aerosol, while younger children can be treated with face masks. If a young toddler cannot tolerate a face mask, put the child on the parent's lap and deliver the aerosol through a paper cup held by the parent. Inhaled adrenergics are also more efficacious than intravenous aminophylline or parenteral beta agonists.

Table 15-4 lists the types and doses of beta agonists available for nebulization. Albuterol (0.5%) and terbutaline are preferable because of increased beta-2 selectivity and increased duration. Frequent small doses (0.05 mg/kg/dose q 20 minutes) of nebulized albuterol (maximum 2.5 mg) are safe and produce an early peak response and a smooth rise in PEFR. *Continuous* nebulized terbutaline is also effective in the severely distressed child. The beta-2 aerosols have a high therapeutic ratio with rare untoward effects. Nonetheless, monitor the pulse in all children receiving these agents and discontinue treatment if heart rate exceeds 180/min.

Anticholinergics (atropine sulfate, atropine methonitrate, ipatroprium bromide) are also potent bronchodilators, although their onset of action is somewhat slower than that of the sympathomimetic agents. Anticholinergics may be more effective initially in children under 1 year of age and may provide additional efficacy in older children when used after maximal bronchodilatation with inhaled beta adrenergics. Use inhaled anticholinergic therapy either as a later

TABLE 15-4. *Recommended Doses for Inhaled Medications*

Medication Generic (Trade Name)	Preparation Available for Aerosolized Use	Dose (mg/kg) (maximum)*	Dose (ml/kg) (maximum)*
Albuterol (Proventil, Ventolin)	0.5% solution†	0.05–0.15 mg/kg	0.01–0.03 ml/kg
	0.083% solution‡ (2.5 mg)	(2.5 mg)	(0.3 ml)
Terbutaline (Brethine)	0.1% solution	0.1–0.2 mg/kg	0.1–0.2 ml/kg
		(1–2 mg)	(1–2 ml)
Metaproterenol (Alupent)	5% solution†	0.5 mg/kg	0.01 ml/kg
	0.4% solution (10 mg)‡	(15 mg)	(0.3 ml)
	0.6% solution (15 mg)‡		
Atropine (generic)	0.1% solution	0.5 mg/kg	0.5 ml/kg
		(2 mg)	(2 ml)

* The maximum is given in *total* ml per dose or *total* mg per dose. Guidelines for maximum recommended dose not established for children under 2 years of age.
† Multiple dose solution.
‡ Unit dose solution.

adjunct to successful beta-adrenergic therapy, or as an alternative to unsuccessful inhaled beta-adrenergic treatment.

ISOPROTERENOL

Consider adding isoproterenol, a powerful beta-adrenergic agonist, in children with impending respiratory failure ($PaCO_2$ > 50 mm Hg) and significant acidemia (pH < 7.20). Isoproterenol may provide sufficient bronchodilatation to avert mechanical ventilation in severely distressed patients. Isoproterenol therapy requires continuous electrocardiographic and hemodynamic monitoring and is administered most appropriately in an intensive care unit. Begin at 0.1 μg/kg/minute, then increase the dose in stepwise fashion by 0.1 μg/kg/minute every 10 to 15 minutes until clinical response and arterial blood gas measurements establish therapeutic success, or until the heart rate approaches 200/min or an arrhythmia develops. Clinical response usually occurs at a dose of 0.3 to 0.4 μg/kg/minute. Doses greater than 1.0 μg/kg/minute may not be safe.

During the intravenous infusion of isoproterenol, continue intravenous aminophylline and corticosteroid therapy. Monitor serum theophylline levels closely. Discontinue all adrenergic aerosols during isoproterenol infusion. Untoward effects of isoproterenol therapy (cardiac arrhythmias, myocardial ischemia, and necrosis) may be potentiated by concomitant use of aerosol beta adrenergics. Progressive ventilatory failure despite isoproterenol therapy necessitates intubation and mechanical ventilation.

INTRAVENOUS FLUIDS

Administer IV fluids to maintain adequate volume status and/or to correct dehydration. Avoid overhydration. The syndrome of inappropriate antidiuretic hormone (SIADH), although uncommon, may occur

TABLE 15–6. *Factors Affecting Theophylline Clearance*

Increased Clearance (decreases theophylline blood level)	Decreased Clearance (increases theophylline blood level)
Low CHO, high-protein diet	High CHO diet
Phenobarbital	Cimetidine
Phenytoin	Erythromycin
Rifampin	Febrile upper respiratory infections
Hyperthyroidism	Liver dysfunction
	Pneumonia
	Obesity

in acute severe asthma. Careful monitoring of serum electrolytes and urine specific gravity is indicated. In the well-hydrated patient, 1,500 ml/M^2/day of IV fluid is adequate replacement for the asthmatic child whose compromised respiratory status restricts oral intake.

AMINOPHYLLINE

Theophylline offers little, if any, additional bronchodilatory benefit to patients in the first four hours of an acute attack when they have received maximally effective doses of inhaled beta-adrenergic agents. *Therefore, this drug has little value in the ED management of asthma.* However, IV aminophylline may be useful for those patients who do not respond well to inhaled beta agonists in the ED and are being admitted to the hospital. Adjust the loading dose to the previous 24-hour oral theophylline dosage and results of a stat theophylline level. If there has been no recent administration of a theophylline preparation, give a bolus of 2 to 6 mg/kg over 20 minutes. Table 15-5 provides the exact dose by age. Infants 2 to 6 months usually require 2–3 mg/kg and infants 6 months to 1 year 4–5 mg/kg for loading. *Ideally, each 1 mg/kg bolus should raise the serum theophylline level by approximately 2 μg/ml in children under 12 months of age.*

Start an aminophylline drip after the initial bolus. Titrate the dose to patient age, weight, clinical status, recent maintenance dose, and other interacting variables. Certain medications, illnesses, and dietary manipulations will influence theophylline metabolism (see Table 15-6). Check theophylline levels 30 minutes after completion of initial and subsequent boluses, six to eight hours after maintenance drip, and every 24 hours while the infusion is continued.

TABLE 15–5. *Recommended Infusion Rates for Aminophylline*

Patient Age	mg/kg/hr*†
<6 weeks	0.16
2–6 months	0.5
6–11 months	0.9
1–9 years	1.0
10–16 years	0.7 to 0.8

* Actual dose must be based on individual's metabolism of aminophylline and may vary within specified age groups.
† Aminophylline dose = theophylline dose/0.80.

TABLE 15-7. *Physical Examination and Laboratory Findings Indicating Need for Hospitalization*

Obvious respiratory exhaustion
Clinical dehydration (especially children < 24 months)
Altered consciousness
Severe airflow limitation (silent chest)
Hypercarbia ($PaCO_2 \geq 40$ mm Hg)
Hypoxia ($PaO_2 \leq 50$ mm Hg)
Significant atelectasis
Extrapleural air (pneumothorax, pneumomediastinum, subcutaneous air)
Presenting FEV1 or PEFR less than 30% of predicted with less than 35% improvement after 1 hour of aggressive therapy
Cyanosis
Other
    Inability to take oral fluids and/or medication
    Social situation

CORTICOSTEROIDS

Use corticosteroids when initial response to inhaled bronchodilator therapy is inadequate, in patients who have received steroids within the past 6 months, in patients who have required previous hospitalization for asthma, and in all patients admitted for acute severe asthma. Corticosteroids improve oxygenation, decrease airway obstruction, and increase response to beta agonists. Early use of steroids also appears to shorten recovery time and to decrease the need for hospitalization. Infection is not a contraindication for steroids.

Administer either methylprednisolone (Solu-Medrol), 1 to 2 mg/kg IV bolus, followed by 0.5 to 0.8 mg/kg every 6 hours if hospitalized or by 1 to 2 mg/kg/day as an oral medication; or alternatively hydrocortisone (Solu-Cortef) 7 mg/kg IV, then 2 mg/kg every 6 hours. Hydrocortisone has a greater mineralocorticoid effect but is less expensive. A five-day course does not require a tapering dose, but some patients will have bronchial rebound, which may require a longer treatment course and a judicious taper. Precipitating factors such as potent viral triggers (RSV in particular) may also necessitate a longer steroid course. There appears to be no increased advantage of parenteral over oral corticosteroid therapy.

CAVEATS

Treatment modalities to avoid include:

1. Chest percussion and postural drainage for uncomplicated asthmatic exacerbation
2. Antibiotics (unless a bacterial infection is documented)

3. Repeated epinephrine or Sus-Phrine injections
4. Any sedating medications that may alter the patient's mental status or ventilatory effort (unless the patient is receiving assisted ventilation in an ICU setting).

Disposition ■

HOSPITALIZATION

Signs of imminent respiratory failure such as respiratory exhaustion, markedly decreased pulmonary function assessed by peak flow, alteration of consciousness, pulsus paradoxus, hypotension, severe hypoxia, and hypercarbia with $pCO_2 > 40$ mm Hg signal the need for immediate hospital admission. Other indications for admission include severe acute asthma unresponsive to four aerosol treatments in the ED; two visits to the ED in a 24-hour period; persistent vomiting of medications; moderate wheezing and underlying cardiopulmonary disease (e.g., bronchopulmonary dysplasia, neuromuscular disease, congenital heart disease); and moderate wheezing with inadequate reliability of home treatment compliance. Table 15-7 outlines the major physical examination and laboratory findings indicating inpatient management.

Patients with respiratory acidosis and those poorly responsive to aggressive ED treatment are best admitted to an ICU capable of handling children or transferred expeditiously to a pediatric critical care center.

DISCHARGE

Successfully treated patients can be discharged with careful instructions for home care and a telephone number for immediate physician contact. The biggest mistakes made in discharging children from the ED are lack of understanding on the patient's part of prescribed discharge medications, the lack of scheduled follow-up, and no contact number for medical advice. On discharge, ensure that the patient with acute severe asthma has regular beta-agonist therapy (inhaled and/or oral), corticosteroid therapy, and theophylline (in selected patients). If inhaled therapy is prescribed, verify that the family has proper ancillary devices for medication delivery (spacer device, nebulizer, etc.) and that the family understands their correct use. Instruct the patient and parents in asthma warning signs and arrange follow-up within 24 hours.

Prevention

Any ED visit reflects a failure of medical management. Patient, family, and physician education must be the mainstay of preventive care. Proper understanding of asthmatic triggers, educated objective pulmonary home monitoring (peak flow metering), and stepwise home treatment plans customized by the primary physician are imperative. Early disease recognition, appropriate prophylactic care, and prompt aggressive management will decrease asthma-related morbidity and mortality.

Bibliography ■

Calant SP: Therapeutic approach to acute asthma in children. In: Tinkelman DG, Falliers CJ, Naspitz CK, eds.: *Childhood asthma pathophysiology and treatment.* New York: Marcel Dekker, 1987.

Godfrey S: Childhood asthma. In: Clark TJH, Godfrey S, eds.: *Asthma.* London: Chapman and Hall, 1983.

Haas A, Stiehm ER, Rachelefsky GS, et al: Status asthmaticus—A house manual. Pediatric Asthma, Allergy & Immunol 1987; 1:231–239.

Kurland G, Leong AB: The management of status asthmaticus in childhood. In: Gershwin ME, ed.: *Bronchial asthma: Principles of diagnosis and treatment.* Orlando: Grune & Stratton, 1986.

Mansmann HC Jr, Bierman CW, Pearlman DS: Treatment of acute asthma in children. In: Bierman CW, Pearlman DS, eds.: *Allergic diseases from infancy to adulthood.* Philadelphia: WB Saunders, 1988.

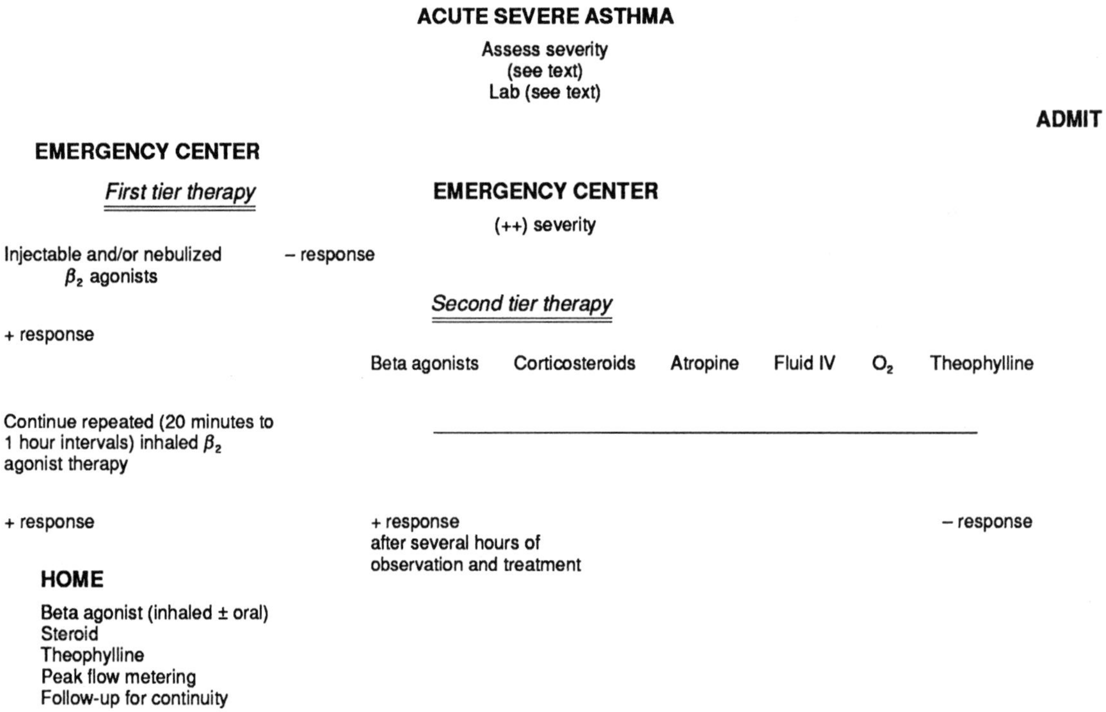

FIGURE 15-1. Emergency department approach to severe asthma.

IV
Emergent Complaints

16 Altered Mental Status

Joseph E. Simon

Altered mental status (AMS) refers to any deviation from a child's normal age-appropriate cognitive responsiveness to environmental stimuli. This chapter focuses on disorders with significant changes in responsiveness, beyond mild lethargy or irritability.

Because *changes in mental status* while under observation have enormous diagnostic, therapeutic, and prognostic implications, the evaluation must first quantify the extent of a patient's AMS. In older patients this can be accomplished using the Glasgow Coma Scale; a modified scale may be more appropriate for younger patients (Table 16-1). Applying these scales requires the repeated use of standard verbal and painful stimuli. For a pediatric patient, shouting the child's name and pinching the child's toe would be examples of appropriate stimuli. The important point is to use the *same* stimuli when the child's mental status evaluation is repeated.

Etiology and Pathophysiology ■

Many pathophysiological pathways lead to the final common pathway of an AMS. Table 16-2 presents an acronym (AEIOU-TIPS-O) for use in organizing the differential diagnosis of the child who presents with an AMS.

Suspect *A*lcohol as a primary or contributing factor in an adolescent presenting with an AMS (see Chapter 67).

*E*ncephalitis includes several infection-related central nervous system problems in addition to encephalitis: meningitis, para-infectious encephalopathies (Reye's syndrome, shigella, post-infectious varicella encephalitis, etc.), and brain abscess.

*I*nsulin problems, either too much or too little, may cause hypoglycemia, hyperglycemia, and diabetic ketoacidosis (see Chapters 23 and 103).

*O*verdose is a very common cause of AMS in children. Though possible at any age, it is particularly common in toddlers (accidental) and adolescents (nonaccidental) (see Chapter 63).

*U*remia is one of many *metabolic* encephalopathies, secondary to organ failure. Table 16-3 presents other organ system disorders associated with AMS. Other metabolic causes of AMS include status postanoxia, electrolyte disturbances, hypothermia and hyperthermia, and inborn errors of metabolism.

*T*rauma, usually head injury, is another very common cause of AMS in the pediatric patient.

*T*umor, presenting with an acute alteration in mental status, is unusual. When it does occur, acute hemorrhage into the tumor is the most likely explanation.

*I*nfarction and *I*ntracranial hemorrhage not secondary to trauma include several unusual diagnoses:

Acute hemiplegia of childhood
Embolism (usually secondary to congenital heart disease)
Intraoral trauma to the carotid artery
Arteriovenous malformation
Hemorrhage secondary to a bleeding diathesis
Venous thrombosis secondary to severe dehydration
Arterial thrombosis secondary to sickle-cell disease.

The last of these diagnoses is the most common; any black child presenting with an AMS should be promptly screened for sickle-cell disease.

The most common *P*sychiatric cause of AMS is hysterical coma. Acute psychoses may also occur in adolescents but are rare (see Chapter 130).

*S*eizures may be subtle in infants. Typical tonic/clonic movements are often *not* present (see Chapter 26). Even more difficult than the diagnosis of subtle seizure activity is the diagnosis of a postictal state in a child who has experienced an unwitnessed seizure. Because one in 20 children will experience a febrile seizure that may be unwitnessed, many children under age 5 who present to the emergency department with an AMS and fever will, in fact, be postictal. A lumbar puncture and spinal fluid analysis may be necessary to rule out CNS infection in these children (see Chapter 110).

*O*ther for AMS in childhood represents at least four diagnoses: *intussusception, hydrocephalus, vasculi-*

TABLE 16–1. *Modified Glasgow Coma Scale*

	Eyes Opening	
	>1 Year	<1 Year
4	Spontaneously	Spontaneously
3	To verbal command	To shout
2	To pain	To pain
1	No response	No response

	Best Motor Response	
	>1 Year	<1 Year
6	Obeys	Spontaneous
5	Localizes pain	Localizes pain
4	Flexion-withdrawal	Flexion-withdrawal
3	Flexion-abnormal (decorticate rigidity)	Flexion-abnormal (decerebrate rigidity)
2	Extension (decerebrate rigidity)	Extension (decorticate rigidity)
1	No response	No response

	Best Verbal Response		
	>5 Years	2–5 Years	0–23 Months
5	Oriented and converses	Appropriate words and phrases	Smiles, coos appropriately
4	Disoriented and converses	Inappropriate words	Cries, consolable
3	Inappropriate words	Persistent cries and/or screams	Persistent inappropriate crying and/or screaming
2	Incomprehensible sounds	Grunts	Grunts, agitated/restless
1	No response	No response	No response

Total **3–15**

TABLE 16–2. *Differential Diagnosis of AMS*

A—Alcohol
E—Encephalitis/meningitis
I—Insulin
O—Overdose
U—Uremia/metabolic encephalopathy
T—Trauma, tumor
I—Intracranial hemorrhage/infarction
P—Psychiatric
S—Seizure
O—Other

TABLE 16–3. *Organ System Disorders Associated With AMS*

Lung
  Hypoxia
  Hypercapnea

Cardiovascular
  Shock

Kidney
  Uremia
  Hypertensive
    encephalopathy

Liver
  Hepatic encephalopathy

Thyroid
  Hyperthyroidism
  Hypothyroidism

Adrenal
  Addisonian crisis

TABLE 16–4. *Clinical Findings and Laboratory Data in Diagnostic Categories for AMS*

Diagnostic Category	Historical Findings	Physical Findings	Laboratory Evaluation	Caveats
A Alcohol	Toddler or teen, no prodrome	Breath odor	Alcohol level	Search for 2nd cause of AMS: another drug, head trauma.
E Encephalitis, meningitis, para-infectious encephalopathy	Prodrome or recent viral illness, fever	Fever, meningismus, rash	LP, NH3, stool culture, CT scan	Caution: LP may carry risk if increased ICP present.
I Insulin (hypoglycemia and hyperglycemia)			Glucose, VBG quantitative	Chemstrip should be done on all blood sent for glucose.
O Overdose	Usually no prodrome, toddler, teen, GI symptoms frequent	Toxidromes (see Section VIII: Toxicology). Pupils, skin color, & temp., VS, secretions	KUB, toxicology screen, carboxyhemoglobin, EKG, anion/osmolar gap	Trial of Narcan should be considered. Consider suicide attempt if older child or teen.
U Uremia, hypoxia, shock, S/P anoxia, hyper/hypothermia, electrolyte abnormalities, dehydration, inborn errors of metabolism, methemoglobinemia, hepatic and hypertensive encephalopathies	Subacute onset typical of most of these	Color, perfusion, BP, temp., dehydration	Electrolytes, BUN, NH3, SGOT, methemoglobin	Hypoxia and shock should be the first consideration.
T Trauma, tumor	For tumor: prodromal history of vomiting, AM headaches, ataxia	Signs of trauma, retinal hemorrhages, focal neuro findings, signs of increased ICP	CT Scan Hct.	This category should remind the clinician of child abuse.
I Infarction, intracranial hemorrhage	SS disease, CHD, recent OM or sinusitis, fever	Focal neuro findings, signs of increased ICP, dehydration, otitis media/mastoiditis	SS screen, mastoid/sinus X-rays, PT, PTT, Plts, CT scan	
P Psychiatric	Teen, psychiatric Hx in teen or family	Response to spirits of ammonia, eye blink challenge, response to pain		
S Seizures/postictal states	Fever, F/H of seizures, acute onset	Tone, eye movements	EEG	Trial of an anticonvulsant occasionally useful. With partial seizures some appropriate responses may be present.
O Other: intussusception, vasculitis, hydrocephalus, hem. shock and encephalopathy syndrome	See text	See text	See text	

tis, and *hemorrhagic shock and encephalopathy syndrome.* Of these, intussusception is the most common. At least 10% of infants with intussusception will present *solely* with a depressed level of consciousness. They will not have the typical prodrome of rhythmic irritability, hematochezia, and vomiting (see Chapter 40). Consider acute hydrocephalus in any child with a ventricular shunt in place and in any child who has had a recent neurological insult such as meningitis or head trauma.

Clinical Findings ■

Table 16-4 presents the pertinent history, physical findings, laboratory data, and caveats for differential diagnosis of AMS. Age is helpful in initially narrowing the possibilities. *For infants,* the diagnostic categories of major importance are meningitis; hypothermia or hyperthermia, electrolyte abnormalities, inborn errors of metabolism, dehydration, and methemoglobinemia; trauma; seizures; and intussusception. *For adolescents,* the major diagnostic categories are alcohol, overdose, trauma, and psychiatric. Recent historical factors of greatest importance are fever, onset/prodrome, trauma and availability of poisons/toxins, recent viral illness (para-infectious encephalopathy), headaches and vomiting (tumor and infarction), and psychological stress factors. Identify known or unrecognized chronic illnesses, particularly diabetes mellitus, seizures, bleeding diatheses, renal disease, and collagen-vascular illness.

Ancillary Data ■

Table 16-4 lists principal laboratory tests. Four deserve special mention. The lumbar puncture is key to many of the diagnoses in the encephalitis category, but several of these diagnoses are complicated by increased intracranial pressure, a *relative* contraindication to a lumbar puncture. Exercise caution, therefore, in the timing and performance of a lumbar puncture in an afebrile child with an AMS. *However, if bacterial meningitis is the most likely possibility, a lumbar puncture should be performed promptly.* In other children with low suspicion for bacterial meningitis, before doing a lumbar puncture obtain a CT scan *quickly* to rule out an increase in intracranial pressure.

In addition to routine blood work (electrolytes, complete blood count, toxicology screen), consider a *serum ammonia* (for Reye's syndrome, inborn errors of metabolism, hepatic encephalopathy), a *carboxyhemoglobin level, clotting studies,* and a *chemstrip.* Hypoglycemia should never be diagnosed by the laboratory before being diagnosed by the clinician with a bedside chemstrip.

An *ECG,* looking for evidence of overdose by cardiac drugs or tricyclic antidepressants (TCA), might be considered in a child with an unexplained alteration in mental status. Major complications of TCA overdose (coma, convulsions, shock) usually occur in the first few hours of hospitalization, before the toxicology screen has been reported. Tachycardia, with a QRS complex widened beyond 0.10 milliseconds, provides a valuable early warning of impending TCA complications.

Treatment ■

The first step is to evaluate *and stabilize* the child's ABCs (see Chapters 6, 8, and 14). Always suspect trauma, including physical abuse and the shaken baby syndrome. The airway of the child with an AMS is vulnerable because of the potential loss of protective reflexes and subsequent aspiration of stomach contents. Therefore, if a gag reflex is absent, consider early, but not necessarily emergent, endotracheal intubation. When increased intracranial pressure is suspected, use a controlled induction sequence for airway management, as outlined in Chapter 49, to minimize further pressure elevations. The breathing of a child with an AMS may appear adequate, but appearances may easily deceive in this situation. Routinely administer supplemental oxygen, apply continuous pulse oximetry, and obtain a pCO_2 (arterial, venous, or capnography, depending on clinical conditions). Next, assess the child's circulation using peripheral circulatory signs (heart rate, pulse strength, capillary refill, temperature and color of the extremities) and blood pressure.

After the ABCs, establish an intravenous line at a to-keep-open rate unless there is clear need for fluid administration based upon evaluation of circulation. A fluid bolus may worsen cerebral perfusion in a euvolemic child with intracranial pressure elevation; on the other hand, if the child has systemic hypoperfusion from hypovolemia, fluid therapy to a euvolemic level is essential to ensure adequate cerebral perfusion. Optimal treatment of significant intracranial pressure elevation also includes endotracheal intubation and hyperventilation. After the IV is in place, administer 25% dextrose in water at 2 ml/kg (<2 years) or 50% dextrose in water at 1 ml/kg (>2 years), if the bedside chemstrip is less than 100 mg%. Give naloxone, 0.4 mg IV in an infant and 1 mg IV in older children, if AMS is accompanied by central nervous system and/or respiratory depression. Further therapy is guided by diagnosis.

Disposition ■

Disposition depends on both the specific diagnosis and the degree of AMS. Any persistent AMS requires hospital admission. Any profound AMS requires admission to an intensive care unit or transfer to a pediatric critical care center. Until admission, the child with an AMS requires both continuous electronic monitoring *and* continuous nursing monitoring. In particular, the child with an AMS should *not* be sent to the radiology department without the benefit of *both* forms of monitoring.

Bibliography ■

Case Reports of the Massachusetts General Hospital (Case 35-1981). *N Eng J Med* 1981; 305:507–514.

Lyon G, Dodge PR, Adams RD: The acute encephalopathies of obscure origins in infants and children. *Brain* 1961; 84:680–708.

Seshia SS, Seshia MMK, Sachena RK: Coma in childhood. *Dev Med Child Neurol* 1977; 19:614.

Solomon GE: Strokes in children. *Pediatr Ann* 1978; 7:813.

Tenebein M, Wiseman NE: Early coma in intussusception: Endogenous opioid induced? *Pediatr Emerg Care* 1987; 3:22.

17 Anaphylaxis

Michael T. Kelley

Anaphylaxis is an acute, life-threatening state that occurs after the interaction of antigen and antibody. Anaphylaxis is also referred to as the immediate hypersensitivity reaction. Anaphylactoid reactions cause similar physical signs and symptoms as anaphylaxis but are not mediated by immunoglobulin E (IgE).

Etiology and Pathophysiology ■

Table 17-1 lists common causes of anaphylaxis in childhood. Hymenoptera or bee stings are the most common.

Antibodies are formed when the immunologic system is exposed to an antigen. This initial process, called sensitization, results in the binding of IgE antibody to the cell membranes of basophils and mast cells. This is normally a protective mechanism that allows the body to defend against foreign substances.

Anaphylaxis occurs after second or subsequent exposures to the sensitizing antigen. When the antigen binds to two or more cell surface antibodies, cellular changes cause the release of *preformed mediators* via mast-cell degranulation. In addition, arachidonic acid and other phospholipid cascades are initiated, resulting in production of *formed mediators* of anaphylaxis. Of the multiple *preformed mediators* of anaphylaxis (Table 17-2), histamine is the most prominent, as it produces the most significant physiologic effects. In the lung, histamine causes bronchoconstriction, bronchospasm, and bronchorrhea. In the vasculature, it produces generalized vasodilatation and increased capillary permeability. In animal models, histamine is also arrhythmogenic, causing ectopic beats and ventricular tachyarrhythmias and lowering the ventricular fibrillation threshold.

There are also multiple *formed mediators* of anaphylaxis (Table 17-2). The leukotrienes, previously known as slow reactive substance of anaphylaxis, are products of the arachidonic acid cascade. They are major mediators of airway anaphylaxis. Leukotriene

D_4, for example, is 6,000 times more potent on a mole-to-mole basis than histamine in producing bronchoconstriction. Further, although histamine produces brief bronchoconstriction, the leukotrienes produce sustained, prolonged bronchoconstriction. In the heart, the leukotrienes decrease coronary blood flow and myocardial contractility. In the vasculature they increase vascular permeability and cause capillary leakage, which contributes to urticaria and angioedema. The hydroxyacids are chemotactic for leukocytes. They also induce the release of lysosomal enzymes and cause bronchoconstriction. Prostaglandin D_2, F_2, and thromboxane A_2 are also bronchoconstricting agents and may decrease coronary artery blood flow.

Platelet activating factor (PAF), a phospholipid formed independently of the arachidonic acid cascade, plays a prominent role in anaphylaxis. In the heart, PAF causes a decrease in coronary blood flow and myocardial contraction. In the pulmonary system, PAF causes a bronchoconstriction that is intermediate in duration between the shorter-acting histamine and the longer-acting leukotrienes.

Clinical Findings ■

Diagnosing anaphylaxis is often difficult. Atopic individuals have a higher incidence of anaphylaxis, but persons who have no history of allergic reactions have anaphylactic reactions. Signs and symptoms range from urticaria and pruritis to cardiopulmonary arrest. Clinical findings may be limited to one system, such as the skin (urticaria), or may involve all systems, as in cardiopulmonary arrest. Table 17-3 presents the clinical spectrum of hypersensitivity reactions, with true anaphylaxis at the extreme.

In frank anaphylaxis, the clinical picture is rarely mistaken. Vasodilatation and capillary leakage cause urticaria, nonpitting edema, angioedema, and hypotension. In the lung, bronchospasm and bronchorrhea cause respiratory distress, leading to diffuse wheezes and decreased oxygenation.

TABLE 17–1. *Common Causes of Anaphylaxis*

Foods	Hormones, Drugs	Insect Stings
Nuts	Insulin	Hymenoptera
Fish	ACTH	Spider venom
Shellfish	Antibiotics	*Miscellaneous*
Eggs	Meperidine	Alpine slides
Fruits	Chymopapain	
Vegetables	Blood products	
Pollen extract	Local anesthetics	
Chocolate	Vitamins	
Chamomile tea	Many others	

TABLE 17–2. *Mediators of Anaphylaxis*

Preformed Mediators	Formed Mediators
Histamine	Leukotrienes
Eosinophil chemotactic factor	Hydroxyacids
Heparin proteoglycan	Thromboxanes
Bradykinin	Prostaglandins
Serotonin	Platelet activating
Chymase	factor

Cardiovascular manifestations of anaphylaxis include arrhythmias and hypotension. Electrocardiographic changes consistent with acute myocardial infarction may be seen.

Abdominal cramping, nausea, vomiting, diarrhea (sometimes bloody), and incontinence are gastrointestinal manifestations of anaphylaxis. Central nervous system manifestations include headache, dizziness, and seizures. These symptoms are presumably a consequence of disturbed cerebral blood flow and/or brain hypoxia. However, hemiparesis and hemiparalysis occur without concurrent changes in oxygenation and blood pressure.

The onset of the signs and symptoms of anaphylaxis is often abrupt, usually within seconds to minutes after parenterally administered antigens. Most cases occur within 20 minutes of exposure, but in some cases anaphylaxis is delayed for many hours. Anaphylaxis from ingested antigens is frequently delayed and recurrent. Other routes of exposure include topical application to mucous membranes and inhalation.

Treatment ■

Anaphylaxis is a medical emergency. Treatment should begin with the ABCs: airway, breathing, and circulation (see Chapter 7). Equally important is to prevent further mediator release and to counteract the effects of the mediators already released (see Figure 17–1).

The release and formation of the mediators of anaphylaxis is decreased by increasing the intracellular concentration of c-AMP. Stimulation of the beta-adrenergic receptor increases intracellular c-AMP and decreases the circulating levels of histamine and the leukotrienes.

The first priority is to protect the airway. Administer 100% oxygen. Intubation is indicated if there is severe bronchospasm or angioedema. If intubation is impossible because of excessive swelling, perform cricothyrotomy.

A single drug, epinephrine, can correct breathing and circulation and prevent further mediator release. It is the most important drug for the treatment of anaphylaxis and should be used for all manifestations of anaphylaxis, from isolated urticaria to severe bronchospasm and hypotension. Its beta-agonistic

TABLE 17–3. *Clinical Spectrum of Anaphylaxis*

Anaphylaxis can present as only one or a combination of all of the following conditions:

Capillary Leakage	Bronchoconstriction	Cardiovascular
Urticaria	Shortness of breath	Hypotension
Periorbital edema	Anxiety	Arrhythmias
Angioedema	Wheezes	Myocardial infarction
Hypotension	Bronchospasm	
Gastrointestinal	Respiratory arrest	
Nausea	*Neurologic*	
Vomiting	Hemiparesis	
Diarrhea	Hemiparalysis	
Abdominal		
cramps		

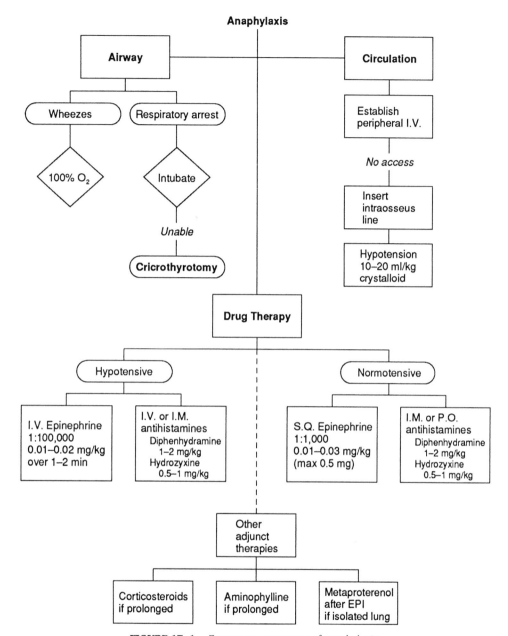

FIGURE 17–1. Emergency treatment of anaphylaxis.

action relaxes bronchial smooth muscle, increases cardiac rate and contractility, and prevents further mediator release. In addition, its alpha-agonist effects cause vasoconstriction, which increases blood pressure and decreases capillary leakage, the cause of angioedema and urticaria.

Epinephrine, however, can have adverse side effects, including hypertension, intracerebral hemorrhage, myocardial ischemia, and ventricular arrhythmias. Arrhythmias typically occur when rates of administration exceed 0.5 μg/kg/min.

The patient's clinical state dictates epinephrine

usage. Adverse effects usually result from overly rapid administration. In normotensive patients, give epinephrine subcutaneously in a dose of 0.01–0.03 mg/kg of a 1:1,000 solution (to a maximum of 0.5 mg). If epinephrine must be given intravenously, as in the hypotensive, hypoperfused patient, dilute the solution to 1:100,000 and infuse 0.01 mg/kg over 1–2 minutes. If intravenous access is not available, a 1:10,000 solution can be administered via an endotracheal tube, or the 1:100,000 solution via an intraosseous line. Repeat the initial dose every 15–20 minutes, or begin an infusion of 0.1 μg/kg/min (maximum, 0.5 μg/kg/min). Note that this is lower than the 1 μg/kg/min dose recommended by the American Academy of Pediatricians.

Treat hypotension with an initial bolus of 10–20 ml/kg of crystalloid solution. Military antishock trousers (MAST) may be helpful, but have unproven efficacy and safety in children.

Antihistamines in the H_1-receptor antagonist class (diphenhydramine hydrochloride 1–2 mg/kg q 6 hr IM or IV, or hydroxyzine hydrochloride 0.5–1 mg/kg q 6 hr IM or IV) are used as an adjunct to epinephrine therapy. Antihistamines should not be used alone, as they have no effect on the pathophysiologic processes of the formed mediators. Even isolated urticaria, if due to an anaphylactic process, should be treated with epinephrine and antihistamines. Antihistamines have no effect on the vasodilatory and capillary-leakage-producing properties of the leukotrienes and platelet activating factor.

Antihistamines in the H_2-receptor antagonist class may help prevent anaphylactoid reactions and may be beneficial in treating chronic urticaria. However, their efficacy in anaphylaxis is unproven in children and they are of no value in resuscitation. They should not be used without concomitant H_1 antihistamines, since histamine may cause profound coronary artery constriction in H_2-receptor blocked hearts. The pediatric dose of cimetidine is 20–40 mg/kg/day in four divided doses.

Corticosteroids are not useful in the immediate treatment of anaphylaxis. In severe reactions where prolonged release of mediators is likely to occur, corticosteroid administration may be beneficial, but its efficacy is unproven.

Beta-agonist inhaled bronchodilators may be beneficial, especially if the reaction is limited to the lungs. Metaproterenol (5%, 0.1–0.3 mg in 3 mls NS) is an effective bronchodilating agent in children who can cooperate. Inhaled beta agonists do not reach high levels in the systemic circulation and may be inadequate to stop the continued release of cellular mediators in areas outside the lung. Even in isolated pulmonary anaphylaxis, epinephrine is the drug of choice.

Theophylline may also be beneficial in cases of prolonged anaphylaxis.

Complications and Caveats ■

Even mild manifestations of anaphylaxis should be treated aggressively, as they can progress to severe life-threatening conditions.

Although rare, profound anaphylactic episodes that may be resistant to epinephrine therapy may occur in children on beta blockers. In these cases, glucagon 0.03 mg/kg (maximum, 1 mg/dose) may be useful.

Bibliography ■

Bach MK: Mediators of anaphylaxis and inflammation. *Ann Rev Microbiol* 1982; 36:371–413.

Barach EM, Nowak RM, Lee TG, et al: Epinephrine for treatment of anaphylactic shock. *JAMA* 1984; 251:2118–2122.

Baumann G, Loher U, Felix B, et al: Deleterious effects of cimetidine in the presence of histamine on the coronary circulation. *Res Exp Med (Berl)* 1982; 180:209–213.

Darius H, Lefer DJ, Smith B, et al: Role of platelet-activating factor-acether in mediating guinea pig anaphylaxis. *Science* 1986; 232:58–60.

Kaliner M, Orange RP, Austin F: Immunological release of histamine and slow reacting substance of anaphylaxis from human lung. *J Exp Med* 1972; 136:556–567.

Meszaros I: Transient cerebral ischemic attack caused by Hymenoptera stings: The brain as an anaphylactic shock organ. *Eur Neurol* 1986; 25:248–252.

Monroe EW: Combined H1 and H2 antihistamine therapy in chronic urticaria. *Arch Derm* 1981; 117:404–407.

Stark BJ, Sullivan TJ: Biphasic and protracted anaphylaxis. *J Allergy Clin Immunol* 1986; 78:76–83.

18 Apnea

John Colin Partridge

Apneic pauses or periodic breathing occurs in 25–50% of premature infants and in 1–3% of full-term infants. It is a heterogeneous entity (see Table 18-1) with a mortality of 2–6%. The more severe of these episodes have been termed apparent life-threatening events (ALTE) and are thought to be related to sudden infant death. After one presenting ALTE, 40–60% of patients experience a recurrent ALTE and 0.4–10% of infants subsequently die from sudden infant death; after 2–3 ALTE episodes, there may be a threefold increase in risk. Sudden infant death syndrome (SIDS) is the leading cause of death in infants between the ages of 1 month and 1 year, accounting for 5–10,000 deaths per year in the United States (see Chapter 126). Apnea of infancy (AI) may be a predisposing condition for subsequent SIDS, but only 2–4% of SIDS cases have had documented apnea of prematurity and less than 7% have had an ALTE.

The objectives for emergency department (ED) evaluation and management of the child with suspected AI include:

1. Establishing the type of breathing abnormality from the subjective description of a frightened parent
2. Preventing a later event by managing an asymptomatic infant with a potentially life-threatening situation or by stabilizing an infant after an ALTE
3. Determining whether hospitalization for observation and further work-up is necessary
4. Dealing with the sudden infant death and resuscitation of the infant (see Chapters 9 and 126).

Pathophysiology ■

Infants presenting with apnea have abnormal breathing patterns, excessive time spent in periodic breathing, short and prolonged apneic episodes (either central or obstructive in origin). They may hypoventilate or have blunted ventilatory responses or arousal responses to hypercarbia and hypoxia. Other infants have alterations in heart rate and variability suggestive of increased sympathetic activity. In some term infants, the brain stem regulation of respiration is delayed and the apneic episodes of preterm infants persist. These abnormalities represent a maturational aspect and/or abnormality of CNS regulation of respiration, exacerbated by chronic intrauterine hypoxia or by repetitive postnatal central or obstructive apneic episodes. Whether apneic pauses are related to ALTE is uncertain.

Epidemiologic risk factors are given in Table 18-2. Premature infants (< 36 weeks gestation) are at increased risk because of immature central and peripheral chemoreceptor respiratory control, obstructive and mixed apnea from hypotonia and airway obstruction during sleep, and decreased lung volumes and airway tone from compliant chest walls. Thirty percent of siblings of SIDS victims demonstrate breathing abnormalities. Eleven percent of these infants, when monitored at home, will subsequently need some form of intervention, whereas none of the siblings with normal breathing studies will require intervention at home.

Clinical Findings ■

Usually, AI presents clinically as visible cessation of respiratory activity, cyanosis, or pallor. ALTEs present with more severe findings and unresponsiveness. In SIDS, the infant is usually found dead in bed, often with blood-tinged secretions in the oropharynx.

Parents' historical accounts are variable and include the following correlations: apnea within 1 hour before or after feeding (54%), sleep (18.8%), cyanosis (7.5%), apnea after crying or agitation (6.3%), awake apnea unrelated to feeding (5.0%), apnea with seizure-like activity (3.8%), apnea with respiratory infection (2.5%), premature infant (2.5%). However, parental historical details may not distinguish the infant at high risk prospectively and are often useful only in retrospect.

History: Obtain important historical data from an eyewitness. Key details include:

Timing of the episode
Relationship to last feeding and position

TABLE 18–1. *Definitions of Apneic Pauses in Infants*

Apnea

Cessation of respiratory air flow. The respiratory pause may be central or diaphragmatic (i.e., no respiratory effort), obstructive (usually due to upper airway obstruction), or mixed. Short (≤15 seconds), central apnea can be normal at all ages.

Pathologic Apnea

A respiratory pause is abnormal if it is prolonged (≥20 seconds) or associated with cyanosis; abrupt, marked pallor or hypotonia; or bradycardia.

Apnea of Infancy

An unexplained and frightening episode of cessation of breathing for 20 seconds or longer or a shorter respiratory pause associated with bradycardia, cyanosis, pallor, and/or marked hypotonia.

SIDS

The sudden death of any infant or young child which is unexpected by history, and in which a thorough postmortem examination fails to demonstrate an adequate cause for death.

Apparent Life-threatening Event (ALTE or "Near-miss" SIDS)

An episode that is frightening to the observer and that is characterized by some combination of apnea (central or occasionally obstructive), color change (usually cyanotic or pallid but occasionally erythematous or plethoric), marked change in muscle tone (usually marked limpness), choking, or gagging. Previously used terminology such as "aborted crib death" or "near-miss SIDS" should be abandoned because it implies a possibly misleadingly close association between this type of spell and SIDS.

Periodic Breathing

A breathing pattern in which there are three or more respiratory pauses of greater than 3 seconds' duration with less than 20 seconds of respiration between pauses. Periodic breathing can be a normal event.

Apnea of Prematurity

Periodic breathing with pathologic apnea breathing in a premature infant. Apnea of prematurity usually ceases by 37 weeks gestation (menstrual dating) but occasionally persists for several weeks past term.

Sleep state
Color changes
Abnormal movements or posturing
Presence or absence of respiratory efforts, emesis, choking, cough
Duration of event
Degree of intervention or resuscitation necessary
Behavior after episode
History of prior episodes
History of feeding difficulties
Past medical history (gestational age at birth and neonatal problems)
Intercurrent illnesses or fever
Family history.

Physical examination: Physical examination must elicit diagnostic clues suggesting a specific etiology. Document height, weight, craniofacial abnormalities, breath sounds, and heart murmurs, and perform a thorough neurologic assessment. Investigate any signs of past or present trauma.

Differential diagnosis: ALTEs can be caused by a variety of identifiable diseases or conditions (see Table 18-3). Provocative risk factors include immaturity (the most common associated factor), hypoxemia, airway obstruction or pulmonary disease, primary CNS conditions (such as seizures or masses), metabolic problems (e.g., hypocalcemia, hypoglycemia, acidosis), gastroesophageal reflux, and hyperbilirubinemia, and intercurrent infection (see Table 18-2). In up to 50% of patients, a cause can be identified and specific treatment will then lead to a resolution of the apnea. In infants with specific treatable causes, immediately start the appropriate therapy (e.g., anticonvulsants for seizure-associated apnea, antibiotic for sepsis, upright positioning and thickened feedings for gastroesophageal reflux).

Infants with subtle abnormalities of cardiorespiratory activity without identifiable causes require hospitalization; therapeutic options after complete evaluation involve supportive care, stimulants, and/or continuous home monitoring of cardiac and respiratory activity.

Ancillary Data ■

Useful ancillary tests are listed in Table 18-4. Specific diagnostic tests to rule out treatable conditions should be based on the history (e.g., bacterial and viral cultures of blood or cerebrospinal fluid in infants

TABLE 18–2. *Risk Factors for Apnea of Infancy and SIDS*

Maternal	Age < 20 years
	Single
	Low socioeconomic status
	Little or no prenatal care
	Antepartum illness
	Prior fetal loss
	Smoker
	Substance abuse
	Short interval between pregnancies
Paternal	Age < 20 years
	Low socioeconomic status
Race	Black > native American > white > Asian
Infant	Prematurity
	Low birth weight
	History of low Apgar scores or resuscitation at birth
	Twin or triplet
	Male > female
	Age < 6 months
Current Problems	History of feeding problems
	Mild gastrointestinal or respiratory illness
Family History	Sibling of SIDS victim
Environmental	Seasonal (winter > summer)

with apnea accompanied by fever, or investigation of the airway in infants with signs of obstruction). An electrocardiogram will rule out primary cardiac disease or right ventricular hypertrophy from chronic hypoxemia. Consider a head sonogram or CT scan in all infants whose spells do not occur just with feeding or who have neurologic signs or symptoms. Barium studies may be diagnostic in infants with feeding problems and vomiting.

Laboratory studies have a low yield. In one study, only 0.5% of 1,278 laboratory measurements performed on 163 patients hospitalized for a "presumed near-miss" SIDS event were useful in diagnosing or treating the apnea episodes. Limit ED screening evaluation until a specific etiology is suspected and specific studies are indicated.

Treatment ■

Management of apneic episodes in infants depends on the cause and the acuity at presentation. Of all spontaneous apneic episodes in infants, ⅓ abort

spontaneously, ½ respond to cutaneous stimulation, and only ¹⁄₁₀ need bag-and-mask ventilation or resuscitation. However, the more severe episodes seen in the ED more often necessitate resuscitation, as follows:

1. Stabilize the airway and ensure adequate ventilation. Attach pulse oximeter or obtain arterial blood gas measurements.
2. Obtain an initial history.
3. Perform a screening diagnostic evaluation (see below).
4. Treat underlying causes, such as pneumonia, airway obstruction, aspiration, sepsis, narcotic depression, metabolic acidosis.
5. Treat hypoxia: increase F_iO_2, stimulate breathing, administer low continuous positive airway pressures (CPAP) or intubate and mechanically ventilate.
6. Avoid causing reflex-associated apnea; increase cutaneous and vestibular afferent input; decrease environmental temperature but avoid hypothermia.
7. Admit the infant if the episode has occurred within two days of presentation.
8. Monitor closely until the infant is admitted to the ward.
9. For obstructive apnea: administer oxygen; if obstruction is not improved by CPAP or nasopharyngeal or endotracheal tube, consider surgical intervention (e.g., tonsillectomy and adenoidectomy, or tracheostomy).

Disposition ■

HOSPITALIZATION

Admit any infant with an apneic spell sufficiently frightening to prompt resuscitation by parents or caretakers or that is associated with pallor, cyanosis, or hypotonia. In-hospital observation, evaluation, and monitoring (for apnea > 15–20 seconds and for bradycardia < 80 bpm) will guide rational therapy and accurate prognosis.

Diagnostic and therapeutic alternatives, after complete evaluation, include *sleep studies, pharmacologic intervention, and home cardiorespiratory monitoring*.

PHARMACOLOGIC INTERVENTION

In full-term or preterm infants with apnea, methylxanthines will eliminate observed spells and laboratory abnormalities of prolonged apnea and periodic breathing. Methylxanthines (caffeine or theophylline) excite CNS rhythm generators for re-

TABLE 18–3. *Differential Diagnosis of Apnea of Infancy**

Neonatal Period	Infancy
Prematurity	Immature respiratory control
Respiratory distress syndrome	Respiratory diseases with hypoxemia
Sepsis, meningitis	Infection
Airway obstruction or anomalies	RSV, enterovirus, parainfluenza, pertussis, botulism
Choanal atresia	Obstructive lesions of the airway
Vocal cord paralysis	Adenoid hypertrophy
Glottic/tracheal mass or web	Hypothyroidism
Tracheo-esophageal fistula	Pierre Robin anomalad
Central nervous system	Glottic/tracheal mass or web
Intracranial hemorrhage	Vascular ring
Seizures	Central nervous system
Meningitis	Seizures
Encephalopathy (bilirubin, asphyxia)	Meningitis, encephalitis
Myopathy	Encephalopathy (bilirubin, asphyxia)
Hypovolemia	Myopathy
Anemia	Tumor
Congenital heart disease	Central hypoventilation
Patent ductus arteriosus	Anemia
Cardiac arrhythmias	Congenital heart disease
Gastroesophageal reflux	ASD, VSD, PDA
Necrotizing enterocolitis	Cardiac arrhythmias
Metabolic causes	Gastroesophageal reflux/aspiration
Hypoglycemia, hypocalcemia, hyponatremia, acidosis	Metabolic causes
Iatrogenic	Hypoglycemia, hypocalcemia, hyponatremia
Hypoxemia	Inborn errors of metabolism
Stimulation of reflex apnea	Breath-holding spells
Thermal	Ingestion or toxic exposure
Drug intoxication	Organophosphate
Opiates	Child abuse
Magnesium sulfate	ALTE or "near-miss" SIDS

* (Adapted from Emmanouilides GC, Baylen BG, eds: *Neonatal cardiopulmonary distress.* Chicago: Year Book Medical Publishers, Inc., 1988, p 78; and Kattwinkel J: Apnea in the neonatal period. *Pediatr Rev* 1980; 2:115–120.)

spiratory control, lower chemoreceptor sensitivity, improve oxygenation and ventilation, and decrease the number of hypoxic episodes. They also produce an increased metabolic rate, cardiac chronotropic and inotropic effects, vasodilatation, increased renal blood flow, skeletal muscle stimulation, and altered endocrine and glucose homeostasis. Pharmacologic therapy may be considered in symptomatic infants with all the following factors:

1. Severe and recurrent central or mixed apnea
   a. Preterm infants—15 secs occurring more than three times in 6 hours, excessive short apnea with bradycardia, periodic breathing for > 10% of sleep time (especially if associated with bradycardia)
   b. Older infants—severe clinical apnea necessitating intervention or associated with pallor, cyanosis, or hypotonia

2. No apparent contraindications (gastroesophageal reflux or seizures)
3. Adequate follow-up.

These drugs are best prescribed by the child's primary care provider. Infants treated pharmacologically must be followed closely with theophylline levels to prevent toxicity and to verify a response to therapy.

Apnea of Prematurity ■

This very common problem in the premature infant resolves with maturation of the central control of respiration. One-fourth of infants less than 1,800 gm have apnea. The ED physician will rarely encounter apnea of prematurity and should consider other etiologies for apneic episodes. The infant should be hospitalized and observed on a cardiorespiratory

TABLE 18–4. *Ancillary Data in Evaluation of Apnea of Infancy*

Complete physical examination, complete neurologic examination
Vital signs and blood pressure
Blood sugar (random or fasting)
Serum electrolytes, calcium, phosphate, magnesium
Complete blood count and differential
Chest x-ray
Transcutaneous oxygen or saturation monitoring
Arterial blood gas analysis

Consider
    Blood culture
    Cerebrospinal fluid analysis and culture
    Viral culture or immunofluorescence
    Lateral neck x-ray
    Direct laryngoscopy or endoscopy
    Electrocardiogram and possibly echocardiogram
    Head sonogram or computerized tomography of head
    Electroencephalogram
    Esophageal reflux studies (scintigraphy, barium swallow, or pH probe study)
    Thermistor-pneumocardiogram or polysomnography

In-hospital observation with monitoring

monitor while treatable primary conditions are ruled out.

Outcome ■

The recurrence risk for ALTE is 43–66%. Of infants discharged from the hospital on a monitor, 12% have at least two episodes of apnea requiring at least vigorous stimulation by parents, and approximately 1% of infants require emergency CPR and subsequent hospitalization. Of infants with a history of apnea in the neonatal period, 5% die who had only one spell; 44% die with more than one spell. There is a subsequent mortality of up to 2% after a previous ALTE.

Bibliography ■

Ariagno RL, Guilleminault C, Korobkin R, et al: "Near-miss" for sudden infant death syndrome infants: A clinical problem. *Pediatrics* 1983; 71:726–730.

Ariagno RL: Evaluation and management of infantile apnea. *Pediatr Ann* 1984; 13:210–217.

Brooks JG: Apnea of infancy and sudden infant death syndrome. *Am J Dis Child* 1982; 136:1012–1023.

Consensus Statement: National Institutes of Health Consensus Development Conference on Infantile Apnea and Home Monitoring. *Pediatrics* 1987; 79:292–299.

Duffty P, Bryan MH: Home apnea monitoring in "near-miss" sudden infant death syndrome (SIDS) and siblings of SIDS victims. *Pediatrics* 1982; 70:69–74.

Kelly DH, Shannon DC: Sudden infant death syndrome and near sudden infant death syndrome: A review of the literature, 1964–1982. *Pediatr Clin North Am* 1982; 29: 1241–1261.

Kelly DH, Shannon DC: Treatment of apnea and excessive periodic breathing in the full-term infant. *Pediatrics* 1981; 68:183–186.

Lewis JM, Ganick DJ: Initial laboratory evaluations of infants with "presumed near-miss" sudden infant death syndrome. *Am J Dis Child* 1986; 140:484–486.

Shannon DC, Kelly DH: SIDS and near SIDS, parts I & II. *Engl J Med* 1982; 306:959–965 and 1022–1028.

Spitzer AR, Fox WW: Infant apnea. *Pediatr Clin North Am* 1986; 33:561–581.

19 Bleeding

Marion A. Koerper

Excessive bleeding in children may be due to either congenital or acquired abnormalities of plasma coagulation factors, platelets, or connective tissue and blood vessels.

The most common congenital bleeding disorders include hemophilia A (incidence 1 in 10,000), hemophilia B (1 in 50,000), and von Willebrand's disease (at least 1 in 10,000). Congenital deficiencies of the other clotting factors (I, II, V, VII, X, XI, and XIII) are very rare, with an incidence of less than 1 in 100,000 each. Congenital disorders of platelet function also are very rare, with a similar incidence of less than 1 in 100,000.

The most common acquired bleeding disorders in children include liver disease, vitamin K deficiency, disseminated intravascular coagulation (DIC), thrombocytopenia, and uremia. Other causes for apparent easy bruising include Ehlers-Danlos syndrome and Henoch-Schönlein purpura.

Etiology and Pathophysiology ■

Hemophilia A (classic hemophilia, factor VIII deficiency, AHF deficiency) and hemophilia B (factor IX deficiency, Christmas disease) are usually inherited in an X-linked manner; von Willebrand's disease and afibrinogenemia (factor I deficiency) are usually inherited in an autosomal-dominant fashion. The other clotting factor deficiencies, as well as platelet function disorders, show an autosomal-recessive pattern of inheritance.

In all the clotting factor deficiencies, a defective gene leads to decreased or absent synthesis of the clotting factor or to synthesis of a structurally aberrant protein that cannot activate the next clotting factor in the sequence leading to formation of a stable clot. These patients do not bleed faster than normal; they merely bleed longer than normal because of their inability to form a clot in the usual amount of time. In patients with defective platelet function, there is either an absent or an abnormal platelet protein re-quired to bind clotting factors to the platelet membrane, or there is absence of the platelet secretory granule proteins required for the irreversible aggregation of platelets into a stable clot. Once again, these platelet abnormalities lead to inability of the blood to clot in the usual amount of time.

In liver disease and vitamin K deficiency, there is *decreased synthesis* of clotting factors (especially II, VII, IX, and X), but in DIC there is *increased consumption* of clotting factors due to platelet activation by viral or bacterial sepsis or by hypoxia, acidosis, or hypotension.

The most common cause of thrombocytopenia is immune thrombocytopenic purpura (ITP), in which a viral-induced antibody attaches to the patient's platelets, which leads to their removal by the patient's reticuloendothelial system. Other acquired causes of thrombocytopenia include decreased bone marrow production due to leukemia, aplastic anemia, or chronic infection of the bone marrow.

In uremia, metabolic byproducts that normally would be cleared by the kidneys accumulate in the blood, thereby interfering with normal platelet function by affecting the binding of von Willebrand factor to platelets. In Ehlers-Danlos syndrome, abnormal connective tissue leads to easy bruising and bleeding. In Henoch-Schönlein purpura, circulating immune complexes produce an allergic vasculitis-type picture with purpuric skin lesions, urticaria, and hematuria.

Clinical Findings ■

HISTORY

A *bleeding history* should include information about the following:

1. *Prior episodes of bleeding or bruising.* Significant bleeding may occur after surgery (including circumcision), trauma (including fractures and lacerations requiring suturing), loss of deciduous or permanent teeth, or dental work. Other significant bleeding symptoms include menorrhagia, epi-

staxis, GI bleeding, excessively large bruises, petechiae, bleeding from the gums, swollen joints or muscles, anemia secondary to blood loss, and blood transfusions necessitated by excessive bleeding. Determine the length of time over which the abnormal bleeding has occurred to ascertain whether this is a lifelong (i.e., congenital) problem or a recently acquired one. The age at onset can give a clue to the severity of the congenital clotting disorder: the more severe present earlier in life (Table 19-1).

2. *Family history of excessive bleeding or bruising.* Determine the same bleeding history outlined above for both parents, both sets of grandparents, and any siblings of the child, parents, and grandparents. Plot the family tree and highlight those individuals with a positive bleeding history to establish whether the disorder is inherited in a sex-linked or an autosomal fashion.

3. *Exposure to drugs or toxins that may cause decreased plasma coagulation factors or affect platelet function or number.* See Table 19-2.

4. *Any recent antibiotic administration or illness* such as diarrhea, hepatitis, or upper respiratory infection that may result in thrombocytopenia, vitamin K deficiency, or liver or kidney dysfunction.

PHYSICAL EXAMINATION

On *physical examination* note:

1. Location, size, and age of petechiae, purpura, or ecchymoses. Note especially whether all the lesions are of the same age or of varying ages and states of resolution. Palpate for tender subcutaneous nodules of blood under the ecchymoses.

2. Swollen, tender joints or muscles or large soft-tissue swelling without ecchymosis, which represents bleeding deep in the subcutaneous tissue.

3. Evidence of bleeding in the fundi, ears, nares, or pharynx, or in the stool, urine, sputum, or vomitus.

4. Signs of liver disease (hepatosplenomegaly, jaundice, spider angiomata, or abnormal venous pattern of the abdomen).

5. Signs of malignancy (adenopathy, cachexia, hepatosplenomegaly, pallor, or palpable tumor mass).

6. Abnormal skin elasticity and hyperextensibility of joints suggesting connective tissue disorder (Ehlers-Danlos syndrome).

7. Purpura plus urticaria, swollen hands and feet, and abdominal or joint pain (Henoch-Schönlein purpura).

Ancillary Data ■

If the abnormal findings on history and physical examination suggest a bleeding disorder, perform four screening tests, including prothrombin time (PT), partial thromboplastin time (PTT), platelet count, and bleeding time (Table 19-3). Based on results of the screening tests, next perform definitive tests to establish the correct diagnosis (Table 19-4). Note that in mild bleeding disorders, especially von Willebrand's disease, all four screening tests may be normal. If the clinical signs and symptoms strongly suggest a bleeding disorder, order definitive tests anyway.

Treatment ■

See Chapter 136. The goals of therapy are to:

1. Stop bleeding by replacing the missing or defective clotting factor(s) and/or platelets.

2. Remove any offending drug(s) (e.g., aspirin) that are producing the bleeding.

3. Correct any hypovolemia and anemia (see Chapter 136 for principles of red blood cell transfusion).

4. Reduce tissue damage and pain due to pressure of blood in an enclosed space.

COAGULATION FACTOR REPLACEMENT

Hemophilia A

One unit of factor VIII per kg body weight will increase plasma factor VIII activity by 2%. The dose for

TABLE 19-1. *Severity of Hemophilia A or B*

Level of Severity	Factor Activity (%)	Usual Age at Presentation	Clinical Manifestations
Severe	<1	Birth–2 yrs	Spontaneous bleeding and bleeding with minor and major trauma and surgery
Moderate	1–5	1–5 yrs	Bleeding with minor trauma, major trauma, or surgery
Mild	5–30	3 yrs–adult	Bleeding with major trauma or surgery

TABLE 19–2. *Drugs Associated With Clinical Bleeding*

Decreased Plasma Clotting Factor Level or Function
Heparin
Warfarin (Coumadin)

Abnormal Platelet Function
Acetylsalicylic acid (aspirin)
Antihistamines
Clofibrate
Dextran sulfate
Dipyridamole (Persantin)
Glycerol guaiacolate
Nonsteroidal anti-inflammatory drugs
Penicillin derivatives
Sulfinpyrazone
Theophylline
Tricyclic antidepressants
Vasodilators

Antibody-Induced Thrombocytopenia
Analgesics
Antibiotics
Anticonvulsants
Cinchona alkaloids
Hypnotics
Nonsteroidal anti-inflammatory drugs
Propylthiouracil
Sedatives
Sulfonamide derivatives
Vaccines

Bone-Marrow Aplasia or Hypoplasia
Anticonvulsants
Antimetabolites
Benzene derivatives
Chloramphenicol
Chlorpropamide
Phenantoin
Phenylbutazone
Propylthiouracil
Sulfamethoxazole
Sulfamethoxypyridazine
Trimethadione
Tolbutamide

an early, mild to moderate bleed (e.g., into a joint, muscle, or soft tissue) is 20–25 units/kg to raise the plasma factor VIII activity to 40–50%. Usually a single dose is sufficient to stop the bleeding. The appropriate loading dose for a severe injury, life-threatening hemorrhage (e.g., central nervous system), or a bleed of longer than 24 hours' duration is 40–50 units/kg to raise the circulating factor VIII level to 80–100%. The maintenance dose for these severe bleeds is half the loading dose, or 20–25 units/kg, given every half-life of 8–12 hours. Judge adequacy of therapy by normalization of the PTT and by trough

factor VIII levels of 50% or greater. The length of time to maintain trough levels greater than 50% depends on the location and severity of the bleed, trauma, or surgery and can vary from 1 to 3 or 4 weeks. Consult a pediatric hematologist for long-term management once the patient is stabilized.

The blood products available for factor VIII replacement therapy are listed in Table 19-5. Calculate the dosage by rounding up to the nearest whole container (e.g., if the child weighs 20 kg, for a dose of 20 units/kg = 20 × 20 = 400 units, round up to 500 units or 20 ml) and administer the entire reconstituted dose.

Starting in 1985, all factor VIII concentrates have been dry-heat-treated to destroy HIV. Newer products available since 1987 include pasteurized, solvent-detergent-treated, and monoclonal-antibody-purified factor VIII concentrates. Each is increasingly safer against transmission of hepatitis B and non-A, non-B hepatitis. Now all factor VIII concentrates are infinitely safer with regard to transmission of these three viruses than either cryoprecipitate or fresh-frozen plasma *and are the preferred treatment when available.*

Cryoprecipitate is also a concentrated form of factor VIII, containing 5–7 units/ml. A single bag of cryoprecipitate is derived from a single donated unit of blood; however, cryoprecipitate cannot be heated or treated in any way to destroy viruses, so that the risk for transmission of HIV and hepatitis B and non-A, non-B is equal to the risk for that particular donor community. Fresh-frozen plasma is not a concentrate at all, but contains the same concentration of factor VIII activity (1 unit/ml) as is found in normal plasma. Volume overload constraints limit the amount of fresh-frozen plasma that can be given at one time to about 10 ml/kg; the maximum increase in factor VIII activity that this volume will produce is 20%, which is not enough to stop bleeding except in the mildest cases (see Table 19-1), where the circulating factor VIII level is already 20–30%. Fresh-frozen plasma has the same risk of transmitting HIV and hepatitis B and non-A, non-B hepatitis as does cryoprecipitate from the same donor community. Unless the patient is already immune, vaccination against hepatitis B is indicated (see Appendix 138). Note that this vaccine must be given SQ in hemophiliacs.

Recombinant factor VIII is under investigational protocol and should ultimately become the treatment of choice for hemophilia A because it will eliminate transmission of viral infections.

For some patients with very mild hemophilia A (factor VIII activity 10–30%), an additional treatment method is available that avoids exposure to blood products. This method involves an infusion of 1-desamino-8-D-arginine vasopressin (DDAVP, desmo-

TABLE 19–3. *Screening Tests for Abnormalities of Hemostasis*

Disorder	Prothrombin Time	Partial Thromboplastin Time	Platelet Count	Bleeding Time*
Hemophilia A, B, C	Normal	Long	Normal	Normal
von Willebrand's disease	Normal	Normal or Long	Normal	Normal or Long
Factor VII deficiency	Long	Normal	Normal	Normal
Factor I, II, V, X deficiency	Long	Long	Normal	Normal
Liver disease, vitamin K deficiency	Long	Long	Normal	Normal
Disseminated intravascular coagulation	Long	Long	Low	Long*
Thrombocytopenia	Normal	Normal	Low	Long*
Qualitative platelet function disorder	Normal	Normal	Normal	Long
Uremia	Normal	Normal	Normal	Long
Ehlers–Danlos syndrome	Normal	Normal	Normal	Normal or Long
Henoch–Schönlein purpura	Normal	Normal	Normal	Normal

* The bleeding time reflects platelet number as well as function and will become prolonged whenever the platelet count falls below 100,000/mm³, even if the platelet function is normal. Thus the platelet count must be obtained before the bleeding time is performed, and if the count is below 100,000, the bleeding time is not done.

pressin acetate, Stimate) at a dose of 0.3 micrograms/kg body weight given intravenously in 30 ml of normal saline over 30 minutes. (Note that this is a much larger dose than is given intranasally to patients with diabetes insipidus.) The drug acts by causing the release of factor VIII stores in the liver. The maximum factor VIII level occurs 1–4 hours after the infusion; it is usually back to baseline by 8–24 hours. The response is uncertain in individual patients. An infusion of DDAVP could be given and a PTT and factor VIII level drawn an hour later, but if the bleed is serious and the delay for lab results could lead to potentially life-threatening hemorrhaging, choose one of the factor VIII replacement products instead.

TABLE 19–4. *Definite Tests For Abnormalities of Hemostasis*

Disorder	Definite Test(s)
Hemophilia A, B, C	Factor VIII, IX, XI activity
von Willebrand's disease	Factor VIII activity, von Willebrand antigen, ristocetin cofactor activity, factor VIII-related multimers
Factor VII deficiency	Factor VII activity
Factor I, II, V, X deficiency	Factor I, II, V, X activity
Liver disease	Factor VII activity, fibrinogen, ALT, bilirubin
Vitamin K deficiency	Factor VII activity, fibrinogen
Disseminated intravascular coagulation	Fibrinogen, fibrin D-dimers (or fibrin split products)
Thrombocytopenia	Platelet-associated immunoglobulin, bone marrow biopsy
Qualitative platelet dysfunction	Platelet aggregation studies
Uremia	BUN, creatinine
Ehlers–Danlos syndrome	Skin biopsy
Henoch–Schönlein purpura	ESR, urinalysis, IgA

TABLE 19–5. *Blood Products Available for Replacement Therapy in Hemophilia A*

Product	Factor VIII Content (units/ml)	Volume per Container (ml)
Factor VIII Concentrate		
Monoclonal purified (Hemofil-M, Monoclate-P)	25–125	2.5, 5, 10
Solvent-detergent treated (Koate HP, Profilate SD)	25–150	5, 10, 25
Pasteurized (Humate P, Koate HS)	25	10, 20, 40
Cryoprecipitate	5–7	15–20
*Fresh-Frozen Plasma**	1	200–250

* The large volume of plasma required to achieve hemostasis would result in circulatory overload. Therefore, fresh-frozen plasma should not be used unless none of the other products is available.

Manage specific bleeds as follows:

1. *Soft tissue, joint, and muscle bleeds:* A single dose of 20–25 units/kg of factor VIII is often adequate to control bleeding, but if pain persists and swelling increases or does not decrease, give a loading dose of 40–50 units/kg followed by maintenance doses of 20–25 units/kg every 8–12 hours until pain and swelling have subsided. The joint may need to be splinted in the position of comfort for 2–3 days, followed by physical therapy to regain range of motion and strength.
2. *Surface wounds:* Small superficial cuts, including venipuncture sites, may require only local pressure for 10–15 minutes. Suturing, if required, must be preceded by a single infusion of 40–50 units/kg of factor VIII. Leave sutures in place for 8–10 days, even on the face, to allow complete healing to take place.
3. *Mouth bleeds:* Loss of deciduous or permanent teeth due to trauma and lacerations of the tongue, frenulum, and soft tissues in the mouth may bleed for weeks unless adequate therapy is given. Achieve hemostasis by infusing a dose of factor VIII concentrate of 40–50 units/kg to raise the circulating factor VIII level to 100%. Then prescribe a plasminogen inhibitor such as epsilon-amino caproic acid (EACA or Amicar) at a dose of 100 mg/kg/dose (maximum dose 6 grams) given every 6 hours around the clock for 10–14 days to prevent digestion of the clot by the proteolytic enzymes of the saliva. Instruct the patient to eat only soft foods while on Amicar to prevent mechanical dis-

lodging of the clot. Amicar should *not* be given if hematuria is present.
4. *Intracranial hemorrhage:* Carefully screen all hemophiliacs following head trauma, as well as patients with severe hemophilia even without known antecedent trauma who present with suspicious neurologic symptoms or signs (such as severe headache). Immediately infuse 40–50 units/kg factor VIII concentrate to raise the circulating factor VIII level to 100%. Perform CT imaging of the head only after adequate factor VIII levels have been achieved. Continue factor VIII replacement for 1–3 days if the scans are negative. See below for managing operative intervention.
5. *Surgery:* Give an initial loading dose of 40–50 units/kg factor VIII just before surgery, and document the actual factor VIII level achieved by a PTT and factor VIII level drawn immediately after the infusion. These can be performed while surgery commences, and additional factor VIII can be given intraoperatively if the initial factor VIII level did not reach 100%. Consult a pediatric hematologist to assist with intraoperative and postoperative management of clotting.
6. *Epistaxis:* See Chapter 35. Cut bullet-shaped pieces of salt pork large enough to fit snugly in the nostril. Insert one piece on each side and hold in place by applying a large piece of tape across the cheeks and nostrils. Remove the tape after approximately 18–24 hours, allowing the pieces of salt pork to slide out of the nostrils without dislodging the clots. If the bleeding is so brisk that the salt pork will not stay in place initially, administer a dose

TABLE 19–6. *Management of Patients With Inhibitors*

Level of Inhibitor	Maximum Inhibitor Titer (BU)	Replacement Therapy
Low	<2	Factor VIII concentrate: increase dose by 25%–50%
Moderate	2–10	Factor IX concentrate, 75–100 units/kg
High	>10	Activated factor Xa (Autoplex or FEIBA), 75–100 units/kg

of factor VIII concentrate of 20–25 units/kg to achieve initial hemostasis before the salt pork is inserted. Use the salt pork even if the bleeding has stopped after the factor VIII infusion, because often it will resume when the patient arrives home.

7. *Hematuria:* History of trauma to the kidneys and/or painful hematuria are indications for radiographic studies to determine the location and extent of the bleeding and whether surgical intervention is indicated (see Chapter 57). If surgery is to be performed or if there is a large subcapsular hematoma, infuse 40–50 units/kg factor VIII; otherwise, give 20–25 units/kg factor VIII and follow the patient closely. For spontaneous, *painless* hematuria, begin oral prednisone at 2 mg/kg/day until hematuria has cleared and then in tapering doses for the next 6 days. Gross hematuria will usually resolve in one day, but microscopic hematuria may persist for 2–3 days after clearing of the gross hematuria. Amicar is contraindicated when there is renal bleeding because it inhibits the urokinase system of the kidney and can result in a clotted kidney.

8. *Inhibitors:* About 10–15% of patients with severe hemophilia A will develop inhibitors to factor VIII, which are antibodies that irreversibly inactivate any factor VIII that is administered. Suspect an inhib-

itor when a large dose of factor VIII (50 units/kg) does not correct the PTT or raise the factor VIII level and when clinically the patient does not improve after several doses of factor VIII concentrate (Table 19-6).

Hemophilia B

Products available for replacement therapy are listed in Table 19-7. One unit of factor IX activity per kg body weight will raise the circulating factor IX level by 1%. Thus, the dose for a mild to moderate bleed is 40–50 units/kg, while the loading dose for a severe bleed, trauma, or surgery is 80–100 units/kg followed by a maintenance dose of 40–50 units/kg given every half-life of 12–24 hours until healing is complete. The same principles of management apply as for factor VIII deficiency. The factor IX products (prothrombin complex concentrates) listed in Table 19-7 are all dry-heat-treated, so that while the risk for HIV transmission has been virtually eliminated, the risk for transmission of hepatitis B and non-A, non-B hepatitis remains.

Fresh-frozen plasma may be used to treat mild bleeding episodes in patients with very mild hemophilia B (factor IX level 20–30%). However, since

TABLE 19–7. *Blood Products Available for Replacement Therapy in Hemophilia B*

Product	Factor IX Content (units/ml)	Volume per Container (ml)
Prothrombin complex concentrate, dry heat-treated (Konyne, Profilnine)	25	20, 40
Fresh-frozen plasma*	1	200–250

* The large volume of plasma required to achieve hemostasis would result in circulatory overload. Therefore, fresh-frozen plasma should not be used unless none of the other products is available.

TABLE 19–8. *Classification of von Willebrand's Disease*

Type	Abnormality
I	Quantitative decrease of normal von Willebrand's factor
II	Qualitatively abnormal von Willebrand's factor with decreased or absent binding to platelets
III	Total absence of von Willebrand's factor

the concentration of factor IX (1 unit/ml) is the same as in normal plasma, volume constraints limit the amount that can be safely administered to approximately 10 ml/kg; this will produce a rise of only 20%, which is not adequate for surgery, major bleeding, or trauma. In these cases, factor IX concentrate must be used. The risk of transmission of HIV, hepatitis B, and non-A, non-B hepatitis by fresh-frozen plasma is the same as the general risk for that donor community.

Do not use factor VIII concentrate or cryoprecipitate for treating patients with hemophilia B, as they do not contain factor IX.

Other Congenital Disorders of Coagulation

1. *Hemophilia C (factor XI deficiency):* Treatment is with fresh frozen plasma, 10 ml/kg given every 6–12 hours.
2. *Von Willebrand's disease:* Von Willebrand's disease is subdivided into type I (quantitative decrease of normal von Willebrand factor), type II (qualitative abnormality of von Willebrand factor), and type III (total absence of von Willebrand factor) (Table 19-8).
   For all patients with type I and most patients with type II von Willebrand's disease, 1-desamino-8-D-arginine vasopressin (DDAVP, desmopressin

acetate, Stimate) is effective in controlling bleeding by releasing stored von Willebrand factor from endothelial cells (Table 19-9). The dose is 0.3 micrograms/kg given intravenously in 30 ml of normal saline over 30 minutes. The maximal effect is seen 1–4 hours after infusion and may persist for up to 7–10 days in some patients. Look for correction of the bleeding time about an hour post-infusion. Repeat the bleeding time every 24 hours to judge when a second infusion is needed. Consult a pediatric hematologist to assist with children who fail to respond.
3. *Factor VII deficiency:* Treat with fresh-frozen plasma, 10 ml/kg for mild disease or 10 ml/kg/hour for severe disease with life-threatening bleeding. Consult a pediatric hematologist for appropriate management.
4. *Congenital afibrinogenemia (factor I deficiency):* Cryoprecipitate is the product of choice for treating fibrinogen deficiency, either congenital or acquired. One bag per 2 kg of body weight will raise the fibrinogen level to normal (250–400 mg/dl); the half-life is 3–4 days. Fresh-frozen plasma contains fibrinogen in the same concentration as normal plasma (2.5–4.0 mg/ml), so that the maximum volume that can be safely infused at one time, 10 ml/kg, will raise the fibrinogen level by about 50 mg/dl. This will achieve adequate hemostasis only in the mildest deficiencies.
5. *Factors II, V, X:* Treat with fresh frozen plasma, 10 ml/kg body weight given every 6–12 hours. Adequacy of treatment can be judged by normalization of the PT and PTT and by achieving factor levels of 40–50%.

Acquired Disorders of Clotting Factors

1. *Liver disease:* Abnormalities of hemostasis may accompany liver disease due to any etiology, including viral hepatitis, passive congestion, and cryptogenic cirrhosis. Decreased synthetic capacity of

TABLE 19–9. *Products Available for Treatment of von Willebrand's Disease*

Product	Dose	Type of VWD
DDAVP (Desmopressin acetate, Stimate)	0.3 mg/kg IV in 30 ml saline over 30 minutes	I, II
Cryoprecipitate	1 bag/2–5 kg	I, II, III
Pasteurized factor VIII concentrate (Humate-P, Koate HS)	Mild bleed: 20–25 units/kg Severe bleed: 40–50 units/kg	I, II, III

TABLE 19–10. *Dosage of Vitamin K to Correct Prothrombin Time*

Route	Dose	Time to Correct PT
PO	5–10 mg	18–24 hr
SQ	1–5 mg	12–18 hr
IM	1–5 mg	8–12 hr
IV*	1–2 mg *slow* (1 hr)	4–6 hr

* When giving intravenously, do not administer more rapidly because flushing, tachycardia, dyspnea, and hypotension may occur.

the hepatocytes leads to deficiency of all the clotting factors except factor VIII. The vitamin K-dependent factors II, VII, IX, and X decline first, followed by XI, V, and fibrinogen. If the fibrinogen level is still normal, give fresh frozen plasma, 10 ml/kg every 6–24 hours, to correct the bleeding tendency. Look for correction of the PT and PTT one hour after the infusion. However, if the fibrinogen is low, the PT and PTT will not be corrected and bleeding will not stop until cryoprecipitate, 1 bag/2–5 kg, is given. In this case, document correction of the fibrinogen level as well as the PT and PTT. Consult a pediatric hematologist for help with this complex problem.

2. *Vitamin K deficiency:* Administration of Vitamin K will correct the prolonged PT and PTT in 4–24 hours, depending on the route of administration. The routes, doses, and times for correction are indicated in Table 19-10.

   For emergency treatment of severe hemorrhage, fresh-frozen plasma at a dose of 10 ml/kg should be immediately administered, followed by Vitamin K, preferably given IV over one hour.

   For hypoprothrombinemia of the newborn:
   a. Prophylaxis: 0.5–1.0 mg IM, SQ or PO.
   b. Therapy: 1–2 mg IM or IV.

   For malabsorption (obstructive jaundice, malabsorption syndromes, chronic diarrhea, malnutrition, chronic antibiotic therapy):
   a. Prophylaxis: Vitamin K 1–2 mg IM or IV every other day.
   b. Therapy: 2–5 mg IM or IV.

   For drug-induced hypoprothrombinemia (warfarin or Coumadin):
   a. Therapeutic doses: Discontinue the drug. Administer Vitamin K, 2–5 mg IM or IV. If PT is greater than 24 sec, or immediate correction is required, give fresh-frozen plasma, 10 ml/kg.
   b. Overdose or accidental ingestion: Give Vitamin K, 25–50 mg IM or IV (3 mg/m^2/min) every 8

hours and follow the PT. Fresh-frozen plasma, 10 ml/kg, will rapidly improve the clotting abnormalities but may not fully correct them. Repeat the PT every 6 hours until stable off therapy for 72 hours.

3. *DIC:* Activation by platelets and disseminated consumption of clotting factors can occur in a variety of disease states, such as sepsis, hypoxia, hypovolemia, acidosis, massive trauma, or burns. Identification and correction of the underlying disorder is the most important step in managing DIC. Consult a pediatric hematologist for assistance with this complex problem.

Platelet Disorders

1. *Thrombocytopenia* may be due to decreased bone marrow production or increased destruction.

   Causes of decreased production include leukemia, lymphoma, neuroblastoma or other malignancy, aplastic anemia, chronic infection, and chemotherapy. In these conditions, give a platelet transfusion, one unit per 5 kg, before surgery if the platelet count is below 50,000, or for symptomatic bleeding at any platelet count. The risk of severe life-threatening (i.e., central nervous system) bleeding increases greatly when the platelet count falls below 10,000, so give platelets prophylactically at that time. Products available for replacement therapy are listed in Table 19-11. Obtain a platelet count 1 hour post-transfusion and then every 24 hours thereafter.

   Thrombocytopenia due to increased destruction of platelets may result from antibody production (immune thrombocytopenic purpura) or from sequestration in a large spleen or hemangioma. In these instances prophylactic administration of platelets will not result in a demonstrable rise in platelet count 1 hour post-transfusion, so avoid prophylactic platelet transfusions. However, if the patient is acutely bleeding, then transfuse 1 unit platelets/5 kg every 6 hours to stop the bleeding, since half the platelets will go to the bleeding site immediately and be incorporated in the clot before they can be removed from the circulation by the spleen.

2. *Platelet function disorders:* Treat only symptomatic bleeding episodes that cannot be managed with local measures (e.g., salt-pork for epistaxis, Amicar for oral bleeding, prednisone and/or bed rest for hematuria) and major trauma, as well as before and after surgery. Transfuse 1 unit platelets/5 kg, test for correction of bleeding time 1 hour post-transfusion and then every 24 hours; consult a pediatric hematologist for long-term management.

TABLE 19–11. *Products Available for Platelet Replacement*

Product	Dose	Expected Rise in Platelet Count
Plateletpheresis unit	1/4 unit (60 ml*)/5 kg	50–100,000
Platelet concentrate	1 unit (60 ml*)/5 kg	50–100,000
Platelet-rich plasma	10 ml/kg	30,000
Fresh whole blood	10 ml/kg	15,000

* For small infants and for patients in whom large volumes may produce cardiovascular overload, a "dry" unit with a volume of 30 ml may be requested.

Caveats ∎

1. Never give aspirin to a patient with a bleeding disorder.
2. Never give intramuscular injections to a patient with a bleeding disorder.
3. Never take rectal temperatures or give suppositories to a patient with a bleeding disorder.
4. Never do fingersticks, heelsticks, jugular sticks, femoral sticks, or arterial sticks in a patient with a possible bleeding disorder.
5. If patient's hepatitis B status is unknown, immunize at time of diagnosis or first exposure to blood products with hepatitis B vaccine, 0.5 ml subcutaneously in the upper arm for a child under age 10, or 1 ml subcutaneously in the upper arm for a child 10 years and older. Repeat in 1 and 6 months.

Bibliography ∎

Biggs R: *The treatment of haemophilia A and B and von Willebrand's disease,* 2nd edition. Oxford: Blackwell Scientific Publications, 1978.

Boone D: *Comprehensive management of hemophilia.* Philadelphia: FA Davis Company, 1976.

Hilgartner MW: *Hemophilia in children.* Littleton MA: Publishing Sciences Group, Inc., 1976.

Lusher JM, Barnhart MI: *Acquired bleeding disorders in children: Abnormalities of hemostasis.* New York: Masson Publishing USA, Inc., 1981.

Lusher JM, Barnhart MI: *Acquired bleeding disorders in children: Platelet abnormalities and laboratory methods.* New York: Masson Publishing USA, Inc., 1981.

Menache D, Surgenor DM, Anderson H: *Hemophilia and hemostasis.* New York: Alan Liss, Inc., 1981.

20 Coma

Thomas K. Koch

Coma is not a disease, but rather a state of central nervous system depression or dysfunction that may result from many different life-threatening conditions. In most situations, the initial evaluation will indicate the anatomic site, suggest the etiology, and allow for the immediate institution of appropriate therapy. This initial therapy is often life-saving.

Definitions ■

Coma is a state of unconsciousness from which the patient cannot be aroused ("unarousable unresponsiveness"). There is no speech, the eyes do not open, and the extremities do not move to command, nor do they appropriately ward off noxious stimuli. Reflex movements may be retained.

Stupor is a state similar to coma except that the patient is arousable only with vigorous stimulation. When the stimulation ceases, the patient immediately returns to an unresponsive state.

Obtundation is a state similar to stupor except that the patient can be aroused with stimulation and can maintain the aroused state after removal of the stimulus.

Anatomy of Consciousness ■

Consciousness requires both *arousal* and *awareness*. Arousal is simply wakefulness, which is clinically manifested by spontaneous or stimulus-induced eye-opening. Activation of the reticular activating system (RAS), which spans the paramedian regions from the midbrain to the level of the midpons, results in arousal. Awareness is the ability to recognize self and the environment. Awareness allows for the accomplishment of goal-directed or purposeful tasks. This ability implies integrity of the cerebral hemispheres. With compromise of either one or both of these structures, the patient will be rendered unconscious. A chronic condition emerging after severe cortical injury, distinct from coma by intact arousal but without awareness, has been termed "persistent vegetative state."

Etiology and Pathophysiology ■

In general terms, the pathophysiologic mechanisms responsible for the production of coma may be considered in three broad categories: *mass lesions, metabolic encephalopathy,* and *seizures.* The goal in evaluating the comatose patient is to arrive at the correct etiologic *category* so that appropriate diagnostic and therapeutic measures may proceed in a timely fashion.

1. *Mass lesions* (tumors, abscesses, hematomas) may be either supratentorial or subtentorial. Supratentorial lesions produce coma by brainstem compression through either central downward or uncal herniation, while subtentorial lesions may cause either intrinsic brainstem damage or extrinsic compression of the brainstem. *Head trauma is one of the most important causes of mass lesions leading to coma in children.* Given a history of closed head trauma, it is imperative to evaluate the patient for intra- and/or extraaxial hematomas. Severe brain swelling termed "malignant hyperemia" may also occur in children after severe head trauma without a mass lesion. Consider the shaken-child syndrome in any child with head trauma and a suspicious history.

2. *Metabolic abnormalities* produce diffuse disturbances of brain function. This is usually symmetric, although it may alternate side to side. Common causes of metabolic coma include hypoxic ischemia, hypoglycemia, toxin or drug ingestion, hepatic failure, Reye's syndrome, uremia, infection, hypothermia, diabetic ketoacidosis, hyponatremia, adrenal failure, and myxedema. *A characteristic feature of metabolic coma is preservation of the pupillary light reflex despite depression of more caudal brainstem functions.* Notable exceptions

to this include glutethimide intoxication, high-dose barbiturates, atropine, profound hypothermia, and anoxia. In children, miotic pupils are often seen in drug ingestions and are distinctly unusual with trauma-related coma.

3. *Seizures* and the postictal state may present as unconsciousness. Although seizures usually are accompanied by some clinical manifestations, on occasion they may be absent. If there is significant clinical suspicion to consider seizures as an etiology, an immediate electroencephalogram (EEG) is necessary. A prolonged postictal state may follow status epilepticus and may occur in patients with a chronic encephalopathy.

Clinical Findings ■

A careful *history* from the parents or caretaker may provide the diagnosis. Fever, antecedent symptoms, exposure to drugs or poisons, past medical history, and possible trauma are key historical features.

The *examination* of the comatose patient may provide important clues as to the etiology of the coma. Pay immediate attention to the vital functions. In addition to airway patency and respirations, blood pressure and heart rate need careful monitoring. An elevated blood pressure may indicate an intracranial hemorrhage or a posterior fossa mass lesion. The fundiscopic examination may reveal papilledema, indicating increased intracranial pressure. When present, retinal hemorrhages imply trauma, acute hypertension, or increased intracranial pressure. Check the head, ears, and nose for signs of trauma, including Battle's sign (hemotympanum), raccoon eyes, and CSF leakage. A stiff neck implies meningeal irritation from infection, subarachnoid blood, or cerebellar tonsillar herniation.

NEUROLOGIC EVALUATION

The neurologic examination of the comatose patient consists of five simple assessments of cortical and brainstem integrity: *level of consciousness, respiratory pattern, pupillary reflexes, extraocular motility,* and *motor response to stimulation.* The patient's response can be correlated with specific levels of brain function and can help establish an anatomic understanding for the patient's coma. Also, the pattern of response is indicative of the pathophysiologic etiology.

1. *Level of consciousness* is best assessed by the ease and degree of arousal. Eye-opening indicates an intact RAS. Eye-opening may occur spontaneously or only in response to either verbal or painful stimulation. In the truly comatose patient, there is *no* arousal.

2. *Respiratory pattern,* when normal, indicates brainstem integrity. Cheyne-Stokes or periodic respirations in which hyperventilation and apnea alternate may be seen with bilateral cortical or upper brainstem (thalamus/upper midbrain) damage. True hyperventilation may be seen with acid-base abnormalities or midbrain damage causing central neurogenic hyperventilation. Ataxic or irregular breathing suggests pontomedullary dysfunction.

3. *Pupillary reflexes* are the single most important feature in the examination of the comatose patient. Symmetric pupils 3–4 mm in diameter that are responsive to light both directly and consensually indicate midbrain integrity. As mentioned earlier, most forms of metabolic coma preserve the pupillary light reflex. Midposition, fixed pupils indicate midbrain failure and usually imply severe, often irreversible brainstem injury. They are commonly called the "pupils of death."

4. *Extraocular motility* can be tested on a reflex level using the oculocephalic (doll's eyes) or oculovestibular response (caloric stimulation). To elicit the oculocephalic reflex, the patient's eyes are opened and the head is rotated from side to side. If full conjugate gaze is elicited, then the midbrain and pons are intact and this essentially excludes a posterior fossa lesion as an etiology. If the maneuver is negative (eyes remain straight ahead within the head) then a stronger stimulus needs to be given. Perform cold water calorics after the integrity of the tympanic membrane is documented. To perform the maneuver, place the head in midline with 30 degrees of elevation. Inject about 30–50 ml of ice water into the ear canal. If the midbrain and pons are intact, there will be tonic deviation of the both eyes toward the side of the cold-water irrigation. If only the ipsilateral eye abducts without the contralateral eye adducting, the patient has an internuclear ophthalmoplegia (INO), indicating a functioning pons but dysfunction to the medial longitudinal fasciculus (MLF) and/or midbrain. No response with either eye indicates pontine damage.

5. *Motor response* to painful stimulation (supraorbital, sternal, or nailbed compression) may be either purposeful withdrawal, abnormal posturing, or flaccid/unresponsiveness. Posturing is either decorticate (flexion of the upper extremities and extension of the lower) or decerebrate (extension of all extremities). Decorticate posturing may be seen with thalamic dysfunction, while decerebrate posturing indicates midbrain damage.

Glasgow Coma Scale

Neurosurgeons commonly grade the severity of coma using the Glasgow Coma Scale (see Table 50-1). This is a helpful way of quantifying coma to follow the patient serially, but because the Glasgow score does not evaluate specific brainstem integrity, it does not replace the neurologic examination.

Anatomic Stages of Coma ■

Four essential neurologic parameters (respiratory pattern, pupillary reflex, extraocular motility, and motor response) establish an anatomic level of nervous system function (Table 20-1). The *early diencephalic* stage corresponds to a level with an intact brainstem without cerebral hemispheric function. With the *late diencephalic* stage there is loss of thalamic function. The *midbrain* stage indicates damage to the midbrain and all rostral structures. The *pontomedullary* stage indicates total brainstem damage.

Differential Diagnosis ■

Clinical features characteristic of a metabolic coma include:

1. A mixed pattern of anatomic stages of involvement (i.e., reactive pupils, absent doll's-eye sign, absent calorics, ataxic breathing, purposeful withdrawal to pain);
2. Pupils that are usually reactive to light (exceptions noted above) despite early depression of consciousness and respirations;
3. Symmetric motor response to pain.

Suspect a supratentorial mass lesion if there is significant asymmetry to the examination and/or there is an evolving rostral-caudal progression to the coma (early diencephalic to late diencephalic to midbrain to pontomedullary stages), indicating a central downward herniation syndrome. Lesions in the medial portion of the temporal lobe may produce an uncal herniation syndrome, in which the patient presents with unilateral pupillary dilatation and diminished response to light. A complete pattern of midbrain dysfunction may develop rapidly due to the direct compression of the midbrain by the herniating uncus. Subtentorial mass lesions present with midbrain and pontine dysfunction. If the patient has not received narcotics, "pinpoint" pupils may reflect pontine damage. This may be further substantiated if an internuclear ophthalmoplegia is present.

Treatment ■

Immediate management of the comatose patient requires careful attention to the vital functions: airway, breathing, and circulation. Protecting the airway is imperative if it appears that the patient cannot maintain an adequate airway or ventilatory drive, followed by intubation and ventilatory support. Next, establish reliable intravenous access. While this is being performed, obtain a serum specimen for bedside dipstick glucose testing. If the dipstick value is below 100 mg%, or if the patient has diabetes or another disorder of glucose, give 1–2 ml/kg of 25% dextrose in water (<2 years) IV, or 1 ml/kg of 50% dextrose in water (>2 years). Last, administer naloxone, an opiate antagonist, 1–2 mg IV, or 0.4 mg in neonates.

TABLE 20–1. *Anatomic Stages of Coma*

	Early Diencephalic	Late Diencephalic	Midbrain	Pontomedullary
Respiratory Pattern	Normal or Cheyne–Stokes	Cheyne–Stokes	Cheyne–Stokes, hyperventilation	Ataxic
Pupillary Reflex	Small, reactive	Small, reactive	Midposition, fixed	Midposition, fixed
Extraocular Motility	Intact doll's/calorics	Intact doll's/calorics	INO*	Absent calorics
Motor Response	Appropriate	Decorticate	Decerebrate	Flaccid

* Internuclear ophthalmoplegia.

Ancillary Data and Disposition ■

Laboratory studies should include blood gases, blood sugar, complete blood count, electrolytes, BUN, creatinine, osmolality, liver functions, urinalysis, toxicology screen, and spinal fluid analysis (exclude mass lesion before doing a spinal tap). If a mass lesion is suspected as an etiology of the coma, perform an emergent computed tomography (CT) brain scan. If seizures are felt to play a role, then anticonvulsant therapy and an EEG are necessary.

Metabolic coma requires careful medical management in an intensive care unit with appropriate supportive care, or transfer to a pediatric critical care center. If infection is a major consideration, the patient needs an immediate lumbar puncture. Continued patient care depends on the results of the ancillary studies.

Bibliography ■

Caronna J, Simon R: The comatose patient: A diagnostic approach and treatment. *Int Anesthesiol Clin* 1979; 17: 3–18.

Edwards R, Simon R: Coma. In: Baker AB and Joynt RJ, eds. *Clinical Neurology*, vol. 2. Philadelphia: Harper & Row, 1979, 17:1–44.

Levy DE, Bates D, Caronna JJ, et al: Prognosis in nontraumatic coma. *Ann Intern Med* 1981; 94:293–301.

Plum F, Posner J: *The diagnosis of stupor and coma,* 3rd ed. Philadelphia: FA Davis, 1980.

Simon R: Coma. In: Berg BO, ed. *Child Neurology: A Clinical Manual.* Greenbrae: CA Jones Medical Publications, 1984; 20:287–301.

21 Cyanosis

Steven C. Cassidy and Scott J. Soifer

Cyanosis occurs in diseases involving different organ systems. It is defined as the blue discoloration of the skin, lips, mucous membranes, and nail beds caused by hemoglobin desaturation. Cyanosis may be acute or chronic, continual or episodic. The degree of cyanosis depends on the nature and severity of the underlying disease (see Table 21-1).

Etiology and Pathophysiology ■

CONGENITAL HEART DISEASE

Cyanosis occurs in congenital heart disease due to decreased pulmonary blood flow, intracardiac mixing of oxygenated and unoxygenated blood, and inadequate supply of oxygenated blood to the systemic circulation.

An obstruction to pulmonary blood flow causes cyanosis by decreasing pulmonary blood flow, leading to the right-to-left shunting of unoxygenated blood through atrial or ventricular septal defects, as in pulmonary atresia and tricuspid atresia with intact ventricular septum. Newborns become acutely cyanotic in the first week of life when the ductus arteriosus closes, restricting pulmonary blood flow. *The onset of cyanosis in the newborn period suggests ductus arteriosus-dependent cyanotic heart disease.* Older patients with these conditions are chronically cyanotic.

The most frequent cardiac cause of acute severe cyanosis is tetralogy of Fallot, a ventricular septal defect with pulmonary stenosis, right ventricular hypertrophy, and an overriding aorta. Cyanosis results from decreased pulmonary blood flow caused by infundibular, valvular and supravalvular pulmonary obstruction and right-to-left ventricular shunting of blood. Hypercyanotic episodes ("spells") can occur at any age in untreated patients but are most commonly seen in the first year of life. These episodes are characterized by hyperpnea, increasing cyanosis, syncope, limpness, and rarely convulsions, stroke, and death.

Cyanosis also occurs when bidirectional intracardiac shunting results in mixing of oxygenated and unoxygenated blood in the systemic circulation, as seen in truncus arteriosus, single ventricle, tricuspid atresia with a ventricular septal defect, and total anomalous pulmonary venous connection. These children are chronically cyanotic and often have congestive heart failure due to increased pulmonary blood flow.

Transposition of the great arteries is the most common cardiac cause of cyanosis in the newborn period. These patients are cyanotic because there are two parallel circulations: pulmonary venous blood is pumped back to the lungs, systemic venous blood is pumped back to the body. These patients are very cyanotic if there is inadequate mixing between the two circulations through a septal defect or a patent ductus arteriosus. Most infants present in the immediate newborn period. They are initially treated by a balloon atrial septostomy until definitive surgical correction.

Cyanosis also occurs when there is inadequate delivery of oxygenated blood to the systemic circulation. Infants who have left-sided obstructive diseases severe enough to cause circulatory failure (critical aortic stenosis, coarctation of the aorta, and interruption of the aortic arch) can be cyanotic if tissue oxygen delivery is severely impaired. Cyanosis results when sluggish blood flow causes increased oxygen uptake and subsequent venous hemoglobin desaturation. Symptoms develop when the ductus arteriosus closes and blood flow to the lower body greatly decreases. Older patients with less severe forms of these defects are rarely cyanotic. Similarly, children with severe arrhythmias (supraventricular tachycardia, complete heart block) or large pericardial effusions (with cardiac tamponade) can be cyanotic.

PULMONARY DISEASES

A variety of lung diseases can cause cyanosis. Cyanosis may be due to inadequate air movement into and out of the lungs, decreased pulmonary blood flow, or inadequate gas exchange across the alveolar-

123

TABLE 21–1. *Common Causes of Cyanosis*

Heart Disease	**Neuromuscular Diseases**
Tetralogy of Fallot	Apnea during seizure
Pulmonary atresia	CNS depression from drugs
Tricuspid atresia	Head trauma
Transposition of the great arteries	Central apnea
Total anomalous pulmonary venous connection	Werdnig–Hoffman disease
Single ventricle	Guillain–Barré syndrome
Truncus arteriosus	Muscular dystrophy
Secondary pulmonary vascular disease	Phrenic nerve trauma
Left-sided obstructive lesions	Ondine's curse
Lung and Airway Diseases	**Hematologic Disease**
Foreign body	Methemoglobinemia
Epiglottitis	Severe anemia
Croup	Sickle-cell disease
Tracheomalacia	Thalassemia
Asthma	
Bronchiolitis	**Gastrointestinal Disease**
Pneumonia	Gastroesophageal reflux
Pleural effusion	Tracheoesophageal fistula
Pneumothorax	Liver disease
Pulmonary embolism	Alagille syndrome
Pulmonary edema	**Miscellaneous**
Adult respiratory distress syndrome	Near-miss sudden infant death syndrome
Cystic fibrosis	Asphyxia

capillary membrane. Inadequate air movement can result from diseases of the airway such as severe croup, epiglottitis, status asthmaticus, intratracheal foreign body, and severe tracheomalacia. Air movement can also be impaired by lung compression due to a pleural effusion or pneumothorax, or by processes that restrict chest movement such as severe scoliosis. Decreased alveolar ventilation in these conditions leads to a mismatch of ventilation and perfusion. If untreated, respiratory failure can develop. Decreased pulmonary blood flow can be caused by a fat embolism after long bone fractures. Cyanosis caused by impaired diffusion of oxygen across the alveolar-capillary membranes occurs in pulmonary edema, pneumonia, and the adult respiratory distress syndrome. These patients may have respiratory distress.

Patients with cystic fibrosis or other chronic lung diseases are frequently seen in the emergency department (ED). These patients are chronically cyanotic from chronic airway obstruction, alveolar damage, and pulmonary hypertension. Worsening cyanosis suggests an acute process such as pneumonia or pneumothorax. These episodes may be life-threatening.

NEUROMUSCULAR DISEASES

Cyanosis occurs in patients with neuromuscular diseases or neurologic events secondary to hypoventi-lation. Central nervous system depression due to drug ingestion or coma can cause hypoventilation resulting in cyanosis. Transient hypoventilation and airway obstruction during seizures can cause cyanosis. Central apnea (Ondine's curse, apnea of prematurity) can cause hypoventilation. Peripheral neuromuscular diseases such as Werdnig-Hoffman disease, phrenic nerve trauma, Guillain-Barré Syndrome, and muscular dystrophy can also cause hypoventilation and cyanosis.

GASTROINTESTINAL DISEASES

Gastrointestinal disease occasionally causes cyanosis. Infants with gastroesophageal reflux may have the acute onset of cyanosis during or immediately after a feeding. These infants are likely to have an exaggerated vagal reflex, protective laryngospasm, and apnea.

HEMATOLOGIC DISEASES

Hematologic diseases may cause cyanosis due to the decreased oxygen-carrying capacity of the blood. Methemoglobinemia, either caused by the absence of hemoglobin reductase or by the presence of abnormal hemoglobin M, can cause cyanosis. Cyanosis occasionally occurs in severe anemia, or in hemoglobinopathies, such as sickle-cell disease or thalassemia major.

Clinical Findings ■

Cyanosis may indicate a life-threatening event or may represent a longstanding process. It is therefore important to start treatment while seeking the cause (see Table 21-2).

History may be key to determining the cause of cyanosis. Obtain information about the presence of any underlying chronic disease. Assess the duration and severity of the cyanosis, the association of any neurologic events, the relationship to feeding, the number of previous episodes, and the degree of respiratory distress.

Physical examination of the patient must first address the adequacy of ventilation. If ventilation is inadequate, institute prompt treatment (see Chapter 14). Record vital signs. Note the presence of arrhythmias, bradycardia, or tachycardia. Note the presence and depth of cyanosis. Examine the chest carefully visually for trauma, asymmetry of movement, retractions, precordial deformity, or previous thoracotomy. Chest percussion may demonstrate dullness caused by a consolidation or a pleural effusion or the hyperresonance of a pneumothorax. Auscultation of the lung fields will usually reveal evidence of airway or alveolar disease in the older child, but may be deceivingly normal in the infant. Medial displacement of the cardiac impulse indicates right ventricular hypertension. Auscultation of the heart for splitting of the second heart sound, extra sounds, or murmurs may be diagnostic. Palpate the pulses in all limbs. Nail clubbing suggests longstanding cyanosis.

Ancillary Data ■

Obtain an arterial blood gas measurement in all patients who are either acutely or severely cyanotic, have inadequate ventilation, or are in respiratory distress. Arterial blood gas analysis allows for rapid evaluation of ventilation, oxygenation, and acid-base status. Rapid treatment is needed in patients who are in respiratory failure or who have severe acidosis. If the arterial blood gas analysis reveals a normal pH and $PaCO_2$, and moderate hypoxemia, evaluation and treatment may proceed more slowly. Pulse oximetry and transcutaneous PaO_2 monitors are valuable for determining the degree of cyanosis and evaluating response to treatment. However, they offer no information about the patient's acid-base status.

Chest X-ray examination will confirm the presence of pulmonary or pleural disease suspected from clinical examination. X-rays may also reveal hyperinflation, suggesting unsuspected airway obstruction or a foreign body. Decreased pulmonary blood flow caused by cyanotic congenital heart disease may be evident. Evaluation of the adequacy of the airway and ventilation is essential before sending any patient to the radiology department. *Do not delay urgent treatment of respiratory failure, airway obstruction, or tension pneumothorax for an X-ray.*

Other imaging techniques may be useful. If congenital heart disease is suspected, perform an electrocardiogram and echocardiogram. Magnetic resonance imaging, computerized tomography, or occasionally barium swallow will diagnose airway obstruction caused by a foreign body or by extrinsic compression by a mass. Bronchoscopy may be needed to treat patients who have airway obstruction by a foreign body.

Differential Diagnosis ■

Although cyanosis is usually correctly diagnosed, confusing signs are occasionally found. Rubor, pallor,

---

TABLE 21–2. *Management of Cyanotic Patients*

Goal	Diagnosis	Therapy
Insure adequacy of airway and ventilation	Look in mouth, auscultation of neck and chest, arterial blood gas analysis	Suction, mechanical ventilation
Improve oxygenation	Arterial blood gas analysis, pulse oximeter	Administer O_2
Improve acid–base balance	Arterial blood gas analysis	Improve circulating volume, sodium bicarbonate, THAM
Improve oxygen-carrying capacity	Measure hemoglobin/hematocrit	Red cell transfusion
Improve circulating volume	Check skin temperature and liver size, measure urine output, central venous pressure	Intravenous fluid
Support blood pressure	Measure blood pressure	Improve circulating volume, inotropic support

and acrocyanosis, especially in infants and children, can mimic true cyanosis. Patients who have poor skin circulation from cold or frostbite can appear cyanotic. The goal of management is to differentiate cyanosis from these other signs.

Treatment ■

GENERAL PRINCIPLES

The ED physician must immediately evaluate the patient's level of consciousness and the adequacy of ventilation. Patients who are cyanotic, unconscious, and not spontaneously breathing require urgent intervention. After checking for neck injury, inspect and clear the airway. Start mechanical ventilation immediately, using mask-and-bag ventilation. Administer oxygen and perform elective tracheal intubation. Assess the adequacy of circulation and initiate cardiopulmonary resuscitation if necessary (see Chapter 6). In patients who are comatose and spontaneously breathing, assess the adequacy of the airway and ventilation using physical examination, arterial blood gas analysis, and pulse oximetry.

Patients present to the ED with different types of respiratory distress. Patients in respiratory distress caused by airway obstruction often have arterial blood gas evidence for respiratory failure (increased $PaCO_2$) before they are cyanotic. In these patients, hypoxemia indicates severe airway disease and demands prompt treatment. Patients in respiratory distress caused by alveolar disease are cyanotic due to impaired alveolar-capillary gas exchange. Administration of supplemental oxygen will often be sufficient to restore normal PaO_2.

Administer supplemental oxygen to all cyanotic patients until the etiology and the duration of the cyanosis is established. Supplemental oxygen may not decrease the degree of cyanosis as much in heart disease as it does in pulmonary disease. Patients with chronic obstructive airway disease should receive no more than 30–40% oxygen because they rely on hypoxic drive for ventilation. Similarly, newborns with congenital heart disease depend on a patent ductus arteriosus for pulmonary blood flow, for mixing, or for lower-body perfusion; therefore administer no more than 40% oxygen to avoid constricting the ductus arteriosus.

The acid-base balance is often disturbed in cyanotic patients. Decreased delivery of oxygen to the tissues causes a shift to anaerobic metabolism and the production of lactic acid. Consider correction of metabolic acidosis. Decreased oxygen-carrying capacity caused by anemia can worsen the ill effects of cyanosis. To improve oxygen-carrying capacity, hypoxemic patients should receive a red blood cell transfusion. The ideal hemoglobin concentration for cyanotic patients is 15–18 mg/dl.

Disposition ■

Admit to the hospital all patients who have acute or worsening severe cyanosis. Admit patients with respiratory distress, airway obstruction, or acid-base disturbance. Hospitalizing these patients will permit extended observation and monitoring as well as initial treatment of the cause of cyanosis.

Specific Conditions ■

CONGENITAL HEART DISEASES

Tetralogy of Fallot Spells

Place the child in the knee-chest position and administer supplemental oxygen. Administer intravenous fluid (10–20 ml/kg bolus of normal saline) to increase ventricular volume and increase pulmonary blood flow. In addition, sedate the patient with morphine sulfate (0.1 mg/kg). If the cyanosis persists despite these maneuvers, administer phenylephrine HCl intravenously (0.01 milligram/kg/dose, then infuse 0.3–0.5 µg/kg/minute). This will increase ventricular volume and systemic vascular resistance, decrease right-to-left shunt, increase pulmonary blood flow, and improve oxygenation.

Other Heart Disease

Cyanotic patients benefit from red blood cell transfusions to increase oxygen-carrying capacity. In newborns, an intravenous infusion of prostaglandin E_1 (0.05–0.1 µg/kg/min) reopens the ductus arteriosus, improves pulmonary blood flow and mixing of blood, and decreases cyanosis. In patients with other congenital heart disease, treatment of congestive heart failure with digoxin, diuretics, and red cell transfusion is beneficial (see Chapter 9).

PULMONARY DISEASES

In patients with upper airway obstruction, respiratory distress and stridor are usually evident. In these patients, careful inspection of the airway is necessary. Remove the foreign body if possible or, rarely, do cricothyrotomy (see Chapter 13). Epiglottitis is a special situation requiring emergency inspection of the airway by a qualified physician in the operating room (see Chapter 115). Anaphylaxis should be rapidly treated with epinephrine, diphenhydramine, cimetidine, steroids, and support of the airway if necessary (see Chapter 17).

Airway obstruction may also occur from croup (see Chapter 115).

Small airway disease causes wheezing, respiratory distress, and respiratory failure. Asthma is the most frequent small airway disease (see Chapter 15). Another small airway disease, bronchiolitis, is caused by infection by respiratory syncytial virus (see Chapter 116).

Patients who have lung compression caused by either pleural effusion or pneumothorax should have immediate evacuation of the fluid or air if ventilation is impaired (see Chapter 139 for procedure).

Pneumonia, pulmonary edema, and adult respiratory distress syndrome can cause cyanosis. Administration of oxygen may relieve cyanosis completely. Diuretic therapy may improve gas exchange and reduce cyanosis due to pulmonary edema caused by congestive heart failure. If the hypoxemia in these diseases is severe, administration of continuous positive airway pressure either by mask or after tracheal intubation may improve oxygenation.

OTHER DISEASES

Treat patients that have methemoglobinemia caused by absence of hemoglobin reductase with ascorbic acid (200–500 milligrams daily in divided doses) to decrease the proportion of circulating methemoglobin (see Chapter 83). There is no specific therapy for patients whose methemoglobinemia is caused by abnormal hemoglobin M.

Complications and Caveats ■

Most patients can tolerate brief periods of mild-to-moderate cyanosis without difficulty. Hypoxemia for longer periods and of greater degree can cause ischemia. The brain, heart, and kidneys are the most susceptible, since injury may occur after only 5 minutes of ischemia. Hypoxemia may cause the patient to have seizures, lose consciousness, or suffer a stroke. Decreased cardiac function or myocardial infarction can occur. Acute renal failure is common following hypoxemic insult. Permanent damage to muscle and skin generally take several hours of hypoxemia. During the initial treatment of cyanosis, the physician must carefully assess all organ systems for the sequelae of the hypoxemic insult.

Bibliography ■

Adams FH, Emmanouilides GC, ed.: *Moss' heart disease in infants, children, and adolescents,* 3rd ed. Baltimore: Williams & Wilkins, 1983.

Kendig EL, Chernick V: *Disorders of the respiratory tract in children,* 3rd ed. Philadelphia: WB Saunders, 1977.

Levin DL, Morriss FC, Moore GC: *A practical guide to pediatric intensive care,* 2nd ed. St. Louis: CV Mosby, 1984.

Rogers MC: *Textbook of pediatric intensive care.* Baltimore: Williams & Wilkins, 1987.

Rudolph AM, Hoffman JIE, eds.: *Pediatrics,* 18th ed. Los Altos, CA: Appleton & Lange, 1988.

22 Dehydration

Ronald A. Dieckmann

Dehydration is a common pediatric emergency. Acute gastroenteritis, the usual cause, accounts for about 5% of all outpatient visits and 3–5% of pediatric hospital admissions. Gastroenteritis in its extreme forms can be life-threatening; it is a leading etiology for reversible shock in infants and children. Early identification of the distressed child and vigilant management with oral and parenteral fluids will avert major complications.

Etiology and Pathophysiology ■

Acute dehydration refers to loss of extracellular water and sodium. Since water diffuses freely between the intracellular space (ICS) and extracellular space (ECS), rapid losses of extracellular water and sodium soon cause intracellular losses of water and the principal intracellular cation, potassium. The duration of the dehydration determines expected relative losses from each space or compartment. For periods of dehydration of 2–7 days, water losses are considered 60% ECS and 40% ICS. Therapy is aimed at replenishing water and cations for both compartments.

Dehydration in children is most often caused by infectious diarrhea, with or without vomiting. In the United States and the developed world, viruses are the usual pathogens, particularly rotavirus or reovirus. Rotavirus alone causes three-fourths of winter diarrhea and about one-fourth of summer diarrhea. Other important pathogens for childhood gastroenteritis are enumerated in Chapter 29. Many of these agents produce disease by directly invading the intestinal mucosal cells, while others elaborate powerful enterotoxins that mediate the intestinal dysfunctions.

In the invasive form of viral gastroenteritis, direct cellular invasion causes an inflammatory response that interrupts sodium resorption and, secondarily, water resorption. In the toxigenic form, enterotoxins bind to mucosal cell plasma membranes without inflammation and impair sodium resorption. In both invasive and toxigenic illness, unabsorbed water and solute are lost as diarrheal stools. Electrolyte losses are typically higher with toxigenic diarrhea.

Other non-diarrheal conditions occasionally produce significant water and electrolyte losses. Table 22-1 lists important conditions that may result in acute dehydration. Insensible losses from the skin are especially important in the very young child (under 6 months) with fever and tachypnea, environmental exposure, or a large burn area.

Clinical Findings ■

Regardless of the exact etiology for dehydration, emergency management must be directed at immediate volume restoration and reversal of circulatory insufficiency. The urgency of volume resuscitation and the composition of fluid and electrolyte administration is based on rapid *clinical* assessment of the degree of dehydration. This assessment is derived from key physical findings, which approximate the acute state as *mild* (3–5%), *moderate* (5–10%) or *severe* (>10%) *dehydration*. Table 22-2 lists clinical features of these three categories. Physical features reflect sequential intrinsic homeostatic adjustments to the decreasing availability of solute and decreasing perfusion. In children, tachycardia and peripheral vasoconstriction are the most sensitive adaptive responses.

In addition to the clinical findings in Table 22-2, evaluation of hydration status also includes body weight and vital signs. If the child's pre-illness weight is known, comparison to weight at presentation is quite useful for calculating water deficit. Abrupt changes in body weight over days are almost always secondary to water loss. Vital signs require adjustments for age (see Chapter 133). Blood pressure, however, is a relatively poor indicator of decreased perfusion. Children compensate for shock for extended periods through increases in heart rate and arteriolar vasoconstriction, then suddenly decompensate. Blood pressure plummets, and they develop irreversible shock. Blood pressure below 70% of

TABLE 22–1. *Nondiarrheal Causes of Dehydration*

Skin Losses
Burns
Open wounds
Sweat

Inadequate Intake
Anorexia
Stomatitis
Pharyngitis

Errors in Formula Preparation

Sepsis, Pneumonia, Meningitis

Polyuria
Renal insufficiency, with salt wasting
Overtreatment with diuretics
Mineralocorticoid deficiency
Diabetes mellitus
Diabetes insipidus

Hemorrhage from Trauma

Poisoning

Hyperthermia

Body Fluid Losses
Colostomy losses
CSF drainage

predicted normal for age (80 + twice age in years) represents a dire cardiovascular state requiring immediate intervention.

The "tilt test" is a better measure of volume status than blood pressure. Serial determinations of heart rate and blood pressure are obtained one minute apart, with the child in the supine, sitting, and standing positions. Increases in heart rate of more than 20/bpm are well correlated with moderate to severe dehydration.

Ancillary Data ■

Laboratory assessment of dehydration is secondary to clinical examination. Its role is to fine-tune evaluation and management. The following tests are helpful: complete blood count, sodium, potassium, chloride, CO_2, BUN, creatinine, calcium, glucose, osmolality, and urinalysis. Arterial blood gases may be worthwhile in severe cases. A moderate-severe dehydration state causes increased hematocrit, increased BUN with normal creatinine, decreased CO_2 and decreased arterial pH. Increased urine specific gravity is quite sensitive to mild dehydration but is relatively nonspecific to degree (see Table 22-2.)

Serum sodium concentration does not indicate degree of dehydration, but does provide the basis for a conventional osmolal classification of dehydration states. This system uses serum sodium level to divide dehydration into *hyponatremic, isotonic,* and *hypernatremic* forms; appropriate rates for volume restoration and the sodium concentration in replacement fluids can then be derived. Serum potassium levels do not reflect body potassium stores. Indeed, serum potassium in moderate-severe dehydration is high because of associated acidosis, despite significant intracellular hypokalemia. This is especially noteworthy in infants where hypotonia, weakness,

TABLE 22–2. *Clinical Spectrum of Dehydration*

	Mild	Moderate	Severe
Weight Loss (% total body weight)	3%–5%	10%	15%
Approximate Deficit	30–5 ml/kg	50%–100%	>1,000 ml/kg
Clinical Features:			
Heart rate	Normal	Usually normal	Rapid, weak
	± tilt test	± tilt test	
Blood pressure	Normal	Usually normal	Decreased (<70% normal)
Respirations	Normal	Deep	Deep, rapid
Mental status	Alert, restless	Lethargic	Obtuned, comatose
Skin	Cold, sweaty	Cold, dry	Cool, doughy
Turgor			
Eyes	Sunken	Sunken	Sunken
Fontanelle	Depressed	Depressed	Depressed

abdominal distention, and hyporeflexia may be manifestations of intracellular hypokalemia.

Metabolic acidosis is often present in dehydration, particularly in hyponatremic forms where hypoperfusion develops early in the process. While metabolic acidosis is quite sensitive as a laboratory indicator of dehydration, it rarely requires treatment, other than volume and electrolyte replacement.

Hypocalcemia is sometimes seen in the profoundly dehydrated child; however, there is no evidence to support routine administration of calcium. Instead, calcium replacement may be considered after initial volume resuscitation. *Hypoglycemia* may occur in the young (under 5 years) dehydrated child. Adding dextrose to replacement fluids is necessary with this age group, after primary stabilization. Occasionally, rapid administration of 1–2 ml/kg of $D_{25}W$ is indicated in the profoundly hypoglycemic child (see Chapter 103).

Characteristics of Osmolal Dehydration States ■

About 75% of dehydration states are *isotonic,* where salt and water are lost in equal proportions. Fifteen percent of cases are *hypernatremic* (serum sodium >150 mEq/l), a condition seen most often in infants with voluminous hypotonic diarrheal losses from viral illness, exacerbated by vomiting and early cessation of oral intake. *Hyponatremic* dehydration (serum sodium <130 mEq/l) comprises 10% of cases in the United States; it often presents in the child who continues to take hypotonic oral solution in the presence of persistent diarrhea.

Clinical characteristics of these different osmolal states are noted in Table 22-3. Hypernatremic dehydration preserves perfusion longer and manifests CNS symptoms earlier.

Treatment ■

After clinical assessment of degree of dehydration, a strategy for volume and solute replacement is initiated. Laboratory analysis, frequent reassessment of response to therapy, and volume of ongoing losses provide modifications to the rehydration plan. All calculations are crude, since homeostatic mechanisms in the brain and kidney effect sensitive internal adjustments, once rehydration is established.

Total volume and solute needs = Deficit replacement + maintenance requirements + ongoing losses.

1. *Deficit replacement:* This is derived from physical assessment of the dehydrated child, as outlined.
2. *Maintenance requirements:* Basic metabolic requirements for water, sodium, and potassium are most simply determined by formulae based on body weight. See Table 22-4. Conditions such as fever, tachypnea, or change of ambient temperature will alter basic requirements.
3. *Ongoing losses:* Abnormal output in vomitus, diarrhea, and polyuria requires careful monitoring and inclusion into fluid and electrolyte recalculation.

METHODS OF WATER AND ELECTROLYTE ADMINISTRATION

If the child has moderate to severe dehydration or cannot tolerate oral fluids, parenteral replacement is

TABLE 22–3. *Clinical Characteristics of Different Osmolal States*

Type of Dehydration	Hyponatremic	Isotonic	Hypernatremic
Serum Sodium	<130	130–150	>150
Clinical features			
Heart rate			
Blood pressure			
Mental status	Seizures	Lethargy	Coma, seizures
Skin	Cold, sweaty	Cold, dry	Cool, doughy
Turgor			
Eyes	Sunken	Sunken	Sunken
Fontanelle	Depressed	Depressed	Depressed

TABLE 22–4. *Basal Requirements for Water, Sodium, and Potassium*

Water*	
First 1–10 kg	100 ml/kg/day
10–20 kg	1,000 ml + 50 ml/kg/day
After 20 kg	1,500 ml + 20 ml/kg day
Sodium	
3 mEq/kg/day	
Potassium†	
2 mEq/kg/day	

* One centigrade degree temperature elevation increases water requirement by 7 ml/kg/day.
† Never administer > 4 mEq/hr in infancy; use oral route when possible; add to IV after observed urination only.

required. Parenteral volume and solute administration requires an ordered implementation scheme that is best implemented in three phases: *emergency stabilization, early replacement,* and *late replacement.*

1. *Emergency stabilization (first hour):* For severely dehydrated patients with signs of circulatory impairment, immediate isotonic volume administration is imperative. Normal saline, lactated Ringer's, or fresh-frozen plasma is acceptable. Administer 20 ml/kg every 10 minutes until vital signs are stable. Fresh whole blood, or saline mixed with packed red blood cells, are necessary if shock persists after 60 ml/kg of isotonic fluid.
2. *Early replacement (hour 1–8):* After stabilization, the infusion is slowed. For hyponatremic and isotonic dehydration, calculate volume infusion so that 50% of water and sodium deficits are replaced in the first 8 hours, then 50% over the following 16 hours. Ongoing losses may require an increased infusion rate. Potassium can be added to the infusion once urination is observed; *potassium deficits should be replaced over 48 hours.* Oral rehydration therapy (ORT) should ordinarily be initiated in this phase. For hypernatremic dehydration, deficit replacement is divided evenly over 48–72 hours, to avoid rapid osmolal shifts and CNS complications from overly aggressive therapy.
3. *Late replacement stage (hours 8–16):* In isotonic or hyponatremic states, 50% of the deficit is replaced during this phase; for hypernatremia, the infusion rate remains constant. Body weight, urine output, vital signs, and physical assessment determine rate adjustments. ORT will ordinarily be well established in this phase.

Oral Rehydration Therapy

ORT is the preferred method of rehydration in children with mild-moderate dehydration who can take fluids orally. Vomiting is not a contraindication, since appropriate use of small-volume ORT can actually enhance gastrointestinal retention. It should not be used in the child with shock, altered mental status, unrelenting vomiting, or severe weakness.

The composition of ORT is set ideally by the World Health Organization (WHO) at 90 mm Eq/l sodium, 20 mEq/l potassium, 30 mEq/l citrate, with a 1–2% glucose concentration. This glucose level will achieve optimal intestinal sodium absorption; solutions greater than 2.5% glucose may worsen diarrhea. Commercial preparations that approximate the WHO ORT recommendations include Pedialyte, Lytren, Resol, and Hydralyte (see Table 29-2).

The safety of ORT in the hyponatremic child is well documented. CNS complications, sometimes seen during parenteral rehydration, are rarely experienced with ORT.

Complications ■

A wide spectrum of complications may develop from dehydration and rehydration, some evolving from shock and hypoperfusion of major organs and others from the rapid water shifts produced by iatrogenic osmolal changes.

The most dreaded complications are CNS ones, including seizures and coma. Moreover, inappropriate rehydration technique, especially in the young hypernatremic child, can result in cavernous sinus thrombosis and intracranial bleeding.

Renal damage from hypoperfusion can manifest as acute tubular necrosis and renal failure. Further, metabolic abnormalities such as hypoglycemia, hypokalemia, and hypocalcemia may accompany dehydration and complicate short-term and long-term organ function.

Disposition ■

Over 91% of mild-moderate dehydration cases can be discharged home from the ED after assessment, initiation of rehydration by oral and sometimes by parenteral methods, and observation of successful ORT. Parental instructions for home care and appropriate follow-up are imperative (see Chapter 143).

A small number of dehydrated patients require consideration for inpatient care. This includes children with any of the following features:

1. Shock or hypotension
2. Severe electrolyte abnormalities (Na <130 mEq/l or >150 mEq/l)
3. Significant acidosis (pH <7.25)
4. >10% dehydration
5. Altered mental status
6. Protracted diarrhea (>10 ml/kg/hr stool)
7. Sustained vomiting
8. Severe fatigue with inability to drink
9. Advanced underlying nutritional deficiencies
10. Unreliable or unstable home situation.

Bibliography ■

Barkin R: Acute infectious diarrheal disease in children. *J Emerg Med* 1985; 3:1–10.

Dieckmann R: Hydration techniques in children. *Critical Decision in Emergency Medicine* 1988; 3:1–7.

Finberg L: Severe dehydration secondary to diarrhea. In: Finberg L, Kravath RD, Fleischman AR, eds.: *Water and Electrolytes in Pediatrics: Physiology, Pathophysiology and Treatment.* Philadelphia: WB Saunders, 1982.

Hirschorn N: The treatment of acute diarrhea in children: An historical and physiological perspective. *Am J Clin Nutr* 1980; 33:637–663.

Martin D, Goldhagen JL: Oral rehydration therapy. In Barkin R, ed.: *The emergently ill child: Dilemmas in assessment and management.* Rockville, MD: Aspen, 1987.

23 Diabetic Ketoacidosis

Byron Y. Aoki and James Hanson

Diabetic ketoacidosis (DKA) is a complex disease that has been associated with significant morbidity and mortality. Improved therapy has resulted in a marked decline in mortality and overall excellent patient outcome. Understanding the pathophysiology of DKA has been key in this achievement, for DKA poses a dilemma: untreated, it will result in death, but treatment without comprehending the pathophysiology can produce complications that also result in death.

Etiology and Pathophysiology ■

Diabetes in childhood is most commonly Type I or insulin-dependent diabetes mellitus. When uncontrolled, it results in DKA. DKA is seen most often in known diabetics with inadequate control or those whose balance has been upset by stress, as infection; it is also often the initial presentation of diabetes mellitus. The key steps in its development are outlined below.

1. The etiology of DKA is absent insulin. Hyperglycemia is one of its results.
2. Hyperglycemia has several consequences:
   a. Water loss: Osmotic diuresis results when the renal threshold for glucose reabsorption is exceeded.
   b. Electrolyte losses: Large quantities of Na, K, Ca, and phosphate are lost during diuresis.
   c. Serum hyperosmolality: Serum osmolality increases as glucose values rise.
3. Since glucose is not available for use, alternative sources of energy are needed. The absence of insulin and the activation of counterregulatory hormones (epinephrine, cortisol, glucagon, and growth hormone) produce several energy sources.
   Glycogenolysis, gluconeogenesis, and polyphagia increase serum glucose further, but this glucose remains unavailable to cells. Proteinolysis and lipolysis provide alternate usable energy

sources. The result is lipemia and ketoacid production. The resulting hyperglycemia, ketonemia, metabolic acidosis, glucosuria, and ketonuria secondary to absent insulin constitute DKA.

Metabolic Disturbances in DKA ■

There is a wide range of metabolic and laboratory derangements in DKA patients. These include:

1. Hyperglycemia: Glucose levels are generally above 200 mg/dl and may reach values above 1,000 mg/dl.
2. Water loss: Large obligatory water losses result once the renal threshold for glucose reabsorption is exceeded. Glucose is a potent diuretic and brisk diuresis continues well into shock; oliguria and anuria are preterminal events. Large amounts of electrolytes are lost in the urine during diuresis.
3. Hyperosmolality and idiogenic osmols: Hyperglycemia raises the serum osmolality; this causes water to move out of the cells to equalize intracellular and extracellular fluid osmolalities. If the osmotic difference is large, the fluid shift can produce brain shrinkage with stretching and tearing of the bridging vessels. The brain, however, has developed a response that reduces its shrinkage in hyperosmolar states: it produces idiogenic osmols that increase intracellular osmolality. While the idiogenic osmols protect the brain during hyperosmolar conditions, they pose a potentially lethal problem during therapy. Because idiogenic osmols break down slowly, with rapid correction of serum glucose and osmolality to normal, intracellular osmolality will be higher than serum osmolality. Fluid will then move from the extracellular compartment into the brain and cerebral edema and herniation can result.
4. Lipemia: The blood may be grossly lipemic in DKA.
5. Ketones: Acetoacetate, acetone, and beta-hy-

133

droxybutyrate are the ketone bodies formed in DKA. With increasing acidosis, formation of beta-hydroxybutyrate is favored; with therapy, decreasing acidosis favors the formation of acetoacetate and acetone. Only acetoacetate and acetone produce a positive reaction with ketone tablets and dipsticks, so increasing ketosis, as determined by these methods, during therapy does not indicate patient deterioration.

6. Acidosis: Acidosis is primarily the result of ketoacid production; lactic acid contributes to acidosis when dehydration develops. Hyperventilation and Kussmaul respirations are compensatory efforts to maintain normal pH. Eventually, uncompensated metabolic acidosis results. In severe DKA, HCO_3 may be less than 5 mEq/L, pCO_2 may be as low as 8–9 torr, and pH as low as 6.7–6.8. The acidotic state in DKA, however, is unique: many DKA patients with pH's in the 6.9–7.0 range have remarkably good mentation and cardiac function. The explanation lies in the fact that acidosis develops over several days so that the CSF, especially, has had a chance to compensate and maintain a near-normal pH in the presence of serum acidosis.

7. Sodium: Initial sodium values are frequently low, but are not of clinical concern. The sodium values are factitiously low because of lipemia and because Na is decreased by 1.6 mEq/L for every 100 mg/dl elevation of glucose. Hyponatremia should steadily correct to normal values during therapy.

8. Potassium: Initial serum K^+ values may be low, normal, or high while total body stores of potassium are invariably depleted. With therapy, K^+ levels fall, sometimes to dangerous levels, as ongoing urine losses are coupled with intracellular movement of K^+ due to the correction of acidosis and provision of insulin.

9. Phosphate: Body phosphate stores are low and initial serum phosphate levels are variable. Phosphate levels usually fall during therapy. The clinical significance of hypophosphatemia in DKA remains uncertain, but treatment of hypophosphatemia is probably indicated.

10. Calcium: Despite calcium losses in the urine, calcium values are usually normal.

11. BUN and creatinine: BUN and creatinine will be elevated from dehydration. The creatinine may be falsely elevated secondary to ketones, which can interfere with true creatinine determination. Enzymatic creatinine determination, however, remains accurate.

12. Amylase: Amylase may be elevated in DKA. It is not of pancreatic origin and has no clinical significance.

13. Leukocytosis: Elevated white blood cells up to 20–30,000 with granulocyte predominance are common. This is most often a catecholamine response and does not indicate infection.

14. Hemoconcentration: Elevation of the Hgb and Hct are found in significant dehydration.

Clinical Findings ■

In early diabetes, few abnormalities may be present on physical examination. A history of polyuria (including enuresis and nocturia), polydipsia, polyphagia, weight loss, and fatigue may be obtained. Laboratory abnormalities are limited to hyperglycemia, ketonemia, glucosuria, and ketonuria; acidosis is absent. Insulin therapy is all that is usually needed.

The moderately ill DKA patient has the above findings plus complaints that may include malaise, difficulty breathing, abdominal pain, nausea, and emesis. Physical examination is remarkable for tachycardia and Kussmaul respirations. The classic odor of acetone may be present in the breath. Signs of dehydration, including diminished perfusion and diminished pulses, may be present. The child is fatigued and lethargic. Abdominal tenderness may be present. In addition to elevated glucose and ketones in both blood and urine, partially compensated metabolic acidosis with the pH as low as 7.1 will be found. Emesis is a red flag, as it heralds the rapid development of dehydration and shock if left untreated.

The severely ill DKA patient will have some or all of the following findings: severe dehydration with cool extremities, poor perfusion; profound Kussmaul respirations; prostration; lethargy/obtundation. Laboratory findings include worsening of previously mentioned lab studies, arterial pH less than 7.1, HCO_3 under 10 mEq/L, hemoconcentration, elevated BUN, and creatinine. In the pre-arrest state, shock, coma, or oliguria or anuria is found. At any stage of illness, coexisting infection, which may have precipitated decompensation, may be present.

Diagnosis ■

The diagnosis of DKA is made on the basis of a history compatible with diabetes mellitus and the laboratory findings of hyperglycemia, ketonemia, glucosuria, ketonuria, and metabolic acidosis. Table 23-2 lists the differential diagnoses.

Ancillary Data ■

Admission lab studies must include glucose, electrolytes, a complete blood count, and urinalysis. A bedside determination of glucose should also be obtained emergently.

In moderate to severe DKA, the following additional lab studies should be obtained: arterial blood gases, BUN, creatinine, phosphate, and calcium. Appropriate studies should be obtained for suspected infection. During emergency treatment for DKA, a lab flow sheet (Table 23-1) is valuable for monitoring problems and progress.

Treatment ■

The therapy for DKA involves more than regulating insulin and glucose. As some of the derangements in DKA are life-threatening, these problems take priority over glucose management in the emergency situation. Specifically, fluid therapy is the single most important concern in the initial management of DKA. Restoring circulation is the first priority of treatment; fluid therapy alone will result in significant clinical and metabolic improvement. Insulin administration and metabolic problems are the other major areas of concern. Table 23-3 presents the key elements in the emergency treatment of DKA.

FLUID THERAPY

1. *Restoring Circulation:* Therapy begins with 20 ml/kg IV push of lactated Ringer's or normal saline in the dehydrated or shocky patient. A total of 40–60 ml/kg of lactated Ringer's or normal saline in 20-ml/kg increments will be required to restore circulation in the severely dehydrated or shocky patient. Lactated Ringer's offers two advantages over normal saline: it has less chloride (hyperchloremic acidosis), and it has lactate, which is gradually converted to bicarbonate. Avoid dextrose-containing lactated Ringer's or normal saline boluses to avoid aggravating hyperglycemia.

TABLE 23-1. *Laboratory Flow Sheet*

Hour	Glucose	Na$^+$	K$^+$	HCO$_3^-$	PO$_4$	Ca^{++}
0	+	+	+	+	+	+
1	+					
2	+	*	*	*	*	*
3	+					
4	+	+	+	+	+	+
5	+					
6	+	*	*	*	*	*
7	+					
8	+	+	+	+	+	+

* = Additional lab tests for severe DKA

TABLE 23-2. *Differential Diagnosis*

Lactic Acidosis
Ingestions (salicylates)
Uremia
Starvation
Pneumonia
Gastrointestinal problems
Reye's syndrome
Other neurologic disease
Inborn errors of metabolism

2. *Rehydration:* 1/2 normal saline plus 20 mEq KCl and 20 mEq KPO$_4$ per L at 2–3 times maintenance rate. The patient with moderate to severe DKA has water deficits amounting to 10–15% body weight in infants and toddlers and 6–9% in older children. A practical IV rate to use after restoring circulation is 2–3 times the maintenance rate. This is usually sufficient to replace the existing fluid deficit and brisk diuretic losses that will continue for the first few hours. Possible IV composition modifications include:

   a. Potassium should be withheld in the anuric patient until K$^+$ values return.
   b. 5% dextrose is added to the solution if serum glucose is 300 mg/dl or less.
   c. Some of the Na (up to 40 mEq/L) may be given as Na-Acetate rather than NaCl in the severely acidotic patient. Acetate is converted to bicarbonate, is compatible with medications such as

TABLE 23-3. *Emergency Treatment of DKA*

Obtain labs: Glucose, Lytes, CBC, U/A; ABG, BUN, Creat., Ca, P04.
Restore circulation: LR or NS push, 20 ml/kg, if needed. May need up to 40–60 ml/kg total in 20-ml/kg increments.
Rehydration: ½ NS + 20 mEq KCl and 20 mEq KPO$_4$ per liter.
   Rate: 2–3 times maintenance rate.
   Hold K$^+$ in anuric patient; await K$^+$ lab value.
Insulin infusion: 50 units insulin in 250 ml NS.
   Dose: 0.1 unit insulin/kg/hr IV = 0.5 ml/kg/hr IV.
Emergency problems
   Blood glucose ≤ 300 mg/dl: add 5% dextrose to rehydrating IV solution.
   K$^+$ < 3.0 mEq/L: give 0.5 mEq KCl/kg IV over 1 hour.
   BP, perfusion worsen: 10–20 ml/kg LR or NS bolus IV.
Treat coexisting problems, as infection.

insulin, and is therefore preferable to bicarbonate. The amount of base provided in this manner will not raise the HCO_3 too rapidly.

INSULIN THERAPY

Insulin therapy (insulin infusion at 0.1 unit/kg/hour) is initiated as soon as, or shortly after, rehydration has begun. Continuous IV insulin is used because it offers many advantages over intermittent injected insulin: availability to tissues is ensured; a steady level of insulin minimizes rapid drops in glucose and K^+; it can be piggybacked onto the maintenance IV line without the need to start another IV. To prepare the IV insulin drip, place 50 units of *regular* insulin in 250 ml normal saline. Synthetic human insulin is preferred. Several milliliters of the solution are flushed through the IV tubing to saturate insulin binding sites, then the infusion is regulated by an IV pump. The solution and set-up are good for 24 hours.

This solution has 0.2 units of insulin/ml. The insulin dose is 0.1 unit/kg/hour = 0.5 ml/kg/hour. Higher doses are rarely needed; up to 0.2 units/kg/hour may be needed in sepsis or severe acidosis. The insulin drip is usually continued until the HCO_3 is greater than 16–18 mEq/L and ketonuria is trace or absent. As hyperglycemia almost always corrects before acidemia and ketonemia, adding up to 10% dextrose to the IV solution is preferable to decreasing the insulin drip rate during the acute phase of DKA therapy.

OTHER MEASURES

1. Supplemental oxygen is provided for shocky, obtunded, or comatose patients.
2. Antibiotics are given for bacterial infections.
3. NPO status is maintained until GI symptoms resolve and mental status is adequate.
4. A heparin lock may be placed for the frequent blood-drawing that is needed to monitor therapy.

Complications and Caveats ■

Life-threatening complications and death can arise during therapy, even in the child who looks stable or even good on admission. The major complications encountered during therapy include hypoglycemia, cardiac dysrhythmias, cerebral edema, and herniation. While some of the complications and deaths arising during therapy are unexplained, most are clearly secondary to mismanagement of the metabolic problems found in DKA. Management of several of the metabolic problems seen in DKA is an exception to usual medical rules.

1. *Monitoring:* Monitoring the DKA patient is essential. Hourly monitoring of vital signs, neurologic status, input and output is needed. Metabolic values must be followed closely and a DKA flow sheet is useful.
2. *Bicarbonate, acidosis:* Rapid correction of acidosis to normal through $NaHCO_3$ administration is contraindicated, as it can precipitate many complications:
   a. Paradoxical CSF acidosis and CNS deterioration;
   b. Cardiac dysrhythmias and dysfunction, as serum K^+ may drop to low values;
   c. Hypocalcemia with tetany;
   d. Tissue hypoxia as the oxygen dissociation curve shifts to the right.

   For these reasons, and the observation that acidotic DKA patients function remarkably well, bicarbonate correction is not provided. If, however, the pH is in the 6.7–7.0 range and cardiac function is compromised, 1 mEq $NaHCO_3$/kg IV may be infused safely over 1 hour; the patient needs to be monitored closely. Serum bicarbonate will rise as the patient improves and it is the best lab indicator of patient improvement. It should be noted that HCO_3 values will rise very slowly when HCO_3 is below 10 mEq/L. Repeat arterial blood gases are not indicated when the child is improving clinically and the HCO_3 is rising.
3. *Potassium:* Serum K^+ values may drop very quickly with therapy and produce cardiac dysrhythmias. For this reason, in the absence of anuria, it is wise to add K^+ to IV fluids early, even when the initial K^+ values are normal to high. Potassium concentration in the IV solution is later adjusted to lab results. If the K^+ falls below 3.0 mEq/L, a 0.5 mEq KCl/Kg IV bolus over 1 hour is recommended; the serum K^+ should be rechecked and the bolus repeated if the K^+ remains less than 3.0. ECG monitoring is indicated during therapy. K^+ in high concentration and at rapid infusion rates can cause severe pain at the IV site. Starting a second IV and giving one-half of the hourly IV fluids in each IV usually eliminates the pain.
4. *Glucose:* Glucose needs to be monitored hourly. Glucose meters are useful, but periodic laboratory confirmation of values is advisable. A rapid drop in serum glucose should be avoided, as it will drop serum osmolality. The presence of idiogenic osmols in the brain will cause fluid to move into the brain and produce cerebral edema and herniation. To minimize this complication, the goal of therapy is to steadily reduce the serum glucose by 70–100 mg/dl/hour, which is usually attained with the recommended insulin infusion dose. When the blood glucose is 300 mg/dl or less, 5% dextrose is added to the rehydrating IV solution. If the glucose drops

to less than 150 mg/dl, dextrose concentrations can be increased up to 10% as needed. If, with 10% dextrose, serum glucose is less than 100–150 mg/dl, the insulin infusion rate may be decreased to 0.05 units/kg/hour. If hypoglycemia develops at any time, the patient should be given 1 mg/kg D50 IV push.

5. *Phosphate:* Low phosphate values commonly occur several hours into therapy. For the theoretical risk of tissue hypoxia, especially cerebral hypoxia, phosphate replacement is recommended.

6. *Fluids:* Polyuria will persist until the serum glucose falls below the renal threshold. Initially, additional pushes of lactated Ringer's or normal saline in 10–20 ml/kg increments may be needed when urine output exceeds fluid intake and circulation deteriorates. Adjustments in the rehydration rate may have to be made.

7. *Sodium:* Initially low Na values should rise with therapy. A normal Na value that falls to subnormal levels, or an initially low Na that does not rise during therapy may be an indication of excessive fluid administration and a harbinger of CNS deterioration. When this happens, the rehydration rate should be decreased.

8. *Neurologic status:* Most patients being treated for DKA have some degree of cerebral edema but remain asymptomatic. A few patients do, however, develop clinical signs of increased intracranial pressure (ICP). When this occurs, the usual progression of symptoms is: headache and irritability; decreasing level of consciousness; urinary incontinence; coma; signs of brain stem herniation—pupil changes, abnormal respirations, posturing, and finally arrest. Identifiable causes include rapid drop in glucose, falling Na (excessive hydration), and tissue hypoxia.

If such signs appear, stat glucose, electrolytes, and arterial blood gases should be checked; deviations from expected values should be promptly treated. If coma or brain stem signs are present, emergency therapy is required. Mannitol 0.5–1.0 gm/kg IV is given and 100% oxygen is provided. If the vital signs are unstable, the patient should also be intubated using increased ICP precautions and hyperventilated. Cerebral edema is the usual etiology, but vascular problems such as thrombosis may be found. When aggressive therapy for cerebral edema is instituted before an arrest occurs, the patient may still do well. After an arrest takes place, the patient prognosis is very poor.

Disposition ■

The child with new onset diabetes mellitus needs to be hospitalized for both therapy and education. As for the established diabetic patient, several factors will determine the need for hospitalization: most children with DKA and vomiting will need admission; the infant and very young child, the child with a concomitant illness (such as pneumonia), and the child without a stable home situation will need earlier admission. These patients may be adequately managed on a general pediatric ward, but PICU admission is indicated when there is shock, significant mental status changes, or profound acidosis metabolic abnormalities.

Bibliography ■

Duck S, Wyatt D: Factors associated with brain herniation in the treatment of diabetic ketoacidosis. *J Pediatr* 1988; 113:10.

Hale PJ, Crase J, Nattrass M: Metabolic effects of bicarbonate in the treatment of diabetic ketoacidosis. *Br Med J* 1984; 289:1035.

Krane E, Rockoff M, Wallman J, et al: Subclinical brain swelling in children during treatment of diabetic ketoacidosis. *N Eng J Med* 1985; 312:1147.

Krane E: Diabetic ketoacidosis: Biochemistry, physiology, treatment, and prevention. *Pediatr Clin North Am* 1987; 34:935.

Van der Meulen J, Klip A, Grinstein S: Possible mechanism for cerebral oedema in diabetic ketoacidosis. *Lancet* 1987; 2:306.

Weigle C: Metabolic and endocrine disease in pediatric intensive care. In: Rogers M, ed: *Textbook of pediatric intensive care.* Baltimore: Williams & Wilkins, 1987: 1058.

24 Fever in the Young Child

Moses Grossman

Fever is a time-honored signal to let parents know their child is ill; it is also the signal that often leads to a physician or emergency department (ED) visit. Some 20% of all pediatric ED presentations have fever as the chief complaint. Fever may be defined as an oral temperature higher than 37.3°C (99.1°F) or a rectal temperature (obtained in children younger than 5 years) higher than 37.9°C (100.1°F). Fever may be accompanied by other symptoms that suggest a diagnosis or at least an organ system, such as headache, earache, cough, or diarrhea. In the absence of other symptoms, examination of the child may reveal physical signs pointing to a diagnosis such as a red, nonmobile eardrum or a swollen, red joint. No specific historical features or localized findings will be elicited in a significant number of children. This chapter will deal principally with children with fever without localizing findings.

Etiology ■

Most febrile illnesses in children have an infectious etiology—viral, bacterial, or fungal. However, remember that there are other causes for fever in children, principally collagen-vascular or autoimmune diseases and malignancies.

Clinical Findings ■

Every child presenting with fever should have a rapid assessment to ensure that children with meningitis, septic shock, or a very high fever will not experience significant delay in diagnosis and therapy. The evaluation of disease severity in febrile children depends on the risk factors outlined in Table 24-1.

Every febrile child requires a carefully performed history and physical examination. It is particularly important to observe and record findings that deal with the child's general state of health, over and above the individual organ system physical findings. Table 3-3 presents observational findings in sick children

that hold useful predictive value in assessing disease severity (the Yale Observation Scale). These observations will enable the physician to make an accurate assessment and provide some documentation in the medical record about how sick the child appears to be. Such observational features may be more sensitive in detecting serious illness than localized physical signs or the height of the fever.

Meningitis is a life-threatening pediatric illness in which early recognition and treatment is most important (see Chapter 114). It is particularly important to check the febrile child's state of alertness, to try to elicit signs of meningeal irritation (stiff neck, Kernig and Brudzinski signs), and to record the findings.

Ancillary Data ■

If the cause of the fever is not clear from clinical findings, the next consideration will be laboratory investigations (Table 24-2).

1. *Urinalysis* is the cornerstone of diagnosing urinary tract infection. In young infants and children, collecting the specimen requires a little effort (see Chapter 122). If the urinalysis is positive, obtain a clear or sterile urine sample for culture before initiating therapy.
2. *White blood cell count (WBC).* Of febrile children with rectal temperature >38.5°C between the ages of 6 months and 2 years, 5–10% will have a positive bacterial culture for *S. pneumoniae* or *H. influenzae.* A WBC greater than 15,000/ml³ or less than 5,000/ml³ has known predictive value for bacteremia. Obtain a WBC on very young infants (<3 months), infants and children with very high fever (over 40°C), those who appear sick by the general observation scales, and those whose degree of illness and fever appear to be excessive for the localized physical findings (e.g., temperature of 40.5°C in a child with mild pharyngitis and otitis).
3. *Differential.* Correlation exists between the total PMN count, the number of nonfilamented PMNs

TABLE 24-1. *Risk Factors for Serious Disease in the Child With Fever*

Age
Height of fever
Compromised immunity
State of alertness
Toxic appearance
Cardiovascular stability
Family epidemiology

TABLE 24-2. *Laboratory Investigation in Febrile Children*

Urinalysis and urine culture
White blood cell count
Differential count
Blood culture
Chest film
Lumbar puncture

(bands), and bacteremia, but the differential adds only minimal predictive value to the total WBC. One exception is Shigella infections, where the total WBC is within normal limits but the differential shifts markedly to the left (increased band count).

4. *Blood culture.* When the height of the child's fever and general observation suggest that bacteremia is likely, perform a blood culture. It is also indicated with localized findings (e.g., pneumonia or otitis), when the degree of the child's illness suggests that bacteremia may be present. Identifying the bacteria from blood culture is usually important for future management; an opportunity to find an organism may be lost once antimicrobial therapy is started.

5. *Chest film.* Pneumonia in young infants may elude recognition by physical examination. When pneumonia is suspected or when a child is extraordinarily ill, a chest film may disclose the diagnosis.

6. *Lumbar puncture (LP) and examination of CSF.* The only way to make a diagnosis of meningitis is by examining the spinal fluid. *Always perform an LP when meningitis is considered or suspected.* Infants younger than 2 or 3 months often fail to show signs of meningeal irritation. In this group, LP is a *routine* part of the "septic workup" for fever.

Treatment ■

1. *Antipyretics.* Febrile children are generally more comfortable and have fewer metabolic requirements if their body temperature is lowered to approach normal. This is best accomplished by administering acetaminophen 5–10 mg/kg p.o. or p.r. On occasion, tepid (not cold!) sponge baths may be indicated.

2. *Hydration.* Stress oral fluid intake.

3. *Antimicrobials.* The vast majority of febrile illnesses in young children are viral in origin and thus are not amenable to antimicrobial therapy. Most series in the literature show that 6–10% of febrile children between the ages of 6 months and 2 years will have a serious bacterial infection, often occult bacteremia. These are likely to be the children with very high fever, toxicity by observation, abnormal WBC with blood cultures performed as part of the visit, and LP performed as outpatients. Some of these children will already be hospitalized and on IV antimicrobials.

For febrile children with suspected bacteremia who are discharged home, the dilemma is whether to prescribe an antimicrobial. Children who receive appropriate outpatient oral antimicrobials and then turn out to have a positive blood culture do better than those who are sent home without antimicrobials.

However, oral antimicrobials *do not* prevent the development of meningitis. The availability of ceftriaxone, a long-acting, third-generation injectable cephalosporin, makes available another treatment option, although no evidence exists that such therapy would indeed prevent meningitis.

Hence, three options are available: no antimicrobials, oral antimicrobials, or injectable, long-acting ceftriaxone (Table 24-3). Whichever option is chosen, *follow-up* of the child is crucial.

TABLE 24-3. *Antimicrobials* for Febrile Young Children Without Localizing Findings*

Generic Name	Brand Name
Oral	
Amoxicillin	
Amoxicillin + clavulinic acid	Augmentin
Cefaclor	Ceclor
Sulfatrimethoprim	Bactrim, Septra
Sulfa-erythromycin	Pediazole
Injectable	
Ceftriaxone	Rocef

* See Chapter 145 for dosage.

Disposition ∎

The decision to hospitalize depends on many medical factors, including the child's age, height of the fever, and degree of the child's illness, as well as some social factors such as the ability to follow a child at home and access of the family to a phone and transportation.

Hospitalize febrile infants younger than 10–12 weeks old, children with fevers higher than 40.6°C, those who require IV medication (fluids or otherwise), and those who appear very ill judged by observational features or cardiovascular instability.

Follow-up ∎

The follow-up of discharged children is crucial. The febrile youngster often leaves the ED *without* a clear diagnosis. A significant number of children with bacteremia will develop localizing findings within 24–48 hours. These may include pneumonia, cellulitis, otitis media, and meningitis; the latter may develop even though the initial LP during the emergency visit was negative. Review daily the laboratory results of cultures obtained for urine, blood, and CSF. Establish a clear, written plan for parents for follow-up. The higher-risk children should be seen; others can be followed by phone. Clarify who bears the responsibility for follow-up—family, the primary-care physician, or the ED physician.

Bibliography ∎

Baron MA, Fink HD, Cicchetti DV: Blood cultures in private pediatric practice: An 11-year experience. *Pediatr Infect Dis J* 1989; 8:2–7.

Crocker PJ, Quick G, McCombs W: Occult bacteremia in the emergency department: Diagnostic criteria for the young febrile child. *Ann Emerg Med* 1985; 14:1172–1177.

Grossman M: Management of the febrile patient. *Pediatr Infect Dis J* 1986; 5:730.

Jaffe DM, Tanz RR, Davis AT, et al: Antibiotic administration to treat possible occult bacteremia in febrile children. *N Engl J Med* 1987; 317:1175–1180.

McCarthy PL, Sharpe MR, Spiegel SZ, et al: Observation scales to identify serious illness in febrile children. *Pediatrics* 1982; 70:802–809.

25 Limp

Ruth Ann Parish

Limp, an uneven, jerky, or laborious gait, is usually recognized readily by parents. Limp in children is a frequent and elusive problem; it may account for up to 7% of office visits to the pediatrician and 0.5–1% of all emergency department (ED) visits. Limp in children may be difficult for the physician to evaluate for a number of reasons. Children often cannot clearly express their symptoms with words; they may have experienced trauma unwitnessed (and therefore unreported) by the parent; and several different entities may be mistakenly identified as "limp" by the parents (limb pain, joint pain, ataxia, or even vertigo).

Etiology and Pathophysiology ■

There are two phases to the human gait: the stance phase (beginning with the heel strike and ending with "toeing off") and the swing phase (bending the knee, flexing the hip, and then extending the knee to allow heel contact for the next stance). Loss of this rhythmic set of movements, pain, or muscular weakness can all produce limp.

There are many varied etiologies of limp (see Table 25-1). Some etiologies are suggested by certain gaits: the *antalgic* gait results from pain in one extremity, such that the patient shortens the stance phase on that side (as if one had a tack in one's shoe). The *Trendelenburg* gait is a downward pelvic tilt during the swing phase due to weakness of the contralateral gluteus medius muscle. Climbing stairs may be difficult for the child with pain or weakness of the quadriceps femoris or gluteus muscle groups.

The child's age is one of the main clues to the diagnosis. If the child is less than 2 years of age, the physician must rule out a septic hip. In the preschool and elementary-age child, Legg-Perthes disease (avascular necrosis of the femoral head) must be considered. In the older child and adolescent (particularly if the child is overweight), consider slipped capital femoral epiphysis (SCFE). Serious conditions that demand recognition at any age include osteo-myelitis, paraspinal abscess, spinal cord tumors, a septic joint, Guillain-Barré syndrome, tick paralysis, meningitis, or encephalitis.

Clinical Findings ■

An accurate history is the single most important factor in diagnosis and disposition. The physician must establish the length of symptoms, the localization of the pain, any underlying disease states, a history of trauma, recent inoculations, new shoes, any hint of psychosocial disturbance, and other important associated symptoms.

Keys to the successful physical examination include establishing rapport with the child, avoiding the painful area until last in the examination, inspecting before palpating, and doing a complete physical examination—the child who complains of knee pain may in fact be experiencing referred pain from the hip. Important physical findings are outlined in Table 25-2. Make a careful note of the child's preferred position at rest; a flexed-hip, flexed-knee, and abducted position at rest suggests that the child does not want to put any stress on the hip capsule, and should lead the examiner to think about either an SCFE, a septic hip, or possibly Legg-Perthes disease (avascular necrosis of the femoral head).

Differential Diagnosis ■

Table 25-1 presents the common causes of limp and their distinguishing features.

Ancillary Data ■

Laboratory tests include a complete blood count (CBC) with erythrocyte sedimentation rate (ESR), a sickle-cell prep in those patients at risk for the disease, blood culture, and X-rays of hips, knees, ankles, or feet. CT or magnetic resonance imaging (MRI) may be indicated. A bone scan is rarely necessary.

TABLE 25–1. *Differential Diagnosis of Limp in Children*

Condition	History	Physical Exam	Comment
Disorders of CNS			
Acute cerebellar ataxia	Recent viral illness	Staggering	LP (May need head CT first) CBC, ESR
Drugs	Drug exposure		Toxic screen
CVA/migraine	Sudden hemiplegia	Localizing CNS findings	CT scan
Tumor	Weight loss, headache, blurred vision		CT scan, CBC
Soft-Tissue Injuries	Trauma history, cellulitis, lymphangitis	Antalgic gait	X-rays, CBC
Joint Abnormalities			
Pyarthrosis	Fever	Position of comfort, point tenderness	X-ray, CBC, ESR, joint aspiration, blood cx (see Chapter 44)
Toxic synovitis			
Osseous Abnormalities		Position of comfort, point tenderness	X-rays, CBC, ESR, blood cx
Trauma			
Osteomyelitis	Fever Systemic sx		
Septic hip	Sickle cell Age <2 yrs		
Legg–Perthes	Age 2–10		
SCFE	Early teens, history of injury		
Peripheral Neurologic			
Guillain–Barré	Preceding viral illness	Staggering	CBC
		Lost DTRs	Free erythrocyte protoporphyrin
Tick paralysis	Tick exposure	Embedded tick	
Poisoning	Heavy metal exposure		Toxic screen
Intraabdominal			
Appendicitis	History of abdominal pain	True guarding	Abdominal x-rays, urinalysis
Abscess		Rectal exam	CBC
Perforated bowel			Surgical consultation

TABLE 25–2. *Important Physical Findings in the Limping Child*

Vital signs including temperature
Preferred position at rest
Inflammation of affected area
Obvious joint distention or limited ROM (compare with normal)
Type of gait disturbance (antalgic, muscular weakness, staggering)
Compressed spine and pelvis
Rectal examination to evaluate coccygeal or colon tenderness
Straight leg raise
Valsalva maneuver to assess ileo-psoas pain
Neurologic examination of lower extremities

TABLE 25–3. *Conditions Requiring Inpatient Evaluation of Limp*

Acute onset of fever
Exquisitely tender joint
Rapid progression of previously insidious illness
Suspected serious infection
Focal neurologic abnormality
Related conditions
  Osteomyelitis
  Paraspinal abscess
  Spinal cord tumor
  Pyarthrosis
  Guillain–Barré
  Tick paralysis
  Cerebral abscess
  Meningitis/encephalitis

Disposition ■

Table 25-3 presents conditions that demand early recognition and inpatient treatment.

Often the child with a limp will go undiagnosed in the ED despite a full evaluation. Outpatient management is usually safe, with close follow-up. Patients with minor trauma or with toxic synovitis (viral process) will continue to limp for a few days, without onset of fever or explosive illness; observation on a daily basis may be safest, until symptoms resolve. Parents should be told to watch for fever, debilitation, sudden onset of more severe pain, or more extensive neurologic problems. Any child whose limp lasts more than 10–14 days will require a more extensive inpatient workup to rule out infection, rheumatoid conditions, or tumor.

Bibliography ■

Bowyer SL, Hollister JR: Limb pain in childhood. *Pediatr Clin North Am* 1984; 31:1053–1081.

Callavan DL: Causes of refusal to walk in childhood. *South Med J* 1982; 75:20–22.

McCarthy PL, Wasserman D, Spiezel SZ, et al: Evaluation of arthritis and arthralgia in the pediatric patient. *Clin Pediatr* 1980; 19:183–190.

Singer JI: The cause of gait disturbance in 425 pediatric patients. *Pediatr Emerg Care* 1985; 1:7–10.

Singer JI: Altered locomotion. In: Barkin RM, ed: *The emergently ill child*. Rockville, MD: Aspen Publications, 1987, pp. 260–269.

26 Seizures

Donna M. Ferriero

A *seizure* is a paroxysmal alteration of brain function consisting of an electrical discharge of neurons. *Epilepsy* is defined as two or more unprovoked seizures. Seventy percent of cases of epilepsy begin in childhood, and about one in 15 children will have a seizure during the first seven years of life.

Whether seizures recur depends on genetic factors or the presence of fixed brain lesions or untreated metabolic derangements. Certain seizure types, such as absence and focal motor seizures, have a greater than 90% chance of recurring.

This chapter will deal first with the life-threatening form of seizures—*status epilepticus*—and then will briefly discuss *neonatal, febrile,* and *recurrent seizures.*

The International Classification of Epileptic Seizures (Table 26-1) presents the different seizure types.

Status Epilepticus ■

When seizures persist for more than 20 minutes or recur repetitively so that the patient does not recover consciousness between seizures, the patient is in *status epilepticus.* Status epilepticus is often the first manifestation of epilepsy in children. Mortality can be as high as 11%, and about half the deaths are a consequence of status itself or its complications (e.g., aspiration pneumonia, cardiovascular failure, hyperthermia). The sequelae of status epilepticus range from no pathology to severe mental retardation.

Convulsive status epilepticus is a series of motor seizures, partial or generalized, without recovery of function. Particularly during this type of status, metabolic disturbances can occur, including hypoxia, acidosis, hypotension, hypoglycemia, hyperkalemia, hyperpyrexia, and raised intracranial pressure.

TREATMENT
General Supportive Measures

1. Place the child in a semiprone position and clear the airway. Insert a plastic oropharyngeal or nasopharyngeal airway and administer oxygen.

2. Use Dextrostix to check for hypoglycemia. If present, treat immediately.
3. Insert a nasogastric tube to empty gastric contents.
4. Remove excess clothing; if the child is febrile, use tepid sponging, cooling blankets, and rectal antipyretics.
5. Avoid overhydration, since brain edema may result.
6. Insert a urinary catheter.

Drug Treatment

The goal of therapy is to stop seizures without causing additional cardiovascular compromise. Follow the following sequence for drug administration:

1. *Diazepam* 0.3 mg/kg IV × 1, not to exceed 10 mg. If IV access is not established, administer diazepam 0.2–0.5 mg/kg rectally with a 5f feeding tube. Proceed immediately to:
2. *Diphenylhydantoin* 15–20 mg/kg IV slow infusion (1 mg/kg/min). If ineffective, repeat to maximum dose of 40 mg/kg. If seizure stops, no further immediate drug therapy is indicated. If seizure continues following total dose, proceed immediately to:
3. *Phenobarbital* 15–20 mg/kg IV slow infusion. If seizure continues, proceed to:
4. *Paraldehyde* 0.3 ml/kg diluted in 2 volumes of mineral oil and given PR or as a 4% solution in normal saline IV. May repeat q 1–4 hours. If seizure continues, proceed to:
5. *Pentobarbital coma:* loading dose 15 mg/kg over 1 hour, maintenance infusion 0.5–2 mg/kg/hour, additional loading doses (5 mg/kg to maximum of 30 mg/kg in first 12 hours) as needed to control seizures or attain burst-suppression.

If pentobarbital coma is necessary, the patient requires ICU admission, intubation and ventilation, and arterial line and EEG monitoring for level of anesthesia. Most status epilepticus does not require intubation in the emergency department (ED) unless the seizure persists after diazepam and 40 mg/kg of diphenylhydantoin.

TABLE 26–1. *International Classification of Epileptic Seizures*

  I. Partial seizures
    A. Simple partial (consciousness retained)
       1. Motor
       2. Sensory
       3. Autonomic
       4. Psychic
    B. Complex partial (consciousness impaired)
       1. Simple partial, followed by impaired consciousness
       2. Consciousness impaired at onset
    C. Partial seizures with secondary generalization
 II. Generalized seizures
    A. Absences
       1. Typical
       2. Atypical
    B. Generalized tonic-clonic
    C. Tonic
    D. Clonic
    E. Myoclonic
    F. Atonic
III. Unclassified seizures

(Adapted from Dreifuss FE, Bancaud J, Henriksen O, et al: Proposal for revised clinical and EEG classification of epileptic seizures. *Epilepsia* 1981; 22:489–501)

NONCONVULSIVE STATUS

Children with absence (petit mal status) or partial complex status may present with an altered state of consciousness or confusion. Most children still can perform purposeful activities and can interact with the environment. The EEG is diagnostic in each case and the drug therapy will be determined by the neurologist.

ETIOLOGY OF STATUS EPILEPTICUS

After the patient has been initially stabilized, obtain blood chemistries for electrolytes; liver function tests, NH_3; blood cultures; complete blood count and platelets. Perform a CT scan without contrast, after neurology consultation, to look for space-occupying lesions, blood, or increased intracranial pressure. If normal, perform an lumbar puncture and appropriate cultures. In endemic areas, obtain CSF titer for cysticercosis antibodies. Send urine for culture and toxicology screen. Specific conditions associated with status epilepticus are presented in Table 26-2.

Febrile Seizures ■

Febrile convulsions usually occur between the ages of 3 months to 5 years, but it is unusual for a first febrile convulsion to appear after age 4 years. Recurrence ranges from 30–40%, but does not increase the risk of epilepsy.

The factors for a high-risk group requiring treatment include the following:

1. Atypical seizures, such as a prolonged focal seizure or a seizure followed by transient or permanent neurologic abnormalities;
2. Positive family history of *non*-febrile seizures;
3. Abnormal neurologic examinations before the febrile seizure.

There is a 13% incidence of developing recurrent afebrile seizures in patients in this high-risk category. Treatment consists of phenobarbital for children under 2 years and valproate for older children. Since phenobarbital causes significant hyperactivity, the primary physician may find it desirable to change to valproate.

TABLE 26–2. *Conditions Associated With Status Epilepticus in Children*

Acute Conditions
Poor compliance with anticonvulsants
Fever
CNS infection
    Bacterial meningitis
    Aseptic meningitis
    Encephalitis
Fluid and electrolyte disturbances
    Hypoglycemia
    Hyponatremia
    Hypocalcemia
Poisoning
    Lead
    Aspirin
    Theophylline
    Antidepressants
    Isoniazid
    Phenothiazines
    Hydrocarbons
    Sympathomimetics (phencyclidine, cocaine, LSD, amphetamine)
Closed head trauma

Chronic Conditions
Posthypoxic
Posthemorrhagic
Postinfectious
Post-traumatic
Degenerative disease

Idiopathic

(From Dieckmann RA: Management of Status Epilepticus in Children. In Barkin RM: The emergently ill child: Dilemmas in assessment and management. Rockville, Md.: Aspen, 1987, p. 209)

TABLE 26–3. *Treatment of Seizures*

Seizure Disorder	Drugs	Usual Daily Dosage		Usual Therapeutic Serum Concentrations
		Adults	Children	
Tonic–Clonic (Grand Mal)				
Drugs of choice	Carbamazepine	600–1200 mg	20–30 mg/kg	6–12 µg/ml
	Phenytoin	300–400 mg	4–7 mg/kg	10–20 µg/ml
	Valproate*	1000–3000 mg	15–60 mg/kg	100–150 µg/ml
Alternatives	Phenobarbital	120–250 mg	3–5 mg/kg	15–35 µg/ml
	Primidone	750–1500 mg	10–25 mg/kg	6–12 µg/ml
Partial, Including Secondarily Generalized				
Drugs of choice	Carbamazepine	600–1200 mg	20–30 mg/kg	6–12 µg/ml
	Phenytoin	300–400 mg	4–7 mg/kg	10–20 µg/ml
Alternatives	Phenobarbital	120–250 mg	3–5 mg/kg	15–35 µg/ml
	Primidone	750–1500 mg	10–25 mg/kg	6–12 µg/ml
Absence (Petit Mal)				
Drugs of choice	Ethosuximide	750–2000 mg	20–40 mg/kg	40–100 µg/ml
	Valproate	1000–3000 mg	15–60 mg/kg	100–150 µg/ml
Alternatives	Clonazepam	1.5–20 mg	0.01–0.2 mg/kg	0.013–0.072 µg/ml
Atypical Absence, Myoclonic, Atonic				
Drugs of choice	Valproate*	1000–3000 mg	15–60 mg/kg	100–150 µg/ml
Alternatives	Clonazepam	1.5–20 mg	0.01–0.2 mg/kg	0.013–0.072 µg/ml

* Not FDA approved unless absence is involved.
(From *Medical Lett Drug Ther* 1986; 723:91)

Perform a lumbar puncture in any child under the age of 2 years to determine if meningitis is present, whether or not a source of infection has been found. Shaken-baby syndrome with subdural hematomas must be considered in any infant presenting with apnea and seizures.

Treatment of Different Seizure Disorders ■

Table 26-3 lists the most common types of epileptic seizures with dosage recommendations and usual serum concentrations.

Differential Diagnosis ■

SYNCOPE

Syncope is usually associated with a feeling of light-headedness, and gray-out of vision does not occur in the supine position except with *cardiac syncope*. The patient is usually pale, cold, and clammy. Loss of consciousness is almost always for under two minutes. Some motor activity (tonic) may be present,

but it is minimal and occurs after the loss of consciousness. Usually there is no "postictal" confusion; if present, it is very brief and *not* associated with lethargy (see Table 27-5).

BREATH-HOLDING SPELLS

Breath-holding spells are seen in children between 6 months and 5 years, with the onset usually in the first or second year of life and diminishing with time. Episodes are usually precipitated by frustration, fear, or pain. Tonic or tonic-clonic jerks may occur briefly as the attack subsides, especially if apnea is prolonged. There is no postictal lethargy or confusion.

NIGHT TERRORS

Children are screaming and difficult to arouse. These spells occur during stage III sleep and, if severe, spells can be aborted with diazepam or imipramine.

ACUTE CONFUSIONAL STATE FROM MIGRAINE

The symptomatology may resemble that of complex partial status, but the EEG lacks seizure activity. There is usually a family history of migraine (see Chapter 43).

OTHER CONSIDERATIONS

1. Hereditary chin trembling
2. Familial choreoathetosis
3. Narcolepsy
4. Pseudoseizures

Bibliography ■

Berg BO: *Child neurology—A clinical manual.* Greenbrae, CA: Jones Publishing Co., 1984.

Dieckmann RA: Management of status epilepticus in children. In: Barkin RM, ed: *The emergently ill child: Dilemmas in assessment and management.* Rockville, Md.: Aspen, 1987, pp. 208–216.

Dreifuss FE, Bancaud J, Henriksen O, et al: Proposal for revised clinical and EEG classification of epileptic seizures. *Epilepsia* 1981; 22:489–501.

Drugs for epilepsy. *Med Lett Drugs Ther* 1986; 723(28):91.

Lechtenberg R: *The diagnosis and treatment of epilepsy.* New York: Macmillan, 1985.

Lowenstein DH, Aminoff MJ, Simon RP: Barbiturate anesthesia in the treatment of status epilepticus: Clinical experience with 14 patients. *Neurology* 1988; 38:395–400.

Oppenheimer EY, Rossman NP: Seizures in childhood: An approach to emergency management. *Pediatr Clin North Am* 1979; 26:845.

Simon RP: Management of status epilepticus. In: Pedly TA, Meldrum BS, eds: *Recent advances in epilepsy,* vol. 2. New York: Churchill-Livingstone, pp. 137–160.

27 Syncope

Jeffrey R. Fineman and Scott J. Soifer

Syncope is a transient loss of consciousness, usually of sudden onset and brief duration, caused by a deprivation of essential substrates (oxygen and glucose) from the brain. This is often the consequence of an impairment in cardiac output with the subsequent reduction of cerebral perfusion. The episode almost always occurs with the patient in an upright position and is usually preceded by warning signs such as dizziness, nausea, perspiration, and pallor. The period of unconsciousness lasts for seconds to minutes and is associated with generalized muscle weakness, pallor, diaphoresis, poorly palpable pulses, and decreased blood pressure. Clonic movements of the limbs and face may occur. With the return of consciousness, the patient, although weak, rapidly becomes alert and aware of the environment.

Syncope is commonly seen in the emergency department (ED); in fact, as many as 15% of children have had a syncopal episode by the end of adolescence. Although the large majority of these patients are hemodynamically stable at presentation, they require a careful and thorough evaluation because a small group of children with syncope have a serious underlying disorder that may lead to subsequent morbidity and mortality.

Etiology and Clinical Findings ■

There are six major causes of syncope in childhood: *vasodepressor, vascular/reflex, cardiac, toxic/ metabolic, neurologic,* and *psychologic* (see Table 27-1).

VASODEPRESSOR SYNCOPE

Vasodepressor syncope (the "vasovagal reaction" or "common faint") is the most common cause of syncope. Often the precipitating events are emotional stresses such as anxiety, a shocking incident, painful stimuli (blood drawing or a dressing change), or a prolonged period in a warm, crowded environment.

The common faint almost always begins with the patient standing or sitting in an erect position. Pallor, diaphoresis, epigastric discomfort, and occasionally blurred vision occur minutes before the loss of consciousness. At this time, patients have pupillary dilatation and tachycardia. During unconsciousness, however, bradycardia is usually present. Placing the patient in a supine position with the head down results in the return of consciousness. Although pallor, diaphoresis, nausea, and weakness may all persist, the child is alert and oriented after consciousness returns.

The pathophysiology of vasodepressor syncope is a marked decrease in peripheral vascular resistance with pooling of blood in the skeletal muscle bed, which decreases ventricular filling and cardiac output. This leads to hypotension and decreased cerebral perfusion (see Table 27-2). The mechanism by which a precipitating event leads to this decrease in peripheral vascular resistance is not well understood.

Most children presenting with vasodepressor syncope are otherwise well and require only reassurance and education. Keep in mind, however, that certain underlying conditions, such as congenital heart disease and anemia, increase the risk of having these episodes.

VASCULAR/REFLEX SYNCOPE

Orthostatic syncope (orthostatic hypotension) is the most common form of vascular syncope. It is characterized by a brief loss of consciousness that occurs when the patient rises rapidly from the recumbent to standing position. When a child stands, normal blood pressure is maintained by arteriolar and venous constriction, leg muscle contractions to increase venous return to the heart, and increased heart rate. Orthostatic syncope occurs upon rising rapidly when there is inadequate cerebral perfusion. Unlike the vasodepressor syncope, there is little prodrome (e.g., pallor, sweating, nausea). Orthostatic syncope occurs in a variety of clinical conditions (see Table 27-3). Consider dehydration and bleeding, as well as the ingestion of certain drugs.

TABLE 27–1. *Etiology of Syncope*

Vasodepressor (common faint)
Vascular/reflex
  Orthostatic hypotension
  Hypovolemia
  Cerebrovascular
Cardiac
  Arrhythmia
  Congenital or acquired heart disease
Metabolic/toxic
Neurologic
Psychologic

TABLE 27–3. *Causes of Orthostatic Syncope*

Volume depletion or venous pooling
  Bleeding
  Dehydration
  Prolonged bed rest
  Pregnancy
Drugs
  Phenothiazines
  Antihypertensives
  Nitrates
  Diuretics
Autonomic nervous system dysfunction
  Primary
  Spinal cord injury or surgery

There are other less common forms of vascular/reflex syncope. *Cerebrovascular syncope,* a rare form of syncope in childhood, occurs when cerebral blood flow is reduced by embolic or thrombotic events resulting in transient ischemic attacks or cerebral vascular accidents. *Cough syncope* refers to the brief loss of consciousness following paroxysms of coughing. The reduction in cardiac output is probably related to decreased venous return from the marked increase in intrathoracic pressure generated during a coughing paroxysm. *Micturition syncope* is a loss of consciousness occurring immediately after voiding. The decrease in intraabdominal volume with bladder emptying may stimulate a reflex decrease in peripheral vascular resistance leading to the syncopal attack. *Carotid sinus syncope* is rare in childhood and occurs with massage of the carotid sinus. *Migraine syncope* is a period of unconsciousness following the aura of a migraine. Upon return of consciousness there is a severe headache, usually in the occipital region.

CARDIAC SYNCOPE

Cardiac syncope occurs when cardiac output decreases, reducing cerebral perfusion. This may occur because of arrhythmias or congenital and acquired heart diseases (see Table 27-4).

Cardiac syncope often occurs during strenuous activity. Exercise may elicit or worsen arrhythmias. Some children who are sensitive to catecholamines develop ventricular arrhythmias during exercise or emotional excitement. Similarly, patients with mitral valve prolapse also develop ventricular arrhythmias. Exercise may induce ventricular arrhythmias, syncope, and even sudden death in children with the prolonged QT syndrome. This syndrome may be congenital or acquired transiently because of drugs, electrolyte imbalance, or myocarditis. An episode of syncope associated with exercise is cause for concern and requires a thorough evaluation.

Certain congenital heart diseases may predispose patients to syncope. In patients with aortic stenosis, cardiac output may not increase adequately to compensate for the decreased peripheral vascular resis-

TABLE 27–2. *Pathophysiology of Vasodepressor Syncope*

Precipitating event
↓
Decreased peripheral vascular resistance
↓
Decreased left ventricular filling
↓
Decreased cardiac output
↓
Hypotension
↓
Cerebral ischemia
↓
Syncope

TABLE 27–4. *Causes of Cardiac Syncope*

Arrhythmias	*Congenital or Acquired Heart Disease*
Supraventricular tachycardia	Aortic stenosis
Atrial fibrillation/flutter	Hypertrophic cardiomyopathy
Wolff–Parkinson–White syndrome	Tetralogy of Fallot
Ventricular tachycardia/fibrillation	Cardiac tamponade
Sinus bradycardia	Pulmonic stenosis
Heart block	Pulmonary embolus
	Pulmonary hypertension
	Myxoma/tumor

TABLE 27-5. *Differentiation of Syncope From Seizures*

	Syncope	Seizure
Preceding Aura	Rare	Common
Period of Unconsciousness	Seconds	Minutes
Tonic–Clonic Movements	Rare	Common
Alertness at Awakening	Common	Rare

tance and increased metabolic needs occur during exercise. Similarly, in patients with hypertrophic cardiomyopathy, the obstruction to left ventricular output may worsen during exercise secondary to increased contractility and decreased ventricular volume. In patients with cyanotic heart disease, worsening hypoxemia may precipitate a syncopal episode (see Chapter 21).

METABOLIC/TOXIC SYNCOPE

Syncope due to metabolic/toxic causes is often associated with other etiologies. Anemia, for example, precipitates orthostatic syncope, and various drugs may cause either orthostatic or cardiac syncope.

Profound hypoglycemia produces confusion, altered consciousness, weakness, and diaphoresis. It may be caused by insulin overdose, various tumors, or pituitary or liver dysfunction. Unlike other causes of syncope, it is of gradual onset and is unrelated to posture. Blood pressure most often is normal. There is a rapid reversal of symptoms with glucose administration (see Chapter 103).

Hypoxia causes syncope by producing cerebral ischemia or as a precipitating event of vasodepressor syncope. Exposure to high altitude is a common cause (see Chapter 101).

NEUROLOGIC SYNCOPE

Seizures cause sudden, transient periods of unconsciousness that may be difficult to distinguish from syncope. Clonic movements may be seen at the end of a prolonged syncopal episode. The presence of an aura, postictal drowsiness, a prolonged period of unconsciousness, incontinence, and normal cardiovasculature parameters all suggest a seizure disorder rather than a syncopal episode (see Table 27-5 and Chapter 26).

History
Physical Exam
Laboratory Tests (EKG, serum glucose, and hematocrit)

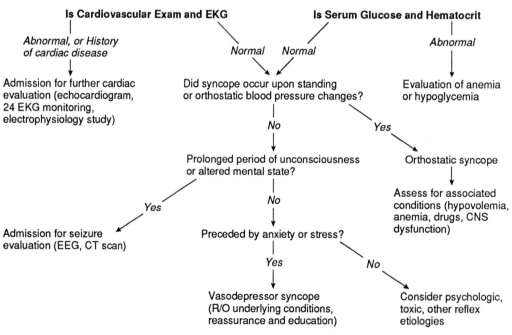

FIGURE 27-1. Diagnostic evaluation of syncope.

TABLE 27–6. *Important Historical Information*

Presence of prodrome
Precipitating event
Body position at onset (supine vs. erect, after sudden
  rising)
Duration of unconsciousness
Presence of tonic–clonic movements
Alertness after recovery
History of previous syncopal episodes
History of cardiac, neurologic, or psychologic disorders
Medication or drug use
Pregnancy

Vertigo also may be confused with syncope, particularly when it is associated with a sudden fall. The fall is the result of a loss of balance, however, and not a decrease in cardiac output or impairment in the level of consciousness.

PSYCHOLOGIC SYNCOPE

Hysterical syncopal episodes occur without true loss of consciousness or organic cause. They are witnessed events where the patient falls gradually without injury. Vital signs are normal. The patient appears unalarmed while describing the episode. In other patients who respond to anxiety with pronounced hyperventilation, symptoms of numb extremities and altered consciousness develop because hypocapnia decreases cerebral perfusion. True loss of consciousness is rare except when the hyperventilation precipitates a vasodepressor reaction. Having the patient breathe into a bag may alleviate the symptoms, but never use this technique in patients who may be hypoxic.

Clinical Findings ■

Since syncopal episodes are of brief duration, most patients will be conscious and hemodynamically stable at presentation. Although the majority of episodes reflect a benign condition, syncope may be a symptom of a serious underlying disease process that may predispose the patient to sudden death. The evaluation, therefore, must be systematic and thorough. The initial assessment of every child presenting with a sudden loss of consciousness should include a detailed history and physical exam as well as an EKG, serum glucose, and hematocrit determination. This will allow the physician to determine the etiology of the syncopal episode and will permit a more directed evaluation (see Figure 27-1).

An accurate, detailed *history* is imperative to es-tablish the etiology of syncope (see Table 27-6). For example, if loss of unconsciousness occurs during exercise in a patient who complains of palpitations, the etiology of the syncopal episode most likely is an arrhythmia and extensive cardiac evaluation is necessary. On the other hand, an adolescent on bed rest for an injury who collapses immediately after quickly rising from bed has orthostatic syncope associated with venous pooling. This patient needs only reassurance. Historical information is also most helpful in differentiating a seizure from syncope (see Table 27-5).

The *physical examination* should include blood pressures obtained in the supine and erect positions. A drop in systolic blood pressure of 20–30 mm Hg upon standing is diagnostic of orthostatic hypotension (see Table 27-3). Perform careful cardiac and neurologic examinations.

Treatment and Disposition ■

Upon the return of consciousness and hemodynamic stability, the therapy for syncope varies depending upon the underlying etiology. Consider hospitalizing children with a cardiac etiology, since they may require urgent pharmacologic or surgical intervention. Children whose apparent syncope is due to a convulsive seizure may also benefit by a hospital admission for urgent evaluation of their neurologic status (see Chapter 26). Children with orthostatic syncope may require treatment for hypovolemia or anemia. Fortunately, however, most syncopal episodes are benign and require only reassurance and guidance to avoid the precipitating events.

Bibliography ■

Beder SD, Cohen MH, Riemenschneider TA: Occult arrhythmias as the etiology of unexplained syncope in children with structurally normal hearts. *Am Heart J* 1985; 109:309–313.

Boudoulas H, Weissler AM, Lewis RP, et al: The clinical diagnosis of syncope. *Curr Probl Cardiol* 1982; 7:7–40.

Day SC, Cook EF, Funkenstein H, et al: Evaluation and outcome of emergency room patients with transient loss of consciousness. *Am J Med* 1982; 73:15–23.

Eagle KA, Black HR, Cook EF, et al: Evaluation of prognostic classifications for patients with syncope. *Am J Med* 1985; 79:455–460.

Goldstein DS, Spanarkel M, Pitterman A, et al: Circulatory control mechanisms in vasodepressor syncope. *Am Heart J* 1982; 104:1071–1075.

Ruckman RN: Cardiac causes of syncope. *Pediat Rev* 1987; 9:101–108.

Sapire DW, Casta A, Safley W, et al: Vasovagal syncope in children requiring pacemaker implantation. *Am Heart J* 1983; 106:1406–1411.

V

Nonemergent Complaints

28 Colic

Sylvia F. Villarreal

The infant's cry is basic to survival. Crying communicates hunger, pain, illness, and the need for attention. Parents, health providers, and others depend on this cry to assess the child's health and well-being.

Quantitative and qualitative differences in crying signal distress in a young infant. The average crying time per day increases from 1 hour at 2 weeks, peaks at 3.5 hours at 6 weeks, and decreases to 1 hour at 3 months. Parents can usually interpret their infant's cry and distinguish hurt from hunger.

In the emergency department (ED) setting, health providers must depend on this interpretation to evaluate illness. Problems arise in the translation when parents are developmentally young, inexperienced, stressed, or psychiatrically impaired, because such parents may have difficulty assessing changes in their infant's cry. Cultural and language differences also influence interpretation of the quality of crying: What may be taken for normal crying in a black family may not be acceptable for a Hispanic or Chinese family.

Figure 28-1 presents a decision algorithm for the diagnosis of a crying infant (under 1 year of age), based on the quality and quantity of crying.

Differential Diagnosis ■

Intussusception can present as crying alternating with quiet periods. Physical exam may reveal a sausage-shaped right upper quadrant mass and abdominal distension (see Chapter 40).

Sepsis in a young infant is a medical emergency. Severely ill infants may present in shock, listless, weak, and with a weakened, high-pitched cry. The child's temperature may be elevated or there may be hypothermia (see Chapter 113). Localized infections may cause crying (e.g., otitis media may present in young infants merely as crying). The physical exam and appropriate ancillary tests such as complete blood count, urinalysis, and cerebrospinal fluid analysis assist in the diagnosis.

Drug-exposed infants are jittery and inconsolable and may be poor feeders. In-utero exposure to "crack" cocaine, heroin, methadone, PCP (phencyclidine), and amphetamines can result in disturbances in normal-state control. By taking a careful history, the in-utero exposure can be elicited from the natural or foster family. Treatment consists of swaddling the infant and placing him or her in a quiet environment; infrequently diazepam, phenobarbital, or methadone is used.

Hydrocephalus with increasing head circumference in early infancy can present with a high-pitched cry. A bulging fontanelle, sunsetting eyes, and positive transillumination in a developmentally delayed infant aids in the diagnosis. An ultrasound or CAT scan will show the increasing ventricular size.

Subdural hematomas and skull fractures in young infants may present as crying, increasing head circumference, and irritability. Consider child abuse.

Intestinal obstruction must be excluded. Anorexia in a previously healthy infant associated with bilious emesis, inconsolable crying, and obstipation suggests the rare entity of midgut volvulus (see Chapter 31).

Constipation is a symptom complex of hard, infrequent stooling and the parents' perception of how the infant moves his or her bowels. Consider an anal fissure (see Chapter 30) if hard, pellet-like stools make the infant draw up his or her legs, turn red in the face, and then release blood-streaked stool. Anal fissures can cause crying with bowel movements.

Cinical Findings ■

While taking the history from the caretakers on an infant who is actively crying, ensure that the physical assessment includes the features noted in Figure 28-2. A thorough eye examination is important but not easy with a screaming baby. Look for eyelashes curled up and causing a foreign body reaction. Consider fluorescein to check for corneal abrasion. Photophobia, increased tearing, and a hazy cornea suggests the rare possibility of glaucoma. Examine the infant's extremities for evidence of strangulation of fingers, toes, or penis by hair or thread. Carefully

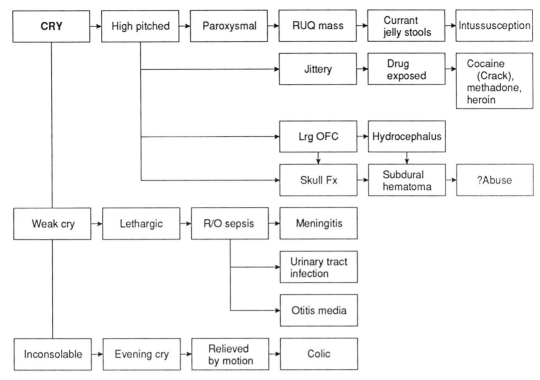

FIGURE 28–1. Evaluation of crying in infancy.

palpate arms, legs, and skull for fractures, crepitation, or swelling. Look for possible DPT reaction sites on arms or legs; these are often red, warm, swollen areas of induration. An open diaper pin in a cloth diaper is occasionally a cause for crying.

Infantile Colic ■

Colic is a diagnosis of exclusion. Inconsolable, paroxysmal crying that is nocturnal is characteristic of infantile colic. The quality of the cry is screamlike. The crying usually lasts more than 3 hours per day, more than 3 times a week and the infant is usually 2 or 3 weeks old. The baby becomes irritable and fussy and cries in a violent, rhythmic fashion. He or she may be hypertonic with stiffening of the extremities, clenching of fists, and legs drawn up over the abdomen. The arms can be flailing, flapping, or batting, the body writhing, twisting, or turning. Parents report that the baby is easily startled or awakened. This child may have daytime wakefulness and may take few if any naps. The infant is otherwise perfectly healthy and happy. The physical exam is normal. The baby's growth and development are normal.

About 10% of all infants are colicky. Colic is often ascribed to sensitive temperaments. *Treatment should be aimed at assuaging the parents' concern and anxiety.* Extensive laboratory tests are likely to make both parents and the health provider more anxious.

A number of treatment approaches are helpful. Try rhythmic motion: carrying the infant in a pack, swing, cradle, waterbed, rocking chair, car, or vibrating chair. Folk remedies such as mint or chamomile teas, massage, or a warm-water bottle to the abdomen are sometimes successful. Gently remind parents that the cry does not necessarily mean hunger, and that overfeeding the infant will not help. Encourage breastfeeding mothers to decrease or eliminate the use of caffeinated beverages and other stimulants. Attempt to modify the infant's daytime sleep pattern; the baby should not sleep more than 3 hours at a time. The infant should be placed on his or her abdomen to sleep.

Provide support and guidance to the family, and ensure follow-up with the primary physician. Other support services are often indicated. A grandmother or babysitter can give the parents time for outside activity to help them maintain their peace of mind.

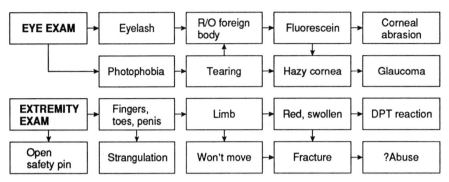

FIGURE 28–2. Physical examination in infantile crying.

Psychiatric referral is occasionally warranted. Colicky babies frustrate parents, and preventing child abuse is an essential concern for all affected families, especially for infants of teen and drug-using parents.

Bibliography ■

Brazelton TB: Crying in infancy. *Pediatrics* 1962; 29:579.

Chasnoff IJ, Lewis DE, Squires L: Cocaine intoxication in a breast-fed infant. *Pediatrics* 1987; 80:836.

Illingworth RS: Infantile colic revisited. *Arch Dis Child* 1985; 60:981.

Oro AS, Dixon SD: Perinatal cocaine and methamphetamine exposure: Maternal and neonatal correlates. *J Pediatr* 1987; 111:571.

Rebelsky F, Black R: Crying in infancy. *J Genet Psychol* 1972; 121:49.

Schmitt BD: *Your child's health: A pediatric guide for parents.* New York: Bantam, 1987:124.

Weissbluth M: *Crybabies.* New York: Berkeley, 1983.

Weissbluth M: *Healthy sleep habits, happy child.* New York: Fawcett Columbine, 1987.

29 Diarrhea

Sylvia F. Villarreal

Diarrhea is a major cause of childhood deaths in developing countries; in the United States, it accounts for 2% of the postneonatal infant deaths. Diarrhea is the excessive loss of fluids and electrolytes in the stool, through either an increase in number of the stools or a softening in their usual consistency. Excessive loss in an infant is usually greater than 20 ml/kg/day; an older child's fecal loss may exceed 200 ml/m²/day. Loss of this fluid results in hypovolemia and hypoperfusion and ultimately, if not treated, in shock (see Chapters 8 and 22).

Acute diarrhea, lasting less than 5 to 6 days, typically results from gastroenteritis. Diarrhea is usually self-limited. The challenge to the health provider is to prevent dehydration and malnutrition and to identify associated serious disorders such as bacteremia, hemolytic uremic syndrome, intussusception, and Hirschsprung's enterocolitis.

Etiology ■

Table 29-1 lists the infectious causes of diarrhea. Rotavirus is responsible for the major morbidity from diarrheal illness in the United States and for one-third of winter hospitalizations in children 4 to 36 months.

Clinical Findings ■

A good *history* is paramount: when did the diarrhea start, how many episodes per day or hour, what color, how much water loss? Inquire about stool odor, episodes associated with crying, abdominal or rectal pain, or vomiting. Is there fever? How often has the diaper been wet (urine and not stool)? Are there tears, is the mouth moist, are the eyes normal and shiny, is the child active and playful, and is the fontanelle or soft spot flat and not sunken? Has the child lost weight? Is a previous recent weight known? Was the child on any medications or antibiotics before the onset of diarrhea? Is the child prone to otitis media?

A dietary history will establish recent changes in formula, breast milk, or diet; any home remedies or folk cures such as herbal teas, rice water, or antidiarrheal agents; and the fluid intake over the past day.

A history of recent travel, especially to mountainous areas or foreign countries, will help in the diagnosis of parasitic or bacterial diarrheas. New pets, others ill with diarrhea, day-care attendance, or family picnics help distinguish food poisoning from viral and bacterial causes. Ask about previous growth and development. Failure to thrive may suggest that the diarrhea is a chronic condition such as cystic fibrosis, celiac sprue, inflammatory bowel disease, or human immunodeficiency virus (AIDS) infection.

Physical examination must assess the severity of dehydration. Obtain a naked weight and compare it to a previous weight if available (see Chapter 22). Pay careful attention to the vital signs, as well as to the skin, mucous membranes, abdominal and rectal examinations.

Ancillary Data ■

Place a urine collection bag on every young infant with diarrhea after weight and vital signs. Hematest the stool for the presence of blood, then examine it microscopically for fecal leukocytes by doing a methylene blue stain. Finding sheets of inflammatory cells indicates a probable bacterial infection such as Campylobacter, Salmonella, Shigella, Yersinia, enteroinvasive E. coli, or Clostridium dificile.

Send a stool specimen for culture and sensitivity when any of the following are present:

1. Heme-positive stools and/or fecal leukocytes
2. Infants one year and younger who are toxic and dehydrated
3. Children with hemoglobinopathies and immunodeficiencies.

Request tests for ova and parasites on children who are recent immigrants, who have a significant travel history, or whose diarrhea lingers more than a week.

TABLE 29–1. *Infectious Causes of Acute Diarrhea*

Agents	Age	Diarrhea	Fever	Blood	Fecal WBC
Rotavirus	<5 yrs	Watery	50%–75%	0	12%
Norwalk	All	45%	Rare	0	0
Campylobacter	Any	Initially watery	80%	90%	85%
Salmonella	Any	Foul-smelling, mucous, loose	75%	80%	75%
Shigella	Any	Odorless mucous	50%–70%	++	84%
E. coli, enterotoxigenic	Any	Profuse watery	20% (low grade)	0	0
Yersinia	Any	Watery	50%–80%	10%	10%–50%
Giardia	Any	Watery, foul-smelling	0	0	0

(Adapted from Nurko S, Walker WA: Acute diarrhea. In Dersheurtz RA, ed: Ambulatory Pediatric Care. Philadelphia, JB Lippincott, 1980: 468)

Children who appear toxic, are >5% dehydrated, or are under 2 months old warrant a urine specific gravity, urinalysis, serum electrolytes, and BUN. A complete blood count is helpful in evaluating sepsis.

Figure 29-1 presents an algorithm for differential diagnosis based on clinical findings and simple ancillary data.

Treatment ■

The major objective in managing diarrhea is to prevent further dehydration, acidosis, and shock. Oral rehydration, which is useful in 95–98% of children, has made a great impact both in the United States and developing countries in the treatment of diarrhea.

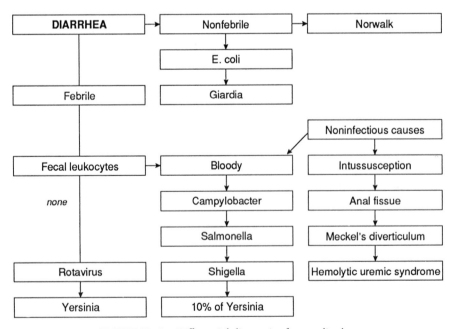

FIGURE 29–1. Differential diagnosis of acute diarrhea.

TABLE 29–2. *Oral Rehydration Solutions*

Solutions	mEq/L			Base	CHO (%)
	Na$^+$	K$^+$	Cl$^-$		
WHO	90	20	80	HCO 30	G 2%
Hydra-Lyte	84	10	59	HCO 30 + Citrate 20	G + S 2%
Lytren	50	25	45	Citrate 20	G 2%
Pedialyte	45	20	35	Citrate 30	G 2%
Resol	50	20	50	Citrate 34	G 2%

Table 29-2 lists the compositions of commercially available oral solutions for use in diarrhea. Breast-feeding infants should continue to feed while taking oral rehydration. Formula-fed infants can be placed on solely oral rehydration fluids and later weaned back to formula. The use of pectin, such as in apples or rice, can be helpful in mild diarrhea. *Kaolin, anticholinergics, antiemetics, or opiates have not been shown to shorten the course of diarrhea and should not be used in young infants with diarrhea.*

Pepto-Bismol may be effective in managing viral gastroenteritis in adolescents. Bismuth is the active ingredient and has no toxicity at recommended doses. Do not routinely use antibiotics and antiparasitics unless the diagnosis is established by stool inspection for ova and parasites or stool culture and antibiotic sensitivity. However, an infant under 1 year who is truly symptomatic with bloody stools and fecal leukocytes may have shigellosis: in such an instance, prescribe trimethoprim/sulfamethoxazole (8–12 mg/kg TMP, or 30–60 mg/kg SMX per 24 hours, divided every 12 hours) empirically, prior to laboratory verification.

Disposition ■

Hospitalize children who meet the dehydration criteria outlined in Chapter 22. Close telephone contact or a return visit is necessary for infants under 6 months old who are discharged with oral rehydration. Advise the parents of older infants and toddlers to return or call the clinic or ED if the diarrhea persists after 3 days of fluid and diet management. Ensure that parents know the warning signs of dehydration and have written take-home instructions (see Chapter 143).

Bibliography ■

Barkin R: Acute infectious diarrheal disease in children. *J Emerg Med* 1985; 3:1.

Brown KH, McLean VC: Nutritional management of acute diarrhea: An appraisal of the alternatives. *Pediatrics* 1984; 73:119.

Carpenter CCJ, Greenough WB, Pierce NF: Oral rehydration therapy: The role of polymeric substrates. *N Eng J Med* 1988; 319:1346.

Ho MS, Glass RI, Pinsky PF, et al: Diarrheal deaths in American children. *JAMA* 1988; 260:3281.

Jason JM, Jarvis WR: Infectious diseases: Preventable causes of infant mortality. *Pediatrics* 1987; 80:335.

Levine MM, Pizarro D: Advances in therapy of diarrheal dehydration: Oral rehydration. *Adv Pediatr* 1984; 31:207.

Listernick R, Zieserl E, Davis AT: Outpatient oral rehydration in the United States. *Am J Dis Child* 1986; 140:211.

Nurko S, Walker WA: Acute diarrhea. In: Dershewitz RA, ed. *Ambulatory pediatric care.* Philadelphia: JB Lippincott, 1988:468.

Tamer AM, Friedman LB, Maxwell SRW, et al. Oral rehydration of infants in a large urban US medical center. *J Pediatr* 1986; 107:14.

30 Constipation

Sylvia F. Villarreal

The ability to defecate easily is a complex interaction. Constipation is a condition of the bowels in which the feces are dry and hardened and evacuation is difficult and infrequent.

Normal stooling patterns for children and adults vary widely. Some newborns may have a stool with every feed (gastrocolic reflex) while others who are breast-fed may have large, soft stools once every seven days. New parents may misinterpret as constipation the normal red face, pulling up of the legs to the abdomen, grunting, and straining of noncrying infants. Children 1 to 4 years old may stool once or twice a day. Ninety-five percent of children have a bowel movement between once every other day and three times a day. In the emergency, acute-care setting, about 3–4% of all visits concern constipation.

Table 30-1 describes the differential diagnosis for constipation in infants 18 months and younger. Table 30-2 addresses constipation in children and adolescents.

Infantile Constipation ■

MECHANICAL

Constipation in a newborn is abnormal. About 90% of infants will stool within one day of life. *Hirschsprung's disease* (congenital aganglionosis) is a relatively uncommon abnormality with absence of ganglion cells in the distal rectum and a variable length of proximal bowel. This segment of the bowel is in tonic contraction, producing a functional obstruction.

Hirschsprung's may clinically present as an infant who fails to pass meconium within 48 hours of life and continues to stool infrequently. Frank obstruction with bilious emesis and abdominal distention may occur at any time. One-third of Hirschsprung's cases go undiagnosed until after 3 months of age; 15–25% are diagnosed at age 5 years or older. Diarrhea in children with Hirschsprung's is an ominous sign of enterocolitis, protein-losing enteropathy, and impending sepsis. A rectal exam usually reveals an empty ampulla and produces transient dilatation of a narrowed rectal segment. The exam may produce an explosive release of stool and gas. A surgical consultation should be obtained. A careful barium enema can reveal a distal narrowed segment with classical saw-toothed contractions, variable degrees of proximal obstruction, and the delayed emptying of barium. If readily available, rectal manometry or suction rectal biopsy can be the initial screen for a nontoxic infant.

Another mechanical variation is the *anterior ectopic anus,* which can be diagnosed on physical exam. An eccentrically situated anus is on the pigmented perineum. It is most common in females and hard straining becomes apparent in the newborn. An anal wink can be demonstrated posterior to the anal orifice. On rectal exam a sharp posterior angle is felt along with a posterior shelf. These infants will need a surgical evaluation.

PAINFUL CONSTIPATION

Anal fissures (see Chapter 32) may be both the cause and effect of constipation. Bright-red stripes of blood on the stool may cause great alarm in parents. A rectal exam done by carefully spreading the buttocks will often reveal the breaks in the mucosa.

Rectal prolapse in infancy is rare; it may be a sign of cystic fibrosis or sexual abuse.

MOTILITY DISORDERS

Motility disorders may be caused by hypothyroidism, hyperparathyroidism, hypercalcemia, renal tubular acidosis, or diabetes insipidus. In an emergency setting, a complete endocrine or metabolic workup cannot be done; routine electrolytes, calcium, phosphorus, and urinalysis are good screening laboratory examinations. The diagnosis is further aided by the fact that many of these infants fail to thrive. Suspect an organic etiology in constipation with poor growth.

NEUROMUSCULAR DISORDERS

Neuromuscular disorders may present with constipation in a floppy or developmentally delayed infant.

TABLE 30–1. *Infantile Constipation*

Definitional
  Breast-fed
  Normal variation

Mechanical
  Hirschsprung's
  Anterior ectopic anus

Painful
  Anal fissure
  Rectal prolapse

Motility Disorders

  Endocrine/Metabolic Disorders
    Hypothyroid
    Hyperparathyroidism
    Hypercalcemia
    Renal tubular acidosis
    Diabetes insipidus

  Neuromuscular Disorders
    Hypotonia
    Werdnig-Hoffman
    Spina bifida
    Cerebral palsy
    Spinal cord tumor

  Infectious Diseases
    Viral illness
    Infant botulism

  Drug-Induced
    Anticholinergics
    Anticonvulsants
    Narcotics
    Iron
    Lead

Compositional Constipation
  Milk excess

Hypotonia, Werdnig-Hoffman disease, spina bifida, cerebral palsy, or spinal cord tumor all have altered neurologic input to the rectal and anorectal sphincter. The rectal exam will reveal a large amount of stool in the ampulla. These babies often require digital stimulation or chronic use of suppositories and stool softeners to ensure regular passage of stool.

INFECTIOUS ETIOLOGIES

Infections may cause transient constipation; viral illness with its associated anorexia and dehydration may cause an acute problem. Infant botulism may present as a breast-feeding young infant with a few days of constipation followed by progressive weakness and symmetrical paresis or paralysis. Send confirmatory stool for toxin or organism of *Clostridium botulinum*, and hospitalize suspected infants.

DRUGS

Anticholinergics, anticonvulsants, narcotics, and iron may cause acute constipation in infants. Lead poisoning, more likely to occur in inner-city infants or those living near battery factories, may present with constipation.

COMPOSITIONAL CONSTIPATION

By far the most common cause of compositional constipation is excessive milk intake, especially whole cow's milk. A diet history will reveal that the young infant may be taking 30–40 ounces of milk a day and nothing else. Improper mixing of concentrated formula may lead to constipation, as well as fluid and electrolyte abnormalities.

TABLE 30–2. *Childhood and Adolescent Constipation*

Functional
  Chronic retentive
  Encopresis

Painful Defecation
  Anal fissures
  Sexual abuse
  Foreign body
  Rectal prolapse
  Proctitis
  Anal stenosis

Mechanical Constipation
  Hirschsprung's disease
  Celiac disease

Motility Disorders

  Neuromuscular
    (see Table 30–1.)
    Repaired imperforate anus

  Drug-Induced
    Anticholinergics
    Anticonvulsants
    Antidepressants
    Iron
    Lead
    Anesthetics
    Aluminum-based antacids
    Narcotics (legal and street)

Idiopathic Slow Transit Constipation

Depression

Anorexia Nervosa

Pregnancy

Childhood and Adolescent Constipation ■

For many children, the onset of toilet training and the normal development of independence marks the onset of constipation. Table 30-2 lists the differential diagnosis for older children and adolescents.

Functional or chronic retentive constipation is more common in males, peaks at age 2 to 4, and is associated with the passage of large stools. Associated urinary-tract problems are common. A rectal exam reveals a large stool mass in the ampulla; otherwise the child has normal growth and development. Send a urinalysis, and refer these children to a primary-care setting or gastroenterologist for bowel rehabilitation.

Encopresis is soiling or incontinence of stool. An oversimplification is that the child is constipated and impacted. The hard stool blocks the passage of more liquid matter, and therefore the soiling may be overflow secondary to the withheld stool. The cause is usually psychogenic. On abdominal exam, hard stools are palpated throughout the sigmoid colon. A rectal exam reveals stool in the ampulla, and on inspection the underwear may be soiled. Refer these children to a primary-care setting or a behavioral clinic.

PAINFUL DEFECATION

Anal fissures may be secondary to hard stools. Constipation may also be the presenting complaint of a sexually abused child. Foreign bodies, rectal prolapse, proctitis, and anal stenosis cause pain and can be found on a routine rectal examination.

MECHANICAL CONSTIPATION

As in infancy, Hirschsprung's disease may present in a child with chronic constipation. A rectal exam reveals an empty ampulla. Celiac disease may present with marked abdominal distention, poor growth, and chronic constipation.

MOTILITY DISORDERS

The same neuromuscular disorders that cause constipation in infancy may also cause chronic constipation in children. A child with a repaired imperforate anus may have chronic problems with constipation. Drugs producing constipation may include antide-pressants, anesthetics, aluminum-based antacids, and narcotics (legal or street drugs).

Idiopathic slow transit constipation presents in teenage girls. A careful history should explore the possibility of pregnancy, parasites, depression, anorexia nervosa, sexual abuse, and a junk-food diet. Preliminary lab tests may include a urinalysis, pregnancy test, and stool for parasites.

Treatment and Disposition ■

Acute constipation in all age groups requires reassurance and understanding. Encourage the parents to avoid aggressive procedures such as rectal dilatations, enemas, and frequent suppositories. Dietary changes are useful, especially decreasing milk consumption. Diluting the milk and decreasing the volume of intake may solve the problem. Dark Karo syrup in formula (½ to 2 teaspoons per bottle) may help in infants less than 6 months old. Diluted prune juice can be used in infants 6 months or older. Bran and fiber introduced into a child's or adolescent's diet is ideal, although difficult to maintain in this fast-food society. Try malt extract (1–4 tablespoons/day) with older children and adolescents.

Severe chronic constipation (longer than one month's duration) is a special problem. Refer these children to a primary-care setting once impaction and pain have been controlled. An aggressive program for bowel clean-out and rehabilitation is indicated.

Bibliography ■

Abrahamian FP, Lloyd-Still JD: Chronic constipation in childhood: A longitudinal study of 186 patients. *J Pediatr Gastroenterol Nutr* 1984; 3:460–467.

Hatch TF: Encopresis and constipation in children. *Pediatr Clin North Am* 1988; 35:2;257–279.

Levine MD: *Current pediatric therapy 12: Constipation and encopresis.* Philadelphia: WB Saunders, 1986;187–190.

Long SS: Epidemiologic study of infant botulism in Pennsylvania: Report of the infant botulism study group. *Pediatrics* 1985; 75:928–934.

Schmitt BD: Constipation. In: *Your Child's Health. A Pediatric Guide for Parents.* New York: Bantam, 1987;483–488.

Weaver LT, Ewing G, Taylor LC, et al: The bowel habits of milk-fed infants. *J Pediatr Gastroenterol Nutr* 1988; 7:568.

31 Vomiting

Colin D. Rudolph

Pathophysiology ■

Vomiting is a complex coordinated activity. The abdominal muscles and diaphragm contract while the pylorus closes and the lower esophageal sphincter relaxes, resulting in the forceful ejection of the stomach contents through the mouth. Vomiting occurs when a region of the reticular formation in the brainstem is activated by a large number of different stimuli. Emetic drugs and toxins act on the "chemoreceptor trigger zone" located in the area postrema. Other neural afferents from the GI tract, pharynx, coronary vessels, peritoneum, bile ducts, and cerebral cortex also impinge on the vomiting center and stimulate vomiting.

Nausea is the sensation that often precedes vomiting. Retching is like vomiting, but gastric contents are not ejected. Nausea and retching often occur before vomiting, but can occur independent of vomiting. Regardless of cause, vomiting can result in aspiration pneumonia, Mallory-Weiss tears, esophageal rupture, or dehydration.

Vomiting must not be confused with regurgitation or gastroesophageal reflux. Non-forceful regurgitation of gastric contents into the esophagus and through the mouth commonly occurs after meals during transient relaxations of the lower esophageal sphincter. This results in regurgitation of food after meals in normal, well infants and toddlers. An approach to gastroesophageal reflux is discussed below.

Clinical Findings ■

The myriad causes of vomiting demand that the evaluation be directed by a careful history and physical exam, which often provide important diagnostic clues. The time of onset of vomiting, relationship to meals, and frequency of vomiting are important to determine. Morning vomiting often occurs with pregnancy or in patients with increased intracranial pressure. The possibility of food poisoning or exposure to infectious agents, toxins, or medications should be explored. Presence of bile in the vomitus or vomitus with a feculent odor indicates possible GI obstruction. The presence of coffee-ground material or gross blood in the vomitus requires evaluation for a cause of upper GI bleeding (see Chapter 32).

Initially, focus the physical exam on the patient's overall status. It is important to determine if immediate rehydration is necessary. Note extra-GI findings of infection including fever, irritability, or cough. Carefully assess the patient's mental status. Irritability or lethargy are common in patients exposed to toxins or drugs. Altered mental status and vomiting are cardinal findings in patients with Reye's syndrome or with increased intracranial pressure due to meningitis or intracranial hemorrhage. Examine ocular fundi for evidence of increased intracranial pressure.

Perform the abdominal exam as if the patient had an "acute abdomen," since vomiting is often the presenting symptom of illnesses such as appendicitis, pancreatitis, and intussusception. Hepatomegaly may indicate hepatitis. In infants palpation of an olive-like mass in the right upper quadrant indicates the diagnosis of pyloric stenosis. In older children, a sausage-shaped mass in the right upper quadrant would suggest the possibility of intussusception, or the genital exam may reveal an incarcerated inguinal hernia.

Vomiting in the Newborn ■

Vomiting in the immediate neonatal period requires careful, rapid evaluation. Most infants regurgitate or "spit up," but real vomiting usually indicates a serious underlying disorder such as a congenital GI obstruction, infection, or metabolic disorder.

GASTROINTESTINAL OBSTRUCTION

Intestinal atresia, which presents with vomiting shortly after birth, is the most common cause of intestinal obstruction in the newborn. Plain abdominal films reveal air fluid levels in the stomach and duodenum ("double-bubble") in the case of duodenal atresia or show multiple dilated loops of bowel with the absence of colonic air. Surgical intervention is mandatory in all cases of intestinal atresia.

Meconium ileus can present with vomiting and findings identical to those of intestinal atresia. Ninety percent of patients with meconium ileus have cystic fibrosis. An associated antenatal perforation is suggested by the presence of ascites and extraluminal calcifications.

Meconium plug syndrome should be differentiated from meconium ileus. A plug of meconium obstructs the distal colon in the newborn, resulting in obstruction and vomiting. Barium enema is usually diagnostic and therapeutic. Patients with Hirschsprung's disease have a high incidence of meconium plug syndrome.

Midgut volvulus can occur at any age but is most common in the first month of life. The infant has bile-stained vomiting and abdominal distention with progressive signs of bowel ischemia, including passage of currant-jelly stools. Abdominal plain films may be normal in appearance or may demonstrate obstruction and distention. Upper GI series demonstrate a twisted "corkscrew" obstruction at the ligament of Treitz. Barium enema may demonstrate a malrotation of the colon but cannot reliably confirm the diagnosis of midgut volvulus. The catastrophic results of late diagnosis demand that any infant with possible midgut volvulus be rapidly evaluated and, if possible, transferred for expert pediatric surgical management.

Hirschsprung's disease or colonic aganglionosis is suggested by the delayed passage of meconium and abdominal distention with bilious vomiting in the first week of life. Barium enema reveals a narrowed distal rectum with a transition to dilated bowel at variable distances from the anus. Suction rectal biopsy or anorectal manometry confirm the diagnosis (see Chapter 30).

Imperforate anus results in lower GI obstruction with vomiting. A careful physical examination should rule out this diagnosis.

Pyloric stenosis causes non-bilious projectile vomiting. It may commence within the first week after birth, but typically the onset is delayed until 4 to 8 weeks of age. Physical examination reveals visible peristaltic waves associated with a palpable pyloric tumor ("olive"). The diagnosis can be confirmed by abdominal ultrasound or upper GI study. After hydration, surgical intervention is necessary.

VOMITING WITHOUT OBSTRUCTION

Sepsis or *meningitis* can cause bilious or non-bilious vomiting. Evaluate and treat infants with suspected GI obstruction for possible bacterial infection before radiologic and surgical evaluation for bowel obstruction.

Congenital metabolic disorders can initially present with vomiting. Usually vomiting occurs after meals and is not bile-stained. Congenital adrenal hyperplasia, phenylketonuria, galactosemia, hereditary fructose intolerance, urea cycle disorders, and other abnormalities in amino and organic acid metabolism should be considered in the newborn with vomiting.

Other causes include renal insufficiency, renal tubular acidosis or obstructive uropathy, subdural hematoma, and withdrawal from maternal drugs of abuse.

Cow's milk or soy formula intolerance is a relatively uncommon cause of vomiting. Vomiting attributed to this condition is more likely common gastroenteritis.

GASTROESOPHAGEAL REFLUX

Regurgitation or "spitting up" occurs in most infants. Typically, curdled milk is expelled from the mouth shortly after feeding. The infant otherwise appears well. Unless the infant is not growing or has problems with aspiration, no treatment is required. Inexperienced parents often present in the emergency department (ED) complaining of vomiting that, in fact, is normal "spitting up." Counseling the parents to give the infant more frequent, smaller feeds and to burp the infant in the middle of feedings is often very useful. Positioning the infant in the prone position with the head elevated also decreases the amount of regurgitation. Changing formulas is not effective. No medications should be administered unless there is clear evidence of poor weight gain, esophagitis, or respiratory problems. Controlled trials do not support the efficacy of the currently available antireflux medications in infants.

Vomiting in Infants and Children ■

Etiologies of vomiting are even more diverse in older infants and children than in the newborn. *GI infection accounts for the overwhelming majority of cases of vomiting.* However, vomiting can be the presenting symptom of many serious disorders.

GI DISORDERS

GI obstruction is suggested by the presence of bile in the vomitus. Midgut volvulus and Hirschsprung's disease are discussed above but can occur at any age. Vomiting may occur with intussusception prior to the passage of bloody stools. Always consider incarcerated inguinal hernias, postsurgical adhesions, and foreign bodies as possible explanations of GI obstruction. If a history of trauma is obtained, obstruction by a duodenal hematoma must be differentiated from post-traumatic pancreatitis. Non-bilious vomiting occurs with pyloric stenosis as noted above. Vomiting is occasionally the presenting complaint of patients with achalasia or esophageal stricture.

Peptic ulcer disease may result in nausea and vomiting. In younger children it may be difficult to obtain a history of typical "ulcer" pain. Periumbilical or generalized abdominal pain is more commonly described, particularly at night.

Pancreatitis is another common cause of recurrent vomiting and abdominal pain.

Appendicitis often begins with a prodrome of nausea and vomiting before the typical pattern of fever and right lower quadrant pain is apparent (see Chapter 40).

Hepatitis is frequently associated with nausea and vomiting during the anicteric phase (see Chapter 105).

OTHER DISORDERS ASSOCIATED WITH VOMITING

Reye's syndrome is characterized by the onset of severe, intractable vomiting followed by alterations in state of consciousness with rapid progression to coma. Characteristically, it occurs in children under 15 years of age after an antecedent viral illness, most commonly chicken pox or a respiratory illness. Laboratory tests reveal markedly elevated transaminases, ammonia, and prothrombin time, with bilirubin less than 3 mg/dl (50 μmol/l). Hypoglycemia is common.

Administer intravenous 10% dextrose to all children suspected of having Reye's syndrome. Comatose patients need emergency treatment consisting of IV 15% dextrose at ¾ maintenance volumes, endotracheal intubation, and hyperventilation. Give 0.5–1 g/kg mannitol every 4–6 hours if there are signs of cerebral edema. Transfer any child with suspected Reye's syndrome immediately to a pediatric critical care center.

Several disorders must be differentiated from Reye's syndrome, including systemic carnitine defi-

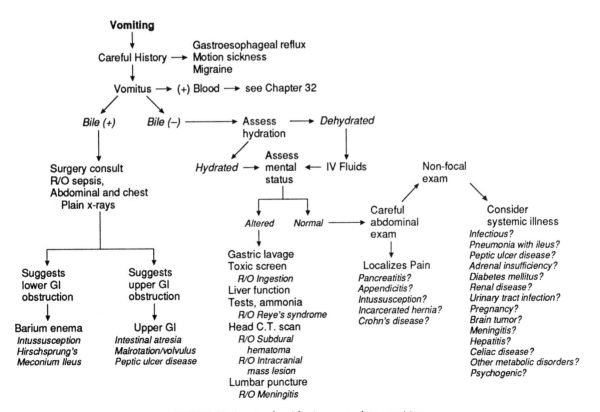

FIGURE 31–1. An algorithmic approach to vomiting.

ciency, acyl CoA dehydrogenase deficiency, and fulminant hepatic failure.

Neurologic disorders, such as subdural hematoma, intracranial mass lesions, encephalitis, and meningitis may present with the chief complaint of vomiting. Perform a complete neurologic evaluation in all patients with unexplained vomiting.

Pneumonia can cause vomiting with or without ileus. This is a commonly overlooked, easily treated cause of vomiting. Coughing may also be associated with vomiting. Usually a careful history can discriminate between cases of coughing causing vomiting versus vomiting resulting in aspiration and coughing.

Urinary tract infection, uremia, and obstructive uropathies result in vomiting.

Electrolyte disturbances resulting from adrenal insufficiency, disorders of calcium metabolism, or diabetes mellitus present with vomiting.

Toxin and drug ingestions commonly presenting with vomiting as a major sign include lead, theophylline, digoxin, aspirin, and iron.

Treatment ■

The diagnostic and therapeutic approach to vomiting in the infant and child are outlined below and in Figure 31-1.

1. Place an intravenous cannula for treatment of dehydration (see Chapter 22).
2. If GI obstruction is present, place a nasogastric tube with intermittent suction to decompress the stomach.
3. Obtain laboratory tests, including electrolytes, complete blood count (CBC) and differential, platelet count, urinalysis, and glucose. If meningitis is considered as a possible explanation for the vomiting, perform a lumbar puncture. Treat for possible bacterial infection as outlined in Chapter 113.
4. Perform radiologic studies including plain x-rays of the abdomen or upper GI or enema studies as

indicated from plain films. In an ill infant with bilious vomiting, consider midgut volvulus and perform an emergency upper GI study regardless of the findings on the plain x-rays of the abdomen. If a subdural hematoma is suspected, obtain a head CT scan.
5. Obtain surgical consultation in the evaluation of the newborn with bilious vomiting.
6. If GI obstruction is not evident on abdominal x-rays, consider another diagnosis listed above. Obtain laboratory tests including serum ammonia, creatinine, liver function tests, and amino acids, urine organic acids, and urine reducing substances.
7. *Antiemetics are rarely indicated in pediatric patients.* Limit ED use of these drugs. Prophylactic use in patients receiving chemotherapy is routine. Compazine, Torecan, and other phenothiazines carry a risk of tardive dyskinesia. For motion sickness, prophylactic treatment with meclizine or with a topical scopolamine patch is effective.

Disposition ■

Instruct patients with probable GI infections or other transient, self-limited causes of vomiting to continue taking fluids despite continued vomiting. In patients without GI obstruction or ileus, the ability to maintain hydration despite vomiting is impressive. Instruct all patients who do not require admission to return for further evaluation if there is a change in mental status, if the vomitus becomes bilious, if the vomitus contains blood or coffee-grounds, or if the infant or child develops signs of dehydration. See Chapter 143 for parental instructions.

Bibliography ■

Greene CL, Blitzer MG, Shapira E: Inborn errors of metabolism and Reye's syndrome: Differential diagnosis. *J Pediatr* 1988; 113:156.

32 Gastrointestinal Bleeding

Colin D. Rudolph

Gastrointestinal hemorrhage occurs when infection or ischemia results in inflammation and ulceration of the bowel mucosal lining. Alternatively, a blood vessel such as a varix or hemangioma can bleed directly into the bowel lumen. *Hematemesis* (vomiting blood) or *melena* (black stool from blood in the colon) usually indicates that the site of bleeding is in the proximal GI tract. *Hematochezia* (frank blood per rectum) usually results from bleeding in the distal small bowel or colon. However, due to the rapid GI transit in children, hematochezia alone can occur after an upper GI bleed.

Clinical Findings ■

The patient's age, general condition, and the amount and type of bleeding all help determine the most likely etiology and the most efficacious evaluation. Painless bleeding is usually not associated with ischemia of the bowel, which occurs during intussusception or volvulus. A history of vomiting, diarrhea, or fever is useful.

On physical exam, evaluate signs of perfusion including pallor, capillary refill, heart rate, and blood pressure. Icterus, ascites, and splenomegaly suggest liver disease and/or portal hypertension. Presence of petechiae or ecchymosis suggest a systemic coagulopathy. Angiomas, telangiectasias, or the mucosal pigmentation of Peutz-Jeghers syndrome are associated with intestinal vascular malformations or polyps.

Next, determine if GI hemorrhage has truly occurred. Occasionally, epistaxis, nasopharyngeal trauma, or hemoptysis can result in vomiting of coffee-ground emesis. A history of recent nosebleeds, recent severe coughing, or oral surgery may indicate that the GI tract is not the source of bleeding. Ingestion of red food colorings, medications, or gelatin desserts can result in passage of red stool, so confirm true bleeding with a Hemocult test of the stool or Gastrocult test of vomitus. Menstrual bleeding or hematuria are occasionally confused with rectal bleeding.

Upper and Lower GI Bleeding in the Newborn ■

ETIOLOGIES

1. *Swallowing maternal blood* during delivery or from a fissured nipple during breast feeding can result in hematemesis or melena in an otherwise well-appearing newborn. The Apt-Downey test differentiates infant from maternal blood by identifying fetal hemoglobin, which if present establishes that the blood is derived from the infant. A small amount of stool is mixed with tap water (1 part to 5 parts), and the mixture is centrifuged. Then, 1 ml of 0.25N sodium hydroxide is added to 5 ml of supernatant pink fluid; after 5 minutes a brown-yellow color indicates the presence of adult hemoglobin, whereas a pink color establishes the presence of fetal hemoglobin.
2. *Hemorrhagic disease of the newborn* can present with melena or hematochezia. Usually there is other evidence of a generalized bleeding disorder such as ecchymoses, petechiae, or umbilical bleeding. Routine Vitamin K prophylaxis has decreased the incidence of Vitamin K deficiency-associated bleeding. Ask if the mother received aspirin, anticoagulants, or anticonvulsants before delivery and determine if there is a family history of a bleeding disorder. Congenital thrombocytopenic purpura can result from a variety of causes. Coagulation studies, including prothrombin time, partial thromboplastin time, and platelet count, are required for diagnosis.
3. *Stress ulcers and hemorrhagic gastritis* are often associated with a history of asphyxia, sepsis, or hypovolemia. A blood transfusion is occasionally necessary. Diagnosis can be made by esophagogastroduodenoscopy (EGD). Antacids provide adequate treatment.
4. *Necrotizing enterocolitis* usually occurs within 7 days of the initiation of feeding. It is uncommon except in premature infants but does occur in full-term infants with congenital heart disease or after

167

exchange transfusions. Abdominal distention, vomiting, and hematochezia progress to perforation with sepsis, disseminated intravascular coagulation, and shock. Diagnosis is often delayed in full-term infants. Abdominal x-rays reveal the pathognomic findings of ileus, moderate distention, pneumatosis intestinales, and gas in the portal system.

5. *Midgut volvulus with malrotation* should be ruled out in any child with bilious vomiting (see Chapter 31).
6. *Neonatal hepatic necrosis or cirrhosis* can initially present with GI bleeding. Liver function tests are usually abnormal.

ANCILLARY DATA

1. Apt-Downey test
2. Coagulation studies: If abnormal, treat with 1 mg intravenous Vitamin K and fresh-frozen plasma (10 ml/kg) after obtaining blood for complete evaluation of bleeding diathesis.
3. Liver function tests
4. Serial hematocrits
5. Nasogastric tube placement and lavage to determine if bleeding originates from upper or lower bowel.
6. Abdominal films: If evidence of obstruction is present, perform an upper GI series emergently and obtain surgical consultation. If bleeding persists, there is no evidence of obstruction, and the remainder of the workup is negative, an endoscopic examination is indicated.

Upper GI Bleeding in Infants and Children ■

ETIOLOGIES

1. *Esophagitis or gastric and duodenal ulceration* are the most common causes of upper GI bleeding in infants and toddlers. A history of frequent regurgitation suggests esophagitis. EGD is often required to make the diagnosis and is preferable to radiographic studies.
2. *Esophageal varices* are uncommon in infants but may develop during the first to second year of life in children with liver disease or portal vein thrombosis. A history of omphalitis or umbilical vein catheterization as a newborn suggests the latter diagnosis. Variceal bleeding can be severe.

   Treatment is IV vasopressin for up to 48 hours to decrease bleeding. In children younger than 5 years, administer 0.1 unit/min IV. Increase the dose by 0.05 units/min to a maximum of 0.2 units/

min. In children less than 12 years, the maximum dose is 0.3 units/min; in adolescents and adults, 0.4 units/min.

Extreme pallor and disappearance of peripheral pulses due to arterial constriction occur frequently and are an indication for discontinuing vasopressin. Hypertension, cardiac arrythmias, and hyponatremia also occur. Emergency upper endoscopy and therapeutic sclerotherapy is the treatment of choice. In patients with esophageal varices, more than 40% of upper GI bleeds are actually due to gastritis or ulcers; therefore, a diagnostic EGD is key to specific diagnosis and treatment.

3. *Mallory-Weiss tears* usually occur after forceful vomiting. Diagnosis is made by EGD. With treatment of the vomiting, bleeding usually ceases.
4. *Foreign body ulceration* of the esophageal or gastric mucosa is a rare cause of GI bleeding in infants and toddlers.

Lower GI Bleeding in Infants and Children ■

ETIOLOGIES

1. *Anal fissure* is the most common cause of hematochezia in an otherwise well infant or toddler. A history of a small amount of blood on the outside of the stool and a history of constipation is common. Symptoms resolve with treatment of the constipation (see Chapter 30).
2. *Allergic proctocolitis* is a common cause of hematochezia. Diarrheal stool usually contains blood and mucous. Inflammation of the small and large bowel results from a sensitivity to the protein contained in cow's milk. One-quarter of infants with a cow's milk protein allergy are also allergic to soy protein. Definitive diagnosis by proctosigmoidoscopy and biopsy is accurate and cost-effective.
3. *Intussusception* usually occurs before 2 years of age. Symptoms include colicky abdominal pain, vomiting, and abdominal distention. Intussusception occurs frequently in children with cystic fibrosis or Henoch-Schönlein purpura (see Chapter 40).
4. *Meckel's diverticulum* most commonly presents with the painless passage of variable amounts of bright-red blood in the stool. Patients are usually less than 2 years old. Bleeding is due to mucosal ulceration by acid secreted from heterotopic gastric mucosa. Initially the quantity of blood loss may be small, but it increases rapidly, leading to shock. A nuclear medicine [99]technetium-per-

technate scan is required for diagnosis, and emergency laparotomy is necessary for treatment.

5. *Infectious diarrhea* is commonly associated with fever and the passage of blood and mucus in the stool. Most infants appear ill. The causes and nuances of presentation are discussed in Chapters 22 and 29. The most common pathogens are Campylobacter, Shigella, Salmonella, Yersinia, Clostridium dificile, and toxigenic E. coli.

6. *Hemolytic-uremic syndrome* is characterized by bloody diarrhea, hemolytic anemia, thrombocytopenia, and acute renal failure. It usually occurs in infants less than 2 years old. Hospitalization and careful observation are required. The colitis can progress to a toxic megacolon with perforation. See Chapter 111.

7. *Polyps* occur at all ages but are most common between 2 and 5 years of age. Bright-red blood is passed in the stool of an otherwise well child. Occasionally anemia results from chronic blood loss. The most common type of polyp is a juvenile inflammatory polyp, which is not associated with malignancy. Adenomatous polyps occur in familial polyposis syndrome and Gardner's syndrome. Hamartomatous polyps of the large and small bowel are associated with pigmentation of the buccal mucosa in patients with Peutz-Jeghers syndrome. Diagnosis is made by air-contrast barium enema or colonoscopy during the investigation of painless rectal bleeding in an otherwise well child.

8. *Hemangiomas and telangiectasias* can cause painless upper or lower GI bleeding at any age. Cutaneous skin lesions are sometimes associated, as in hereditary hemorrhagic telangiectasia syndrome (Rendu-Osler-Weber syndrome). Diagnosis is made by endoscopy or angiography.

9. *Henoch-Schönlein purpura (HSP)* causes hematochezia and is associated with severe colicky abdominal pain, joint swelling, a purpuric hemorrhagic skin rash (characteristic), and renal involvement. The abdominal pain and GI bleeding can precede the appearance of the skin rash. Submucosal hemorrhage can be seen endoscopically or is suggested by "thumbprinting and scalloping" on upper or lower GI radiographic studies. Rarely, intussusception occurs in patients with HSP. Barium enema may be diagnostic and therapeutic.

10. *Inflammatory bowel disease (Crohn's disease and ulcerative colitis)* is associated with abdominal pain, upper and lower GI bleeding, diarrhea, and poor growth. There is large variability in the presentation and prognosis. *Consider inflammatory bowel disease in all children with chronic GI bleeding.* Some children present with severe colitis and can have significant acute blood losses requiring aggressive inpatient management. Occasionally patients initially present with a toxic megacolon. Patients already diagnosed with inflammatory bowel disease may also develop this serious complication. Consider toxic megacolon

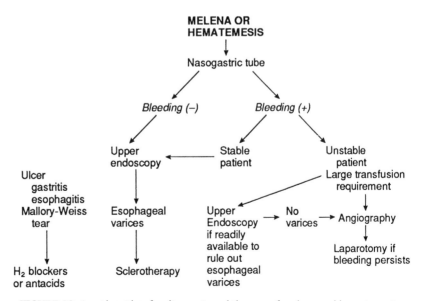

FIGURE 32–1. Algorithm for diagnosis and therapy of melena and hematemesis.

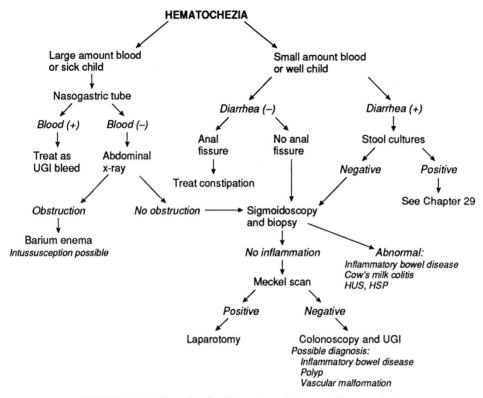

FIGURE 32-2. Algorithm for diagnosis and therapy of hematochezia.

when a patient with a history of inflammatory bowel disease or the recent onset of symptoms of colitis has a rapid worsening of symptoms associated with fever, abdominal distention and tenderness, and leukocytosis. Abdominal radiographs will reveal a distention of the transverse colon of over 5 cm.

When toxic megacolon is suspected, obtain an emergency surgical consultation and admit the patient to an intensive care unit. Treat dehydration aggressively and place a nasogastric tube for small bowel decompression. Administer IV ampicillin, gentamicin, and metronidazole, plus hydrocortisone (10 mg/kg/day).

11. *Hemorrhoids* are relatively rare in children, although they do occur in patients with portal hypertension.

A diagnostic and therapeutic approach to GI bleeding in the infant and child are outlined in Figure 32-1.

Treatment ■

Admit all patients with upper GI bleeding for observation and evaluation. In the well patient, diagnostic evaluation and treatment of hematochezia can usually be performed as an outpatient. In the ill-appearing patient, perform diagnostic evaluation only after the patient is stable. Emergent surgery is sometimes necessary to determine the source of bleeding.

The following management sequence is appropriate for any child with significant GI hemorrhage (Fig. 32-2):

1. Evaluate for cardiovascular stability, orthostasis, tachycardia.
2. Obtain history regarding amount of blood loss.
3. If a large amount of blood loss has occurred, place a large bore (at least 18G) IV cannula.
4. Type and cross-match blood and obtain baseline hematocrit, platelet count, prothrombin time, creatinine, BUN.

5. Infuse 0.9% saline or Ringer's lactate as required for shock (see Chapter 8). Rarely, with severe blood loss and hypotension, transfuse type O, Rh-negative blood. Otherwise, with a more stable patient, wait for type-specific or fully cross-matched blood.

6. Place a large-caliber nasogastric tube and lavage to determine if the bleeding originates from the upper or the lower GI tract. There is no advantage to lavage with ice-cold saline versus room temperature saline. *Iced lavage solutions can cause hypothermia in infants and are therefore contraindicated.*

7. Administer IV vitamin K (5 to 10 mg) after blood is obtained to rule out a bleeding diathesis.

8. If the patient's cardiovascular status is stable and blood requirements do not exceed 10 ml/kg/hr, diagnostic workup can proceed. If blood loss is more rapid, obtain surgical consultation and consider angiography. If blood replacement requirements are greater than 40 ml/kg in a 4-hour period, emergency surgery is necessary to determine the site and to control bleeding.

Bibliography ■

Cox K, Ament, ME: Upper gastrointestinal bleeding in children and adolescents. *Pediatrics* 1979; 63:408.

Hyams JS, Leichtner AL, Schwartz AN: Recent advances in diagnosis and treatment of gastrointestinal hemorrhage in infants and children. *J Pediatr* 1985; 106:1.

Roy CC, Morin CL, Weber AM: GI emergency problems in pediatric practice. *Clin Gastroenterol* 1981; 10:225.

Sherman NJ, Clatworthy HW: GI bleeding in neonates: A study of 94 cases. *Surgery* 1967; 62:614.

33 Swallowed Foreign Body

Colin D. Rudolph

Swallowing of foreign bodies is common in children between the ages of 6 months and 5 years. A large variety of objects are accidentally ingested, including coins, marbles, bones, toy animals, pins, and stones. Ingestion of foreign bodies by older children and adolescents usually results from intentional suicide gestures or attempts at "circus-like" pranks.

Clinical Findings ■

The approach to the patient who has swallowed a foreign body depends on a careful history. If the specific object ingested can be described in detail, the relative risk is more easily assessed. Sharp, long objects have a higher risk of perforation than dull, round objects. Objects with a diameter of less than 20 mm usually pass without incident. Objects containing mercury or lead must be removed if possible to prevent poisoning. Alkaline "button" batteries contain a 45% potassium hydroxide mixture and often perforate the esophagus; urgent removal is required. Foreign bodies may lodge in the esophagus, the stomach or small bowel, or the colon or rectum.

Esophageal Foreign Bodies ■

The esophagus is the most common location of acute foreign body obstruction. Fifty to sixty percent of foreign bodies lodge in the cervical esophagus, 25% at the aortic arch and 25% at the lower esophageal sphincter. Obstruction with meat is most common above a strictured region or in patients with esophageal motility disorders. Symptoms of esophageal obstruction include mild to severe retrosternal pain and the inability to swallow with hypersalivation. *The perceived location of obstruction often does not correlate with the actual site of obstruction.* Physical exam is usually normal, but crepitus over the neck or anterior chest wall is an ominous sign suggesting perforation.

Radiographic studies should include anterior-posterior (AP) and lateral soft-tissue films of the neck and chest. Foreign bodies in the esophagus tend to align with the wide dimension best seen in the AP direction, whereas foreign bodies in the trachea tend to align with the wide dimension facing laterally. Since many foreign bodies (including aluminum pull-tabs and wooden toys) are radiolucent, remember that normal radiographic studies do not rule out a foreign body. If symptoms persist, further evaluation by endoscopy is necessary. Avoid barium studies, which tend to obscure the view during later endoscopic efforts to retrieve objects.

TREATMENT

All esophageal foreign bodies require removal. "Button" batteries and sharp foreign bodies are more likely to cause esophageal perforation and therefore require immediate removal. The National Button Battery Ingestion Study has a 24-hour telephone emergency line available to provide advice: (209) 625-3333. On the other hand, if the foreign body (including "button" batteries or sharp objects) is dislodged into the stomach, further treatment is often not required.

1. Meat or other impacted foreign bodies may dislodge after the esophagus relaxes with the administration of intravenous glucagon, 0.2 mg/kg (maximum 1 mg). A single trial of glucagon is reasonable. However, aspiration of the dislodged foreign body can occur, so the patient must be alert and upright. Enzymatic digestion with papain has been utilized to dislodge meat, although reports of papain aspiration have decreased the attractiveness of this approach.

2. Retrieval of dull foreign bodies, particularly coins, may be accomplished by passing a Foley catheter, 10F or 12F, into the stomach with fluoroscopic guidance. The catheter balloon is then inflated with 4 ml of Gastrografin and slowly pulled back with fluoroscopic guidance. The foreign body is dislodged and pulled back into the mouth. This method carries significant risk of aspiration of the foreign body, since the object is free in the pharynx during the retrieval process.

3. *The safest method of retrieving foreign bodies is fiber-optic endoscopy.* Sharp objects are best removed by this method because an oversheath can be used to protect the esophagus from further damage as the object is pulled back. An experienced endoscopist must perform the procedure. Uncooperative patients may require general anesthesia.

Gastric and Small Bowel Foreign Bodies ■

More than 90% of swallowed foreign bodies that reach the stomach pass through the remainder of the GI tract without difficulty. Objects less than 20 mm (quarter-sized) tend to pass through the pylorus except in very small children. Objects should be removed if they remain in the stomach for more than three days: It is unlikely that they will pass after this time, and removal becomes more difficult as the object becomes embedded in the gastric mucosa. In such cases, consult a gastroenterologist.

Sharp or long foreign bodies that pass through the pylorus can become lodged in the duodenum or je-junum and can cause intestinal obstruction. A common site of obstruction is in the region of the ileocecal valve.

Sharp objects such as razor blades and needles may also be managed conservatively. Observe these children in the hospital for signs of obstruction and perforation such as fever, abdominal pain, vomiting, or GI bleeding. Daily abdominal radiographs determine if the object is moving. If an object does not move for two to three weeks or if there is evidence of obstruction or perforation, obtain surgical consultation for operative removal.

Colonic and rectal foreign bodies are discussed in Chapter 105. Swallowed foreign bodies, even razor blades, that enter the colon usually pass through the anal sphincter without difficulty.

Bibliography ■

Gracia C, Frey CF, Blazas BJ: Diagnosis and management of ingested foreign bodies: A ten-year experience. *Ann Emerg Med* 1984; 13:30.

Webb WA, McDaniel L, Jones L: Foreign bodies of the upper gastrointestinal tract: Current management. *Southern Med J* 1984; 77:1093.

34 Cough

Sylvia F. Villarreal

A cough is a child's mechanism to clear foreign matter or secretions from the respiratory tract. Cough receptors are located from the larynx to the bronchioles. If stimulated, the afferent impulse moves along the vagus nerve to the brain stem and pons. Efferent signals communicate the cough to the larynx, intercostals, diaphragm, and musculature of the abdomen and pelvic floor.

Cough is a frequent complaint in the emergency department (ED) and acute-care setting. A logical approach to diagnosis will usually avert an extensive workup with expensive lab tests and X-rays. First, define the cough as acute or persistent (lasting 2 to 4 weeks). Next, use the child's age to narrow the differential diagnosis to congenital anomalies, infectious etiologies, foreign bodies, and pulmonary pathologies. Consider other organ systems that interact with the lungs such as the gastrointestinal tract, cardiovascular, central nervous system, and the psyche.

Whenever possible, treat the cause, not the cough.

Etiology ∎

INFANTS AND TODDLERS

A cough in an infant less than 4 months old usually suggests either a congenital malformation or an infection. Figure 34-1 presents an algorithm for diagnosis of cough in a young infant. Feeding difficulties are often the presentation of *congenital malformations* of the airway, such as cysts, laryngeal clefts, tracheoesophageal fistulas, or vascular rings. Obtain barium swallow, endoscopy, and surgical consult to confirm these diagnoses. *Gastroesophageal reflux* can cause persistent cough and regurgitation of milk through the mouth and nose.

Pulmonary infections must be excluded. A *staccato cough* associated with conjunctivitis, wheezing and sneezing, eosinophilia, and hyperinflation on X-ray may signal the presence of chlamydia pneumonia. *Paroxysmal cough* may be caused by adenovirus or Bordatella pertussis. These infants are often quite ill with cyanosis and apnea. *Wheezing* infants may have

bronchiolitis, with respiratory syncytial virus and prolonged cough that may progress to reactive airway disease.

Failure to thrive is a serious indicator of chronic illness in a coughing infant. Infants with human immunodeficiency virus infection (HIV) may present with failure to thrive and a cough indicative of chronic lymphocytic infiltrative pneumonia, tuberculosis, or Pneumocystis carinii pneumonia. *Infants with cystic fibrosis* may have a paroxysmal cough, steatorrhea, and failure to thrive.

TODDLERS AND PRESCHOOL CHILDREN

Figure 34-2 presents a diagnostic algorithm for cough in this age group. Consider *foreign body aspiration,* which may be an unwitnessed event in the recent past or an acute episode witnessed by the parent (see Chapter 13 for discussion of diagnosis and treatment). *Reactive airway disease* may present with persistent cough, with or without wheezing (see Chapter 15). Associated exercise-induced or nighttime cough may lead parents to bring their child to the ED.

Children with *failure to thrive* are worrisome. *Cystic fibrosis* and *HIV* infection must be considered in the diagnosis. *Tuberculosis,* especially in inner-city children or recent immigrants, may produce chronic cough. Consider *sinusitis* in the differential of chronic cough. *Passive smoking* cough may be elucidated in a history of parental smoking, a wood-burning stove, or environmental pollution.

SCHOOL-AGE CHILDREN AND ADOLESCENTS

Figure 34-3 presents a diagnostic algorithm for chronic cough in this age group. *Mycoplasma pneumonia* may cause a persistent cough from one to three months after the acute episode. *Reactive airway disease* may present with exercise or cold-induced bronchospasm, nocturnal cough, and wheezing. *Smoking* (cigarettes, marijuana, or "crack" cocaine) may lead to the adult type of chronic bronchitis and sputum color change. *Passive pollution* is

174

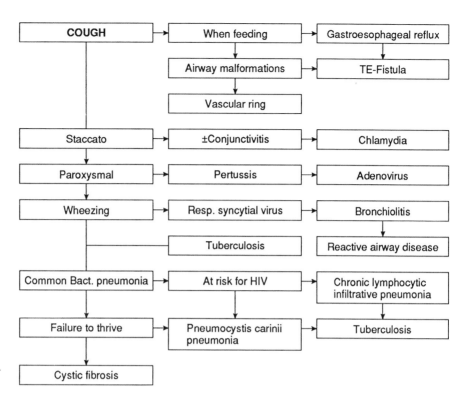

FIGURE 34–1. Diagnosis of cough in infants.

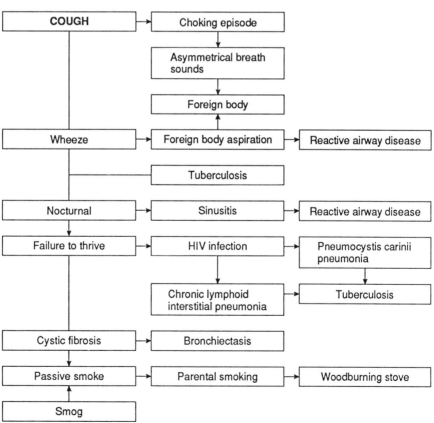

FIGURE 34–2. Diagnosis of cough in toddlers and preschool children.

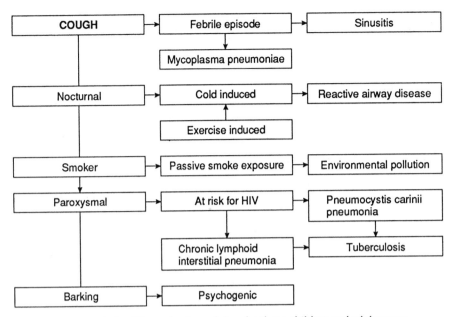

FIGURE 34–3. Diagnosis of cough in school-age children and adolescents.

common. *Psychogenic* coughing sounds like the barking of a seal or a dog. It is usually nonproductive, does not awaken the patient at night, and causes quite a disruption at home or in school. Teens at risk for *HIV infection* may present with Pneumocystis carinii pneumonia. Consider *tuberculosis* in groups at risk and in recent immigrants who present with a productive cough.

Ancillary Data ■

Obtain a chest film in the child or adolescent who has had a truly persistent cough for two to four weeks and who on physical exam has rales, differential breath sounds, and poor growth. Order a sweat chloride test in children with failure to thrive and a persistent cough. Place TB skin tests, either multiple puncture or Mantoux (PPD), on recent immigrants or others at risk for exposure to tuberculosis. Consider bronchoscopy when foreign body aspiration is suspected.

Treatment and Disposition ■

Treatment is based on diagnosis. Usually simple measures are adequate. Humidification, avoidance of cigarette smoke or other pollutants, herbal teas, and lemon and honey (not under 1 year of age) may help. A chronic postinfectious disruptive cough, especially at night, can be suppressed with codeine or dextromethorphan in the older child. Use codeine in children older than 3 years at 0.6 to 1 mg/kg/day in three to four divided doses, not exceeding 60 mg/day. Use dextromethorphan for infants older than 1 year at 0.2 mg/pound or 0.45 mg/kg/day in three to four divided doses. Many proprietary medications contain these ingredients. *Never* suppress a purulent cough.

For children with reactive airway disease, consider a diagnostic and therapeutic trial of a bronchodilator such as metaproterenol sulfate or albuterol. Refer these children to a primary-care setting or an allergist.

Bibliography ■

Alario AJ, McCarthy PL, Markovitz R, et al: Usefulness of chest radiographs in children with acute lower respiratory tract disease. *J Pediatr* 1987; 111:187–93.

Eigen H: The clinical evaluation of chronic cough. *Pediatr Clin North Am* 1982; 29:67–78.

Schmitt BD: Cough. In: *Your child's health.* New York: Bantam, 1987, pp. 469–473.

Starke JR: Modern approach to the diagnosis and management of tuberculosis in children. *Pediatr Clin North Am* 1988; 35(3):441–465.

35 Epistaxis

Ronald A. Dieckmann

Epistaxis is nosebleeding. It is a common condition of childhood and is usually secondary to minor trauma.

Etiology and Pathophysiology ■

The nasal mucosa is richly vascularized and is easily subject to injury. Since the nasal orifice is readily accessible to the probing finger of the young child, the nose is the most frequent site of spontaneous bleeding in pediatric patients. Minor trauma from nosepicking or blunt injury becomes commonplace at 2–3 years and continues through adolescence. Factors that increase mucosal edema or dry the sensitive nasal membranes predispose to epistaxis.

Over 90% of epistaxis in childhood originates from the anterior aspect of the nasal septum, within the vascular anastomosis called Kiesselbach's plexus. Occasionally, hemorrhage develops from the posterior areas supplied by ethmoid and sphenopalatine vessels and poses a more complicated diagnostic and management problem. Important associated conditions are noted in Table 35-1. Recurrent simple epistaxis is usually secondary to rhinitis and repeated picking or scratching of the nose.

Clinical Findings ■

Assessment of epistaxis requires a directed history, emphasizing mechanism of injury and patient or family history of bleeding disorders. Previous bleeding or easy bruisability, family hemorrhagic disease, allergies, foreign bodies, or chronic nasal obstruction should alert the physician to possible underlying disease. Sometimes, the initial complaint is hematemesis or hemoptysis; rarely, bleeding is severe, care is delayed, and the initial presentation is hemorrhagic shock.

An important consideration in later childhood is snorted recreational sympathomimetic agents, particularly cocaine. These drugs dessicate the mucosa and increase susceptibility to nasal bleeding.

Adequate physical examination necessitates proper equipment. Preparation of the patient and equipment will enhance success. Before attempting to visualize the bleeding site, reassure the child and family, explain the procedure, and enlist parental assistance whenever possible. Soft restraints or sedation are rarely needed. Use the following approach to examination:

1. Note vital signs. Orthostatic hypotension is an important clue to moderate to severe volume loss.
2. Inspect for signs of hemorrhagic disease (e.g., ecchymoses, petechiae, organomegaly, telangiectasia).
3. Complete the physical exam and leave the nose for last.
4. Have the child sit upright in a comfortable position and lean forward.
5. Ensure that functional equipment is at hand and an assistant is identified and instructed. Table 35-2 lists minimal equipment and supplies.
6. Have the patient blow his or her nose, then evacuate remaining clots, blood, or foreign material through the nasal speculum with suction.
7. Good lighting and careful inspection usually reveals the bleeding site in the anterior septum. Infrequently, a posterior bleed is signaled by inability to identify the bleeding site and continued oozing of blood into the pharynx, despite treatment.

Ancillary Data ■

No additional data is ordinarily required, if trauma is minor and the history and physical exam show a stable patient with little probability of underlying disease. When the hemorrhage is severe, obtain a complete blood count with hematocrit and platelet count, type and crossmatch and coagulation studies—prothrombin time, partial thromboplastin time (see Chapter 19). Facial or nasal radiographs may be indicated with significant trauma (see Chapter 52).

TABLE 35–1. *Conditions Associated With Epistaxis*

Trauma

Bleeding Disorders
Hemophilia
Leukemia
Thrombocytopenia
Von Willebrand's disease
Rendu–Osler–Weber (telangiectasias)
Aspirin use

Inflammatory Conditions
Allergic rhinitis
Upper respiratory infection

Masses
Juvenile nasal angiofibroma
Foreign body
Polyp
Furuncle

Treatment ∎

The most effective treatment of epistaxis is holding the nose firmly squeezed together with the thumb and index finger for 10 minutes (on the clock!). If this is unsuccessful, take additional steps outlined in Table 35-3. When a bleeding disorder is suspected or known (e.g., hemophilia), do not cauterize the nose, since this will temporarily stop the hemorrhage but will cause later sloughing and more severe rebleeding (see Chapter 19). In these patients, whenever possible, treat epistaxis with salt pork from the grocery store, using the following technique:

1. Slice the pork into 2 × 1 × 0.5 cm pieces and insert into anterior nares.

TABLE 35–2. *Equipment and Supplies for Treatment of Epistaxis*

Adequate movable light source
Experienced assistant
Strong suction with Frazier tip
Nasal speculum
Topical anesthetic agent
    2% tetracaine and epinephrine 1:1,000
    or 4% lidocaine with epinephrine
    or 4% cocaine
    or benzocaine-tetracaine spray
Silver nitrate stick or chromic acid bead for cautery
Petrolatum-soaked ¼ inch nasal packing

TABLE 35–3. *Treatment of Epistaxis*

Anterior Bleed
1. Hold nose firmly for 10 minutes.
2. If bleeding continues, apply topical vasoconstricting agent (see Table 35–2). Soak cotton pledget with solution and apply to bleeding site or as far posterior as possible.
3. If bleeding continues, use cauterizing agent.
4. Pack nose completely with well-lubricated, plain, or antibiotic-impregnated gauze packing as far posterior as possible.

Uncontrollable Anterior Bleed or Posterior Bleed
1. Establish intravenous access.
2. Send blood clot to blood bank for type and crossmatch.
3. Consult otolaryngologist. Surgical ligation may be necessary.
4. Insert posterior pack (commercial pneumatic or hydrostatic device, Foley catheter, or gauze pack)
5. If gauze pack is employed:
    a. Roll two or three 2 × 2 inch gauze sponges.
    b. Tie three long silk sutures around roll.
    c. Insert 5 or 8F feeding tube through nose into pharynx, grasp end of catheter with hemostat, and tie two sutures to end of catheter.
    d. With patient's mouth wide open, pull catheter back through nose, drawing roll retrograde firmly into posterior choana.
    e. Tie two suture ends around gauze roll in front of nostril.
    f. Bring third suture out through mouth and tape to cheek.
6. Admit to hospital.

2. Remove the pork in 48–72 hours. The salt and pork will provide hemostasis, and the fat will facilitate removal.

When nasal masses are identified, consult a pediatric or general otolaryngologist. If hypertension is present, particularly in the adolescent who has been exposed to a potent sympathomimetic, follow guidelines for care presented in Chapter 75.

CAVEATS

Do not pack the nose in the presence of known or suspected cribriform plate fracture. Ensure that packing is removed within 2–3 days to avert infectious complications.

Disposition ∎

Patients with posterior epistaxis require hospital admission and otolaryngologist consultation. Intravenous hydration, bed rest, monitoring of rebleeding, antibiotics, and analgesia are usually indicated.

Almost all patients with anterior epistaxis can be discharged home with nasal packing. The primary physician or emergency physician can remove the packing in 2–3 days. Instruct the patient in signs of infection and the need for immediate follow-up.

Preventing epistaxis requires several simple measures at home:

1. Lubricate the nasal mucosa with petrolatum several times each day.
2. Treat allergic rhinitis.
3. Ensure adequate home humidity, especially in the winter with dry inside heat.
4. Teach the child and parent the technique of squeezing the nose.

Bibliography ■

DeWeese DD, Saunders WH, eds: Nosebleed. In: *Textbook of otolaryngology.* St. Louis: CV Mosby, 1982.

McSwain NE: Nasal hemorrhage. *Emerg Med* 1989; 3:120.

36 Neck Mass

Ellen Taliaferro

Neck masses in children are common and usually represent reactive adenopathy (palpable lymph nodes) or adenitis (adenopathy associated with erythema, warmth, and tenderness). A true emergency is rare and exists when the mass compromises a vital adjacent structure such as the airway, the carotid artery, or the spinal cord.

Etiology and Pathophysiology ■

Neck masses may occur secondary to inflammation, infection, severe allergic reactions, trauma, or congenital anatomic defects (see Table 36-1). Cervical lymphadenopathy is common in children. Infectious adenitis is the most common cause. Most cases of cervical adenitis in children are associated with viral upper respiratory infections or bacterial infections of the teeth, the tonsils, or other areas in the head and neck. About two-thirds of all the bacterial infections are caused by Staphylococcus aureus or Group A streptococci.

Clinical Findings ■

INITIAL ASSESSMENT

Rarely, neck masses are acutely life-threatening. A distressed child with a neck mass requires immediate assessment of airway stability and hemodynamic function. In the first few minutes, a quick but ordered appraisal must include:

1. Airway. Noisy breathing may be obstructed breathing. Stridor, hoarseness, dysphagia, or drooling are signs of possible impending respiratory failure. By looking and listening, assess the patient's ability to speak and move air freely.
2. Breathing. Observe the child's color. Evaluate rate and effort of breathing, including grunting, nasal flaring, and retracting of intercostal muscles. Auscultate for quality and symmetry of breath sounds.

3. Circulation. Evaluate mental status. Look for signs of hypoperfusion such as cool, dry skin; tachycardia; and capillary refill > 2 seconds.

If any of these findings are detected, postpone further assessment and initiate resuscitation and stabilization.

HISTORY

A thorough history must include:

Duration of the mass
Presence of a recent upper respiratory tract infection, sore throat, earache, fever, skin lesions, or dental infections
Exposure to cats
Exposure to persons with tuberculosis or atypical tuberculosis
Travel to areas of specific endemic diseases such as histoplasmosis
Recent fever, night sweats, or weight loss
Allergies
Trauma.

Next, determine the reason for seeking emergency care: Does the presence or unsightliness of the mass alarm the parent? Do the parents fear a malignancy? Does the family perceive a cosmetic problem needing reconstructive surgery? Often, reassuring the parents that the mass is benign is the physician's primary therapeutic action.

PHYSICAL EXAMINATION

During the physical examination, look for sources of infection that might result in lymphadenopathy. Focus on areas of drainage into neck lymph nodes (scalp, neck, face, mouth, teeth, tongue, gums, pharynx). Indicate size, shape, consistency, tenderness, and fluctuance of nodes, as well as adherence to underlying tissue. Measure all abnormal lymph nodes and map them on the patient's record. Note whether adenopathy is generalized (defined as the enlargement of two or more noncontiguous lymph node

TABLE 36-1 *Differential Diagnosis of Neck Masses*

Adenopathy

  Cervical
    Reactive adenopathy to local infection
    Adenitis, with primary infection of the node

  Generalized lymphadenopathy
    Infectious mononucleosis
    Viral hepatitis
    Cytomegalovirus

Granulomatous Diseases
  Cat scratch disease
  Atypical mycobacteria
  Mycobacterium tuberculosis
  Histoplasmosis
  Toxoplasmosis

Malignancy
  Leukemia
  Hodgkin's disease
  Non-Hodgkin's lymphoma
  Neuroblastoma
  Rhabdomyosarcoma

Nonmalignant Tumors
  Goiter

Congenital
  Hemangioma
  Cystic hygroma
  Branchial cleft cyst
  Thyroglossal duct cyst
  Sternocleidomastoid tumor

Trauma
  Hematoma
  Subcutaneous emphysema

groups) or localized. Examine for masses in other parts of the body. Specifically note spleen and liver size, contour, tenderness, and consistency.

Most but not all pediatric neck masses represent lymphadenopathy. Other etiologies include trauma, malignancy, granulomatous disease, and congenital abnormalities. Table 36-1 presents the broad differential diagnostic possibilities.

Lymph Node Characteristics

Lymphadenopathy accounts for most neck masses, but the difference between normal and abnormal lymph nodes is not always clear-cut. These guidelines help:

1. Lymph nodes under 3 mm in diameter are normal.
2. Lymph nodes up to 1 cm in diameter are normal up to age 12 years.

3. Palpable lymph nodes in newborns are abnormal.
4. Lymphoid mass is maximum at 4–5 years of age.

Worrisome lumps have a high risk factor for malignancy. Five risk factors suggest the presence of malignancy:

1. The appearance of a neck lump or mass in the neonatal period.
2. A history of rapid and progressive growth.
3. The presence of skin ulceration.
4. Fixation to or location beneath the fascia.
5. A size greater than 3 cm in longest dimension, and a firm or hard consistency.

Ancillary Data ■

LABORATORY

Obtain the following tests in the child with an abnormal neck mass:

Complete blood count, with differential
Monospot for infectious mononucleosis
Appropriate serological studies for viral disease
Platelet count, prothrombin time, and partial thromboplastin time for suspected bleeding disorders.

Other laboratory tests, such as thyroid function studies, may be indicated to investigate specific diseases such as goiter or thyroid disorders. Arterial blood gas measurements may be useful in determining the degree of oxygenation compromise in suspected or demonstrated airway obstruction.

CULTURES AND SKIN TESTS

Pharyngeal cultures for streptococcus and gonococcus are useful. Skin tests for tuberculosis, fungi, and cat-scratch disease may be appropriate.

RADIOLOGY

A *chest X-ray* may indicate possible etiologies such as lung cancer, tuberculosis, sarcoidosis, acute infection, pneumomediastinum, or a pneumothorax. Other useful radiographic studies include a *lateral neck film* to elicit causes of airway obstruction and *cervical spine films* to detect fractures or dislocations. *Radiography of the paranasal sinuses* may also be useful.

SCANS, CONTRAST STUDIES, AND MRI

Contrast studies such as barium swallow, sialography, angiography, and/or a thyroid scan may be indicated to demonstrate the presence of obstruction or ectopic thyroid tissue. Magnetic resonance imaging has many advantages: it has increased soft-tissue sensitivity and can contrast normal and inflammatory tissues. Additionally, it provides no ionizing radiation.

LYMPH NODE ASPIRATION AND BIOPSY

If no readily identifiable source is established, attempt *lymph node aspiration*. When properly performed, lymph node aspiration is safe and has a high diagnostic yield. Aspirate the largest and/or most fluctuant lymph node. After the overlying skin is cleansed and anesthetized, the aspirate is taken with a sterile 20-ml syringe. If no purulent material is aspirated, inject 1 to 2 ml of sterile nonbacteriostatic saline into the node and reaspirate. All aspirated material should be gram stained, acid-fast stained, and cultured. Perform both aerobic and anaerobic cultures.

Biopsy of the neck mass may be necessary. This may be a "skinny-needle" biopsy, which requires only local anesthesia, or an open excisional biopsy under general anesthesia, depending on clinical circumstances. Expedite arrangements for biopsy when risk factors listed above are present.

Treatment ■

Because most neck masses represent cervical adenitis, treatment is usually straightforward:

1. Treat bacterial infections with appropriate antibiotics (usually dicloxacillin) pending culture results.
2. Provide reassurance.

3. Emphasize supportive care (antipyretics and analgesics) in cases secondary to viral pharyngitis.

Disposition ■

Immediate consultation and hospitalization is required for children with toxicity or life-threatening emergencies, such as airway compromise or dyspnea. Pediatric intensive care admission is appropriate in such cases. Children with mediastinal adenopathy or children with serious systemic symptoms and enlarged peripheral nodes require hospitalization for further evaluation and treatment.

For cervical adenitis in childhood, advise patients and parents that previously infected nodes may take many months to diminish, even though prompt resolution of signs and symptoms usually occurs with antibiotic therapy. Follow-up evaluation for reassessment and remeasurement of neck nodes is best arranged with the primary pediatrician or family physician, within one month.

Bibliography ■

Barton LL: Childhood cervical adenitis. *Am Fam Physician* 1984; 29(4):163–166.

Damion J, Hybels RL: The neck mass: 1. General concepts and congenital causes. *Postgrad Med* 1987; 81(6):75–93.

Knight PJ, Mulne AF, Vassy LE: When is lymph node biopsy indicated in children with enlarged peripheral nodes? *Pediatrics* 1982; 69(4):391–396.

Knight PJ, Reiner CB: Superficial lumps in children: What, when, and why? *Pediatrics* 1983; 72(2):147–153.

Schmitt BD: Cervical adenopathy in children. *Postgrad Med* 1976; 60(3):251–255.

37 Red Eye

William V. Good

Etiology and Pathophysiology ■

The red eye is one of the most common problems encountered in emergency ophthalmology. Redness is caused by vascular dilatation. Distribution of dilated vessels and ancillary physical findings help in the differential diagnosis:

1. Ciliary injection occurs when vessels 2–4 mm behind the corneoscleral limbus become dilated. This usually signifies intraocular inflammation (i.e., iritis).
2. Papillary conjunctival reaction usually signifies bacterial conjunctivitis. Small dots are apparent on the palpebral conjunctiva.
3. Follicular conjunctivitis signifies viral conjunctivitis. Large bumps representing accumulated inflammatory cells are visible on the palpebral conjunctiva. Conjunctivitis due to Neisseria gonorrhea also causes follicles.
4. Chemosis, or swelling of conjunctiva, associated with redness signifies allergic conjunctivitis.
5. Blue-red discoloration of the bulbar conjunctiva often signifies scleritis.

Clinical Findings ■

An assessment of visual acuity is paramount. Distraction of the young patient will facilitate adequate examination. If visual acuity can be measured with the Snellen chart, this should be recorded. In preverbal children, measure vision by observing for fixation and tracking with each eye individually. Measure pupillary responses. The presence of unequal pupillary reaction implies a disorder affecting anterior visual pathway input.

Check the cornea for clarity. Infections of the cornea cause a loss of transparency.

Important structures to examine in the workup of red eye include:

1. Eyelids
2. Conjunctiva
3. Sclera
4. Cornea
5. Anterior chamber

Table 37-1 presents the differential diagnosis of unilateral red eye.

Disorders of the Conjunctiva ■

BACTERIAL CONJUNCTIVITIS

Etiology

The most common cause of a red eye in childhood is conjunctivitis.

Bacterial conjunctivitis is characterized by papillary conjunctival changes. The palpebral conjunctiva has a velvet appearance. Little dots can be distinguished, but "bumps" are not visible. Bacterial conjunctivitis causes a more pronounced exudative response than does viral conjunctivitis.

Important causes of bacterial conjunctivitis in childhood include Hemophilus influenzae, Staphylococcus aureus, and Streptococcus pneumoniae. H. influenzae is characterized by a blue discoloration of the upper and lower eyelids. S. pneumoniae often causes subconjunctival hemorrhaging. Moraxella species cause maceration of the lateral canthus.

Rule out Neisseria gonorrhea. Typically, Neisseria gonorrhea causes a hyperacute conjunctivitis, with massive exudative response. Pre-auricular nodes are present. Neisseria can penetrate intact corneal epithelium, causing a rapidly progressive keratitis.

Ophthalmia neonatorum represents a special subset of the red eye. Conjunctivitis in the newborn occurs 6 hours to 4 weeks after birth. Silver nitrate prophylaxis causes early-onset redness. Bacterial conjunctivitis (S. pneumoniae, S. aureus) causes conjunctivitis in the first week of life. Neisseria gon-

TABLE 37–1.	*Differential Diagnosis of Unilateral Red Eye*

Bacterial conjunctivitis
Chlamydia infection
Molluscum contagiosum
Oculoglandular disease
Iritis
Scleritis
Trauma or foreign body
Phlyctenule

orrhea causes an acute purulent conjunctivitis. Chlamydia causes so-called inclusion conjunctivitis up to age 4 weeks; pneumonia occurs in 30% of cases, often later in infancy.

Inclusion conjunctivitis causes a red eye in adolescence. The chlamydia organism is sexually transmitted and typically affects only one eye. Follicles are present. Pre-auricular nodes are usually present. The condition lasts up to several months and can cause conjunctival scarring.

Treatment and Disposition

Treatment of bacterial conjunctivitis is usually empiric. If bacterial conjunctivitis is suspected, obtain cultures and begin topical antibiotics. Erythromycin covers S. pneumoniae and S. aureus; when H. influenzae is suspected, systemic antibiotics may be necessary as well.

Neisseria gonorrhea requires hospital admission, and systemic antibiotics (cephalosporins) are indicated because topical antibiotics alone are ineffective. Bacitracin drops are usually prescribed at 2-hour intervals.

Chlamydia infection also requires systemic treatment. Prescribe erythromycin, 40 mg/kg/day for 2 weeks. Topical antibiotics are more likely to be effective in younger children. In adolescents and adults, topical antibiotics add little to systemic treatment.

VIRAL CONJUNCTIVITIS

Viral conjunctivitis causes follicles that appear as bumps on the lower palpebral conjunctiva. Pre-auricular lymph nodes are usually palpable. Discharge is scant compared to bacterial conjunctivitis.

Etiology

The differential diagnosis of follicular conjunctivitis is listed in Table 37-2. Follicles do not occur in the first 6 months of life. Adenovirus is the most common cause, but herpes simplex, medicamentosa, entero-

TABLE 37–2.	*Differential Diagnosis of Conjunctival Follicles*

Chlamydia infection
Adenovirus
Picornavirus
Herpes simplex virus
Molluscum contagiosum
Toxic effects of medication

virus, picornavirus, and molluscum contagiosum also cause follicular conjunctivitis. Follicles also occur in chlamydial infections.

Most cases of follicular conjunctivitis are self-limited. Adenovirus (serotype 3, 8, and 18) causes epidemic keratoconjunctivitis. This conjunctivitis is protracted with focal keratitis causing photophobia and decreased vision lasting up to 6 months.

Treatment

Three types of follicular conjunctivitis are treatable: molluscum contagiosum, herpes simplex, and chlamydia.

Molluscum contagiosum conjunctivitis causes a unilateral red eye. A careful search for a molluscum body should be made when a unilateral follicular conjunctivitis is present. The molluscum body can be needled or otherwise manipulated, with resolution.

Herpes simplex conjunctivitis should be treated with topical Viroptic, 1% eye drops, five times a day.

Chlamydial infections must be treated with systemic antibiotics. A serologic test for syphilis is recommended when chlamydia is diagnosed.

Laboratory studies in follicular conjunctivitis of less than 2 weeks' duration are not necessary. The presence of a vesicular rash (see Figure 37-1) or corneal dendrites indicates herpes infection. Follicular conjunctivitis of longer than 2 weeks' duration requires workup. Giemsa stains may reveal intracytoplasmic inclusions, which indicate chlamydial infection. Chlamydia can also be cultured.

PARINAUD'S OCULOGLANDULAR SYNDROME

A conjunctival granuloma is occasionally associated with a large pre-auricular lymph node, causing a unilateral red eye. The differential diagnosis includes cat-scratch fever, lymphogranuloma venereum, tularemia, sarcoid, and tuberculosis. Excision of the granuloma is usually curative.

ALLERGIC CONJUNCTIVITIS

Allergic conjunctivitis is bilateral. Chemosis is marked. Itching is a prominent symptom. There may

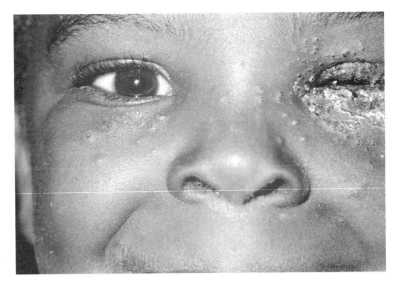

FIGURE 37-1. Herpes simplex infection of the eyes.

be scant mucoid discharge. A Denny's fold under the lower lid is usually present, and the lids may be slightly swollen. There should be no lymph nodes. There may be other signs and symptoms of allergies.

Symptoms of allergic conjunctivitis are often seasonal. Treatment consists of cold washcloths as needed, topical antihistamines, and rarely topical steroids. Because topical steroids can cause glaucoma and cataracts, they should be used sparingly.

VERNAL CONJUNCTIVITIS

A disorder of adolescence and young adulthood, vernal conjunctivitis causes bilateral eye redness and scant discharge. Again, itching may be a prominent symptom. Large cobblestone papillae form on the upper palpebral conjunctiva. Chemosis may be present. Follicles may occur at the corneoscleral limbus. Occasionally, a central corneal ulcer (sterile) is present.

Treatment consists of topical cromolyn 4%. A short course of topical steroids (Pred Forte 1% q2h for 1 week) may also be helpful. Vernal conjunctivitis is usually self-limited. Occasionally corneal scarring will occur.

ATOPIC CONJUNCTIVITIS

Children with atopy may also develop conjunctivitis. Eyelashes often show fibrin accumulation and redness is bilateral. Conjunctival irritation can lead to corneal scarring. Treatment consists of topical cromolyn; occasional treatment with topical steroids is also of value.

Disorders of the Eyelids ■

Ocular adnexa conditions can cause red eyes. Blepharitis is perhaps the most common cause of red eyes in adolescents and adults. Blepharitis can be divided into two types: seborrheic and bacterial.

Seborrheic dermatitis causes bilateral red eyes associated with oily skin. Scurf consists of fibrin accumulation at the base of the eyelashes. Treatment consists of eyelid hygiene and short-term topical antibiotics (i.e., erythromycin ointment b.i.d for 3 weeks).

S. aureus causes so-called collarettes, rings of fibrin that encircle the lashes. Bilateral red eyes will also occur. Treatment consists of eyelid scrubs and appropriate topical antibiotics.

Chalazia occur in the setting of blepharitis. When the meibomian ducts at the eyelid margin become plugged, glandular secretions back up and acute swelling occurs. There may be redness of the eye and pain. A lump is usually noted in the upper or lower eyelid. Treatment consists of hot soaks and topical antibiotics; drainage may be indicated if this treatment fails.

Disorders of the Cornea ■

CORNEAL ABRASION

Corneal abrasion causes a unilateral red eye. In most cases, there is a history of eye trauma, but spontaneous corneal abrasions can occur. A condition termed "map-dot dystrophy" presents as spontaneous corneal abrasion and is caused by abnormal adherence of corneal epithelium to its basement membrane. Previous corneal abrasions may also lead to abnormalities of corneal epithelium and can cause "spontaneous" erosions.

A corneal abrasion is diagnosed with a fluorescein test in which fluorescein dye is placed in the inferior conjunctival cul-de-sac. Denuded epithelium will stain bright green and is best seen with a blue light. Treatment is described in Chapter 52.

Keratitis also causes a unilateral red eye. Usually there is a history of antecedent trauma. The cornea appears white and there is considerable pain and redness of the affected eye. Immediately refer the patient to an ophthalmologist, who will perform cultures and treat with topical and subconjunctival antibiotics, based on the infecting organism.

Prolonged eyelid closure (e.g., coma, patching) can cause filamentary keratitis. Strings of corneal epithelium traverse the cornea (Figure 37-2) and cause redness with pain. The condition is not infectious and can be managed with debridement or topical artificial tears.

PHLYCTENULE

A phlyctenule is focal redness of the eye caused by a type 4 immune reaction. The usual cause is S. aureus; tuberculosis, lymphogranuloma venereum, and coccidiomycosis are rare causes. The patient experiences redness, discomfort, and photophobia. After cultures are obtained, administer topical antibiotics. Low-dose steroids may be beneficial.

SUPERFICIAL FOREIGN BODY

Small flecks of dust, eyelashes, sprays, and pieces of metal can strike the eye and cause unilateral redness. Occasionally the foreign body will embed in the cornea, but usually the inciting agent is rinsed away by tears. Unilateral eye redness should prompt a search for a foreign body. Topical anesthetics are the key to examination and removal. Ensure that the globe is not perforated. Remove corneal foreign bodies, if possible, with a wet cotton-tipped swab or a small needle. Eyelashes on the conjunctival surface should also be removed. The redness resolves on its own in 1 or 2 days. Sometimes, analgesia and eye patching are necessary. When foreign bodies in the cornea cannot be easily removed by simple measures, consult an ophthalmologist to evaluate the need for immediate extraction or next-day follow-up.

IRITIS

Iritis presents as eye redness, pain, and photophobia. The redness is usually unilateral and is in a ciliary

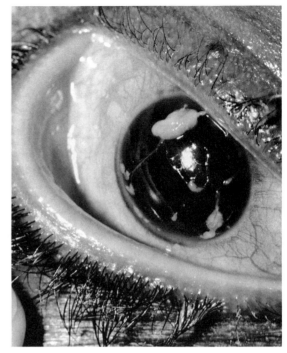

FIGURE 37–2. Corneal abrasion.

distribution (i.e., redness is present 2–4 mm behind the limbus). Photophobia is a prominent symptom. Eye pain is characterized as deep and boring. A careful slit-lamp examination will reveal the presence of cells and flare in the anterior chamber of the eye. Clumps of white blood cells may precipitate on the corneal endothelium.

The differential diagnosis of iritis includes HLA-B27 related conditions, syphilis, sarcoid, juvenile rheumatoid arthritis, herpes iritis, and idiopathic. Treatment usually consists of topical steroids and cycloplegic agents. A search for an underlying etiology is recommended but is often unrewarding.

Bibliography ■

Allansmith MR: Vernal conjunctivitis. In: Duane TD, Jaeger EA: *Clinical ophthalmology,* vol. 4. New York: Harper & Row, 1986.

Beauchamp GR, Gillette TE, Friendly DS: Phlyctenular keratoconjunctivitis. *J Ped Ophthalmol Strabismus* 1981; 18: 22.

Duke-Elder S: Diseases of the outer eye. Part I. Conjunctiva. In: *System of ophthalmology,* vol. 8. St. Louis: CV Mosby, 1965, pp. 498–527.

Hammerschleg MR, Cummings C, Roblin PM, et al: Efficacy of neonatal ocular prophylaxis for the prevention of chlamydial and gonococcal conjunctivitis. *N Engl J Med* 1989, 320:769–772.

38 Vaginal Bleeding

Nicolette S. Horbach

Assessment of the pediatric patient with vaginal bleeding can be facilitated by dividing patients into two groups: premenarchal and postmenarchal girls. In childhood, vaginal bleeding is most commonly due to organic causes, especially foreign bodies. In postmenarchal girls the most common cause is dysfunctional uterine bleeding due to disorders of the hypothalamic-pituitary-ovarian axis. The differential diagnosis of the two groups is presented in Tables 38-1 and 38-2.

Premenarchal Girls ■

ETIOLOGY AND CLINICAL FINDINGS

The diagnosis is evident when blood is observed coming from the genital area. The mother may have noted blood-stained underwear or may report the child's complaint of vulvar irritation. A history of injury or possible sexual abuse necessitates examination of the pelvis to determine the extent of injury.

Neonatal Hormone Withdrawal

Neonatal hormone withdrawal may occur normally in neonates less than 1 week old. Refer the patient for evaluation if she is more than 1 week old.

Foreign Body

The peak incidence of foreign-body insertion occurs between ages 5 and 9. Bleeding is usually minimal and associated with a vaginal discharge that may be foul. A history of insertion is rarely obtained. Soft material, such as paper or cloth, is the most commonly seen foreign body.

Vulvovaginal Infections

Vulvovaginal infections occur most commonly between ages 5 and 7. Acute infections or allergic reactions may result in a bloody or blood-tinged vaginal discharge. Vulvar or vaginal pain may be present. Allergens (chemical or physical agents) must be sought. Nonspecific bacterial or fungal infections are most common. Consider Neisseria gonorrhea.

Tumors

Pain is an unusual complaint. Bleeding may be minimal but may progress to frank hemorrhage in the advanced stage. Condylomata accuminata or prolapsed urethral mucosa may be confused with sarcoma botryoides. Condylomata involve the vulva and lower vagina and are usually larger lesions. Sarcoma botryoides involves multiple areas of the vagina, especially the upper vagina, and is usually painless. Manipulation of prolapsed urethral mucosa elicits pain. Clear cell adenocarcinoma of the vagina and cervix is often associated with a history of maternal ingestion of hormones (estrogen) during pregnancy.

Trauma

Lacerations or vulvovaginal hematomas may be secondary to accidental injury or sexual abuse. A high index of suspicion is necessary. The most common injury is a straddle injury. Although bleeding may be profuse, requiring immediate attention, minimal bleeding or lacerations do not rule out significant vaginal or intra-abdominal injury. A complete evaluation, including rectovaginal examination, may necessitate an examination under general anesthesia. Ensure that the urinary tract is intact by the patient's ability to void and by at least a urinalysis.

ANCILLARY DATA

Perform a wet mount and vulvovaginal cultures in patients with bloody discharge or a history of sexual abuse. Serial complete blood counts may detect the presence of an expanding hematoma or intra-abdominal injury. A nasal speculum or vaginoscopy using a laparoscope or urethroscope may allow iden-

TABLE 38-1. *Causes of Vaginal Bleeding in Premenarchal Girls*

Foreign body
Vulvovaginal infections
Allergic vulvitis with excoriations
Neonatal hormone withdrawal
Exogenous estrogen ingestion
Tumors
    Benign
    Malignant
Prolapsed urethral mucosa
Trauma
    Accidental
    Sexual abuse
Isosexual precocious puberty
Transitory sexual precocity

tification of a foreign body or may detect evidence of upper vaginal trauma.

TREATMENT

Foreign Body

Obtain proper instruments and establish patient cooperation before removal is attempted. The use of vaginoscopy or a nasal speculum may allow removal while the patient is awake. Irrigation of the vagina with an angiocath or pediatric Foley catheter may also be helpful. If an adequate examination cannot be performed while the patient is awake, general anesthesia may be necessary. If vaginitis is present secondary to the foreign body, institute appropriate local treatment.

Vulvovaginal Infections

See Chapter 121.

Tumors

If visual or bimanual examination reveals a possible tumor, refer the patient to a gynecologist to confirm the diagnosis by biopsy. Biopsies should be performed only in the operating room because of the risk of profuse bleeding, especially in the patient with sarcoma botryoides. Condylomata accuminata may be treated by applying 65–85% trichloroacetic acid twice weekly for 2 to 3 weeks. Protect the surrounding skin with zinc oxide, and blot off the excess acid with a paper towel. Resistant or extensive cases may require referral for CO_2 laser vaporization or electrocautery.

Trauma

Cleanse the area with soap and water. Minimal abrasions or small lacerations without significant bleeding do not require repair.

Lacerations of the external genitalia may be repaired in a cooperative patient using local anesthesia. Repair skin lacerations of the vulva with absorbable interrupted or running subcuticular sutures (3-0 or 4-0 dexon) to avoid the discomfort of removing sutures in apprehensive children or adolescents. Repair lacerations of the distal vaginal mucosa with an absorbable suture (3-0 chromic or dexon) in a continuous locking fashion.

Adequate repair of intravaginal lacerations will require anesthesia to ensure adequate exposure. Use a vaginal pack temporarily to provide hemostasis prior to surgery.

Treat a nonexpanding hematoma with ice packs and sitz baths. An expanding hematoma requires evacuation and exploration.

Postmenarchal Girls ■

ETIOLOGY AND CLINICAL DIAGNOSIS

Obtain a menstrual, sexual, and contraceptive history. Test for thyroid disease, galactorrhea, hirsutism, abdominal pain or masses, or coagulation defects after a thorough pelvic examination.

Dysfunctional Uterine Bleeding

Although dysfunctional uterine bleeding accounts for 95% of postmenarchal girls who present with vaginal

TABLE 38-2. *Causes of Vaginal Bleeding in Postmenarchal Girls*

Dysfunctional uterine bleeding	Tumors
Pregnancy-related	Benign
complications	Malignant
Abortion	Hormone-
Ectopic pregnancy	secreting
Infection	Hematologic disorders
Vulvovaginitis	Contraceptive
Cervicitis	complications
Pelvic inflammatory disease	Endocrinologic
Systemic infections	disorders
Trauma	Thyroid disease
Accidental	Prolactinomas
Sexual abuse	Systemic disorders
	Renal disease
	Liver disease
	Nongenital source

bleeding, it is a diagnosis of exclusion. Typically, there is a history of irregular cycles. The bleeding may be similar to normal flow (10 tampons or six perineal pads per cycle) or very heavy, leading to severe anemia or hypovolemic shock. Rule out exogenous hormone ingestion.

Pregnancy-Related Complications

See Figure 38-1. Denial of sexual activity does not exclude this diagnosis. *Threatened abortion* presents as mild to moderate vaginal bleeding, often associated with mild lower abdominal cramping. The patient may report morning sickness, breast tenderness, and urinary frequency consistent with the symptoms of pregnancy. The uterus is usually enlarged, soft, and nontender. The cervical os is closed by digital examination, and no tissue has been passed.

Once the cervical os has opened and/or tissue may have been passed, an *inevitable or incomplete abortion* has occurred. A *complete abortion* is diagnosed once all tissue has been passed, bleeding and cramping is minimal, the cervical os is closed, and the uterus is considerably smaller.

Consider any pregnant patient with vaginal bleeding and lower abdominal pain or an adnexal mass to have an ectopic pregnancy until proven otherwise.

Hematologic Disorders

Up to one-fifth of adolescents who present with acute menorrhagia (Hgb < 10 mg) and one-third of patients requiring transfusion are ultimately found to have a coagulation disorder. Consider von Willebrand's disease, thrombocytopenic purpura, and leukemia.

TREATMENT

Dysfunctional Uterine Bleeding

The goal is to control the bleeding without performing a D&C. Successful management depends on the ability to transform an estrogen-primed endometrium into a progesterone or progestin-type endometrium.

For mild to moderate bleeding of less than 10–14 days' duration, treatment with progesterone is beneficial. Alternatives include medroxyprogesterone (Provera) 10–20 mg daily for 5 to 7 days; norethindrone (Norlutin) 20–40 mg daily for 3 to 5 days; or norethindrone acetate (Norlutate) 10–20 mg daily for 3 to 5 days. Progesterone alone is effective in 70% of cases.

In patients with heavier or more prolonged bleeding, stabilization of the endometrium with an estrogen-progesterone combination may be required: norgestrel 0.5 mg and ethinyl estradiol 50 mg (Ovral) 1 pill q.i.d. for 3 days, then t.i.d. for 3 days, then b.i.d. for 3 days, then daily for one complete cycle. Occasionally, parenteral therapy may be necessary: estradiol valerate (Delestrogen) 10 mg and medroxyprogesterone acetate (Depo-Provera) 50 mg intramuscularly weekly for 3 weeks. Ninety to ninety-five percent of patients will respond to the combination estrogen-progesterone regimes.

Bleeding should cease 48–72 hours after beginning treatment. Withdrawal of the medication results in a "medical" curettage with sloughing of the endometrium. Withdrawal bleeding following parenteral therapy should occur 2 weeks after discontinuing the medication.

PROFUSE VAGINAL BLEEDING: Patients bleeding up to a pad or more per hour or with a Hct < 30% require

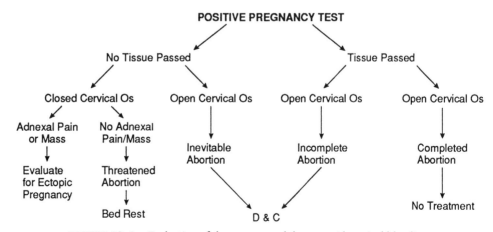

FIGURE 38–1. Evaluation of the pregnant adolescent with vaginal bleeding.

hospitalization for observation and treatment. A Hct < 30% may require transfusion.

Intravenous conjugated estrogen (Premarin) 20 mg every 4 to 6 hours for 24 hours may be effective. Bleeding should significantly decrease in 6–12 hours. Once bleeding is controlled, begin the patient on either progesterone therapy or a combination of estrogen and progesterone so that withdrawal bleeding does not occur for at least 3 to 4 weeks. This enables the patient's blood count to stabilize before her next menses. If the initial one or two doses of intravenous Premarin do not produce a response, subsequent doses will also be ineffective. In patients who fail to respond to intravenous Premarin, or in patients who are acutely hemorrhaging, obtain a gynecologic consultation. A D&C will usually remove endometrial tissue and produce prompt hemostasis.

Prostaglandin inhibitors such as mefenamic acid (Ponstel) 500 mg orally initially, then 250 mg every 6 hours, may decrease blood loss in patients with anovulatory bleeding.

Pregnancy-Related Complications

THREATENED ABORTION: Provide pregnancy counseling and information regarding family planning services to the patient. Recommend bed rest and abstinence from sexual intercourse for 24 to 48 hours. Hormonal treatment is not indicated. An ultrasound may be helpful to confirm a viable intrauterine pregnancy. If the pregnancy is desired, provide referral for prenatal care.

INEVITABLE OR INCOMPLETE ABORTION: Evacuation of the products of conception is mandatory to secure hemostasis and to prevent infection. The preferred method is suction curettage, which can be performed by a trained physician in the emergency department under a paracervical block with or without intravenous sedation: narcotic (Fentanyl 100 mg IV) and/or Valium. An occasional patient will require general anesthesia.

Dilatation and sharp curettage is an alternative method of evacuation, but is more traumatic to the endometrium and increases the possibility of postabortion intrauterine adhesions.

Give patients who are febrile, or who have a tender uterus, intravenous antibiotics prior to the procedure.

POSSIBLE ECTOPIC PREGNANCY: Obtain gynecologic referral for possible ectopic pregnancy for any bleeding patient who is experiencing concomitant abdominal pain, adnexal tenderness, or an adnexal mass and a closed cervical os. Evaluation of these patients may include serial HCG levels, pelvic ultrasound, or operative intervention.

HEMATOLOGIC DISORDERS

Treatment is presented in Chapter 19.

Bibliography ∎

Gidwani G: Vaginal bleeding in adolescents. *J Reprod Med* 1984; 29:417.

Huffman JW, Dewhurst CJ, Capraro VJ, et al, eds: *The gynecology of childhood and adolescence.* Philadelphia: WB Saunders, 1981.

Nilsson L, Rybo G: Treatment of menorrhagia. *Am J Obstet Gynecol* 1971; 110:713.

Radman H: Blood dyscrasia as causative factor in abnormal uterine bleeding. *Am J Obstet Gynecol* 1960; 79:1.

Speroff L, Glass RH and Kase NG, eds: *Clinical gynecologic endocrinology and infertility,* 3rd ed. Baltimore: Williams & Wilkins, 1983, p. 225.

VI
Pain Syndromes

39 Management of Pain in the Emergency Department

Robert H. Levin

Pain is a subjective experience, but it should never be ignored in patients of any age. A number of drugs may be employed, in a number of pharmacologic classes. Each has its advantages and disadvantages for particular procedures.

Basic Principles ■

The route of administration of analgesics and sedatives depends on the quickness of response desired. The IV route (onset of effect is usually within 5 minutes) should be reserved for patients in severe acute pain, or those already with IVs for other reasons who can be carefully monitored. The IM and SC routes, with an onset of effect of about 10–30 minutes, are the most common for treatment of moderate to severe acute pain. The oral route, with an onset of effect of more than 20 minutes, is most appropriate for mild to moderate pain. The topical route can also be used. Local anesthetics, in addition to being infiltrated into tissues, may be applied topically. A common combination now being used as a topical solution to suture wounds in children is tetracaine, epinephrine, and cocaine (TEC or TAC) as discussed in Chapter 62.

Using more than one agent to achieve the desired effect is a common practice. The dose of a narcotic, for instance, can be lowered if a sedative agent is also given. Some combinations, however, may produce an untoward amount of side effects; for instance, the combination of Demerol, Phenergan, and Thorazine (DPT or the "lytic cocktail"), although popular, has no real advantages over other preparations and causes a higher incidence of respiratory depression and hypotension. When Phenergan is added to Demerol, it reduces the analgesic effects of the Demerol, which is probably why the Thorazine was added. *The combination of morphine or meperidine with hydroxyzine or diphenhydramine alone are superior in effects and cause fewer side effects than the DPT combination.*

Analgesia for Different Procedures ■

PAINFUL BUT WITHOUT UNDUE ANXIETY

Examples: incision and drainage of an abscess; routine wound care. (See Chapter 62 for local anesthetics.)

For *severe* pain, use a narcotic (e.g., morphine or meperidine).

For *moderate* pain, use codeine with aspirin or acetaminophen.

For *mild* pain, use aspirin or acetaminophen.

PAINFUL WITH ANXIETY

Examples: burn wound management, minor surgery.

For *severe* pain, use a narcotic plus a benzodiazepine or a phenothiazine.

For *moderate* pain, use a narcotic plus a benzodiazepine or an antihistamine.

For *mild* pain, use codeine plus a benzodiazepine or antihistamine.

ANXIETY ONLY

Examples: X-ray (e.g., IVP).

For *severe* anxiety, use a barbiturate, chloral hydrate, or a benzodiazepine.

For *moderate* anxiety, use a benzodiazepine or antihistamine.

For *mild* anxiety, use an antihistamine.

SEDATION OR SLEEP REQUIRED

Examples: procedures such as an EEG or ECG.

For *severe* anxiety, use a barbiturate, chloral hydrate, or a benzodiazepine.

For *moderate* anxiety, use a benzodiazepine or antihistamine.

TABLE 39–1. *The Rational Use of Medications for Sedation and Analgesia*

Commonly Used Drugs*	Route of Administration	Initial Dose†	Frequency of Use (hrs)	Maximum Dose‡ (mg)	Onset of Effects (min)	Duration of Effects (hrs)
Analgesics						
Narcotics						
Morphine (Morphine)	IV	0.1 mg/kg	q 3	15	5–10	3
	IM	0.1–0.2 mg/kg	q 4	15	10–20	4
	PO	0.1–0.2 mg/kg	q 4–6	30	20–30	4–6
Meperidine (Demerol)	IV	1 mg/kg	q 1–2	100	1–2	1–2
	IM	1–2 mg/kg	q 2–3	150	10–15	2–3
	PO	2–3 mg/kg	q 3–4	300	15–30	3–4
Codeine (Codeine)	IM	0.5 mg/kg	q 4–6	30	15–30	4–6
	PO	0.5–1 mg/kg	q 4–6	60	15–30	4–6
Hydromorphone (Dilaudid)	IV	0.01 mg/kg	q 3–5	2	5	4
	IM, SC	0.01–0.02 mg/kg	q 4	2	15	4–6
	PO, PR	0.02–0.04 mg/kg	q 4–6	6	15–30	4–6
Fentanyl (Sublimaze)	IV, IM	2–20 µg/kg	1 dose	150 µg/kg	5–15	1–2
Agonist/antagonist						
Pentazocine (Talwin)	IV	0.25–0.5 mg/kg	q 3–4	30	2–3	3
	PO	1–2 mg/kg	q 3–4	60	15–30	3
	SC, IM	0.5–1 mg/kg	q 3–4	60	15–20	3
Nonsteroidals§:						
Propionic Acids						
Ibuprofen (Motrin)	PO	5 mg/kg	q 8	800	30	4–6
Naproxen (Naprosyn)	PO	10 mg/kg	q 12	500	1	6–8
Indoles‖						
Indomethacin (Indocin)	PO	1 mg/kg	q 8	50	30	4–6
	PO (SA)¶	1 mg/kg	q 12	75	30	4–6
Salicylates						
Aspirin	PO, PR	10–15 mg/kg	q 4–6	650	30	4–6
Other Analgesics						
Acetaminophen (Tylenol, et al)	PO, PR	10–15 mg/kg	q 4–6	650	30	4–6
Barbiturates						
Pentobarbital (Nembutal)	IV	2–4 mg/kg	1 dose	100	1	3–4
	IM, PO	2–4 mg/kg	1 dose	100	10–15	3–4
Secobarbital (Seconal)	PO	3–6 mg/kg	1 dose	100	10–15	3–4
Benzodiazepines						
Diazepam (Valium)	IV	0.04–0.1 mg/kg	q 6–8	0.2 mg/kg	1–3	4–6
	IM	0.1–0.2 mg/kg	q 6–8	0.6 mg/kg	10–20	4–6
	PO	0.1–0.2 mg/kg	q 6–8	0.6 mg/kg	30–60	4–6
Lorazepam (Ativan)	IV	0.01–0.02 mg/kg	q 8	0.04 mg/kg	15–20	4–6
	IM	0.02–0.04 mg/kg	q 8	0.05 mg/kg	60–120	4–6
Midazolam (Versed)	IV	0.035 mg/kg	1 dose	0.1 mg/kg	2–4	0.5–1
	IM	0.08–0.1 mg/kg	1 dose	0.2 mg/kg	2–4	0.5–1
Antihistamines						
Diphenhydramine (Benadryl)	IV	0.05–0.1 mg/kg	q 4–6	2 mg/kg	10–20	3–6
	IM	1 mg/kg	q 4–6	2 mg/kg	20–30	3–6
	PO	1 mg/kg	q 4–6	2 mg/kg	30–60	3–6
Hydroxyzine (Vistaril)	IM	1 mg/kg	q 4–6	2 mg/kg	20–30	3–6
	PO	1 mg/kg	q 4–6	2 mg/kg	15–30	3–6
Promethazine (Phenergan)	PO	0.5–1 mg/kg	q 6	2 mg/kg	15–30	4–6
	IM, PR	0.25–0.5 mg/kg	q 6	2 mg/kg	15–30	4–6

(continued)

TABLE 39-1. *The Rational Use of Medications for Sedation and Analgesia* (*continued*)

Commonly Used Drugs*	Route of Administration	Initial Dose†	Frequency of Use (hrs)	Maximum Dose‡ (mg)	Onset of Effects (min)	Duration of Effects (hrs)
Other						
Chloral hydrate (Noctec)	PO	50–100 mg/kg	q 4–6	2 g	30–60	60–90
	PR	50–100 mg/kg	q 4–6	2 g	30–60	60–90

* Many other drugs are available, but this table includes only those that are commonly used in children for sedation and analgesia. Local anesthetics are in Chapter 62.
† This is the initial dose for children over 1 month of age.
‡ This is the maximum adult dose.
§ The doses, onset of effects, and duration of effects are for the analgesic effects of the NSAID drugs.
‖ Tolmetin (Tolectin) is in this class but is used only for JRA, not as an analgesic agent.
¶ This is the sustained-release preparation.

For *mild* anxiety, use an antihistamine.
For specific drug treatments, see Table 39-1.

Drugs for Specific Indications ■

DRUGS FOR ANALGESIA

Treat acute severe pain with adequate doses of narcotics to prevent the breakthrough of pain. In most cases, morphine or meperidine is the drug of choice. Titrate the patient very quickly, then continue on a scheduled hourly basis in contrast to a p.r.n. schedule. A p.r.n. schedule is more appropriate for mild to moderate pain treated with codeine in combination with a non-narcotic agent. For ambulatory patients in mild to moderate pain, with or without inflammation, use oral agents such as aspirin, or a nonsteroidal anti-inflammatory drug (NSAID) (e.g., ibuprofen or naproxen). The NSAIDs are particularly useful in children with muscle, bone, or joint injury or inflammation, and in adolescents with dysmenorrhea. Patients in mild to moderate pain without inflammation or those who cannot take aspirin should be given acetaminophen. Acetaminophen is the equivalent of aspirin, milligram for milligram, for treating pain or temperature elevation.

DRUGS FOR SEDATION

Many drugs have been used for sedation. The benzodiazepines, such as diazepam or lorazepam, are generally safe drugs to use parenterally or orally in children. Midazolam, which is only given parenterally for major or minor surgical procedures in children, may produce profound respiratory depression and must be used very cautiously. Antihistamines producing significant sedation (e.g., diphenhydramine, hydroxyzine, or promethazine) are well tolerated by children. They are also antiemetic and have anticholinergic effects. The phenothiazines (e.g., chlorpromazine) have been used for their sedative effects. Chlorpromazine, however, has significant orthostatic hypotensive effects and should be used with caution in dehydrated patients or those with cardiovascular instability.

ANTIEMETIC DRUGS

As mentioned above, the antihistamines may be used, particularly in children 8 years and under who are more sensitive to the phenothiazine-induced torticollis. For more severe vomiting, use phenothiazines (e.g., chlorpromazine or prochlorperazine) in children over 8 years of age. More potent antiemetics are used in different combinations for treating chemotherapy-induced nausea and vomiting (e.g., metoclopramide with diphenhydramine, plus dexamethasone; and lorazepam, or droperidol and/or the cannabinoids dronabinol or nabilone).

ANTICHOLINERGIC DRUGS

The principal agents used in this class are atropine or scopolamine. These are the most efficacious agents, but the antihistamines, such as promethazine or hydroxyzine, may also be used.

Bibliography ■

Amadio P: Peripherally acting analgesics. *Am J Med* 1984; 17:17.

American Pain Society: Principles of analgesic use in the treatment of acute pain or chronic cancer pain. *Clin Pharm* 1987; 6:523.

Anand KJS, Hickey PR: Pain and its effects in the human neonate and fetus. *N Engl J Med* 1987; 317:1321.

Nahata MC: Sedation in pediatric patients undergoing diagnostic procedures. *Drug Intel Clin Pharm* 1988; 22: 711.

Schecter NL: Pain and pain control in children. *Curr Probl Pediatr* 1985; 15:1.

Selbst SM: Managing pain in the pediatric emergency department. *Pediatr Emerg Care* 1989; 5:56.

40 Abdominal Pain

Ronald A. Dieckmann

Abdominal pain is a common complaint of childhood and a frequent presenting problem in the emergency department (ED), pediatric office, or clinic. Causes are multiple and include local and systemic processes both in the abdomen and in other anatomic locations. Functional etiologies are frequent among patients with recurrent pain patterns. The *acute abdomen* is a potentially life-threatening intra-abdominal emergency, requiring immediate surgical intervention; pathologic processes usually originate in the gastrointestinal system and involve either inflammation, obstruction, perforation of a viscus, hemorrhage, or vascular interruption. Recognition of the acute abdomen is sometimes difficult in the young child, but early diagnosis is imperative to avoid unnecessary morbidity and mortality.

Etiology and Pathophysiology ■

Pain in the abdomen may be *visceral, somatic, or referred,* depending on its anatomic origin. *Visceral pain,* which originates in visceral organs, is caused by distention of a viscus or organ capsule, or from spasm or colic of intestinal muscularis fibers due to inflammation or ischemia. It is transmitted via sympathetic autonomic pathways from T6 to L1 spinal levels to the brain. Visceral pain is ill-defined, poorly localized, deep, and achy or crampy in quality.

Somatic pain develops from irritation of the parietal peritoneum or of more superficial muscle or skin; it travels by somatic or segmental afferent pathways, usually from T6 to L1. The pain is sharp, discrete, and well localized. Often, abdominal muscle reflex spasm is present in the affected dermatome.

Referred pain originates in visceral or somatic anatomic sites, but is felt elsewhere. Shared afferent sympathetic pathways to the brain provide the pathophysiologic basis for referred pain sensations. For example, referred pain from the diaphragm is felt in the shoulder, ureteral pain in the testicle, and biliary pain in the scapula.

The etiologies of abdominal pain may be surgical, medical, or functional. *The probabilities for certain diagnoses are strongly associated with the age of the patient.* Table 40-1 presents the common etiologies for abdominal pain, vis-a-vis the patient's age.

Clinical Findings ■

Abdominal pain is difficult to evaluate in the infant and young child, who may not be able to provide a useful history or characterize the quality of pain. It is particularly problematic to diagnose visceral pain in the very young child, since interpretation and description of these sensations requires brain maturation at least at the age level of the older toddler. Clinical evaluation of abdominal pain requires a careful history from parents, caretaker, or patient and a complete physical examination.

HISTORY

Important features include:

1. Nature of onset of pain (eg., sudden, gradual, intermittent)
2. Time of onset and duration of pain
3. Quality and severity
4. Location
5. Presence of fever
6. Anorexia, vomiting, or diarrhea and relation to onset of pain
7. Character of vomitus or diarrhea
8. Changes in bowel habits, and consistency and color of stool
9. Alleviating or exacerbating factors
10. Treatments provided
11. History of trauma or arthropod bites
12. Gynecologic history, when indicated
13. Symptoms of nonabdominal or systemic problems (e.g., fever, lethargy, rash, cough, dyspnea, sore throat, dysuria or hematuria)
14. Past medical history, especially sickle-cell disease, diabetes, renal disease, lactose intolerance,

TABLE 40–1. *Common Etiologies for Abdominal Pain by Age Group*

Under 2 Years	2–5 Years	Over 5 Years
Colic	Appendicitis	Appendicitis
Constipation	Constipation	Ectopic pregnancy
Gastroenteritis	Gastroenteritis	Gastroenteritis
Hirshsprung's disease	Incarcerated hernia	Inflammatory bowel disease
Intussusception	Meckel's diverticulitis	Peptic ulcer disease
Incarcerated hernia	Neoplasm	Pneumonia
Volvulus	Pneumonia	Salpingitis
Neoplasm (e.g., neuroblastoma)	Sickle-cell crisis	Trauma
Sickle-cell crisis	Strep throat	
Viral syndrome	Urinary tract infection	
	Viral syndrome	

endocrine disease, gynecologic disorders, inflammatory bowel disease, and exposure to heavy metals (e.g., lead).

PHYSICAL EXAMINATION

A thorough physical examination requires reassurance, gentleness, and finesse. Whenever possible, enlist parental assistance to calm and hold the child. Delay possibly painful components of the exam until last. A complete physical assessment includes:

1. *Observation of the child.* The infant or young child with visceral pain may withdraw and become listless, irritable, inattentive to the environment, and poorly consolable; during episodes of colic or somatic pain, the child often cries out and becomes restless and agitated.
2. General appearance. Note skin color, turgor, and perfusion. Look for rashes. Assess posture, guarding, and ease of movement.
3. Vital signs. *Ensure that a temperature is obtained.*
4. Head, eyes, ears, nose, and throat. Examine for inflammatory and infectious processes such as pharyngitis, otitis media, and nuchal irritation.
5. Chest. Observe for effort and rate of breathing. Listen carefully for adventitial breath sounds that might point to a pneumonic process.
6. Abdomen. *If the child is in obvious pain, provide analgesia before examination.* This will permit a more accurate examination and will not cloud significant findings. One effective pharmacologic combination is meperidine, 1–2 mg/kg and hydroxyzine, 1 mg/kg intramuscularly, or intravenously.

    After appropriate sedation, *inspect* for shape, visible bowel loops, masses, or external trauma. Look for splinting of muscles and presence of inguinal hernia. Ask the patient to cough; cough tenderness suggests rebound. Flex, extend, and rotate the hip to evaluate irritation of the psoas or obturator muscles. *Listen* for bowel sounds: a silent abdomen suggests ileus; obstruction produces active sounds first, then hypoactive sounds later. Next, *palpate.* Begin where there is no tenderness and move to the most tender area last. Touch gently to assess for quality and location of guarding. Search for the area of maximal tenderness and for masses. Feel for inguinal hernia. Finally, evaluate rebound tenderness. Use gentleness in force of palpation.

7. Rectum. All children with abdominal pain require a rectal examination to assess areas of tenderness, masses, and stool characteristics. Use the fifth digit, ample lubricant, and a slow entry into the rectum. Note the consistency, color, and guaiac testing of stool.
8. Genitourinary system. Inspect the genital area for trauma, discharge, or inflammation. Percuss the costovertebral angle for tenderness of kidneys. In adolescents, perform an internal pelvic exam to evaluate for trauma, infection, inflammation, uterine size, and masses. In younger females, assess pelvic structures by rectal exam.

ANCILLARY TESTS

Laboratory determinations are often necessary, including:

1. Complete blood count (CBC) with differential, serum electrolytes, creatinine, blood urea nitrogen (BUN), and glucose.
2. Urinalysis, with pregnancy test when appropriate.
3. Sickle-cell screen in susceptible patients.
4. Blood clot for type and crossmatch in patients with acute abdomen or significant trauma.

    Radiographic studies include:

1. Chest roentgenography to exclude primary chest pathology.

2. Abdominal film. Plain films can disclose free air, distended bowel, air-fluid levels, appendicolith, mass effect, or loss or psoas shadow from focal inflammation.

3. *Abdominal ultrasound is often the best ancillary procedure.* This painless bedside test can assess for organomegaly, gallstones, abscesses, hematomas, and pelvic pathology. It also has some value in detecting appendicitis and focal inflammatory conditions.

4. Barium enema is useful in cases of suspected intussusception.

5. Abdominal computerized axial tomography (CT) or magnetic resonance imaging (MRI) are extremely sensitive modalities useful in the stable patient without obvious acute abdomen, where ultrasound is nondiagnostic.

Differential Diagnosis, Treatment, and Disposition ■

Table 40-2 presents likely anatomic origins of abdominal pain, based on the location of pain. For infants and young children, localizing pain for the physician is often difficult or impossible. Also, an untreated focal inflammatory process may present with *diffuse* abdominal tenderness and rigidity once peritonitis is well established from irritation by pus, bowel contents, or blood. Differentiate the acute abdomen from nonsurgical conditions; if in doubt, consider hospitalization for careful and frequent observation.

Table 40-3 indicates the clinical and ancillary findings in common disease entities producing abdominal pain in children. Disease entities are divided into

---

TABLE 40–2. *Likely Anatomic Origins for Acute Abdominal Pain by Site of Pain*

Upper Epigastric Pain
Stomach
Duodenum
Biliary tree
Pancreas

Periumbilical Pain
Small bowel
Appendix
Proximal colon

Hypogastric Pain
Distal colon

Sacral Pain
Rectum

---

infectious conditions, inflammatory conditions, obstructive conditions, and masses. Intussusception, appendicitis, incarcerated hernia, and chronic abdominal pain are discussed below; other common diagnoses are colic (Chapter 28), gastroenteritis (Chapter 29), constipation (Chapter 30), and pelvic inflammatory disease and conditions of pregnancy (Chapter 107). Traumatic conditions, such as liver and spleen injury and retroperitoneal hematoma, are discussed in the section on trauma (Chapters 48–62).

ACUTE APPENDICITIS

This condition is common in adolescents and young adults, *but appendicitis must be excluded in every patient of any age with acute abdominal pain.* The presentation may be atypical, or findings may be deceptive in the very young or in the early stages of inflammation.

1. At the onset, pain is usually visceral in quality and epigastric or periumbilical in location. As inflammation extends through the appendix to the peritoneum, pain localizes to the anatomic location, typically the right lower quadrant; this takes about 12–24 hours in most cases. The appendix may be in the pelvis, the retrocecal area, or the upper or left quadrants.

2. As inflammation continues, pain worsens until rupture occurs. Rupture produces transient relief, then pain returns with increasing intensity as local, then generalized, peritonitis develops. Progression to rupture may be rapid.

3. Anorexia is almost universal; if it is not present, the diagnosis is unlikely. Vomiting is common. *Anorexia and vomiting develop after pain starts,* in contrast to gastroenteritis. Diarrhea or constipation are present in about 15% of patients with acute appendicitis.

4. On examination, the child is mildly febrile; temperatures above 39°C suggest rupture or another inflammatory process, such as pyelonephritis. A limp may be present on walking. The posture is often supine, with legs flexed. Abdominal tenderness occurs with movement, cough, or percussion. Palpation reveals local tenderness, usually at McBurney's point (midway between the umbilicus and anterio-superior iliac spine). Guarding and rebound tenderness are easily elicited.

5. The rectal exam may disclose tenderness or mass, when the appendix is located in the pelvis. External rotation of the flexed hip will produce pain (obturator sign) when the appendix lies close to the internal obturator muscle. Extension of the

TABLE 40–3. *Common Nontraumatic Causes of Abdominal Pain*

Clinical Entity	Diagnostic Findings	Ancillary Data	Comments
Infectious Conditions			
Influenza	Signs and symptoms of viral illness	Nonspecific findings	Treat symptoms
Pneumonia	Fever, dyspnea, cough, +/− chest pain	Leukocytosis, +CXR	Treat pathogen
Pyelonephritis or cystitis	More frequent in females, congenital abnormalities common, costovertebral angle tenderness	Urine has +WBCs, + bacteria	Needs urology consult & IVP
Inflammatory Conditions			
Appendicitis	Starts as periumbilical pain, then pain in RLQ, followed by anorexia +/− emesis	WBC 10–18,000, urine: +WBCs, +RBCs, − bacteriuria	Needs immediate operation, may rupture early
Meckel's diverticulitis	Often indistinguishable from appendicitis, recurrent GI bleeds occur	Nonspecific anemia nuclear scan	Similar to above, may need blood
Salpingitis	Pelvic exam shows cervical motion tenderness and adnexal tenderness, +/− vaginal discharge	Leucocytosis	Requires admit and antibiotics
Obstructive Conditions			
Hirschsprung's disease	Infants do not pass meconium in 24 hours, due to aganglionic colon and rectum, diarrhea +/− emesis, abdomen distended, no rectal stool	Abd film shows proximal distention	Decompress stomach, barium enema, rectal biopsy
Intussusception	Child usually under 2 years, with colicky pain, RUQ mass present, with no bowel in RLQ, currant-jelly stool frequent	Nonspecific early, abd film shows obstruction	Barium enema imperative, surgical consult
Volvulus	Sudden cramps with tenderness and distention, sigmoid volvulus common, gastric, midgut and transverse volvulus less common, obstruction marked	Abd film shows distention and obstruction	Fluids needed, surgical consult, barium enema
Masses			
Ectopic pregnancy	Lower quadrant pain and tenderness, with amenorrhea, pelvic exam shows adnexal tenderness	Anemia, + preg test, culdocentesis useful; ultrasound best	Transfuse early, obstetric consult
Incarcerated inguinal hernia	Tender mass in inguinal area of infant, erythema suggests strangulation. Bowel gangrene possible	Leukocytosis common, early abd film normal	Surgical consult
Tumor	May have minor symptoms or chronic pain, neuroblastoma, Wilms' tumor, and lymphoma are most common	Ultrasound, IVP, CT usually needed	Oncology consult

+/− denotes with or without

right leg with the patient in left lateral decubitus position evokes pain (psoas sign) when the inflamed appendix lies close to the iliopsoas muscle.

6. Laboratory analysis shows moderate leukocytosis (10,000–18,000/mm^3) with leftward differential shift. Leukocyte and differential counts may be normal; counts above 18,000 suggest perforation.

7. Urinalysis may disclose ketonuria and high specific gravity. Hematuria and pyuria are present when the inflamed appendix lies close to the urinary collecting system. *If bacteriuria is also detected with pyuria, consider pyelonephritis.*

8. Abdominal films demonstrate a calcified fecalith (appendicolith) in about 10% of cases; this is diagnostic of appendicitis. Other radiographic findings are noted in Table 40-4.

9. Important entities to distinguish are gastroenteritis, pneumonia, urinary infection, salpingitis, primary peritonitis, Henoch-Schönlein purpura,

TABLE 40-4. *Radiographic Findings in Acute Appendicitis*

Calcified fecalith (appendicolith)
Free subdiaphragmatic air
Loss of right psoas shadow
Focal ileus
Thick cecal wall
Right lumbar scoliosis
Mass from abscess formation

and foreign body perforation. Acute mesenteric adenitis, regional ileitis, and Meckel's diverticulitis may also mimic acute appendicitis but are rarely excluded prior to laparotomy.

10. When the diagnosis is suspected but uncertain, arrange for immediate hospitalization and surgical consultation. Begin intravenous fluid hydration, give nothing by mouth, and withhold antibiotics. Serial examinations with sedation, repeat CBCs, and occasionally ultrasound or intravenous pyelogram may be necessary. *Ultrasound in experienced hands has become especially helpful in equivocal cases.* A barium enema has limited value.

11. *When diagnosis is probable, early operative intervention is the conservative approach.* The morbidity and mortality from negative exploration are low compared with the high complication rate from a perforated appendix. A negative exploration rate of 10% is expected.

12. When the diagnosis of acute appendicitis is unlikely and discharge is planned, give the parents careful, specific take-home instructions for immediate return to the ED.

13. When the appendix ruptures, the patient may have abscess formation or generalized peritonitis. Children do not "wall off" perforations as readily as adults and are at greater risk for diffuse peritonitis. Patients with generalized peritonitis are toxic in appearance, shocky or profoundly dehydrated, acidotic, and septic.

14. With the child who has a ruptured appendix, operative care is not as imperative as aggressive reversal of immediate pathophysiology. This includes oxygen, rapid volume restoration, blood product administration when indicated, nasogastric suction, and bladder catheterization to monitor perfusion and volume requirements. A detailed approach to hypovolemic shock is outlined in Chapter 8.

15. When rupture is diagnosed, initiate appropriate antimicrobials, such as intravenous ampicillin, 50

mg/kg; gentamycin, 1.5–2.5 mg/kg; and clindamycin, 10 mg/kg, pending operative management.

INTUSSUSCEPTION

Intussusception is the invagination or telescoping of one segment of bowel into another. The usual location is the ileocecal valve. Jejuno-jejunal, ileo-ileal, colo-colic, and ileo-colic types are less frequent. The condition may develop in utero or in late adulthood, but most commonly occurs between 3 and 12 months of age and almost always before 2 years. The cause is usually unknown, although there is a relationship to adenovirus infections, summer infectious diarrhea, and winter respiratory infections. Hypertrophied Peyer's patches are often seen histologically. About 5–10% of cases occur in the presence of Meckel's diverticulum, foreign bodies, Henoch-Schönlein purpura, appendiceal stump, tumor, intestinal duplication, bowel hematoma, and cystic fibrosis.

1. History often indicates preceding diarrhea or respiratory infection.

2. Pain is recurrent in nature, with asymptomatic intervals of 5–30 minutes.

3. Vomiting is present in half the cases, *after the onset of pain.* Vomitus may contain bile.

4. In about one-third of cases, a normal bowel movement is followed by passage of "currant jelly" stools, with bloody mucus. These children are typically sicker and sometimes shocky.

5. An early physical exam may be normal except for intermittent colic.

6. A later exam in the majority of cases reveals fever, tachycardia, and lethargy. A sausage-shaped mass may be felt, usually in the right upper quadrant. The right lower quadrant has few bowel loops (Dance's sign), suggesting telescoping of the ileo-colic area into transverse bowel.

7. In advanced cases, an abdominal exam reveals exquisite tenderness or rigidity from peritonitis or vascular insufficiency. The overlying bowel segment, however, usually prevents gross spillage of intraluminal contents. The child is grossly toxic.

8. A rectal exam may indicate a mass. Stool is often bloody and mucoid, with a "currant jelly" appearance.

9. Laboratory analysis shows leukocytosis.

10. Abdominal films reveal a soft tissue density and evidence of mechanical obstruction, with distended loops of small bowel and air-fluid levels.

11. Immediate management is determined by the patient's clinical status. Toxic and dehydrated patients require immediate treatment with oxygen,

volume restoration, nasogastric suction, and bladder catheterization. Sedation with meperidine, 1–2 mg/kg and hydroxyzine, 1 mg/kg is indicated. *Ensure the availability of crossmatched blood.*

12. Obtain immediate surgical consultation once the diagnosis is suspected. The surgeon must oversee attempts at reduction of intussusception with barium enema and provide operative intervention for perforation or gangrenous bowel or if hydrostatic reduction is unsuccessful.

13. Obtain a barium enema to establish the diagnosis and to attempt reduction. This is successful in 75–85% of cases and is indicated regardless of the duration of intussusception, unless frank peritonitis is present.

14. *Barium enema technique*: When the child is stable, place barium in warm saline in the rectum via a Foley or larger catheter; wrap the legs together and approximate the buttocks with tape; sedation may be necessary. Elevate the barium canister no more than 100 cm and monitor the flow fluoroscopically. Reduction is signaled by reflux of barium into the ileum and expulsion of flatus and stool. If reduction fails two or three times, surgical reduction is necessary.

15. Recurrence is 2–5%.

INCARCERATED INGUINAL HERNIA

Inguinal hernias occur in about 2% of children, 85% of them male. Hernia is a weakness of overlying supportive structures, primarily muscle, allowing evagination of intra-abdominal contents (usually bowel). In about 10% of cases, usually in the child under 3 years, incarceration develops; this is more frequent in females. Incarceration is entrapment of viscera in the hernial pouch. In females, the hernia may contain an ovary, fallopian tube, uterus, or bladder. Almost one-third of incarcerations become strangulated, posing an immediate danger of vascular interruption. Gangrene develops in about 5%.

1. Diagnosis of incarcerated hernia is not difficult. A firm, often tender, irreducible mass is present in the inguinal canal, extending to the scrotum or labia.

2. Strangulation is suggested by erythema and edema over the mass.

3. Untreated strangulated hernia evolves to intestinal obstruction, at which point clinical findings include abdominal distention and tympany, variable pain, vomiting, anorexia, and cessation of defecation.

4. Abdominal films demonstrate air-fluid levels, dis-tended small bowel, and a gasless rectum. The air-filled incarcerated bowel may be evident.

5. Laboratory analysis may be normal early, but with continued obstruction, strangulation and vascular insufficiency, lab data reflect increasing dehydration, peritoneal irritation, and sepsis.

6. Important entities that must be differentiated from incarcerated hernia include spermatic cord hydrocele (a painless, nontender mass in males that transilluminates) and inguinal lymphadenopathy (tender, discrete lymph nodes, enlarged secondary to local infection of the rectum, leg, or foot).

7. Treatment of incarcerated inguinal hernia includes sedation with intramuscular meperidine, 1–2 mg/kg and hydroxyzine, 1 mg/kg, or intravenous morphine, 0.1 mg/kg; attempted manual reduction; and surgical consultation.

8. Reduction of incarcerated bowel is usually successful if strangulation has not occurred. Apply firm but gentle pressure on the incarcerated portion of bowel with one hand, while compressing the proximal bowel at the internal ring with the other hand to manipulate it through the inguinal opening. This is termed *reduction by taxis*. Do not persist if the child complains of pain. A second attempt is indicated after additional narcotic sedation and careful reassurance.

9. Another reduction technique consists of elevating the foot of the bed 30 degrees and placing the child in a head-down position. This decreases pressure on the incarcerated bowel and facilitates reduction by taxis. Sedation is also required. In the very young child, the head-down position is best secured by wrapping the feet in a cotton gauze roll and tying the gauze to the foot of the bed.

10. Hospitalization is indicated in all cases. Early definitive surgical correction is imperative; in boys, delaying the operation for 24 hours permits edema resolution and minimizes iatrogenic injury to the vas deferens and spermatic cord.

11. Reduction in the ED fails in about 25% of cases; suspect strangulation in these cases. Obtain immediate surgical consultation, insert a nasogastric tube, establish intravenous hydration, and admit the child to the pediatric ward for possible operative reduction and rarely for surgical resection of gangrenous bowel.

CHRONIC ABDOMINAL PAIN

Chronic or recurrent abdominal pain may be functional or organic. Functional pain may be associated with school avoidance, or disordered psychosocial

TABLE 40–5. *Causes of Chronic Abdominal Pain*

Functional Causes	Renal Causes
Psychosocial disturbances	Kidney stones
School phobia	Uremia
	Urinary infection
Gastrointestinal Causes	**Miscellaneous Causes**
Cholecystitis	Abdominal epilepsy
Constipation	Diabetic ketoacidosis
Chronic gastroenteritis	Heavy metal poisoning
Hepatitis	(e.g., lead)
Hiatal hernia	Henoch–Schönlein
Hirschsprung's disease	purpura
Inflammatory bowel	Neoplasm
Irritable bowel	Porphyria
Lactose intolerance	Sickle-cell disease
Peptic ulcer disease	Trauma
Meckel's diverticulitis	
Gynecologic Causes	
Dysmenorrhea	
Endometriosis	
Mittelschmerz	
Salpingitis	

circumstances may be causative. These presentations are often especially perplexing if the physician has not previously assessed the patient. When ED workup is negative, longitudinal care of such patients is best orchestrated by the pediatrician or primary physician.

Sometimes, chronic pain is organic in etiology, and ED evaluation may either identify the condition or initiate definitive diagnosis. Do not assume that recurrent pain is functional without an unbiased assessment. Table 40-5 lists the most frequent causes of chronic abdominal pain. In most of these conditions, outpatient disposition and referral is appropriate.

Bibliography ■

Hatch EI: The acute abdomen in children. *Pediatr Clin North Am* 1985; 32:1151.

Gierup J, Jorulf H, Livaditis A: Management of intussusception in infants and children: A survey based on 288 consecutive cases. *Pediatrics* 1972; 50:535.

O'Shea JS, Bishop ME, Alaro AJ, et al: Diagnosing appendicitis in children with acute abdominal pain. *Pediatric Emerg Care* 1989; 4(3):172.

Roy CC, Morin CL, Weber AM: Gastrointestinal emergency problems in pediatric practice. *Clin Gastroenterol* 1981; 10:225.

Ruddy RR, Ludwig S: Abdominal pain in children. *Critical Decisions in Emergency Medicine* 1985; Vol 1, No. 10.

41 Chest Pain

Mark A. Schiffman

Chest pain in children represents a minor condition in the vast majority of cases. The pain usually emanates from the structures of the chest wall or the gastrointestinal tract. However, a very small number of children with chest pain, or associated symptoms such as palpitations, lightheadedness, syncope, or dyspnea on exertion, have a serious or even life-threatening cardiovascular or pulmonary disorder. These children require rapid identification. The key to diagnosis and therapy is a brief but *carefully focused* history and physical examination, plus the judicious use of a few readily available ancillary tests.

Etiology and Pathophysiology ■

Chest pain can arise from the many structures of the thorax or abdomen, or the chest wall itself. Table 41-1 outlines the multiple sites of origin for chest discomfort in children. In general, structures of the chest wall give rise to sharp and relatively well-localized painful sensations, whereas intrathoracic and intra-abdominal structures give rise to so-called visceral pain, which is felt deeply and diffusely and is often difficult for the patient to pinpoint. Common causes of chest pain in children are listed in Table 41-2.

Clinical Findings ■

Patients presenting with chest pain may look entirely well and may be without significant physical or ancillary findings; rarely they may be critically ill with cardiopulmonary failure and a host of findings related to cardiopulmonary disease. Table 41-2 presents the wide spectrum of clinical presentations and their associated clinical, laboratory, radiographic, and electrocardiogram (ECG) features.

The emergency department (ED) workup of children and adolescents with chest pain requires the following clinical assessments:

1. Immediate cardiopulmonary assessment, concentrating on disturbances of *rate, rhythm, perfusion, and oxygenation status.* When significant abnormalities are detected, follow resuscitation and stabilization guidelines presented in Chapters 6 and 12.
2. Exclusion of serious and life-threatening diseases that can cause chest discomfort in children but appear benign on initial presentation. These entities are usually detected through careful history and occasionally through ancillary testing. Table 41-3 lists clues to diagnosis of serious causes of chest pain.
3. An ordered approach to the diagnosis of chest pain in the typical child who does not appear to be seriously ill on admission, presents no historic risk factors, and has a benign process that requires minimal diagnostic and therapeutic intervention.

Ancillary Data ■

The most important ancillary tests are the ECG and the chest X-ray. In certain cases the erythrocyte sedimentation rate (ESR) or cardiac enzymes may be useful. Finally, in cases of suspected serious structural cardiac disease, and following a pediatric cardiology consultation, an echocardiogram or cardiac catheterization may be required.

TABLE 41-1. *Sources of Chest Pain*

Intrathoracic	Chest Wall	Abdominal
Heart	Ribs	Stomach
Pericardium	Costal cartilages	Small bowel
Great vessels	Intercostal muscles	Liver
Lungs	Skin	Gallbladder
Pleura	Nerve roots	
Diaphragm	(radicular pain)	
Trachea		
Esophagus		

TABLE 41–2. _Differential Diagnosis of Chest Pain_

Diagnostic Category	Symptoms	Physical Findings
Chest Wall Pain	Sharp, well-localized pain and tenderness; possible history of trauma	Point tenderness exactly reproduces pain
Rib fracture	Local rib pain with movement	Chest compression tenderness
Costochondritis	Costochondral pain	Costochondral tenderness
Radicular pain	Pain may be related to neck/back	± reproduce pain by movement
Pleuritic Chest Pain	Sharp, well localized pain; worse on deep inspiration	Splinting respirations, apparent respiratory distress
Pneumonia	Localized dull or pleuritic chest pain, cough, fever, dyspnea	Fever, cough, respiratory distress
Pulmonary embolism/infarction (includes sickle-cell chest crisis)	Pleuritic chest pain, dyspnea	Dyspnea, possible cyanosis or cardiovascular collapse
Pleural effusion	Pleuritic chest pain, dyspnea	Dullness to percussion, diminished breath sounds
Pneumothorax	Pleuritic chest pain, dyspnea	Tympanitic to percussion, diminished breath sounds
Peptic Esophagitis	Burning retrosternal pain; often transiently improved by eating, and worse late at night	Often relieved by treatment with antacids and viscous lidocaine
Organic Heart Disease		
Ischemic Coronary Artery Disease	Crushing, central pain widely radiating into neck, back, arms, associated nausea, diaphoresis, dyspnea	Anxious, cool, clammy
Anomalous origin of coronary arteries	As above for ischemic coronary artery disease	As above
Coronary arteritis	Kawasaki Disease presentation. May have few cardiac symptoms.	Skin signs of Kawasaki disease
Coronary artery spasm		
Cocaine/stimulant abuse	Similar to ischemic pain	Tachycardia, mydriasis, hypertension
Myocarditis	Pleuritic or constant central chest pain ± fever	Pericardial rub (may be intermittent)
Pericarditis	Pleuritic or constant central chest pain ± fever	Pericardial rub (may be intermittent)
Pneumomediastinum	Pleuritic or constant central chest pain	Pericardial rub or crunch
Structural Cardiovascular Disease Hypertrophic cardiomyopathy	Occasional exercise-induced anginal pain or syncope	Variable LV outflow murmur
Mitral valve prolapse	Unpredictable "atypical" pain	Occasional MI murmur
Aortic stenosis	Exercise-induced anginal pain or syncope	Harsh aortic outflow murmur
Aortic aneurysm	Atypical chest pain	None
Eisenmenger's syndrome	Dyspnea, syncope or chest pain on exertion	Possible cyanosis; loud S1
Dysrhythmia	Palpitations, dizziness, syncope, anginal chest pain	Rapid, slow, or irregular pulse

+/− means finding may or may not be present

Laboratory Findings	ECG Findings	CXR Findings	Other Tests
None	Normal	Possible rib fracture or pulmonary contusion	
None	None	Rib fracture present	
None	None	None	
None	None	None	CT, myelogram; nerve conduction
None	None	Possible pulmonary pathology	
Decreased pO_2, elevated WBC; +/− blood culture, +/− sputum culture, gram stain	None	Pulmonary infiltrate(s)	
Possible pulmonary consolidation; decreased p02	Acute right ventricular strain	"Cutoff" sign (rare); associated pleural effusion	Abnormal V/Q scan
Pleural tap with gram stain, culture, chemistries	None	Pleural effusion	Pleural tap
None	None	Pneumothorax	
None	None	None	UGI series or endoscopy
CPK may be elevated. Lab often normal	ST and T wave changes, abnormal Q waves; may be normal initially	Cardiomegaly with pulmonary vascular congestion; may also be normal	Stress ECG. Cardiac catheterization
As above	As above	None	Cardiac catheterization
Elevated ESR	Variable	None	Echocardiogram
+ toxicology screen	Tachycardia; ST-T wave changes	None	Rule out myocardial infarction
Possible elevated ESR	Flat or inverted T waves; ST-segment changes	Possible enlarged heart shadow	
Possible elevated ESR	ST elevations in most leads; T wave inversions; low voltage; PR depression	Possible enlarged heart shadow	Echocardiogram
None	Minimal	Pericardial air	Cross-table lateral CXR shows air best
None	LVH, septal Q waves, T wave inversions in L precordial leads	Normal heart size	Echocardiogram
None	Variable T wave inversions in inferior leads	Normal	Echocardiogram
None	LVH, LV "strain" pattern	Normal or enlarged heart	Echocardiogram
None	None	Possible widened aortic shadow	Echocardiogram, aortography
Low pO_2	RVH	Enlarged pulmonary artery	Cardiac catheterization
None	Abnormal cardiac rhythm or rate	Possible enlarged cardiac shadow	Holter monitor

TABLE 41–3. *Clues to the Diagnosis of Serious Chest Pain*

Historical Features
  Corrected or uncorrected congenital heart disease
  Sickle-cell anemia
  Family history of premature sudden death
  Recent exposure to stimulant drugs (e.g., cocaine or amphetamines)

Physical Features
  Chest pain features
    Exertional
    Associated nausea and diaphoresis
    Radiation in typical coronary pain distribution
  Dyspnea
  Cyanosis
  Palpitations
  Dizziness/syncope (particularly with chest pain or on exertion)
  Fever
  Presence of murmurs, clicks, thrills, or rubs

Ancillary Examinations
  Abnormal ECG findings: ST or T wave segment abnormalities, abnormal Q waves, tachycardia or other cardiac dysrhythmias
  Abnormal CXR findings: cardiomegaly, pneumothorax, pleural effusion

TABLE 41–4. *Immediate Management of the Acutely Ill Patient with Chest Pain*

1. Put the patient at rest, in a supine or semi-Fowler's position.
2. Institute oxygen at 2–3 l/min by nasal cannula.
3. Begin continuous electrocardiographic monitoring.
4. Place a secure intravenous line. Start normal saline. When volume overload and pulmonary congestion is suspected, start 5% dextrose in water at low infusion rate.
5. Manage shock with crystalloid fluids and pressors (see Chapter 8).
6. Consider the use of antiarrhythmic therapy for dysrhythmias (see Chapter 12). Position a defibrillator at the bedside.
7. Use sublingual nitroglycerine and intravenous morphine sulfate in cases of possible ischemic coronary pain, where perfusion is adequate.
8. Admit the child expeditiously to a critical care unit or monitored ward bed.
9. If the patient has probable ischemic cardiac chest pain, obtain immediate cardiologist consultation to consider urgent thrombolytic therapy with tissue thromboplastin activator or streptokinase.

The ECG cannot be relied on in the ED to rule out ischemic cardiac pain or malignant dysrhythmias, which may be absent at the time the ECG is obtained. The ECG, however, may unexpectedly reveal a striking abnormality, such as diffuse ST segment elevations in acute myocarditis or pericarditis, or deeply inverted T waves in hypertrophic cardiomyopathy.

Treatment and Disposition ■

If the patient is unstable or presents signs of serious disease, implement the sequence of interventions in Table 41-4, and admit the patient to the intensive care unit or arrange for transfer to a pediatric critical care center, after pediatric cardiologist consultation.

In most instances, outpatient treatment is symptomatic and combined with reassurance of the patient and family of the benign nature of the problem. Often, a nonsteroidal anti-inflammatory agent, such as ibuprofen or aspirin, or antacids are all that is required, along with careful instruction on indications for appropriate follow-up evaluation with the primary physician.

Bibliography ■

Brenner JI, Ringel RE, Berman MA: Cardiologic perspectives of chest pain in childhood: A referral problem? To whom? *Pediatr Clin North Am* 1984; 31:1241–1258.

Fikar CR, Amrhein JA, Harris JP, et al: Dissecting aortic aneurysm in childhood and adolescence: Case report and literature review. *Clin Pediatr* 1981; 20:578–583.

Glew RH, Varghese PJ, Krovertz LJ, et al: Sudden death in congenital aortic stenosis: a review of eight cases with an evaluation of premonitory clinical features. *Am Heart J* 1969; 78:615–625.

Hamilton W, Rosenthal A, Berwick D, et al: Angina pectoris in a child with sickle-cell anemia. *Pediatrics* 1978; 61: 911–914.

Maron BJ, Roberts WC, McAllister HA, et al: Sudden death in young athletes. *Circulation* 1980; 62:218–229.

Selbst SM, Ruddy RM, Clark BJ, et al: Pediatric chest pain: A prospective study. *Pediatrics* 1988; 82:319–323.

Shappel SD, Marshall CE, Brown RE: Sudden death and the familial occurrence of mid-systolic click, late systolic murmur syndrome. *Circulation* 1973; 46:1128.

Strong WB, Steed D: Cardiovascular evaluation of the young athlete. *Pediatr Clin North Am* 1982; 29:1325–1339.

42 Earache

Kevin P. Coulter

Earache is a common complaint of children. The pain either arises from disease within the ear (otogenic) or is referred from a site extrinsic to the ear (nonotogenic). Otogenic pain in childhood is usually caused by otitis media or otitis externa. Nonotogenic pain often arises from an inflammatory process of the head or neck. Careful attention to visualization of the tympanic membrane and external ear canal and systematic examination of the head and neck will usually uncover the cause of an earache.

Etiology and Pathophysiology ■

Table 42-1 lists various causes of otogenic and nonotogenic ear pain.

Clinical Findings ■

The presenting features of ear pain in a child are age-dependent. Younger, preverbal children tend to have nonspecific symptoms of irritability, lethargy, and gastrointestinal disturbances. Poor sleeping with frequent crying through the night is a common early symptom of ear pain in infants. Older children are much more specific and can accurately describe their pain.

In general, severe constant ear pain is otogenic. Nonotogenic ear pain is more likely to be intermittent, mild, and overshadowed by symptoms elsewhere (e.g., sore throat).

Auricular pathology will be readily apparent on exam. Hematomas of the auricle are firm, tender swellings distorting the normal external ear architecture. Auricular cellulitis produces a red, warm ear lobe, usually with an apparent traumatic source (abrasions, pierced ear lobe). Atopic dermatitis may also involve the auricle and commonly causes cracking and fissuring along the attachment of the ear to the skull.

Otitis externa usually occurs in the summer, when swimming is most frequent. Symptoms include severe ear pain and itching. Ear discharge is common and can be purulent or serous. The pain is increased by traction on the pinna or pressure on the tragus. The external canal is erythematous, coated with purulent debris, and edematous. The edema may obliterate the external canal. The tympanic membrane appears abnormal in 20% of patients with otitis externa. Cervical adenitis may also be present. Culture usually reveals *Staphylococcus aureus* or *Pseudomonas aeruginosa.*

Malignant otitis externa produces severe ear pain, hearing loss, purulent otorrhea, and edema. Granulomatous tissue appearing as a red polyp is usually present in the external canal.

The pain of otitis media is acute in onset, severe, constant, and associated with hearing loss. Pus may rupture through the tympanic membrane, producing purulent ear discharge and a decrease in the pain. *Streptococcus pneumoniae* and *Hemophilus influenza* are the most common pathogens, although *Branhamella catarrhalis* is increasing in incidence. *Streptococcus pyogenes* is less common.

Otoscopy reveals an opaque white tympanic membrane bulging outward, resulting in loss of visible ossicles. Erythema of the tympanic membrane is a common finding in AOM, but is not nearly as sensitive a finding as loss of normal tympanic membrane landmarks. *Decreased movement of the tympanic membrane, demonstrable by pneumatic otoscopy, is a sensitive means of detecting bulging of the tympanic membrane.*

Facial nerve paralysis may develop acutely during an episode of AOM. Vertigo and sensorineural hearing loss may develop if inflammation spreads into the inner ear and causes serous or suppurative labyrinthitis.

Children with AOM may be afebrile or have mild to moderate fever. High fever (>40°C) should alert the physician to the possibility of a more serious underlying infection, such as sepsis and/or meningitis. Children with AOM always have coexistent infection

TABLE 42–1. *Causes of Ear Pain*

Otogenic	Nonotogenic
External Ear	*Upper Respiratory Infections*
1. Trauma	1. Pharyngitis
2. Foreign body, impacted cerumen	2. Tonsillitis
3. Inflammation, infection	3. Peritonsillar abscess
a. Otitis externa	4. Gingivostomatitis
b. Auricular cellulitis	5. Sinusitis
c. Abscesses of external canal	6. Parotitis
d. Herpes infection	*Dental Disease*
e. Furuncle	1. Impacted molar
Middle and Inner Ear	2. Dental abscess
1. Infection	*Lymphadenitis of the Head or Neck*
a. Otitis media	
b. Mastoiditis	*Temporomandibular Joint Dysfunction*
2. Eustachian tube dysfunction	
a. Serous otitis media	
3. Trauma (perforation)	
4. Neoplasm	
5. Bell's palsy	

of mastoid air cells; infection of the bony structure produces clinical mastoiditis. The mastoid area becomes red, tender, and swollen. The auricle is then pushed laterally and downward.

A careful exam of the head and neck will usually reveal the sources of nonotogenic pain, such as oropharyngeal infection, dental abscesses, impacted molars, and adenitis of the head and neck.

Consider temporomandibular joint syndrome (TMJ) when no other source of pain is apparent. The pain is usually unilateral and intense, lasting about 5 minutes and recurring several times daily. Most patients with TMJ have missing teeth, recent orthodontic treatment, bruxism, malocclusion, or crossbite. Tenderness may be elicited by palpating over the TMJ or inserting the finger along the inside of the cheek to the angle of the jaw and palpating the pterygoid muscle.

Ancillary Data ■

Children with uncomplicated ear disease usually require no lab work or X-rays.

The bacteriology of otitis media has been clearly defined. Tympanocentesis is indicated only when unusual organisms may be present (e.g., in neonates or immune-suppressed patients) or if AOM is complicated by sepsis or meningitis. In suspected fungal otitis externa, a KOH slide preparation may confirm diagnosis.

Plain films of the mastoid in children with mastoiditis will show opacification of air cells. A CT scan, however, is the diagnostic evaluation of choice, as it detects small collections of fluid and better defines the septae of the mastoid air cells.

A CT scan is very helpful in evaluating middle and inner ear trauma.

Treatment and Disposition ■

TRAUMA

Aspirate hematomas of the auricle with a 16- or 18-gauge needle. While maintaining negative pressure on the syringe, puncture the hematoma at its most prominent point and aspirate blood. Following aspiration, cover the ear with a pressure dressing and recheck in 24 hours. Suture simple lacerations of the auricle immediately. Complex lacerations into cartilage may require repair by a plastic or ENT (ear, nose and throat) surgeon. External canal lacerations usually require no treatment other than antibiotic drops if there is concern of secondary infection.

Small perforations of the tympanic membrane usually heal spontaneously within 2 weeks. Large perforations may require referral to an ENT surgeon for tympanoplasty. If the perforation is secondary to penetrating trauma of the tympanic membrane, obtain ENT consultation regarding possible injury to middle and inner ear structures.

FOREIGN BODIES

Remove foreign bodies in the external canal; avoid injury to the canal. In children, adequate restraint is critical. Sedation may be necessary. After visualizing the foreign body with an otoscope, direct a curette through the scope past the foreign body, then carefully "rock" it out. Alternatively, grasp the foreign body with a forceps or float it out by filling the external canal with water. Kill insects in the external canal by instilling ½ ml of 1% or 2% lidocaine solution into the external canal, then grasp the insect with a forceps to remove it.

INFECTION

Auricular cellulitis is usually caused by *S. aureus*; treat with penicillinase-resistant antibiotics. Oral antibiotics (dicloxacillin, cephradine) usually suffice. If the infection spreads throughout the ear lobe and into surrounding tissues, intravenous therapy with nafcillin is indicated.

TABLE 42–2. *Dosage of Antibiotics and Activity Against Usual Pathogens in Acute Otitis Media*

Drug	Dosage	*Streptococcus Pneumoniae*	*Hemophilus Influenzae*	*Branhamella Catarrhalis*	*Streptococcus Pyogenes*
Amoxicillin	45 mg/kg/d, tid	+	±	±	+
Trimethoprim–sulfamethoxazole	8 mg trimethoprim per kg/d, bid	+	+	+	–
Erythromycin–sulfisoxazole	40 mg/kg/d, tid	+	+	+	+
Amoxicillin–clavulanate	40 mg/kg/d, tid	+	+	+	+
Cefaclor	40 mg/kg/d, tid	+	+	±	+

± = inactive against strains producing β-lactamase.

Treat otitis externa by gentle irrigation with saline to promote cleaning and remove debris. Treatment with drops containing a steroid and an antibiotic (e.g., Cortisporin otic suspension) for 5 to 7 days will hasten recovery. If the canal is obliterated by edema, gently place a wick to permit entry of medication by capillary action. Treat fungal otitis externa with tolnaftate (Tinactin) drops.

Malignant otitis externa requires hospital admission for intravenous antibiotic therapy directed against *Pseudomonas* as well as debridement of necrotic tissue.

Antimicrobial therapy is indicated for the treatment of otitis media. Amoxicillin remains the treatment of choice. Consider alternative antibiotics if the child has been treated for AOM with amoxicillin within the past month; the prevalence of β-lactamase-producing organisms in the community is high; or the child is at risk for an unusual organism. Table 42-2 lists the antibiotics commonly used for AOM, dosage, and their activity against the usual pathogens. Treat uncomplicated AOM for 10 days.

Infants under 8 weeks of age with AOM are at increased risk for invasive disease. If fever is present or the infant appears ill, hospitalization, full evaluation for sepsis and meningitis, and treatment with intravenous antibiotics active against *S. aureus* and gram-negative organisms is indicated.

When facial nerve paralysis accompanies AOM, a wide myringotomy and intravenous antibiotics is the preferred treatment.

Treat mastoiditis in the same manner as osteomyelitis. Myringotomy with culture of middle ear fluid will guide the choice of intravenous antibiotics. Drainage of the mastoid may be required.

Treat TMJ pain with acetaminophen and hot compresses to the pre-auricular area. Repetitive opening and closing of the mouth following heat treatment is also helpful.

Refer to the appropriate chapters of the text for therapy of the other nonotogenic causes of ear pain.

Bibliography ∎

Bluestone CD: Management of otitis media in infants and children: Current role of old and new antimicrobial agents. *Pediatr Infect Dis J* 1988; 7:6129.

Kramer I, Kramer CM: The otalgia masquerade: TMJ dysfunction. *Cont Pediatr* 1988; 5:96.

Pelton S, Klein JO: The draining ear. *Inf Dis Clin North Am* 1988; 2:117.

Potsic WP: Earache. In: Fleisher GR, Ludwig S, eds: *Textbook of pediatric emergency medicine,* 2nd ed. Baltimore: Williams & Wilkins, 1984, p. 139.

Potsic WP: The ear. In: Rudolph AM, Hoffman J, eds: *Pediatrics,* 18th ed. Norwalk, Conn.: Appleton & Lange, 1987, p. 861.

Tunnessen W: Earache. In: Tunnessen W, ed: *Signs and symptoms in pediatrics,* 2nd ed. Philadelphia: JB Lippincott, 1988, p. 157.

43 Headache

Donna M. Ferriero

Headache is a very common symptom in childhood: almost 50% of children have at least one headache before reaching 15 years of age. In the evaluation of childhood head pain, it is necessary to determine whether the headache is an acute or chronic complaint. All acute (and especially severe) new onset headaches must be evaluated for the presence of a mass lesion.

Etiology ■

Headache has a variety of etiologies: it can be of vascular, inflammatory, toxic, or convulsive origin. In the setting of *acute headache,* exclude treatable causes (e.g., meningitis, encephalitis, toxic exposure, and vascular malformations) (Table 43-1).

Clinical Findings and Ancillary Data ■

In all cases of acute severe headache, it is *essential* to:

TABLE 43-1. *Causes of Acute Headache*

Meningitis
  Fungal
  Bacterial
  Viral
Encephalitis
Sinusitis
Toxins
  Solvents
  Nitrates
  CO
Vitamin excess (especially Vitamin A)
Drug withdrawal
  Amphetamines
  Caffeine
  Phenothiazines
Medications
  Progestational agents
Vascular malformations

1. Determine mental status: alertness, orientation, and age-dependent appropriate behavior.
2. Visualize the fundi; search for papilledema and vitreal or subhyaloid hemorrhage (seen in intracranial hemorrhage).
3. Perform a complete neurological examination, looking for focal abnormalities of the sensory and motor systems, especially ataxia.
4. If there are no signs of increased intracranial pressure or mass lesion and infection is suspected, perform a lumbar puncture. Send cerebrospinal fluid for cell count, glucose, protein, IgG index (IgG index is the CSF IgG/CSF albumin divided by serum albumin/serum IgG; if elevated, this is an index of central nervous system inflammation), viral serology, bacterial and fungal cultures, VDRL, and cryptococcal antigen. If the glucose is very low, send cultures for acid-fast bacilli as well.
5. Perform a CT scan *without* contrast to look for blood from subarachnoid or intraparenchymal hemorrhage caused by arteriovenous malformations (AVM) or aneurysm, calcifications (neurocysticercosis), or mass lesion.

Differential Diagnosis and Treatment of Chronic Headache ■

RECURRENT HEADACHE

Tumor is more likely to present as an acute *recurrent* headache syndrome. A history of severe morning headache relieved by vomiting is sometimes obtained. *Any headache that awakens a child from sleep*

TABLE 43-2. *Craniofacial Pain Syndromes*

Temporomandibular joint
Glossopharyngeal neuralgia
Trigeminal neuralgia
Occipital neuralgia
Talosa–Hunt

210

TABLE 43–3. *Drug Prophylaxis for Migraine*

Drug	Dosage	Comments
Propranolol	1–2 mg/kg/d divided bid	Doses up to 320 mg/d are tolerated; contraindicated in children with asthma, cardiac disease, diabetes.
Ca^{++} channel blockers (verapamil)	1 mg/kg/d divided tid	Use in older children.
Cyproheptadine HCl	0.3 mg/kg/d divided tid	Contraindicated in asthma and pulmonary disease.
Amitriptyline	1–2 mg/kg/d	Especially useful if child also is depressed.
Phenobarbital or phenytoin	2–4 mg/kg/d divided bid	
Ergotamine tartrate (Cafergot, Wigraine)	1–2 tablets (1 mg) at onset, than 1 every 30 minutes until headache resolves or nausea occurs	Limit to 3 mg for children under 12; limit to 6 mg in 24-hour period regardless of age.
Suppository	1 per headache if under 12; over 12, no more than 2	
Sublingual (Wigrettes, Ergomar)	1 tablet (2 mg) at onset	May repeat twice in patients over 12 years.

must be investigated. Search for evidence of hypothalamic-pituitary malfunction (short stature, polydipsia, weight loss), as many tumors are diencephalic in origin. Trauma, migraine, and craniofacial pain syndromes (Table 43-2) may all present as acute recurrent headache.

MIGRAINE

The criteria for *migraine* diagnosis is recurrent headache and at least three of the following:

1. Photophobia or sonophobia
2. Nausea or vomiting
3. Aura (usually visual)
4. Recurrent abdominal pain with or without headache
5. Throbbing or pounding pain
6. Pain restricted *at times* to one side of the head
7. Relief by periods of sleep
8. Family history of migraine.

TABLE 43–4. *Chronic Progressive Headaches*

Tumor
Partially treated meningitis
Vasculitis
Fungal meningitis
Pseudotumor cerebri
Hydrocephalus
Cerebral abscess
Subdural hematoma

The treatment of acute migraine in older children can be accomplished in the emergency department by giving 5 mg prochlorperazine intravenously (to prevent nausea from dihydroergotamine), then 0.75 mg dihydroergotamine intravenously. After 30 minutes, if the patient has not had significant pain relief, give an additional dose.

If migraine is intermittent (only a few episodes a month) and is accompanied by an aura, ergots are effective. If the headache is frequent, prophylaxis is necessary and should be continued for at least six months (Table 43-3), under supervision of the primary physician or pediatric neurologist.

CONVULSIVE HEADACHES

Seizure headaches are usually diffuse or bifrontal, begin *abruptly* at any time, have no precipitating factors, and can continue for hours but usually last less than a day. They are followed by a *distinct* phase of lethargy and sleep. There is a favorable response to anticonvulsants. These headaches may occur at night during sleep. EEG shows spike and wave discharges with occasionally rhythmic theta bursts and bilateral spikes.

CHRONIC PROGRESSIVE HEADACHES

In the progressive form of chronic headache (one that worsens over several days to weeks), suspect

TABLE 43–5. *Benign Intracranial Hypertension: Etiologic Factors and Related Disorders*

Endocrine and Metabolic Disorders
Obesity and menstrual irregularities
Pregnancy and postpartum (without sinus thrombosis)
Menarche
Female sex hormones
Addison's disease
Adrenal steroid withdrawal
Hypoparathyroidism

Intracranial Venous Sinus Thrombosis
Mastoiditis and lateral sinus thrombosis
After head trauma
Pregnancy and postpartum
Oral progestational drugs
"Marantic" sinus thrombosis
Cryofibrinogenemia
Primary (idiopathic) sinus thrombosis

Drugs and Toxins
Vitamin A
Tetracycline
Nalidixic acid
Chlordane (Kepone)

Hematologic Disorders
Iron deficiency anemia
Infectious mononucleosis
Wiskott–Aldrich syndrome

High Cerebrospinal Fluid Protein
Spinal cord tumors
Polyneuritis

"Meningismus" With Systemic Bacterial or Viral Infections

Empty Sella Syndrome

Miscellaneous
Sydenham's chorea
Familial
Lupus erythematosus
Rapid growth in infancy

Idiopathic

Symptomatic Intracranial Hypertension Without Localizing Neurologic Signs Simulating BIH
Mass lesions
Obstructive hydrocephalus
Chronic meningitis (sarcoid, fungal, or meningeal neoplasia)
Hypertensive encephalopathy
Pulmonary encephalopathy due to paralytic hypoventilation, chronic obstructive pulmonary disease, or pickwickian syndrome

(Adapted from Fishman RA: Cerebrospinal Fluid in Diseases of the Nervous System. Philadelphia: WB Saunders, 1980, p. 129)

tumors with secondarily increased intracranial pressure. The common causes of chronic progressive headache are listed in Table 43-4.

Almost all patients with a brain tumor as the cause of headache will show neurologic signs within four months of headache onset. Partially treated meningitis, fungal disease, and vasculitis from systemic lupus erythematosus are all causes of chronic headache. Lumbar puncture and erythrocyte sedimentation rate are helpful in determining these etiologies.

PSEUDOTUMOR CEREBRI

Suspect *pseudotumor cerebri* in any child with *visual loss* and headache, especially if the child is female and obese. The differential diagnosis of pseudotumor is found in Table 43-5.

There is no absolutely effective therapy for pseudotumor. The goal of therapy is to preserve visual function. Treating underlying conditions is mandatory. Acetazolamide is the mainstay of therapy. Consult a pediatric neurologist when this condition is suspected.

MALINGERING

Occasionally, a child presenting with headache will be malingering. This diagnosis is one of exclusion. Rule out all possible etiologies, especially causes of acute headache (Table 43-1), craniofacial pain (Table 43-2), benign intracranial hypertension (Table 43-3), chronic progressive headache (Table 43-4), as well as school avoidance and psychiatric problems.

Bibliography ■

Dalessio DJ: A clinical classification of headache. In: Dalessio DJ, ed: *Wolff's headache.* New York: Oxford University Press, 1980.
Fishman RA: *Cerebrospinal fluid in diseases of the nervous system.* Philadelphia: WB Saunders, 1980, p. 129.
Hanson RR: Headaches in childhood. *Sem Neurology* 1988; 8:51–60.
Prensky AL: Differentiating and treating pediatric headaches. *Contemp Pediatr* 1984; 1:12.
Rothner DA: Diagnosis and management of headache in children and adolescents. *Neurol Clin North Am* 1983; 1:511–526.
Swaiman KF, Frank Y: Seizure headaches in children. *Dev Med Child Neurol* 1978; 20:580–585.

44 Joint Pain

Ruth Ann Parish

Arthritis is inflammation (tenderness, swelling, heat, redness) of a joint; *arthralgia* is subjective joint pain without physical findings of inflammation. *Effusions* are fluid collections *in the joint space itself.* They may be traumatic, with serosanguineous material, or malignant, with serous fluid; when effusions have blood in the joint space (as in hemophilia), they are termed *hemarthrosis. Synovitis* is inflammation of the synovial membrane, the fibrous capsule surrounding a joint space. *Tenosynovitis* is the inflammation of synovial sheaths around tendons.

The child with joint pain in the emergency department can be a diagnostic dilemma, for a number of reasons:

1. Children under age 5 can rarely give an accurate account of the pain, either in duration or location.
2. Many of the clinical entities that create joint pain in children involve referred pain from other anatomic sites.
3. Few children like to be examined, especially when they are uncomfortable, and have few social inhibitions about letting the physician know that.

Pathophysiology ■

Joints are composed of the ends of two bones held together in a fibrous capsule called the synovial membrane, or synovium. Synovial fluid is a plasma dialysate, with hyaluronic acid added. The hyaluronic acid content determines the viscosity of synovial fluid and is the basis for the "string test" for bedside determination of infection in the joint space. (Place a drop of synovial fluid between thumb and finger and attempt to create a "string" of synovial fluid by slowly separating the thumb and finger; synovial fluid from an infected joint space will not "string.")

Outside the synovium are ligaments, which attach to both bony metaphyses, and bursae, fluid-filled spaces designed to lessen traumatic impact to the joint itself. Tendons, with their own synovial sheaths, cross joints and provide further stability.

At the ends of the bones in children, the periosteum forms a thick cuff around the physis (cartilaginous growth plate) called the perichondral ring. This ring binds the epiphysis to the diaphysis (shaft of the bone). The ligaments of a child's joints, which attach one bone to another (outside the synovial capsule), have greater mechanical strength than the perichondral rings and calcified epiphyseal plates. Therefore, children's joints are the most stable element of the bone-joint-bone biomechanical structure, meaning that trauma in children rarely causes dislocations, or ligamentous sprains. Osseous fractures are more common.

Trauma may result in serosanguineous fluid or frank blood in the joint space, which will then inflame the synovial capsule. Free-floating antigen-antibody complexes may also inflame the joint space, and certain antibodies will cross-react with "antigenic" molecules that are fixed on the surface of the synovial membrane, again causing a general picture of inflammation to the joint.

Traumatic or inflammatory injury may involve other structures surrounding the joint space, such as bones, tendons, and bursae, causing pain that may easily be mistaken for true joint pain. Joint pain may be either a local process (as in trauma or localized infection) or a manifestation of a systemic process (sepsis, rheumatic diseases, bacterial endocarditis).

Clinical Findings ■

Table 44-1 identifies the key historical and physical features in the patient's assessment. The child's age

TABLE 44–1. *Clinical Evaluation of Joint Pain*

History
  Duration of pain
  Trauma involved?
  Fever? Previous or underlying illness (especially
    bleeding disorders or valvular heart disease)
  Rash or signs of vasculitis?
  Signs of bone marrow depression (bleeding, pallor,
    recurrent infection)?
  Family history of arthritis or collagen–vascular disease?
  True deformity of the joint? Stiffness in the morning?
  Pattern of onset of joint pain
    Migratory (rheumatic fever, systemic infection,
      serum sickness)
    Progressive (JRA)
    Polycyclic (hydroarthrosis, JRA, gout)
  Distribution, number and type of joints involved
    Monoarticular (septic arthritis, gonococcal
      arthritis)
    Polyarticular (JRA)
    Symmetric (JRA)
    Large joints (rheumatic fever, leukemia)
    Smaller joints (JRA)
  Drug exposure (e.g., hydralazine)

Physical Examination
  General medical condition
  Fever, signs of sepsis
  Pulmonary signs
  Heart murmur
  Genitourinary signs (discharge, vaginitis)
  Rashes, petechiae, purpura, nodules, erythema
    marginatum
  Unusual neurologic signs (e.g., chorea)
  Joint (compare with normal side, but examine last)
    Position at rest (flexion suggests effusion)
    Deformity, asymmetry
    Redness
    Effusion/ecchymosis
    Edema
    Range of motion/joint stability
    Heat (joint usually 1–2° cooler than middle of
      long bones)
    Tenderness
    Fluid wave
    Associated structures
      Tendons
      Synovial sheath
      Ligaments
    Number of joints involved

is often a key variable in evaluating diagnostic possibilities. Thorough examination begins by establishing rapport with the child and parent and is guided by the sequence: look first, palpate later. Save the joint examination for the last part of the physical assessment.

The differential diagnosis of joint pain in children is extensive, and most of the workup is inappropriate in the ED. Life-threatening or joint-threatening conditions must be excluded first before the evaluation for chronic problems is initiated. Table 44-2 presents the complete differential diagnosis. The four most common groups are infections (especially *Staphylococcus aureus, Hemophilus influenza,* and gonococcus), malignancy, noninflammatory conditions (traumatic arthritis or contusion accounts for 90% of joint pain in the ED), and rheumatic conditions.

Ancillary Data ■

The following tests are useful for ED diagnosis and disposition:

1. Cultures (blood, stool, urine, vaginal/urethral swabs)
2. Synovial fluid analysis (see Table 44-3)
3. Hematology (CBC with differential and platelet counts, ESR)
4. Serology (rheumatoid factor (RF), antinuclear antibodies (ANA), antistreptolysin O/streptozyme, muscle enzymes)
5. X-rays (affected joints, chest, sacro-iliac region; films of the contralateral "normal" side may be helpful)
6. Miscellaneous (purified protein derivative test for tuberculosis, bone scan, bone marrow aspiration).

Treatment ■

When a child arrives in the ED with a chief complaint of joint pain, the immediate concern is to ascertain how serious the pain is, and whether any life-threatening process is occurring. Pain control is often the first consideration, to facilitate examination (see Chapter 39). As a general rule, the more gradual the onset of pain, the less likely the etiology is to be a life-threatening disorder. Check vital signs, including blood pressure. A quick assessment should follow the guidelines in Table 44-1. Treatment is directed first at systemic support, when indicated, then by ED diagnosis.

Disposition ■

Inpatient evaluation and treatment are indicated for joint pain associated with conditions listed in Table 44-4. Most patients can be discharged after initiation

TABLE 44–2. *Differential Diagnosis of Joint Pain*

Condition	History	Physical Exam	Comment
Trauma	Recent injury	Ecchymosis, hemarthrosis, abrasions, usually one joint	R/o penetrating injury to joint; consider: tendonitis, fracture, bursitis, myositis
	Hemophilia		
Infection	Fever	Heat, erythema	Joint tap required
	Systemic illness Age <2 years	Tenderness, usually one joint	See Table 44–3
Toxic synovitis	Preceding viral illness	No arthritis	Normal ESR
Hepatitis	History of exposure	Jaundice, no arthritis, arthralgia present	Abnormal LFTs
Henoch–Schönlein purpura	Recent onset purpuric rash, bloody diarrhea	Purpuric lesions +/− arthritis	Check BP, guaiac stool
Reactive arthritis	Gastroenteritis	Sterile effusion	Stool culture helpful
Malignancy	Weight loss, abnormal bleeding	True arthritis/ hemarthrosis	CBC, ESR, x-ray joint
Avascular necrosis	Bone pain, 4–10 years common for Legg–Perthes	No arthritis	X-ray joint
Genetic disorders	Known disorders: Marfans, Ehler-Danlos Hurlers, Morquios diseases, congenital hip dislocation	Congenital abnormalities	R/o trauma, X-ray joint
Rheumatic disorders			
RF	Preceding strep infection	Migratory arthritis, rash, nodules, chorea, fevers	Elevated ESR, throat culture
SLE	Nephritis, family history	Arthritis, malar rash	CBC, ESR, urinalysis
Vasculitides	Muscle weakness	Vasculitic rash	CBC, ESR
Drug reactions	Ingestion history	CNS depression +/− arthritis	Toxic screen
Juvenile rheumatoid arthritis (JRA)			
Polyarticular	Insidious onset, morning stiffness	>3–4 joints, listless, fever	Elevated WBC, elevated ESR, positive ANA (25%), positive RF (15%)
Pauci articular	Few symptoms, age 7–8 years	1–2 joints (knee), iridocyclitis (25%)	ED lab normal, positive ANA (25%)
Still's disease	Acute systemic illness, 1–3 years	Fever, rash, joints variable, lymphadenopathy	Elevated WBC, elevated ESR, negative ANA, negative RF

+/− means with or without finding

of a diagnostic plan and appropriate follow-up with the primary physician. Occasionally, rheumatology or orthopedic consultation from the ED will assist in disposition. Open debridement of the septic joint or open joint fracture requires immediate orthopedic consultation and surgical management.

Home treatment for the painful joint includes aspirin or a nonsteroidal anti-inflammatory agent, rest,

TABLE 44-3. *Synovial Fluid Analysis*

Total protein
    Relative increase in albumin/globulin ratio
    Elevated protein in inflammation, due to increased
       permeability
Glucose
    Normal = 10 mg% less than serum glucose
Leukocytes
    Normal = 10–200 WBC/mm^3
    Differential count

	Range	Average
PMNS	0–25	6.5
Lymphocytes	0–78	24.6
Mononuclear cells	0–71	47.9
Phagocytes	0–21	4.9
Synovial lining	0–12	4.3

Gram stain
Culture and sensitivities
Acid fast-bacillus staining
Antigen studies
    Latex agglutination for *H. influenzae*
Crystals (rule out gout, pseudogout)

TABLE 44-4. *Conditions Requiring Hospitalization*

Septic child, any toxic-appearing child
Fever and acute joint swelling, with equivocal or
    unsuccessful joint tap
Child with bacterial arthritis (proven by joint tap)
Child with malignancy
Child who needs traction to correct a deformed fracture
Severe pain

Bibliography ■

Bowyer SL, Hollister JR: Limb pain in childhood. *Pediatr Clin North Am* 1984; 31:1053–1081.

Carroll WL, Balistreri WH, Brilli RC, et al: The spectrum of salmonella-associated arthritis. *Pediatr* 1981; 68:717–720.

McCarthy PL, Wasserman D, Spiezel SZ, et al: Evaluation of arthritis and arthralgia in the pediatric patient. *Clin Pediatr* 1980; 19:183–190.

Passo MH: Aches and limb pain. *Pediatr Clin North Am* 1982; 29:209–219.

Sherry DD, Weisman R: Psychologic aspects of childhood reflex neurovascular dystrophy. *Pediatr* 1988; 81:572–578.

Wedgewood R, Schaller J: The pediatric arthritides. *Hosp Practice* 1977; 23:56–61.

and splinting to provide comfort. Physical therapy may be necessary. Follow-up is best arranged with the primary physician, or occasionally with a rheumatologist or pediatric orthopedic specialist.

45 Scrotal Pain

Jack W. McAninch

Scrotal pain can create difficult diagnostic problems. The source is either the intrascrotal contents or the scrotal wall.

Intrascotal Abnormalities ■

SPERMATIC CORD TORSION

Acute scrotal pain in childhood is most often secondary to spermatic cord torsion. It is most common in adolescents but can occur in boys of any age, even neonates (or in utero). Torsion of the cord results in vascular obstruction and testicular ischemia. Unless treatment is instituted promptly, testicular necrosis may occur within 4–6 hours.

Etiology and Pathophysiology

Most cases are caused by a congenital abnormality of the tunica vaginalis. This residual portion of the peritoneum is voluminous and inserts well up on the spermatic cord, leaving the testicle suspended in a surrounding cavity (bell-clapper deformity) and prone to rotation. The initiating factor seems to be a spasm or sudden contraction of the cremaster muscle, which inserts obliquely on the cord. This causes the patient's left testicle to rotate counterclockwise and his right testicle to rotate clockwise (as observed from the foot of the bed). The site of rotation is just above the upper pole of the testicle. With vascular occlusion, testicular and epididymal ischemia follow. Complete ischemia (720-degree torsion) will cause testicular necrosis within 4–6 hours. Many patients have only partial ischemia, and immediate correction within 24 hours may result in testicular salvage.

Clinical Findings

The diagnosis is suggested when a boy suddenly develops severe pain in one testicle. Swelling of the organ, lower abdominal pain, nausea, and vomiting ensue. However, some patients experience little or no pain and only moderate scrotal swelling.

On physical exam, the testicle is retracted upward in the scrotum, enlarged, and extremely tender. The overlying scrotal skin may appear mildly erythematous. Scrotal elevation or movement results in increased pain; in contrast, the pain caused by epididymitis is decreased by scrotal elevation. Actual identification of the epididymis by palpation in a patient with torsion may be very difficult.

Ancillary Data

Mild leukocytosis may be present but most often the leukocyte count and pattern are normal. Urinalysis reveals no white cells and the patient is afebrile. Torsion can be differentiated from epididymitis with limited success with the Doppler stethoscope in conjunction with ultrasound. The most definitive test appears to be nucleotide scanning, which can be accurate in 90–100% of cases.

Treatment and Disposition

If the patient is seen within a few hours of onset, attempt manual detorsion. Success requires patient cooperation; the best results are in adolescents. Consult a urologist to perform or assist in the detorsion maneuver. Local anesthesia (1% lidocaine) around the spermatic cord at the level of the pubic bone will result in pain control sufficient to allow detorsion. Rotate the testicle in the direction opposite the torsion (i.e., the right testicle counterclockwise and the left testicle clockwise, as observed from the foot of the bed). Pain relief is immediate. Even when manual detorsion is successful, the urologist must undertake surgical correction.

When detorsion cannot be achieved manually, an operative exploration of the scrotum is immediately necessary to accomplish detorsion and to perform orchiopexy. A similar anatomic abnormality is often present in the contralateral testicle, which likewise will require orchiopexy.

Early recognition and detorsion have resulted in salvage rates as high as 93%. Delay in treatment beyond 6 hours may result in testicular atrophy; beyond 24 hours, atrophy is certain. In such cases, the testicle will slowly decrease in size over a period of months.

ACUTE EPIDIDYMITIS

Epididymitis is seldom seen before puberty. It can mimic spermatic cord torsion and must be carefully differentiated in order not to miss torsion.

Etiology and Pathophysiology

Epididymitis is seen more commonly in the sexually active adolescent. In most circumstances, urethritis or a urinary tract infection precedes or is coincident with it. Bacteria access the opening of the ejaculatory ducts and the vas deferens and infection spreads in a retrograde fashion to the epididymis, which provides a congenial medium for bacterial growth. Enterobacteriaceae (*E. coli*) may be present when cultures are positive. More often, *Chlamydia trachomatis* (and occasionally *Neisseria gonorrhoeae*) is the cause.

Clinical Findings

Epididymitis has a rather slow, insidious onset over several days; rarely, pain may be sudden. Testicular pain may be severe and may extend into the lower abdomen. The patient may have dysuria, but may not complain unless asked specifically. Direct questioning may elicit a history of urethral discharge. Urethral instrumentation or urethral surgery can be related. The patient may have a low-grade fever, but this is not always present.

On physical exam, the testicle and epididymis are enlarged, firm, very tender, and usually in the dependent lower portion of the scrotum. At times, isolated tender swelling of the epididymis is present. Relief of pain after scrotal elevation is an unreliable sign, but pain relief (or cessation) in the supine position is typical of epididymitis.

Ancillary Data

Urine from the first 30 ml voided will usually reveal more than 8 white blood cells per high-power field. Mid-stream urines are usually normal. Positive urine cultures will identify the enterobacteriaceae. The more common causative agent (*C. trachomatis*) will not show a positive culture with standard laboratory techniques. When no bacterial growth is noted, one should assume Chlamydia is the infecting organism. Scrotal sonography can be helpful at times to establish the diagnosis.

Treatment and Disposition

Institute treatment once the diagnosis is confirmed. Tetracycline (in adolescents, 1–2 g/day divided q.i.d. for 14 days) is the drug of choice because it is effective against all offending organisms. Strict bed rest and elevation of the scrotum are essential for 5–7 days. Ice packs to the area decrease pain. High fever and sepsis require hospital admission and intravenous antibiotics.

Epididymitis typically is slow to resolve. However, in the patient in whom pain and swelling persist for longer than 14 days, consider chronic epididymitis or abscess formation. Ultrasonography may help to distinguish these complications.

TORSION OF THE APPENDIX TESTIS

Appendages of the epididymis and testicle located at the upper pole are remnants of the Wolffian and Müllerian ducts and are present in 90% of boys.

The appendix testis commonly undergoes torsion. Typically, the patient experiences sudden pain at the upper pole of the testicle, which may not be severe, but persists. There is no fever and the scrotum appears normal. The testicle is in a normal position and is slightly tender. Careful palpation at the upper pole will reveal exquisite tenderness of the enlarged mass (5–10 mm), which is usually mobile. On occasion, complete infarction of the appendage may be apparent through the scrotal skin (blue dot sign), which makes diagnosis easy. Urinalysis and other laboratory data are normal.

Treatment is expectant in most cases. The pain slowly disappears and infarction is complete within 5 to 7 days. When the diagnosis is ambiguous and differentiation from other testicular torsion is uncertain, undertake surgical exploration.

Scrotal Wall Abnormalities ■

IDIOPATHIC FAT NECROSIS

Idiopathic fat necrosis is an uncommon problem seen in prepubertal boys. The cause is unclear, although a detailed history may reveal minor trauma. There is painful and often erythematous swelling of the scrotal skin, but no open lesions. The testes are palpable and normal, but the scrotal wall is swollen and tender. Sonography will reveal normal testes with a distinct mass.

No therapy is indicated. Observe the patient carefully to detect other conditions such as spermatic cord torsion. The pain will resolve completely in a few days and the mass will disappear within a few weeks. Complications are uncommon.

ACUTE SCROTAL WALL EDEMA

This rare problem, seen in young boys, may involve one or both hemiscrotal compartments. The skin is thickened, edematous, and erythematous and violaceous. The intrascrotal contents are palpable and free of involvement. Often the findings may suggest an insect bite, but its true cause is unknown. It must be distinguished from other acute intrascrotal conditions.

The problem usually resolves within 48 hours. No treatment is necessary, and no complications have been noted.

NECROTIZING INFECTIONS OF THE SCROTAL WALL

Small and superficial abrasions of the scrotum, if left unattended, can lead to localized infection. On rare occasions, severe bacterial infection develops secondary to both aerobic and anaerobic organisms. These infections can progress rapidly and create severe local sepsis and skin death.

On examination, the scrotum will be diffusely involved. Severe erythema and swelling will be present, with at times spontaneous purulent drainage. As the condition progresses, areas of skin necrosis may be apparent. Crepitation secondary to gaseous production from bacteria may be palpable.

This is a true infectious emergency for which broad-spectrum antibiotics and immediate surgical debridement are necessary. Once treatment is initiated, the problem can be controlled and any area of skin loss can undergo reconstruction. Loss of scrotal skin is the major complication, but the spermatic cord and testicles are usually spared.

Bibliography ■

Berger RE, Alexander ER, Harnisch JP, et al: Etiology, manifestations and therapy of acute epididymitis; Prospective study of 50 cases. *J Urol* 1979; 121:750.

Cattolica EV, Karol JB, Rankin KN, et al: High testicular salvage rate in torsion of spermatic cord. *J Urol* 1982; 128:66.

Holland JM, Graham JB, Ignatoff JM: Conservative management of twisted testicular appendages. *J Urol* 1981; 125:213.

46 Sore Throat

Kevin P. Coulter

Sore throat is usually the result of upper respiratory infections, most of which are viral in etiology, are self-limiting, and require only supportive care. However, bacterial infections of the upper airway are important causes of morbidity and can be life-threatening. Oropharyngeal trauma is also common. Table 46-1 lists the common causes of sore throat in children.

Etiology and Pathophysiology ■

INFECTIONS

Infections of the mouth and pharynx cause mucosal inflammation and ulceration, resulting in pain that is exacerbated by swallowing.

Viruses are the most common etiologic agents of infection in the mouth and throat. Herpesvirus type I is a common cause of gingivostomatitis in young children. Enteroviruses, particularly Coxsackie virus, cause erythema and vesicular lesions in the pharynx. Other viruses associated with pharyngitis include adenovirus, influenza, parainfluenza, rhinovirus, Epstein-Barr virus, and respiratory syncytial virus (RSV).

The most common bacterial pathogen is Group A *Streptococcus.* Membranous pharyngitis caused by *Corynebacterium diphtheriae* is now rare in the United States. *Corynebacterium hemolyticum* has been associated with a syndrome of pharyngitis and erythematous rash in adolescents. *Neisseria gonorrhoeae* can infect the pharynx of sexually active teens and victims of sexual abuse. Anaerobes, in combination with fusobacterium species, cause an acute necrotizing gingivitis known as Vincent's angina when the tonsils are involved. *Mycoplasma pneumoniae* may also cause pharyngitis, but usually this is associated with more prominent lower respiratory tract findings. *Hemophilus influenzae* B may cause an acute uvulitis.

Candida albicans commonly infects the mouth of infants (thrush). In older children, it is commonly found in conjunction with immunosuppression or topical steroid therapy.

Tonsillar infections with Group A *Streptococcus* may extend into the surrounding tissue, causing peritonsillar cellulitis or abscess. Less commonly, this complication of tonsillitis can be caused by *H. influenzae, Staphylococcus aureus, Streptococcus pneumoniae,* or anaerobes.

Retropharyngeal abscess is a rare and life-threatening infection that may present as sore throat. It is usually caused by Group A *Streptococcus* and *S. aureus.* This disease usually develops when infection spreads from the pharynx, middle ear, vertebra, or a penetrating injury to the pharynx. The infected lymph nodes of the tissue space between the pharynx and vertebra become enlarged and may progress to abscess formation.

Sore throat is also associated with epiglottitis (see Chapter 115).

INFLAMMATORY DISORDERS

Noninfectious inflammatory disorders of the mouth and throat are less common causes of sore throat. Painful ulcerations of the oropharyngeal mucosa occur with aphthous stomatitis, Stevens-Johnson syndrome, and Behcet's syndrome. Children with allergic rhinitis may experience sore throat because of irritation caused by a posterior pharyngeal drip.

Cyclic neutropenia, or neutropenia associated with drug therapy, may be associated with painful ulcerations of the mouth and pharynx.

TRAUMA

Foreign bodies may lodge in the posterior pharynx and cause severe sore throat. Direct penetrating trauma to the pharynx or palate can occur as children fall with sharp objects (e.g., pencils, forks) in their mouths. Hot fluids, acids, or alkalis can cause direct injury to the mouth and pharynx. Microwaving formula before feeding may cause palatal burns in infants.

TABLE 46–1. *Causes of Sore Throat*

Infection
  Gingivostomatitis
  Oral candidiasis
  Pharyngotonsillitis
  Peritonsillar cellulitis, abscess
  Retropharyngeal abscess
  Epiglottitis
  Laryngotracheitis
  Uvulitis

Allergy
  Allergic rhinitis

Oropharyngeal Trauma
  Burns
  Foreign bodies

Miscellaneous
  Aphthous stomatitis
  Stevens-Johnson syndrome
  Neutropenia

Clinical Findings and Treatment ■

GINGIVOSTOMATITIS

Herpes simplex type I causes multiple small vesicles with surrounding erythema on the lips, buccal mucosa, tongue, gingiva, and palate. It generally occurs in young children (ages 1–3). The lesions are quite painful and cause a high fever (39–40°C) and tender submandibular adenopathy. The child may refuse all oral intake and become dehydrated. The lesions typically persist 7 to 10 days.

Infants with oral candidiasis usually have decreased feeding and cry while drinking. The infection appears as white plaques on the tongue and buccal mucosa, with underlying erythema. Microscopic examination of a scraping of a plaque suspended in KOH will disclose fungal hyphae.

Aphthous ulcers are painful, shallow ulcers of the mouth that usually present initially in adolescence. (See Chapter 47 for diagnosis and treatment.)

Stevens-Johnson syndrome is the severe form of erythema multiforme, in which the lips are covered with a hemorrhagic exudate. Vesicles or bullae develop in the mouth that may rupture, leaving ulcerations covered by a pseudomembrane. Oral findings often occur with conjunctivitis, urethritis, and the skin lesions of erythema multiforme that may progress to bullae. The onset can be abrupt, with significant fever, chills, and toxicity.

The treatment of gingivostomatitis in children is generally supportive, primarily aimed at alleviating discomfort. Local anesthesia can be provided with a solution containing equal parts of Maalox, diphenhydramine, and 2% viscous lidocaine. Children should not consume more than 15 ml of viscous lidocaine every 3 hours. To prevent aspiration, do not allow children to drink for 1 hour after use of the solution.

Treat oral candidiasis with nystatin oral suspension, 1 ml in each side of the mouth 4 times/day for 5 days.

Treat acute necrotizing gingivitis and Vincent's angina with oral penicillin V 40,000 units/kg/day divided t.i.d. for 10 days.

Children with Stevens-Johnson syndrome generally require hospitalization and prompt therapy with intravenous steroids. Intravenous hydration and good nutritional support are essential.

PHARYNGITIS

The most common causes of pharyngitis in children are viruses and Group A *Streptococcus.* A careful history and physical exam help determine which etiology is more likely (Table 46-2). These clues can guide who to culture and in which children to begin empiric therapy before culture results. Observe the following caveats:

1. Streptococcal pharyngitis in children under 3 years old is relatively uncommon. Streptococcal respiratory infections in these children tend to present as a chronic, mucopurulent rhinitis with excoriation of the nares, low-grade fever, and cervical adenopathy.
2. Tonsillar exudate is a nonspecific finding. *M. pneumoniae,* adenovirus, and Epstein-Barr virus can also cause this finding. Children under 3 years old with tonsillar exudate, in fact, are more likely to have a viral infection.
3. Children with streptococcal pharyngitis can have significant abdominal pain and headache that may distract the physician from the pharyngeal findings.
4. Palatal petechiae are associated with Epstein-Barr virus and streptococcal pharyngitis.
5. Scarlatiniform rash is virtually diagnostic of streptococcal infection (see Chapter 104).
6. Vesicular lesions or erythematous macules in the soft palate and tonsillar pillars are indicative of enteroviral pharyngitis. These may be found with similar lesions on the hands and feet in children with Coxsackie virus infection.

Less common causes of pharyngitis also need to be considered. A history of sexual activity or possible sexual abuse may indicate *N. gonorrhoeae.* Pharyngeal gonorrhea is typically asymptomatic, however. *C. hemolyticum* pharyngitis usually occurs in children more than 10 years old and is associated with an er-

TABLE 46–2. *Clinical Clues to Diagnosis of Pharyngitis*

	History	Physical Findings
Streptococcal	Recent exposure to streptococcal infection	Scarlatiniform rash
	Abrupt onset of symptoms	Cervical adenitis
	Throat pain	Palatal petechiae
	Fever	Tonsillar exudate
	Headache, abdominal pain	Child > 3 years old
	Lack of cough, rhinorrhea	
	Winter and spring months	
Viral	Mild to no throat pain	Palatal vesicles or enanthem
	Presence of cough, rhinorrhea	Conjunctivitis
	Summer months	Child < 3 years old

ythematous, scarlatiniform exanthem. Infection with Epstein-Barr virus (infectious mononucleosis) typically presents with fever, sore throat, and posterior cervical lymphadenopathy. The tonsils may be covered with a shaggy white exudate and palatal petechiae may be present. Splenomegaly, hepatomegaly, and rash (particularly when treated with ampicillin) are further indications of infection with Epstein-Barr virus.

Diagnosis

Throat cultures remain the most practical and reliable means of diagnosing streptococcal pharyngitis. A variety of diagnostic kits are available for the rapid detection of streptococcal antigens from throat swabs. These rapid assays are generally quite specific, but they lack the sensitivity of throat cultures.

Throat cultures are *not* cost-effective in the following situations:

1. Children under 3 years old
2. Children over 3 years old with copious rhinorrhea, cough, and conjunctivitis
3. Children with recognizable viral lesions of the oropharynx (e.g., herpetic vesicles, enteroviral exanthem)

Also, culture symptomatic family members. If a child under 3 years old is suspected to have streptococcal infections, culture the nasopharynx.

The white blood cell count (WBC) may be elevated with streptococcal pharyngitis, but this is a nonspecific finding. The WBC may also be increased with Epstein-Barr virus infection, and the blood smear will show 10–20% atypical lymphocytes. Children over 4

years old with infectious mononucleosis will develop heterophile antibodies 1–2 weeks into the course of infection in 30% of cases. Heterophile antibodies are significantly less common in children under 4 years of age.

Treatment

Supportive therapy can help the discomfort of viral or bacterial pharyngitis. Acetaminophen and salt-water gargles help control pain. Oral penicillin remains effective therapy for streptococcal pharyngitis (Table 46-3). If given within 7–9 days of the onset of illness, it will prevent rheumatic fever and avert other infectious complications.

Institute antibiotic therapy at the time of the exam if the child is likely, by clinical criteria, to have streptococcal pharyngitis (Table 46-2). The duration of symptoms will be shortened if treated presumptively rather than waiting for culture results.

A positive rapid antigen test is also an indication to begin treatment. A negative antigen test may be misleading, however, so obtain a throat culture for confirmation if warranted clinically.

Erythromycin is effective alternative therapy for children who are allergic to penicillin. It has the additional benefit of efficacy against *M. pneumoniae* and *C. hemolyticum.*

Parenteral benzathine penicillin in a single dose is also effective. It is particularly useful in noncompliant patients. The pain may be lessened if used in a mixture with procaine penicillin; the dosage is still based on the amount of benzathine penicillin.

TABLE 46–3. *Treatment Regimens for Streptococcal Pharyngitis*

Antibiotic	Dosage	Duration
1. **Penicillin V**	40,000 U/kg/day PO in 2 or 3 divided doses	10 days
2. **Erythromycin**		
Ethylsuccinate	50 mg/kg/day PO in 2 or 3 divided doses	10 days
Estolate	20 mg/kg/day PO in 2 or 3 divided doses	10 days
3. **Benzathine**	Children <60 lbs: 600,000 U/IM	
Penicillin G	Children >60 lbs: 1,200,000 U/IM	1 dose
		1 dose

PERITONSILLAR ABSCESS

The child will experience an abrupt onset of severe sore throat. Fever is usually present. As the infection progresses, the voice becomes muffled, and trismus and drooling become apparent. The child often appears quite toxic.

This infection is typically unilateral. In the initial stages, there is edema and erythema of the soft palate and tonsil (peritonsillar cellulitis). With progression to a peritonsillar abscess, the tonsil and soft palate on the affected side bulge medially, causing deviation of the uvula away from the abscess. With continued progression of the disease, a lateral pharyngeal abscess may develop. This serious complication may manifest as fullness and tenderness of the lateral neck with torticollis. Infections can spread into the mediastinum, causing life-threatening airway compromise.

In the initial stages of peritonsillar cellulitis, the child can be treated as an outpatient with high doses of penicillin and careful follow-up. With progression of the disease, particularly if uvular deviation is present, hospitalize the child and start intravenous antibiotics. Arrange consultation with an ear, nose, and throat (ENT) surgeon. Aspiration of the abscess can be therapeutic and also helpful in guiding antibiotic therapy.

Begin intravenous antibiotic therapy with penicillin G 250,000 units/kg/24 hours divided q 4 hours. Administer nafcillin 150 mg/kg/24 hours divided q 6 hours if *S. aureus* is suspected.

Delay decisions on incision and drainage or definitive tonsillectomy until after ENT consultation.

RETROPHARYNGEAL ABSCESS

The patient will usually give a history of recent pharyngitis or otitis media. The onset of symptoms is abrupt and includes high fever, severe throat pain, difficulty in swallowing, drooling, gurgling respirations or stridor, and hyperextension of the head. Meningismus may be present.

On examination, a posterior pharyngeal wall mass may be apparent. A lateral neck X-ray will show widening of the tissue space between the posterior pharyngeal wall and the prevertebral fascia.

Prompt intervention is mandatory; without treatment, serious complications will occur. The mass may obstruct an airway as it increases in size. Rupture of the abscess will result in aspiration pneumonia. The infection may dissect downward into the mediastinum.

Hospitalize the child immediately and institute intravenous antibiotics (nafcillin 150 mg/kg/24 hours, divided q 6 hours). The airway may need stabilization. Consult an otolaryngologist immediately. Should the mass become fluctuant, expedite incision and drainage in the operating room.

EPIGLOTTITIS AND LARYNGOTRACHEITIS

Children with epiglottitis experience severe pain with swallowing associated with other signs of upper airway obstruction. See Chapter 115 for treatment recommendations.

OROPHARYNGEAL TRAUMA

Significant penetration of the oropharynx may damage deep structures of the neck and may require surgical exploration.

Ingestion of strongly alkaline or acidic substances can burn the oropharynx. Such burns usually appear as areas of erythema or ulceration. Their significance lies more as indicators of possible esophageal burns, although the lack of oral burns after a caustic ingestion does not rule this out. See Chapter 73 for detailed discussion of caustic ingestions.

Foreign bodies in the pharynx or esophagus may present as sore throat, frequently with drooling. See Chapter 33 for treatment.

Children with pharyngeal foreign bodies may have severe airway compromise. Laryngoscopy and immediate intubation may be required. If there is no immediate threat to the airway, a lateral neck film may help localize a hypopharyngeal foreign body. The object may be removed with a forceps or by fiberoptic endoscopy if the child is cooperative (see Chapter 13).

Bibliography ■

Breese BB: A simple scorecard for the tentative diagnosis of streptococcal pharyngitis. *Am J Dis Child* 1977; 131: 514.

Handler S: The pharynx. In: Rudolph AM, Hoffman JIE, eds: *Pediatrics,* 18th ed. Norwalk, Conn.: Appleton & Lange, 1987, p. 879.

Markowitz M: Streptococcal infections: Group A β-hemolytic streptococci. In: Rudolph AM, Hoffman JIE, eds: *Pediatrics,* 18th ed. Norwalk, Conn.: Appleton & Lange, 1987, p. 537.

McCracken G: Diagnosis and management of children with streptococcal pharyngitis. *Pediatr Infect Dis* 1986; 5:754.

Todd JK: The sore throat. *Inf Dis Clin North Am* 1988; 2: 149.

47 Toothache

Merle E. Morris and Raymond L. Braham

Toothache is a common childhood complaint. Its causes are multiple and include conditions of the teeth and the surrounding hard and soft tissues. Usually the problem is benign, with pain as the principal concern, and requires only analgesia and referral to a dentist. Occasionally, more severe disorders present as toothache. Inadequate dental hygiene and noncompliance with regular dental care are often preventable factors in toothache. This chapter will address toothache and related problems of the mouth; Chapter 53 addresses dental trauma.

Clinical Findings ■

The quality of the toothache is the key to diagnosis. Major categories of toothache include:

1. *Pain after eating.* The child can pinpoint the source of the pain.
2. *Toothache caused by hot or cold foods or liquids.*
3. *Toothache caused by hot foods or liquids but relieved by cold.* The child can localize the pain only to the affected dental arch or side of the mouth.
4. *Intense toothache of brief duration, with no apparent triggering mechanism.* The child cannot pinpoint the source.
5. *Intense spontaneous pain that may persist for hours.* This most commonly occurs at night and is usually of a throbbing nature. The patient can localize only the dental arch or affected side.
6. *Toothache with a history of pain and spontaneous relief.* Clinical examination of the affected tooth and related gingival tissue reveals an associated gumboil or chronic abscess.
7. *Intense constant mouth pain.* Examination discloses cellulitis, a diffuse swelling of the maxilla or mandible with extension to the alveolar bone. In the maxilla, there is marked swelling and edema of the palate and infra-orbital tissues, while the mandible exhibits induration of the adjacent sub-

lingual tissues. The pain involves more than one tooth.

Differential Diagnosis and Treatment ■

In *pain after eating,* the child usually can indicate which teeth are involved. Careful examination will, in most cases, reveal the presence of food impacted between the teeth. Removing this debris with a dental explorer will usually provide immediate relief. A radiograph of the teeth may show a carious lesion or lesions in the approximating area of the teeth, which will provide a retentive area for the food debris. Commonly, the cause of the food impaction is inadequate contact between the teeth.

Pain caused by eating or tooth-brushing or digital exploration is frequently attributable to one or more *aphthous ulcers.* (Other causes of soft-tissue lesions in the mouth are described in Chapter 46.) The disease has a predilection for adults but may appear in children as young as 2 years old. Aphthous ulcers may be precipitated by psychological or physical stress, oral trauma, fever, and endocrinologic disturbances. The onset characteristically involves a period of localized hyperemia and paresthesia and occasionally a burning sensation. This is followed by the development of one or more mucosal papules with regular margins surrounded by a distinct erythematous margin. The mucosal papule undergoes erosion, which creates a small ulcer covered by a gray or yellow membrane. The lesions are most painful once they have ulcerated. They heal without scarring in 10–14 days.

Treatment is symptomatic: Orabase with hydrocortisone ointment applied topically two or three times daily. Chlorhexidine gluconate 0.12% mouthwash (Peridex), ½ fl oz undiluted, has been recently approved by the Food & Drug Administration in the

225

United States and is an excellent alternative or additive agent.

Toothache caused by hot or cold food or fluids is usually short in duration. The examination may reveal discolored teeth and carious lesions. Obtain dental radiographs of suspect teeth. Unfortunately, a common finding is that there is no carious lesion and no other apparent cause for the sensitivity to hot and cold.

If caries are detected, refer the patient to a dentist for possible restorative dentistry or extraction, depending on the degree of involvement. If the transient pain persists, refer the patient to a dentist to evaluate traumatic occlusion or high spot on a filling, since these can result in hyperemia of the dental pulp and accompanying symptoms. These conditions are not usually acute emergencies and can wait until the morning or the following Monday. Treat with mild pain medication.

In the case of toothache *caused by hot food or fluids and relieved by cold fluids or ice,* obtain dental radiographs of the suspect teeth. Apply a point source of heat (warm gutta-percha) to the tooth in question. If pain is elicited, try a little ice on the tooth. Relief indicates that the dental pulp is undergoing lique-factive necrosis. Additional diagnostic evidence may be obtained by applying intrusive pressure to the suspect tooth. Do not tap on the tooth with a dental mirror or other instrument, just apply firm pressure. The child will indicate which tooth is the most sensitive. Watching the child's eyes is a good diagnostic tool, since a sudden dilating of the pupil is indicative of pain. After the intrusive pressure, apply the gentle force in a buccal and lingual direction, with the fingers. Sensitivity indicates inflammation of the periodontal ligament.

On an emergency basis, pain medication alone will hold the patient until morning when a dentist can perform a pulpectomy or root-canal therapy. However, if the clinical crown of the tooth is destroyed or the root has undergone major resorption, the tooth will have to be extracted.

Occasionally seen is a *toothache that is fairly intense but of relatively brief duration,* in which there is no apparent triggering mechanism. The child can only localize it to the appropriate side or sometimes the mandible or maxilla. When there is no obvious dental cause for pain in the posterior maxillary teeth, consider the possibility of sinus infection (see Chapter 117). A classic diagnostic sign of sinusitis pain is that it is increased when the patient touches his or her toes or stamps the foot hard. In the case of mandibular pain, eliminate possible causes, such as caries and trauma, and then observe.

In the case of *spontaneous, intense, throbbing pain, usually nocturnal,* that may persist for several hours, the child may be able to point out only the dental arch involved. This pain may be referred along the branches of the trigeminal nerve. Examine all the teeth, both mandibular and maxillary. Apply digital pressure, including intrusive and lateral manipulation. Obtain dental radiographs. Positive responses to all these tests are indicative of congestive, irreversible pulpitis or a pulpal abscess.

Refer the patient to a dentist for immediate removal of the infected pulp or pulps or possible extraction. Establishing pulpal drainage of the infected teeth will usually relieve the pain.

Sometimes the patient may give a history of *toothache with a history of pain and spontaneous relief.* Examination often will reveal a swelling of the gingival tissue adjacent to the tooth. The swelling is usually on the buccal aspect of the tooth. However, in some teeth the apices of the roots are deeply situated and the tracking plane for the pus is to the lingual or palatal aspect. In such cases, gentle pressure will usually express pus from the crevice between the crown and free gingival tissue. The pain is due to the pressure that built up before the abscess perforated the alveolar process; perforation of the alveolar bone releases the pressure and relieves the pain.

No emergency treatment is necessary since the condition has attained a chronic status and any pain experienced will be very slight. Refer the patient to a dentist for definitive treatment.

Intense constant mouth pain is a signal of serious infection. Cellulitis will usually be apparent because of obvious facial asymmetry caused by expansion of the alveolar process with accompanying edema of the adjacent tissues. Fever may be present, with signs of systemic toxicity (see Chapter 117). Identifying the affected tooth is less important than initiating aggressive infection control. Gentle palpation of the swollen area usually indicates the extent of the edema. If the problem is in the mandible, palpate the floor of the mouth and the submandibular region to determine the extent of the infectious process. Tracking across the midline indicates Ludwig's angina with its attendant risk of airway obstruction.

Protecting the airway is paramount. If the airway is obviously endangered, establish a definitive airway as outlined in Chapter 13 for airway obstruction. If partial obstruction is present, hospitalize the patient for incision and drainage under general anesthesia. Once the patient is stabilized and the cellulitis resolved, refer him or her to a dentist for definitive treatment of the offending tooth.

If the airway is safe, hospitalize and initiate antibiotic therapy with penicillin while waiting for the results of the culture and sensitivity. If the patient has a history of penicillin sensitivity, use alternative antimicrobials as presented in Chapter 117. Oral erythromycin or a cephalosporin is suitable for localized processes that do not require hospitalization. A more specific antibiotic can always be substituted later if necessary.

Bibliography ■

Sanger RG, Casamassimo PS, Belanger GK, et al: Oral manifestations of systemic diseases. In: Stewart RE, Barber TK, Troutman KC et al: *Pediatric dentistry: Scientific foundations and clinical practice*. St. Louis: CV Mosby, 1982.

VII
Trauma

48 Initial Resuscitation of the Child with Multiple Injuries

Grace Young and Martin R. Eichelberger

Trauma is the leading cause of death in children over one year of age in the United States. In children aged 0 to 19 years, 71,370 deaths were documented in 1985 by the United States National Center for Health Statistics. Of these, 16,200, or 23%, died from injuries. The single largest cause of all trauma-related deaths is motor vehicle accidents; these totalled 9,796, or 60% of trauma-related deaths. Other causes of traumatic injury in children are burns, drownings, poisonings, firearms, falls, and abuse, in order of decreasing frequency.

Evaluation and treatment of the pediatric trauma victim is a continuum that begins in the prehospital setting (Chapter 2) and continues through the emergency department, in-hospital, and rehabilitation phases. Increasingly, a key component of the care continuum is interfacility transportation of the critically injured child (Chapter 5), after primary resuscitation and stabilization, to a general trauma center, pediatric trauma center, or pediatric critical care center. Better organization of the trauma and critical care systems appears to be improving outcome (Chapter 1).

In children who die soon after injury, the primary mechanisms that cause death are *airway compromise, hypovolemic shock,* and *central nervous system damage.* The focus of this chapter is recognition, rapid assessment and frequent reassessment of the ABCDEs, and appropriate initial resuscitation of the child in the ED.

The pediatric trauma team, a trauma-response team with clearly delineated roles and responsibilities, is an interdisciplinary group designed to meet the anticipated needs of the pediatric trauma patient. A pediatric surgeon or pediatric emergency medicine specialist is the team leader. Additional team members are the neurosurgeon, orthopedic surgeon, radiologist, clinical laboratory, and social worker.

EDs with fewer resources should also develop a pediatric trauma plan, with group paging, defined personnel roles, pre-established treatment protocols, and transfer guidelines. Timely transportation of childhood trauma victims to definitive pediatric trauma centers or general trauma centers, after resuscitation and initial stabilization, averts unnecessary morbidity and mortality.

Overview of Trauma Resuscitation ■

AIRWAY AND CERVICAL SPINE IMMOBILIZATION

The goal of airway management in the injured child is optimal ventilation and oxygenation with protection of the cervical spine (Figure 48-1). Assume any child who sustains significant trauma has a cervical spine injury. A mortality of 42% is associated with traumatic spinal injuries in children. Careless manipulation of a damaged cervical spine leads to spinal cord injury. Manage the cervical spine of all injured children by cervical in-line immobilization with the head in neutral position. Stabilize the spine with a rigid cervical collar, sandbags and tape, or manual immobilization. Obtain a roentgenogram of the lateral cervical spine that clearly delineates all seven cervical vertebrae. In a hemodynamically unstable child, however, when cervical roentgenograms cannot be obtained immediately, immobilize the neck for transport or until further spinal evaluation.

The pediatric airway is easily obstructed, especially in the child with multiple injuries and an altered level of consciousness. Loss of muscle tone in the oropharynx causes the tongue to fall posteriorly, obstructing the airway. Other causes of airway obstruction are the presence of blood, vomitus, secretions, or foreign objects in the oropharynx, larynx, or trachea; severe fractures of the mandible or facial bones; and crush injuries of the larynx or trachea. Compared to the adult, the child's tongue is proportionally larger in a smaller oral cavity, the glottic opening is more

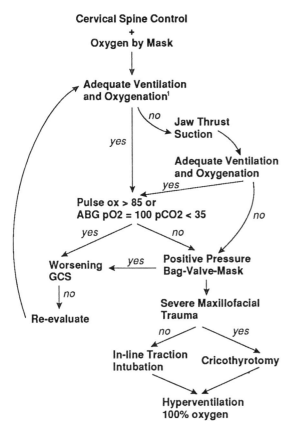

FIGURE 48–1. Adequate ventilation includes symmetrical chest expansion, equal breath sounds, appropriate mental status, and $pCO_2 < 35$ Torr. Adequate oxygenation includes pink skin, pulse oximetry > 85, $pO_2 \geq 100$ torr.

anterior and cephalad, and the trachea is shorter and narrower. These anatomic differences make the pediatric airway more difficult to manage and more prone to iatrogenic injury by less-experienced personnel. Symptoms of upper airway obstruction are dyspnea, diminished breath sounds despite respiratory effort, retractions, dysphonia (e.g., hoarseness, stridor), dysphagia, and drooling.

Treatment

To manage the obstructed airway acutely, perform the jaw thrust maneuver and administer 100% of supplemental oxygen (5–10 L/min). To perform the jaw thrust, place your fingers behind the angle of the mandible and push the mandible anteriorly. Avoid hyperextension or flexion of the neck. Next, remove materials that may cause obstruction from the mouth

and oropharynx, either manually or by strong suction. Oral or nasopharyngeal airways are poorly tolerated by the semiconscious child, and they may induce gagging and vomiting. Oral and nasal airways are only temporizing measures. *A child who tolerates the oral or nasopharyngeal airway usually has compromised protective reflexes and requires definitive airway management with an endotracheal tube.* Ventilate by bag-valve-mask with 100% oxygen until the child is intubated. However, bag-valve-mask has a high potential for gastric distention, increasing the risk of vomiting and aspiration. An oral or nasogastric tube appropriately placed following endotracheal intubation alleviates this complication.

Orotracheal intubation is the preferred approach in the injured child. Rarely are cricothyrotomy or tracheostomy necessary (exceptions are tongue hematomas and severe maxillofacial or laryngeal injury. A controlled intubation sequence or rapid sequence induction (Table 48-1 and Chapter 49) facilitates the atraumatic placement of the endotracheal tube, and minimizes intracranial pressure elevation. Once the child is intubated, provide muscle relaxation intermittently with pancuronium (0.1 mg/kg).

BREATHING

Of children who sustain multiple trauma, only 4.5% have thoracic injuries; however, when chest injury occurs, associated mortality is 25% (see Chapter 55).

Children rarely sustain rib or sternal fractures because of the relative elasticity of their chest walls. *Open pneumothorax* (sucking chest wound) and *flail chest* (paradoxical chest-wall motion with multiple rib fractures) are uncommon. *Tension pneumothorax* profoundly affects ventilation and perfusion. Signs of tension pneumothorax include acute respiratory distress or cyanosis despite adequate airway, tracheal deviation, unilateral absence of breath sounds, or diffuse breath sounds over the chest and abdomen.

TABLE 48–1.   *Controlled Intubation Sequence*

---

1. Maintain cervical in-line immobilization.
2. Clear and suction airway.
3. Ventilate with 100% oxygen by bag-valve-mask for 3–5 minutes.
4. Apply cricoid pressure.
5(A). Administer Surital (4 mg/kg) and pancuronium (0.1 mg/kg) (only if cardiovascular system is stable)
    OR
  (B). Administer thiopental (4–6 mg/kg) and succinylcholine (1–2 mg/kg).
6. Intubate by way of orotracheal route.

Penetrating chest injury may also cause *hemothorax,* especially when major intrathoracic vascular structures (e.g., the aorta) or extra-thoracic systemic arteries (e.g., the intermammary artery) are disrupted.

Blunt chest trauma can also cause *pulmonary contusion* with parenchymal hemorrhage and edema. Significant pulmonary contusion leads to hypoxia, increased intrapulmonary shunting, and respiratory failure.

Treatment

To assess for adequate ventilation, observe symmetric chest expansion, auscultate equal breath sounds bilaterally, and evaluate mental status. Adequate oxygenation is present if the skin is pink centrally and oxygen saturation is 85% or greater by pulse oximeter. Arterial blood gas ($pO_2 = 100$, $pCO_2 < 35$) confirms the adequacy of ventilation and oxygenation, but clinical evaluation is quicker. If ventilation or oxygenation is inadequate, reassess airway and breathing. Check for the correct placement and patency of the endotracheal tube; consider the presence of pneumothorax, hemothorax, or other thoracic injury.

When breathing remains inadequate after positive-pressure ventilation, perform needle thoracentesis to exclude pneumothorax. *Decompression by needle thoracentesis requires tube thoracostomy for definitive treatment.* To treat open pneumothorax, apply petrolatum-impregnated gauze and a sterile dressing over the defect; this re-establishes chest wall integrity. After an open pneumothorax is covered, a tube thoracostomy prevents the development of a tension pneumothorax. In the unusual event of an unstable chest wall from a flail chest, ventilation improves with endotracheal intubation.

If breathing is still inadequate, a significant hemothorax may be present and may require evacuation by thoracostomy tube placement.

CIRCULATION

Once ventilation and oxygenation are established, assessing circulation is the next priority. Early signs of shock are subtle in children. Normal blood volume in a child varies from 7–8%, or 70–80 ml/kg body weight. A volume loss that is considered small in an adult can induce shock in a child.

Early shock from acute blood loss of up to 25% of blood volume, or 20 ml/kg body weight, is generally well tolerated in healthy children. Children in early compensated shock may have normal blood pressure. Table 48-2 displays early and late manifestations of hemorrhagic shock. Rapid assessment of heart rate, pulse pressure, capillary refill, and peripheral perfusion indicates the relative degree of shock (see Chapter 8).

Treatment

Initiate aggressive fluid resuscitation during early compensated shock, before the child becomes hemodynamically unstable (Figure 48-2). Hypotension may not occur until after more than 25% of blood volume is lost. In late uncompensated shock, immediate fluid replacement is imperative. In losses of more than 50% of blood volume, profound hypotension and vasoconstriction result. Infuse boluses of 20 ml/kg of Ringer's lactate for any signs of shock; repeat as needed, even in the case of head injury. Clinically apparent shock and hypotension is often irreversible

TABLE 48–2. *Signs of Shock*

	Manifestations	
	Cardiovascular	CNS
Early signs	Normal blood pressure	Agitation
	Mild tachycardia (>130/min)	Lethargy
	Mild peripheral vasoconstriction	Hypotonia
	Mild dyspnea or tachypnea	
Late signs	Hypotension (<80 Torr)	Obtunded
	Persistent tachycardia	Unconscious
	Prolonged capillary refill (>2 sec)	Unreponsive
	Decreased urine output (<1 ml/kg/hr)	

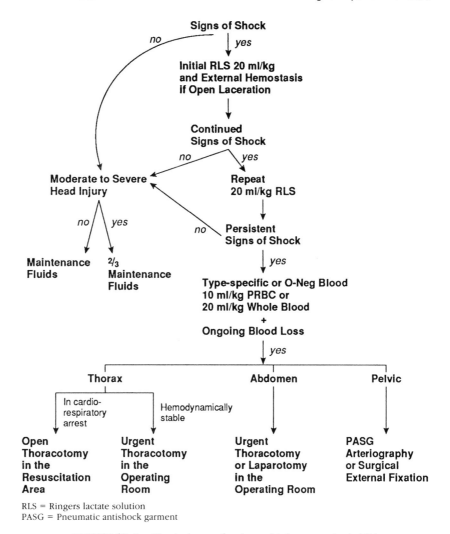

FIGURE 48–2. Shock therapy for the multiply traumatized child.

and resistant to any resuscitative efforts. It leads to multiple organ system failure and death.

Intravenous access is often difficult in injured children, especially those in shock. In the hemodynamically unstable child, obtain intravenous access within the first few minutes of resuscitation. Cannulate the largest vein without interrupting resuscitation. For optimal flow, establish two short, large-diameter catheters (18 or 20 gauge). The antecubital, saphenous, and femoral veins are the usual sites for percutaneous cannulation. The saphenous and femoral veins are the preferred sites for surgical cutdown (Chapter 139). When intravenous access is delayed, intraosseous cannulation (Chapter 139) is effective. All medications and fluids, including blood, that are usually given intravenously can be infused into the intraosseous space.

Control active sites of external bleeding with direct pressure. A deep scalp laceration, in particular, requires proper hemostasis because it often leads to hemodynamically significant blood loss in younger children. Avoid clamping bleeding vessels because of the risk of damage to adjacent structures.

Rarely, ongoing blood loss and persistent shock require the use of pneumatic antishock garments (PASG), also known as military antishock trousers

(MAST). PASG trousers increase both venous return and myocardial afterload. The major indication for the prehospital use of PASG trousers in injured children is hypotension unresponsive to aggressive volume replacement. Inflation of the leg compartments alone is preferable, with the abdominal compartment used only if there is ongoing hemorrhage from a pelvic fracture. Complications that may result from improper use of PASG trousers include:

1. Respiratory insufficiency when inflation of the abdominal portion impedes diaphragmatic excursion
2. Limited access to venous cannulation
3. Ischemia of the extremities secondary to compression
4. Pulmonary edema due to increased preload and afterload
5. Increased bleeding and clot lysis.

Children who require inflation of the abdominal compartment may need endotracheal intubation and positive-pressure ventilation.

Open thoracotomy is infrequently indicated in children (Figure 48-2). Perform immediate open thoracotomy in the emergency resuscitation area if the child is in shock unresponsive to fluid resuscitation, is in cardiorespiratory arrest, or has a penetrating wound to the heart or adjacent vessels. A needle pericardiocentesis (Chapter 139) will provide immediate decompression if cardiac tamponade is suspected and open thoracotomy is delayed.

Rarely, blunt chest trauma causes myocardial contusion. This may lead to pump failure or dysrhythmias. Treat pump failure with inotropic agents (Chapter 8) and ventricular dysrhythmias with lidocaine (1 mg/kg bolus, followed by 50 ug/kg/min infusion).

CARDIORESPIRATORY ARREST FROM TRAUMA

If the child is in cardiorespiratory arrest despite adequate airway (endotracheal intubation) and breathing (oxygenation), immediate insertion of bilateral thoracostomy tubes and simultaneous large fluid bolus infusion are crucial. If the child does not improve with these maneuvers, perform pericardiocentesis, especially if narrow pulse pressure or neck vein distention is present. These measures rapidly treat the mechanical causes of cardiorespiratory arrest. A child who fails to respond to such aggressive treatment will likely have irreversible shock, traumatic myocardial injury with central pump failure, or severe central nervous system injury. These are indications for discontinuation of the resuscitation.

HEAD INJURY

The younger child's head is particularly vulnerable to injury, especially acceleration-deceleration injuries. In the child, the head is relatively larger than the body and has less musculoskeletal support. The scalp has a much greater surface area with an abundant vascular supply. Though the child has a more compliant skull, *increased intracranial pressure (ICP) from diffuse brain injury is more common than intracranial hematoma or hemorrhage.* Cerebral hyperemia and associated increased intracranial blood volume contribute to the higher incidence of increased ICP. Of children with multiple injuries, 51% experience head trauma; of those 1 year or less in age, 66% have associated head injury. Overall, the mortality is 4%; for severe head injury (Glasgow coma score less than 8), the mortality is 32%. Many children, however, make good to excellent recovery.

Half of the deaths secondary to head trauma occur within the first two hours after the injury. Direct injury to brain tissue can occur within milliseconds of the event and may be irreversible. Secondary cerebral injury results from anoxia or ischemia and is associated with profound hypotension and intracranial hypertension. Prevention and treatment of secondary cerebral injury requires adequate ventilation, oxygenation, and treatment of shock.

The Glasgow coma score (GCS) provides an excellent basis for serial assessment of the child's neurologic status (Chapter 16). The GCS evaluates the injured child's best motor, verbal, and eye-opening responses. Management of head injury is guided by severity: the lower the GCS, the more extensive and invasive the treatment.

The best diagnostic tool for head injury is the CT scan. This radiograph outlines anatomic defects with a high degree of resolution and reliability. For mild head injury (GCS 14–15), obtain a CT scan if the child deteriorates neurologically during the observation period or has persistent vomiting or lethargy. In the child with moderately severe or severe head injury (GCS 12 or less), initial resuscitation and stabilization is imperative before evaluation by CT scan. Early diagnosis by the CT scan prompts earlier interhospital transport and better neurologic outcome of children with lesions requiring surgical intervention or proper monitoring in a pediatric trauma center.

Treatment

To manage increased ICP, maintain arterial pCO_2 in the range of 20–25 torr and arterial pO_2 at 100 torr by controlled mechanical hyperventilation. These parameters preserve cerebral perfusion pressure, reduce cerebral vasodilation, and decrease intracranial hypertension. Therefore, intubate the child with increased ICP, even though the child may have a good airway and is hyperventilating spontaneously. Endotracheal intubation secures the airway, ensures optimal oxygenation, and avoids the risk of aspiration. Since "awake" intubation exacerbates intracranial hypertension, a rapid induction sequence is necessary (Table 48-1). If the child is hemodynamically stable and does not have a spinal injury, treatment of increased ICP includes elevating of the head of the bed to 30 degrees, maintaining the head and neck in a midline neutral position, and restricting fluids to ⅔ maintenance. In more severe head injury, an intracranial pressure monitor permits ongoing assessment of ICP changes. With persistent intracranial hypertension or acute brain herniation, administer an osmodiuretic agent (mannitol, 0.25–1.0 mg/kg) if perfusion is adequate.

ABDOMINAL TRAUMA

Intraabdominal trauma most commonly involves the spleen and liver and less commonly the pancreas, duodenum, and kidney (see Chapter 56). Abdominal distention, tenderness, or rigidity are the usual signs of possible intraabdominal injury. Clinical examination alone, however, is occasionally inadequate to assess intraabdominal injury. *In a younger child, the abdominal examination may be misleading in the presence of an altered mental status, gastric distention, or injury to the chest or abdominal wall, pelvis, or spine.* Also, the patient simply may not cooperate.

Hematuria, either gross or microscopic, is a nonspecific marker for injury to the liver, spleen, other intraabdominal organs, retroperitoneum, or the genitourinary tract. Injury to the liver, spleen, or pancreas occurs in 77% of children with hematuria and normal kidneys and in 65% of children with renal or bladder injury.

The duodenum, pancreas, and kidney are relatively protected because of their retroperitoneal location. Injuries of the duodenum include intramural hematoma or perforation; injuries of the pancreas include disruption or contusion. These occur especially after direct blunt trauma, such as bicycle handlebar injury, seat belt injury, or abuse by the human fist or foot.

Treatment

The single best diagnostic method for intraabdominal trauma in children is the contrast-enhanced CT scan. Both structure and function of most abdominal organs can be evaluated rapidly and accurately. Chapter 56 discusses use of CT scanning in detail.

Nonoperative management, especially of splenic and hepatic injuries, is favored in the hemodynamically stable child whose systolic blood pressure remains stable and transfusion requirement does not exceed 50% of the estimated blood volume. Resolution of splenic and hepatic injuries in children who do not undergo surgery is excellent. Definitive management is based on clinical and physiologic status, not findings on CT scan. If nonoperative management is chosen, close continuous monitoring is essential in a pediatric trauma center.

Indications for exploratory laparotomy in children include:

1. Exsanguinating or persistent hemorrhage
2. Penetrating trauma
3. Evidence of gastrointestinal perforation
4. Acute deterioration during or after resuscitation
5. Systolic blood pressure less than 80 torr despite fluid resuscitation
6. Transfusion requirement greater than one-half of blood volume or 40 ml/kg body weight.

GENITOURINARY TRAUMA

The genitourinary examination consists of inspecting the perineal area, assessing pelvic stability, and performing a rectal exam. Signs of potential genitourinary trauma or severe pelvic fracture include blood at the urethral meatus; a high riding prostate; gross hematuria; and labial, scrotal, or perianal ecchymosis or hematoma. Any of these signs is a contraindication for insertion of an indwelling bladder catheter. The vast majority (80–85%) of renal injury is either contusion or laceration. Children who are clinically stable are best managed nonoperatively (see Chapter 57). The child benefits from observation and nonemergent evaluation by Doppler ultrasonography, isotope renal scan, or excretory urography. These tests more specifically detect structure, perfusion, and function of the genitourinary tract.

SPINE AND EXTREMITY TRAUMA

Assessment for spinal injury includes history of transient neurologic dysfunction, such as paresthesia or weakness; important physical findings are localized tenderness and symmetric voluntary movement (see Chapter 54). While injury to the cervical spine is relatively uncommon in children (1%), injury to the lumbar spine occurs in 2% of children with multiple injuries. These include lumbar facet dislocation, fracture of transverse process, or anterior compression fracture of the lumbar vertebral body. Evaluate vertebral injury with anteroposterior and lateral radiographs of the spine. Although asymptomatic intraabdominal injury is infrequent, associated perforation of the bowel or bladder does occur. Initial management of the multiply injured child with any suspected spinal trauma includes cervical spine immobilization and a long back-board for thoracolumbar spine support.

The final component of initial resuscitation is assessment of the neurologic and vascular status of all extremities. Examine all limbs for gross deformity, hematoma, or ecchymosis. Closed fractures require reduction and immobilization. Open fractures, amputations, compartment syndrome, or neurovascular compromise require immediate surgical intervention in the operating room.

Bibliography ■

Brick SH, Taylor GA, Potter BM, et al: Hepatic and splenic injury in children: Role of CT in the decision for laparotomy. *Radiology* 1987; 165:643–646.

Bushore M: Children with multiple injuries. *Pediatrics in Review* 1988; 10:49–57.

Chameides L, ed: *Textbook of pediatric advanced life support.* Dallas: American Heart Association, 1988.

Eichelberger MR, Mangubat EA, Sacco WJ, et al: Outcome analysis of blunt injury in children. *J Trauma* 1988; 28: 1109–1117.

Eichelberger MR, Pratsch GL, eds: *Pediatric trauma care.* Rockville, Md.: Aspen, 1988.

Eichelberger MR, Randolph JG: Pediatric trauma: An algorithm for diagnosis and therapy. *J Trauma* 1983; 23:91–97.

Eichelberger MR, Randolph JG: Progress in pediatric trauma. *World J Surg* 1985; 9:222–235.

Taylor GA, Eggli KD: Lap-belt injuries of the lumbar spine in children: A pitfall in CT diagnosis. *Am J Roentgen* 1988; 150:1355–1358.

Taylor GA, Eichelberger MR, Potter BM: Hematuria: A marker of abdominal injuries in children after blunt trauma. *Ann Surg* 1988; 208:10–15.

Taylor GA, Fallat ME, Eichelberger MR: Hypovolemic shock in children: Abdominal CT manifestations. *Radiology* 1987; 164:479–481.

49 Emergency Anesthesia

Kenneth Drasner and James D. Marks

At major trauma centers, an anesthesiologist is routinely available to provide emergency airway management, to assist in the resuscitation of patients in shock, and to advise on the preoperative preparation of patients requiring anesthesia and surgery. But at centers without in-house anesthesia coverage, the emergency department (ED) physician or occasionally the primary-care physician may need to provide these services. This chapter will address for the non-anesthetist the clinical problems and therapeutic options faced by the anesthetist in the management of the pediatric trauma patient. Because anesthetic considerations and options are largely determined by the severity of the injury, the chapter is divided into two sections, *minor trauma* and *major trauma*.

Minor Trauma ■

Minor trauma is an injury that does not significantly alter systemic physiologic function. Specifically, there is no significant injury to the airway, and hypovolemia, if present, is readily correctable. However, even with a minor injury, the risk for anesthetic-related morbidity and mortality is greater than with elective surgery. The increased risk results primarily from failure to obtain an adequate preoperative database, inadequate preoperative management of acute or underlying medical conditions, and the potential for aspiration of gastric contents. The following sections will detail measures to minimize these risks.

PREOPERATIVE EVALUATION

Although time may be a critical factor, it is rare that an adequate history and physical exam cannot be obtained before induction of anesthesia. Whenever possible, include the following information in the preoperative assessment:

History

1. *Last oral intake:* Because injury can delay gastric emptying, it is important to know not only the nature and time of the last oral intake, but also the relationship between the last oral intake and the time of injury.
2. *Previous surgery and/or anesthesia:* Most patients (or their parents) will be aware if an unusual event or complication occurred during previous anesthesia. Such information, as in the case of malignant hyperthermia, can be life-saving. If time permits, and the medical record is available, a review of the previous anesthetic record can provide useful information including the response to drugs, the relative difficulty in performing mask ventilation and intubation, and the correct endotracheal tube size.
3. *Medications:* A wide variety of commonly prescribed drugs have significant side effects or interactions with the routinely administered intraoperative agents.
4. *Asthma:* The placement of an endotracheal tube, particularly under light anesthesia, is a potent stimulus for bronchoconstriction. The anesthesiologist must be prepared to deal with this potential complication, and in some cases may elect to pretreat the child with bronchodilators or use an induction agent that has bronchodilating properties (e.g., ketamine).
5. *Bleeding abnormalities:* Placing a nasal airway or a nasotracheal tube in a patient who has abnormal clotting can produce a hemorrhage into the airway, with disastrous consequences.
6. *Family history of an adverse reaction to anesthesia:* Several important and potentially life-threatening disorders (e.g., malignant hyperthermia, succinylcholine sensitivity) have a familial tendency.

Physical Exam

1. *Weight:* The initial dose of most intraoperative drugs is selected on the basis of patient weight. If weighing the child is impractical, estimate.
2. *Vital signs (including orthostatics):* In spite of the "vital" nature, these are too often obtained by examining the patient's record rather than the patient.

237

Most anesthetic agents decrease venous return and are potent myocardial depressants. Induction of anesthesia in a hypovolemic patient can result in life-threatening hypotension (see below).

3. *Level of consciousness:* It is critical to establish whether the child is sufficiently alert to protect the airway from aspiration. If not, intubation should proceed without delay. While this can be a difficult judgment, as a general rule the child who has his or her eyes open, or the older child who will follow commands will protect the airway.

4. *Airway:* Assess the degree of difficulty in intubation. Key factors include the size of the chin, the extent of mouth opening, and the degree of neck mobility. Determine the condition of the oral cavity, particularly whether any loose teeth are present.

5. *Cardiopulmonary:* Assess whether bronchoconstriction is present.

Ancillary Data

1. *Hematocrit*
2. *Urinalysis:* Obtaining a urinalysis is a relatively low priority, but if one has been obtained, note the specific gravity. High specific gravities correlate with the development of intraoperative hypotension.

PREOPERATIVE MANAGEMENT OF UNDERLYING CONDITIONS

For elective surgery, optimize underlying medical conditions before the induction of anesthesia. In an emergency, weigh the benefit of postponing surgery against the risk of delaying the procedure. This decision requires knowledge of which injuries need immediate surgical intervention.

Medical conditions that benefit from preoperative treatment include *hypovolemia, bronchospasm, congestive heart failure, and hyperkalemia.* Hypovolemia is particularly important because it is relatively common, is easily treated, and is a leading cause of anesthesia-related morbidity and mortality during emergency anesthesia. In patients with minor trauma, it is rarely necessary to induce anesthesia before correcting hypovolemia.

PREVENTING ASPIRATION PNEUMONITIS

In the setting of elective surgery, difficulties with the airway are the single most important cause of anesthesia-related death and disability. In the setting of emergency surgery, airway management is further complicated by the presence of food or fluid in the child's stomach. With induction of anesthesia, protective airway reflexes are lost, placing the child in a vulnerable state for pulmonary aspiration. Although the percentage of surgical cases performed as emergencies is small, *26% of all pediatric anesthesia-related deaths have been attributed to aspiration of vomitus or blood.*

The clinical significance of an aspiration is determined by the following factors:

1. *Acidity and volume of the gastric fluid:* Recent data suggest that aspiration of gastric contents will be well tolerated, provided the volume of the aspirate is less than 0.4 ml/kg and the pH is greater than 2.5. Unfortunately, these parameters are so often exceeded that over half the children presenting for *elective* surgery would be considered at risk.

2. *Presence of particulate matter.* Aspiration of particulate matter is poorly tolerated. Pulmonary sequelae will depend on the quantity aspirated and the size of the food particles. Smaller particles may result in a wide clinical spectrum, ranging from focal edema and/or hemorrhage followed by a later granulomatous reaction, to more widespread obstruction, atelectasis, bronchospasm, and edema leading to significant hypoxemia. Large particles can completely obstruct the airways.

3. *Bacterial contamination.* Aspiration of bacterially contaminated gastric contents, as may occur in patients with significant bowel obstruction, carries with it the highest mortality.

The following preoperative measures are aimed at decreasing the risk of aspiration pneumonitis either by elevating gastric pH or decreasing gastric contents:

1. *Delay surgery.* The time required for gastric emptying is determined by the child's age and the severity of the injury. The severity of injury is a more reliable predictor of the volume of gastric contents than the duration of fasting. In addition, other factors such as severe pain, anxiety, or narcotic administration can result in similar delays in gastric emptying. When the nature of the acute pathology permits, delay surgery to allow gastric emptying. In general, children should be fasted for as long as they normally go between meals (i.e., four hours for the infant fed on a four-hour schedule and eight hours for the adolescent). It is crucial to recognize that while fasting may decrease the risk of aspiration, there is no guarantee that the stomach will be free of gastric contents.

2. *Accelerate gastric emptying.* Metoclopramide may significantly reduce gastric volume when administered to children two hours before induction of anesthesia for emergency surgery. However, despite this reduction, 38% of the children studied

had gastric volumes of more than 0.5 ml/kg. Furthermore, metoclopramide does not significantly elevate gastric pH. Thus, although some protection is afforded, the use of metoclopramide does not guarantee an empty stomach.

3. *Remove gastric contents.* Some clinicians advocate evacuating the stomach by placing a nasogastric tube in all children scheduled for emergency surgery. Unfortunately, removing gastric contents is inconsistent even with the use of a large-bore tube. Thus, the potential benefit of this procedure may not outweigh the trauma to the child. However, always insert a nasogastric tube in intestinal obstruction; this will decrease the elevated intragastric pressure and will reduce the probability of passive regurgitation during induction of anesthesia.

4. *Raise the gastric fluid pH.* Cimetidine, an H_2 receptor antagonist, reduces both gastric volume and acidity in children undergoing elective surgical procedures. However, H_2 receptor antagonists have no effect on gastric fluid already present in the stomach and therefore are of limited use in the emergency setting. Gastric contents can be neutralized by administering an oral antacid. The nonparticulate antacid sodium citrate has an advantage over particulate antacids in that it will not produce pulmonary lesions if aspirated. It has had limited use in the pediatric population, perhaps because of its unpleasant taste.

Since none of the above maneuvers are 100% effective, assume the trauma patient has a full stomach and is at risk for aspiration of gastric contents. Appropriate anesthetic techniques for these patients include *regional anesthesia, awake intubation of the trachea,* or *a rapid sequence induction with application of cricoid pressure.*

Regional Anesthesia

Except for very minor procedures, the full stomach issue cannot be avoided by the use of regional anesthesia. Most regional techniques require the use of significant quantities of local anesthesia, and an accidental intravascular injection can result in loss of consciousness. Further, the level of sedation required for the younger child to tolerate a surgical procedure is quite likely to be associated with the loss of protective airway reflexes.

Awake Intubation

Awake intubation of the trachea after topical anesthesia of the oropharynx is a very useful technique in the adult, but because of lack of cooperation it is less successful in children.

Rapid Sequence Induction

The most frequently used technique for preventing aspiration during induction of anesthesia is a rapid sequence induction with the application of cricoid pressure (see Table 48-1). In addition, this technique is frequently used in the ED by emergency physicians, anesthesiologists, and primary-care physicians. The essential elements are as follows:

1. *Proceed only if the airway appears straightforward.* The major concern during a rapid sequence induction is a failed intubation, which carries a high risk of aspiration and/or hypoxemia. If intubation appears difficult, use a different technique to secure the airway (see "Major Trauma" below).

2. *Plan ahead.* Ensure the ability to deliver oxygen under positive pressure. Have available two laryngoscopes, appropriate-sized styletted endotracheal tubes, and powerful suction. Estimate the correct endotracheal tube size from the child's age using the following formula: Endotracheal tube size (internal diameter) = (16 + age)/4; or select a tube equal in diameter to the child's fifth digit. Except in infants and young children, use a cuffed endotracheal tube. This eliminates the need for repeat laryngoscopies to select an endotracheal tube that will provide a proper seal to prevent aspiration.

3. *Preoxygenate.* Denitrogenate the lungs by administering 100% oxygen for 3–5 minutes. This will allow a period of apnea of up to 10 minutes before desaturation in older children; in younger children, this period is significantly less.

4. *Induction.* Administer a short-acting intravenous induction agent (usually thiopental 4–6 mg/kg) and a short-acting paralytic drug (usually succinylcholine 1–2 mg/kg) to establish unconsciousness and optimal relaxation for intubation simultaneously. The use of short-acting agents, combined with preoxygenation, will generally enable the patient to awaken and resume spontaneous ventilation after a failed attempt at intubation.

5. *Cricoid pressure.* An assistant applies posterior pressure against the cricoid cartilage. This compresses the cervical portion of the esophagus between the cartilage and the 6th cervical vertebrae, which prevents gastric contents from regurgitating into the pharynx. This technique, first described by Sellick in 1961, is equally efficacious in the pediatric population, preventing reflux in infants at intraesophageal pressures as high as 100 cm H_2O,

even in the presence of a nasogastric tube. Maintain cricoid pressure until tracheal intubation is verified by auscultation.

6. *Tracheal intubation.* Perform laryngoscopy and intubate the trachea. Ventilating the child with a face mask before intubation may distend the stomach. However, properly applied cricoid pressure is effective in preventing gastric distention during mask ventilation in infants even in the presence of a nasogastric tube. Although rarely necessary in the adult, ventilation may be required in the child because cooperation with preoxygenation is often difficult, and because the younger child has a higher oxygen consumption and will therefore desaturate earlier.

Major Trauma ■

Major trauma is associated with injuries to the airway and/or the potential for significant blood loss. The need for acute intervention requires that assessment and resuscitation be carried out simultaneously.

APPROACH TO THE DIFFICULT AIRWAY

Direct your initial attention at ensuring an adequate airway. Indications for immediate tracheal intubation include apnea, inadequate ventilation, significant airway obstruction, obtundation, or hypoxemia that does not respond to supplemental oxygen. Also intubate patients with hypotension unresponsive to volume resuscitation, because they are at risk for hypoxia and aspiration should they lose consciousness.

Choose a technique for tracheal intubation by the difficulty anticipated in performing direct laryngoscopy. Expect difficulty with pre-existing anatomic abnormalities or with significant mandibular, maxillofacial, or neck trauma. In the absence of these conditions, secure the airway using a rapid sequence intubation with cricoid pressure.

When the airway is complicated and spontaneous ventilation is adequate, avoid muscle relaxants. Instead, do an awake intubation using either an oral, blind nasal, fiberoptic, or retrograde transtracheal technique. In situations where this is not possible, perform a cricothyrotomy (see Chapter 139). The specific technique depends on the nature of the pathology, the patient's age, the patient's level of consciousness, and the urgency of intubation.

Alternatives to direct laryngoscopy are more lim-

ited in the infant or younger child. Fiberoptic intubation is limited primarily to older pediatric patients because the smallest flexible bronchoscopes can pass easily only through endotracheal tubes with internal diameters of 5.0 mm or more. A blind nasal intubation can be performed in the infant or young child but is technically more difficult and bleeding is more likely to occur. Similarly, a cricothyrotomy is more difficult to perform and is associated with a higher incidence of serious complications.

Additional constraints exist in the presence of maxillofacial or cervical spine injury. With maxillofacial injury, a blind nasal intubation is relatively contraindicated due to the risk of intubating the sinuses or the cranial vault. With cervical spine injury, manipulation of the neck during rigid direct laryngoscopy may result in further damage to the cord. Suspect this type of injury in all children who have suffered blunt head or neck trauma; it is present in 0.5% of children involved in motor vehicle accidents. If intubation is urgent and the anatomy appears favorable, do a rapid sequence intubation with an assistant applying axial traction. If the airway does not appear straightforward, attempt a blind nasal intubation or cricothyrotomy.

When time permits, obtain radiographic examinations of the cervical spine before intubation. If a cervical spine lesion is identified, immobilize the neck and select a technique for intubation that does not require manipulation of the cervical spine (nasal intubation or cricothyrotomy). If alternative techniques cannot be completed expeditiously, proceed with endotracheal intubation with an assistant using manual in-line axial traction to minimize cervical spine movement. *Never delay intubation of a patient with hypoxia, unstable airway, or ventilatory insufficiency based on fear of spinal injury.* Assume the cervical spine is injured and proceed with the most minimal neck manipulation.

HEMODYNAMIC MANAGEMENT

After an adequate airway is ensured, focus your attention on establishing hemodynamic stability. Place multiple large-bore intravenous lines in all patients who have suffered major trauma. In those cases involving significant abdominal trauma, put at least one intravenous line in the neck or an arm due to the possibility of discontinuity of the inferior vena cava or the iliac veins. Correct hypovolemia before inducing anesthesia. If surgery cannot be delayed or hypovolemia cannot be corrected (i.e., the rate of blood loss exceeds the capacity to transfuse), achieve intubation without an anesthetic; *all anesthetic agents can produce disastrous hemodynamic effects in the presence of hypovolemia.*

Bibliography ■

Gibbs CP, Modell JH: Aspiration pneumonitis. In: Miller RD, ed: *Anesthesia,* 2nd ed. New York: Churchill Livingston, 1986:2023.

James IG: Emergencies in paediatric anaesthesia. *Clinics in Anaesthesiology* 1985; 3:657.

Salem MR, Wong AY, Fizzotti GF: Efficacy of cricoid pressure in preventing aspiration of gastric contents in pediatric patients. *Br J Anaesth* 1972; 44:401.

Sellick BA: Cricoid pressure to control regurgitation of stomach contents during induction of anaesthesia. *Lancet* 1961; 2:404.

Striker TW: Anesthesia for trauma in the pediatric patient. In: Gregory GA: *Pediatric anesthesia.* New York: Churchill Livingston, 1983:899.

50 Head Injury

Lawrence H. Pitts, Samuel F. Ciricillo,
Henry M. Bartkowski, Julian T. Hoff

Head injuries occur often in children; one out of 10 children suffers a significant head injury during the childhood years. Fortunately, of the nearly 5 million head injuries annually, less than 10% are serious. Most are scalp lacerations or minor injuries.

Epidemiology ■

During the toddler years, a short fall is the most frequent cause of head injury. In older age groups, trauma occurs more often from automobile/pedestrian accidents. Thus, while acceleration/deceleration forces produce most injuries in children less than 10 years of age, injuries from direct impact become more important in adolescence.

In most patients who die from the effects of trauma, three or more body areas are involved. Brain injury is the cause of death in 50% of multiply injured patients who die. Thus, prompt and accurate diagnosis and management of the head injury is of critical importance to the outcome of the pediatric trauma victim.

Types of Head Injuries ■

Head trauma in children, as in adults, includes a diverse group of soft tissue, bony, vascular, and parenchymal injuries, as summarized in Table 50-1. Figure 50-1 illustrates the corresponding anatomic landmarks.

Clinical Findings ■

HISTORY

After initial resuscitation, a rapid but thorough history is essential. Important items include the mechanism of injury, speed of collision or height of fall, initial level of consciousness and subsequent changes, oc-

currence of seizures, apnea, vomiting, history of drug or medication use, and any other medical condition that may affect subsequent management. Whenever the history does not adequately explain the severity of neurologic dysfunction, suspect child abuse.

PHYSICAL EXAMINATION

After adequate ventilation and circulation are established, perform a rapid and complete physical examination to identify and treat potentially fatal multisystem injuries. Thoracic, intraabdominal, pelvic, and extremity injuries occur often and must be ruled out. (For further details, see Chapter 48).

1. Face and soft-tissue neck injuries may lead to oropharyngeal or tracheal compression, leading to airway obstruction.
2. Thoracic and lumbar spine injuries may be managed with careful patient transfer and logrolling to maintain spine alignment. Assume cervical spine injuries in all comatose patients until excluded by cervical spine films.
3. Chest injuries can impair lung function and lead to hypoventilation, hypoxia, hypercarbia, and increased venous pressures, all of which can further injure the brain.

BASELINE NEUROLOGIC EVALUATION

Cerebral hemispheric function is best characterized by alterations in level of consciousness. A simple tool for describing the level of consciousness is the Glasgow Coma Scale (GCS) (Table 16-1), which provides a semiquantitative measure of hemispheric function by observing patient performance in three areas: eye opening, motor response, and verbal response. The coma score is the sum of these three responses.

Assess upper brainstem function by observing the function of cranial nerves III through VIII.

1. *Pupillary light reflexes* measure sensory input by way of the optic nerve (II) and pupillary constric-

tion by way of the parasympathetic motor component of the oculomotor nerve (III).

2. *Extraocular motion* requires function of multiple cranial nerve nuclei and peripheral fibers, including cranial nerves III, IV, and VI, linked by the medial longitudinal fasciculus (MLF). This system may be tested either by the "doll's eyes" maneuver (oculocephalic response; done only after excluding cervical spine injury) or by cold-water caloric testing (oculovestibular response).

3. The *corneal reflex* requires intact corneal sensation via the trigeminal nerve (V) and orbicularis oculi motor response via the facial nerve (VII).

Assess lower brainstem function by examining cranial nerves IX through XII.

1. Medullary respiratory centers control respiratory rate and patterns. Specific respiratory patterns correlate poorly with location of brain damage, except that irregular (ataxic) breathing signifies medullary damage.

2. *Gag and cough reflexes,* evoked by pharyngeal and tracheal stimulation respectively, verify the presence of intact pathways of sensory and motor responses of cranial nerves IX, X, and XI in the medulla.

3. Hypoglossal function (XII), which may be assessed by observing tongue function in an awake patient, cannot be reliably assessed in comatose patients.

ANCILLARY DATA

Laboratory studies include:

1. Serial hematocrits
2. Arterial blood gas measurements. Bedside pulse oximetry is useful after initial arterial blood gases.
3. Serum glucose and electrolytes
4. Toxicologic examinations of blood and urine if intoxication is suspected

Radiographic studies are often indicated (see Table 50-2):

1. Obtain *cervical spine radiographs* in all comatose children or when a child appears to have neck pain, extremity numbness, or weakness. A lateral cervical X-ray must show the C7 vertebral body since C6-7 fracture dislocations are not uncommon. If a fracture is identified, protect the spinal cord from further injuries by sandbagging and taping, or by axial cervical traction using either a halter or skeletal-fixation device.

2. *Chest X-rays* are important in head-injured patients to exclude intrathoracic injuries, which can cause hypoxia and hypercarbia, with secondary injury to the traumatized brain.

3. *Computed tomography* (CT) has revolutionized the diagnosis and management of craniocerebral trauma. The presence or lack of specific cranial and brain injuries is readily and rapidly demonstrated. A CT scan is of utmost importance in patients with severe head injuries or in patients with less severe trauma who are clinically deteriorating, as shown in Table 50-2.

4. *Cerebral angiography* may be used in cases of head injury when CT scans are not available. Digital venous or arterial angiography is somewhat faster than a conventional angiogram. Either digital or conventional angiograms can successfully demonstrate both extracerebral and intraparenchymal hematomas by displacement of cerebral blood vessels away from the inner table of the skull or from their usual locations.

5. *Magnetic resonance imaging* (MRI) may prove valuable in the workup of the head-injured patient. Although superior to CT in demonstrating soft-tissue injury and hemorrhage, MRI fails to give the bony detail available with CT. In addition, the strong magnetic field prohibits the use of ventilatory support or monitor devices, limiting the usefulness of MRI in all but the most stable trauma patients.

6. For head-injured patients who require emergency surgery for life-threatening abdominal or thoracic injuries before cranial studies can be performed, a twist-drill air or contrast ventriculogram in the operating room can provide information regarding shifts of midline structures, and intracranial pressure (ICP) can be measured via the ventricular catheter.

Lumbar puncture has no role in the evaluation of head injury! It should be done only when meningitis is suspected (e.g., in the setting of a basilar skull fracture or penetrating trauma) and only after mass lesions and elevated ICP have been excluded by physical evaluation, usually in concert with CT imaging.

Treatment ■

RESUSCITATION

Focus immediate attention on ensuring adequate ventilation and blood pressure in order to prevent secondary brain insults from hypoxia, hypercarbia, and ischemia.

1. All comatose patients require prompt intubation to ensure airway protection and to prevent detrimental effects of elevated ICP. Immobilize the neck with sandbags and tape the head to a carrying

TABLE 50-1. *Clinical Spectrum of Head Injury*

Type of Head Trauma	Description	Mechanism of Injury	Signs & Symptoms	Comments
Extracranial Injury				
Facial injuries	Bony or soft tissue	Penetration, blunt or sharp	Bony or soft-tissue deformities	Occurs in 15% of severe head injuries
Scalp				
Subgaleal hematoma	Collection of blood between pericranium and galea	Blunt trauma leading to rupture of vessels	Soft to firm mobile lump under scalp	Frequent bony fracture in child less than 1 year of age
Cephalohematoma	Collection of blood under pericranium	Shearing force between skull and periosteum	Immobile mass limited by suture lines, usually parietal	Rare bony injury; resorbs after 2–3 weeks
Simple laceration	Linear cut	Sharp		May cause considerable blood loss or shock
Stellate laceration	Irregular gaping wound	Blunt trauma		Edges require debridement prior to closure
Avulsion	Occurs between galea and pericranium	Tangential pull on hair	Skin or scalp loss	Rotation flaps, replantation, or skin grafting often required
Burns	See Chapter 61	Thermal, chemical, electrical	Loss of hair, skin appendages and skin tissue, bone and pericranium	Conservative rx, irrigation/neutralization, debridement
Bony Injury				
Linear fracture	Lucency seen on radiograph	Elastic deformation of bone with impact	Radiographic diagnosis	May cause epidural hematoma if crosses sinus or meningeal artery
Closed				
Open	Overlying laceration			
Depressed fracture	Bony fracture with or without scalp laceration	Direct impact	Depression of skull palpable	Elevation in OR if >3–5 mm
Closed				
Open				
Diastatic fracture	Separation at suture line	Impact	Radiographic diagnosis	More common in infants; fracture edge remains separated
Basilar fracture	Fracture of basilar skull bones	Direct impact	Clinical diagnosis: hemotympanum, Battle's sign, raccoon eyes, pneumocephalus	X-rays not helpful; usually occurs at petrous temporal bone or frontal bone

Intracranial Injury				
Dural laceration	Rent or tear in dura	Penetration by foreign body or bone	May bleed through open fracture	Operative inspection and closure necessary
Subarachnoid hemorrhage	Blood in subarachnoid space	Direct impact, with tearing of bridging veins	Headache, nausea, vomiting, stiff neck	Most common hemorrhage
Epidural hematoma	Blood between skull and dura, either arterial or venous	Tear in middle meningeal artery or skull fracture	Focal neurologic deficit, loss of consciousness w/crescent on CT	Death from expanding mass lesion, seen 4–6 hours after injury
Subdural hematoma-acute, subacute, chronic	Blood between dura and arachnoid	Associated with fracture and underlying focal brain lesion	Focal deficit, behavior change, altered mental status	Frequent underlying cortical damage, mortality 60–70%
Contusion	Bruise to neural parenchyma with extravasation of RBCs under pia	Impact coup-contracoup	Headache, seizures	Most often located in frontal-temporal poles
Laceration	Physical disruption in brain parenchyma	Penetration by bone, foreign body, or marked brain movement	Manifestations of acute mass lesion	Requires operative debridement and repair
Intraparenchymal hemorrhage	Discrete collection of blood in parenchyma on CT	Movement on impact	Focal deficit, aphasia, loss of consciousness	Majority in frontal and temporal poles
Diffuse axonal injury	Reactive axonal swelling, microglial clusters	Rotational acceleration, shearing forces on nerve fibers	Loss of consciousness, brain edema	Poor prognosis

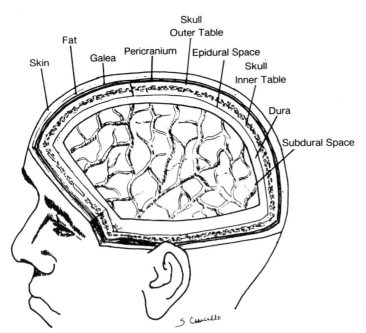

Skin
Fat
Galea
Pericranium
Skull Outer Table
Epidural Space
Skull Inner Table
Dura
Subdural Space

S Cuviello

FIGURE 50-1. Basic anatomy of the skull and brain.

board. During intubation, apply careful axial traction to maintain the cervical spine in a neutral position. Use rapid sequence induction with a short-acting barbiturate and neuromuscular blockade (see Table 48-1 and Chapter 49). Indications for intubation are shown in Table 50-3.
2. Shock significantly increases head-injury mortality and must be reversed as quickly as possible. Control external bleeding with direct pressure, and consider sources of internal hemorrhage, as described in Chapter 48. *Hypovolemic shock can occur rapidly in young children from head injury alone.* This occurs in children under 1 year of age who sustain a linear skull fracture with an epidural hematoma. The epidural blood can dissect into the subgaleal or subperiosteal space, resulting in substantial blood loss before neurologic deterioration occurs. In infants with ventriculoperitoneal shunts, large volumes of intracranial blood can accumulate without evidence of elevated ICP, as the expanding hemorrhage displaces CSF through the shunt. Significant blood loss can also occur from scalp lacerations in children.

TABLE 50-2. *Indications for Radiographic Studies*

Emergent CT
  Severe head injury
  Moderate head injury without improvement in symptoms after 1–2 hours
  Minor head injury with progressive neurologic signs or symptoms (e.g., headache, focal weakness, dysphasia)

Skull X-rays
  Penetrating injury suspected
  Palpable fracture
  Injury caused by blunt object (e.g., stick, bat, rock)

Spine X-rays
  Comatose patients
  Complaint of pain along spine
  Complaint of numbness or weakness

TABLE 50-3. *Indications for Intubation in Head Trauma*

Symptoms of increased intracranial pressure (ICP)
Pulmonary insufficiency
  $PaCO_2 > 45$ with elevated ICP
  $PaO_2 < 60$ on room air
Absent cough/gag reflex
Anatomic airway obstruction
Spontaneous hyperventilation
  $PaCO_2 < 20$
Progressive decreased neurologic status

(Adapted from *Pediatric Neurosurgery: Surgery of the Developing Nervous System,* Grune & Stratton, 1982, p. 772)

3. Treat metabolic abnormalities after diagnostic studies are initiated.
   a. Administer intravenous glucose (under 2 years, 2 ml/kg of 25% dextrose in water; over 2 years, 1 ml/kg of 50% dextrose in water) if Dextrostix analysis shows evidence of hypoglycemia (serum glucose < 100 mg %). Recent data indicate that hyperglycemia, even at moderate levels, causes increased cerebral dysfunction due to the production of lactate by ischemic cells. *Thus, avoid unnecessary dextrose.*
   b. Administer naloxone (0.4 mg IV in infants, 2 mg IV in children) for possible narcotic overdose to patients with depressed consciousness.

INCREASED INTRACRANIAL PRESSURE

If increased ICP is suspected clinically or on the basis of radiologic studies, immediately implement measures to reduce ICP and increase cerebral perfusion:

1. Hyperventilation is the most effective means of rapidly decreasing ICP. Intubation is required, and the pCO_2 should be lowered to 25 to 30 Torr. Paralyzing agents (e.g. pancuronium 0.1 mg/kg every 30–60 min) may be necessary.
2. Elevate the head 15–20 degrees to facilitate cerebral venous return. Keep infusion rates at ⅔ maintenance fluid requirements.
3. Administer mannitol (initial dose 0.5–1 gm/kg) to elevate serum osmolality to 320–330 mosm.
4. For traumatic coma, give phenytoin (20 mg/kg over 20 minutes) or phenobarbital (20 mg/kg over 10–20 minutes) to prevent seizures.
5. Facilitate neurosurgical consultation and appropriate OR or ICU admission. Effective monitoring of the patient with severe to moderate head injuries is impossible in the ED, where untoward consequences may result from delays in consultation and admission. Transfer of the child to a general trauma center, pediatric trauma center, or pediatric critical care center may be indicated.
6. Once elevated ICP is identified, further treatment modalities, including sedation, enhanced diuresis, and barbiturate coma, are guided by a direct ICP monitor placed in the OR.

Complications and Caveats ■

Seizures are not uncommon after severe head injury, particularly when prolonged unconsciousness, early seizures, or intracranial hematomas are present.

1. Immediate epilepsy, a generalized seizure developing within minutes of a mild head injury, occurs infrequently and does not predispose to subsequent seizures. Thus, it does not require treatment.
2. Early post-traumatic epilepsy is defined as one or more seizures occurring within a week of head injury. Initiate anticonvulsant therapy immediately using phenytoin or phenobarbital, and maintain therapeutic levels for a seizure-free period of 9 to 12 months after injury. Carbamazepine may be substituted, as it has a lower incidence of significant side effects than phenytoin or phenobarbital in children.
3. Late post-traumatic epilepsy refers to seizures occurring more than a week after head injury. The likelihood of developing late seizures increases with increasing severity of head injury, extent of focal damage and prolonged coma, and proximity to the central sulcus. Initiate anticonvulsant therapy at high therapeutic levels once late epilepsy begins.

The *post-traumatic syndrome* refers to symptoms of headache, dizziness, forgetfulness, irritability, anxiety, and impaired concentration following head injury. Symptoms, which may last for weeks to months, almost always resolve with time, but may be partially alleviated by mild analgesics, anxiolytics, antidepressants, and medication to control dizziness and vertigo. Severe head injury typically requires a prolonged convalescence, and incomplete recovery may be attended by permanent memory deficits, emotional disturbances, seizures, and focal motor, speech, or visual abnormalities.

Delayed hydrocephalus can occur after head trauma. Patient deterioration should prompt repeat CT scanning to exclude delayed intracranial hemorrhage or hydrocephalus.

Focal motor, speech, or visual deficits in children often improve dramatically with time and appropriate convalescent care. Rehabilitation, including cognitive, speech, occupational, and physical therapies, is a valuable part of patient and family evaluation and retraining, and should be initiated as soon as practical after head injury.

Disposition ■

Not all children with head injuries require hospital admission or extensive radiographic evaluation. Admission is warranted for:

1. Severe or moderate head injuries. Severe head injury is defined as an injury producing coma (i.e., failure to speak, to open the eyes with any stimulus, and to follow commands). Moderate head injury implies significant neural dysfunction including loss of consciousness for brief periods, nausea, vomiting, altered mental status lasting for hours, and transient focal neurologic deficits such as dysphasia or hemiparesis.

2. New skull fractures or cases with unclear mechanism of injury (for example, in possible child abuse or neglect)
3. Unstable or unreliable home situation with mild-to-moderate injury. Parents and caretakers may be unable to comprehend or carry out simple home-care instructions.

A mild head injury, producing transient neurologic abnormalities that resolve completely, does not necessarily require hospitalization. Lethargy and confusion lasting 10 to 15 minutes, amnesia about the injury impact, and headaches lasting hours to days are commonly seen after minor injury.

Parents of children sent home following evaluation of head injury should receive instructions in home observation and indications for return to the hospital (see Chapter 143 for a sample head-trauma instruction sheet).

Bibliography ■

Berger MS, Pitts LH, Lovely M: Outcome from severe head injury in children and adolescents. *J Neurosurg* 1985; 62:214–219.

Brink JD, Imbus C, Woo-Sam J: Physical recovery after severe closed-head trauma in children and adolescents. *J Pediatr* 1981; 97:721–727.

Bruce DA, Alavi A, Bilanuik L, et al: Diffuse cerebral swelling following head injuries in children: The syndrome of "malignant brain edema." *J Neurosurg* 1981; 54:170–178.

Bruce DA, Schut L: The value of CT scanning following pediatric head injury. *Clin Pediatr* 1980; 19:719–725.

Gentry LR, Godersky JC, Thompson B: MR imaging of head trauma: Review of the distribution and radiopathologic features of traumatic lesions. *AJR* 1988; 150:663–672.

Goldstein FC, Levin HS: Epidemiology of pediatric closed head injury: Incidence, clinical characteristics, and risk factors. *J Learn Disabil* 1987; 20:518–525.

Luerssen TG, Klauber MR, Marshall LF: Outcome from head injury related to patient's age. A longitudinal prospective study of adult and pediatric head injury. *J Neurosurg* 1988; 68:409–416.

Mayer TA, Walker ML: Pediatric head injury: The critical role of the emergency physician. *Ann Emerg Med* 1985; 14:1178–1184.

Mayer T, Walker ML, Johnson DG, et al: Causes of morbidity and mortality in severe pediatric trauma. JAMA 1981; 245:719–721.

Pitts LH, Martin N: Head injuries. *Surg Clin North Am* 1982; 62:47–60.

51 Maxillofacial Trauma

M. Anthony Pogrel and Leonard B. Kaban

Maxillofacial injuries rarely occur in children; all studies report a far lower incidence than in adults. Children up to 12 years of age sustain approximately 5% of all maxillofacial injuries; those below the age of 5 years sustain only 1%. Fractures of the middle third of the face are particularly rare and make up less than 0.5% of all maxillofacial injuries.

The general management principles for maxillofacial injuries in children require modifications for anatomic, physiologic, and psychological reasons. Management encompasses both emergency department (ED) treatment of the acute fractures as well as treatment in relation to subsequent facial growth.

Mechanisms of Injury and Pathophysiology ▪

Most childhood maxillofacial injuries result from falls, blows from blunt objects, and motor-vehicle accidents. Child abuse rarely causes maxillofacial injuries but must be considered, especially in patients with repeated trauma.

Fractures of the nasal bones and those of the mandible account for nearly 50% and 25%, respectively, of maxillofacial injuries in children. In the mandible, condylar neck fractures are the most common, followed by the parasymphysis region. The mandibular body is rarely fractured. Young children do not usually sustain midface fractures because of the protection afforded the midface by the prominent calvaria. Pediatric patients with these fractures often exhibit severe craniocerebral trauma and high mortality rates.

Clinical Findings ▪

Three-quarters of patients with mandible fractures and one-quarter of those with midface injuries have associated injuries. These most commonly consist of other hard and soft tissue facial, cranial, cervical spine, and extremity injuries. Patients who suffer trauma to the chin and mandibular symphysis are at particular risk of cervical spine injuries, which usually result from sudden hyperflexion/hyperextension of the neck. These patients require cervical immobilization until the cervical spine is cleared radiographically (see Chapter 54).

MAXILLOFACIAL EXAMINATION

Facial examination is performed systematically from the orbits down or the mandible up. Periorbital ecchymosis and edema indicate a midface, nasal, orbital, or zygomatic complex fracture. Anesthesia distribution to the infraorbital nerve also suggests a midface, orbital, or zygomatic complex fracture. Anesthesia of the lower lip may indicate a fracture of the mandibular body on that side. Intraoral (particularly sublingual) and submandibular ecchymoses denote a mandibular fracture. A laceration over the point of the chin may indicate a parasymphysis fracture and/or unilateral or bilateral condylar fractures.

Maxillary or mandibular fractures may result in malocclusion. In some cases, the malocclusion may be subtle, and the patient can provide important evaluation of the bite (i.e., whether it has changed). Decreased range of motion of the mandible usually indicates a fracture of the condylar neck or of the zygomatic complex impinging upon the coronoid process of the mandible.

Ancillary Data ▪

Although important for diagnosing pediatric maxillofacial fractures, radiographs may be difficult to obtain in the hysterical child. In addition to facial films, lateral and anterior-posterior films of the neck are necessary whenever a cervical injury is suspected. When a laryngeal injury is suspected, soft-tissue films of the neck are indicated.

Radiographs for diagnosis of facial fractures include:

1. Water's view (occipitomental) for the orbits, zygomas, and midface

2. Posterior/anterior (PA) view of the skull and mandible
3. Lateral view of the skull and mandible
4. Panoramic view, which provides the best view of the mandible

If a panoramic view is unobtainable because of a bedridden patient or lack of equipment, lateral oblique, PA, and Towne's (fronto-occipital) views of the mandible are acceptable.

This standard series proves less helpful in children than in adults for two reasons. First, an uncooperative patient may result in poor-quality films. Second, overlapping deciduous and permanent tooth buds and the relative underdevelopment of the sinuses in a young child make interpretation difficult. *CT scans are more important in diagnosing facial fractures in children than in adults.*

Treatment ■

The first priority is to protect the airway. Airway compromise may occur secondary to posterior displacement of the mandible or maxilla or to the presence of oropharyngeal foreign bodies (teeth or blood in the mouth, pharynx, or larynx). Hemorrhage may occur from the nasomaxillary complex, mandibular fractures, or direct laryngeal injuries. Because children have a small larynx with a narrow inlet, edema of the soft tissues easily creates airway distress. With neck trauma, maintain a high index of suspicion for laryngeal injury.

Although potentially dramatic, hemorrhage from maxillofacial structures is rarely life-threatening and is controllable with pressure dressings. Isolated maxillofacial injuries almost never result in hypotension. Nasal and ethmoidal injuries may necessitate anterior or posterior nasal packs (see Chapter 35).

Definitive treatment of facial fractures is usually delayed until the patient is stable and swelling is decreased (1–5 days post-injury). All patients should have specialist follow-up by an oral surgeon, plastic surgeon, or otolaryngologist.

The ED management of midface injuries includes *antibiotic* therapy, since most of these fractures are compounded into the sinuses and nasal or oral cavity, and *tetanus prophylaxis,* if appropriate. Penicillin covers most oral organisms and is the antibiotic of choice. The airway, nose, and sinuses are often congested; both local and systemic decongestants are generally indicated (Neo-Synephrine spray, Sudafed). The patient must maintain a clear liquid diet to prevent chewing, which may be very painful and may drive microorganisms into the deeper structures. Systemic analgesics are permissible, provided they do not mask neurologic signs.

An Erich arch bar secured to the teeth with 26-gauge stainless-steel wire can temporarily immobilize any loose teeth or very mobile dentoalveolar segments containing teeth. On a cooperative child, this can be done under local anesthesia. If definitive treatment is impossible, immobilization may be achieved through intermaxillary fixation by wiring the teeth together with two or three stainless-steel wires in the molar or premolar regions (Figure 51-1). A Barton-type bandage placed around the

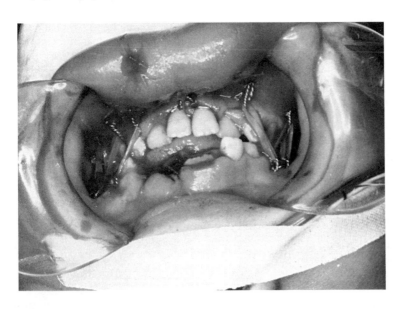

FIGURE 51–1. Intermaxillary fixation by means of 26-gauge stainless steel wires.

mandible may prevent excessive lengthening of the midface before definitive treatment.

Specific Conditions ■

MANDIBULAR FRACTURES

In children, mandibular fractures most commonly result from falls. The chin is the most frequent area of direct trauma, and the resulting spectrum of injury ranges from chin lacerations to unilateral or bilateral condylar neck fractures and/or symphysis fractures. Fractures of the ascending ramus are second most common; those of the mandibular body occur least often in children.

A patient with a unilateral condylar fracture presents with limitation of opening and deviation of the mandible toward the fractured side. The patient often exhibits a cross-bite and premature occlusion of the posterior teeth on the affected side. Bilateral subcondylar fractures result in shortening of the ramus of the mandible on both sides with premature contact on the posterior teeth, an anterior open bite, and mandibular retrognathism (retruded jaw and chin) (Figure 51-2).

Subcondylar fractures produce tenderness over the condyle, and the anterior wall of the external auditory canal may reveal a laceration or bleeding. A condyle displaced from the glenoid fossa creates a palpable depression over the temporomandibular joint (TMJ). By inserting the little finger in the patient's external auditory canal and asking the patient to open the jaw, the physician may detect movement of the condylar head. If movement of the condylar head is not palpable, the patient most likely has a subcondylar fracture. The dental arches may exhibit a step at the site of a mandibular fracture in the tooth-bearing region, and ecchymoses may be present in the floor of the mouth, particularly under the tongue. When the fracture occurs in the mandibular body, damage to the inferior alveolar nerve results in paresthesia of the lip.

Treatment

Management of mandibular fractures varies depending on the site of injury. If the fracture involves a tooth-bearing area, the patient requires antibiotics since the fracture is potentially compounded into the oral cavity via the teeth. Systemic penicillin is the antibiotic of choice. The patient also requires a clear liquid diet to keep wounds as clean as possible and to discourage mandibular movement. The only ED treatment necessary is placement of a Barton bandage to provide mandibular relief and support. When de-

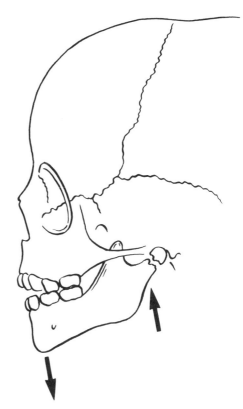

FIGURE 51–2. Bilateral fractures of the mandibular condyle. Note the foreshortening of the mandibular ramus, resulting in downward and backward rotation of the chin, and the appearance of an anterior open bite with only the posterior teeth in contact.

finitive treatment may not occur for several days, one or more eyelet wires placed under local anesthesia will provide temporary intermaxillary fixation.

Intermaxillary fixation in children requires careful technique. Deciduous teeth are shaped differently than permanent teeth but do narrow at the neck of the tooth. Wires placed around the neck provide good fixation. Intermaxillary fixation wires are difficult to place around semi-erupted permanent teeth, although satisfactory results can be achieved by using all available teeth.

MAXILLARY FRACTURES

Maxillary fractures are divided into three types. A *LeFort I* fracture occurs above the roots of the teeth and involves the maxillary alveolus, palate, and floor of the nose. A *LeFort II* fracture separates the maxilla and nose from the rest of the midface. The fracture

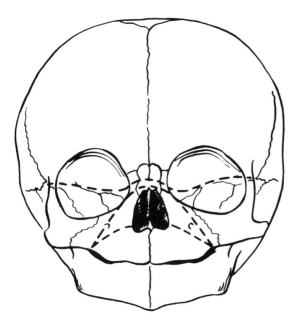

FIGURE 51-3. LeFort I, LeFort II, and LeFort III fracture lines of the midfacial regions.

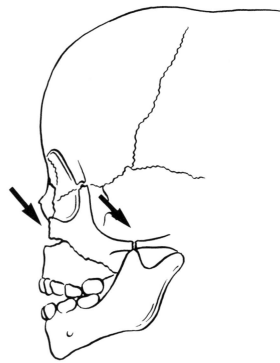

FIGURE 51-4. Severe midface fractures. There is backward and downward displacement of the middle third of the face, resulting in facial lengthening with an anterior open bite and only the posterior teeth in contact.

lines extend across the nasofrontal suture and through the infraorbital foramina beneath the zygomatic buttress to the pterygo-maxillary fissure. A *LeFort III* fracture results in separation of the midface from the cranial base. Fracture lines extend across the orbits and zygomas to the pterygo-maxillary fissure (Figure 51-3).

Children experience periorbital ecchymoses and edema in all three types of LeFort fractures because of the small dimensions of the middle third of the face. They rarely exhibit the typical "dish-face" deformity that occurs in midface fractures in adults. More commonly, a lengthening of the middle third of the face, with resultant anterior open bite and abnormal facial proportions, occurs (Figures 51-4, 51-5 A and B). Because the bridge of the nose is relatively flat in children, fractures in this area may be disguised but are discernible by palpation. Intraoral examination includes palpation of the palate to reveal a midline split, lacerations, and broken, loosened teeth.

All bony margins require palpation. Crepitus may be present around the orbits and nose, and steps may be palpable at the fronto-zygomatic suture or infraorbital rim. To determine the level and mobility of a midface fracture, mobilize the dentomaxillary segment with one hand while palpating the fracture lines with the other. By grasping the anterior maxilla firmly between the fingers and thumb of one hand, the other hand may palpate both fronto-zygomatic sutures, the bridge of the nose, and the infraorbital rim. In this way, it is possible to assess which fracture lines move with the dentoalveolar segments. A CT scan confirms the level of fracture.

ZYGOMATIC COMPLEX FRACTURES

Young children rarely sustain zygomatic complex fractures, probably because of the relative underdevelopment of the zygomatic complex in relation to the size of the cranium. Caused by direct trauma, a zygomatic complex fracture includes fracture of the fronto-zygomatic suture, infraorbital rims, zygomatic arch, and zygomatic buttress intraorally. Symptoms include paresthesia over the cheek, bleeding from the nose, and limited mandibular opening.

Periorbital ecchymoses and subconjuctival hematoma are often present. Detachment of the lateral

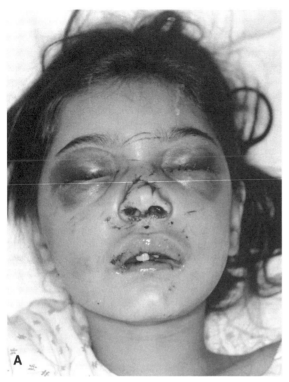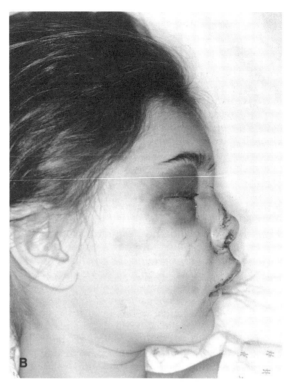

FIGURE 51-5(A) and **(B)**. A child with midfacial fractures. There is ballooning of the face, facial lengthening, anterior open bite, and relative mandibular retrusion. (From Kaban LB: Pediatric Oral and Maxillofacial Surgery. Philadelphia: WB Saunders, 1990:227)

canthal tendon produces an antimongoloid (downward) slant to the eyelid.

Zygomatic complex fractures normally require no emergency management. Definitive treatment by open or closed reduction occurs 4–7 days post-injury.

ORBITAL FRACTURES

Orbital fractures may occur as isolated injuries from direct trauma or as part of a zygomatic complex or LeFort II or III fracture (see Chapter 52).

NASAL FRACTURES

Nasal fractures, probably the most common facial fractures in children, are usually treated on an outpatient basis. The poorly developed nasal dorsum and the plasticity of the nasal bones, which masks crepitation, make diagnosis difficult in children. Nasal bleeding may occur, and a nasal speculum examination may reveal septal hematoma or septal deviation. Radiographs include a lateral nasal projection

and Water's view. Nasoethmoidal fractures warrant special attention due to the complication of telecanthus.

Most pediatric nasal fractures are treated by closed reduction. Hospitalization is not normally required. Follow-up with a maxillofacial specialist is recommended.

SOFT-TISSUE INJURIES

Facial soft-tissue trauma is associated with injuries to adjacent and underlying facial structures: adnexa of the eyes, salivary glands, trigeminal and facial nerves, and skeleton.

Unless major vessels are injured, facial bleeding responds well to simple pressure; further methods of hemostasis are typically unnecessary. Once reasonable hemostasis has been obtained, other soft tissues can be examined for injury.

Any laceration overlying the parotid gland raises the index of suspicion for *facial nerve injuries.* Perform facial nerve function tests early in the examination before soft-tissue swelling and pressure affect nerve function and before the patient receives any local anesthesia. To test the major trunks of the facial nerve, have the patient alternately wrinkle the forehead, close the eyes tightly, smile broadly, and try to whistle. Note any weakness or asymmetry. If facial nerve weakness is demonstrated, the child deserves appropriate surgical consultation as soon as possible.

The *parotid duct* lies on a line from the tragal cartilage to the oral commissure. It runs from the center of the parotid gland to open in the oral cavity opposite the region of the first molar tooth, which erupts at the age of 6 years. The buccal branch of the facial nerve runs in close proximity to the parotid duct, and any injury in this area may damage both structures. A parotid duct injury is likely if clear fluid emanates from the wound and saliva cannot be milked from the orifice intraorally.

Soft-tissue injuries around the medial canthus of the eye may damage the *nasal lacrimal apparatus*. The two puncta lie 2 mm lateral to the medial canthus, just inside the upper and lower lids. The puncta lead into the upper and lower nasolacrimal canaliculi, which drain into the nasolacrimal sac and hence to the nasolacrimal duct, which opens into the inferior meatus of the lateral nasal wall. Approximately 90% of tears drain into the lower puncta and canaliculus. In practice, because only 10% of tears drain into the upper puncta and canaliculus, damage to the upper canaliculus causes few problems. Injuries around the lower punctum, however, warrant immediate consultation and exploration.

Treatment

Soft-tissue injuries are best repaired as soon as possible. The blood supply to the facial soft tissues is so good that virtually all soft-tissue wounds can be closed primarily with minimal to no tissue removal. The "golden period" for closure of facial soft tissue wounds is about eight hours. If the patient is on antibiotics, primary closure may occur as late as 36 hours post-injury without danger. Seemingly nonviable tissue may survive.

Thorough cleansing of the wound within the first few hours is extremely important if it contains extensive dirt or other foreign matter. General anesthesia may be necessary. Elimination of tattooing from foreign debris is almost impossible after healing has occurred. Human bites and gunshot wounds (because of contamination and tissue necrosis, respectively) are the only facial wounds that require delayed primary suturing.

Cosmetic concerns are fundamental to ED care of maxillofacial injuries. Growing children experience worse scarring than adults, and secondary revision surgery is frequently necessary. Use a resorbable suture of approximately 4-0 diameter for deep tissues and a 5 or 6-0 monofilament suture for the skin. Remove sutures after 4–5 days; Steri-Strips can maintain tension on the wound for three weeks. Primary Z-plasties or other soft-tissue closure techniques are inappropriate in the ED management of these wounds since they may compromise later scar revisions.

In the area of the upper and lower lips, it is of paramount importance to obtain proper approximation of the vermilion border of the lip by marking it as soon as possible after injury before gross swelling occurs. When young children need extensive soft-tissue repair, it is best to consult a plastic or maxillofacial surgeon. General anesthesia may allow proper debridement and meticulous closure under optimal conditions of light, sterility, and instrumentation.

Disposition ■

Maxillofacial fractures require careful treatment to restore facial form and function. In children, maxillofacial trauma may affect subsequent growth. Growth retardation occurs after condylar fractures when bony or fibrous ankylosis results in decreased mandibular motion. Midface hypoplasia following midface trauma is rare unless the patient suffered an avulsion injury or extensive damage to the nasal septum. For these reasons, however, patients with condylar fractures or extensive midface injuries warrant at least annual follow-up until growth has ceased.

If necessary, serial dental models or radiographs can be taken to assess facial growth and harmony. Fractures involving teeth and tooth-bearing areas also need follow-up until all teeth in the area have undergone definitive testing for vitality and long-term prognosis and until unerupted permanent teeth have fully developed.

Most extensive soft-tissue injuries in children require hospitalization and, occasionally, general anesthesia for repair. Some dentoalveolar fractures and many subcondylar fractures can be handled on an outpatient basis, but most other maxillofacial fractures require hospitalization for both emergency and definitive management. All maxillofacial injuries, except for small, superficial lacerations, warrant evaluation by a maxillofacial specialist.

Bibliography ■

Donaldson KI: Fractures of the facial skeleton: A survey of 335 patients. *N Z Dent J* 1961; 57:55.

Kaban LB: *Pediatric oral and maxillofacial surgery.* Philadelphia: WB Saunders, 1989 (in press), Chapters 11 & 12.

Kaban LB, Mulliken JB, Murray JE: Facial fractures in children. *Plast Reconstr Surg* 1977; 59:15.

McCay FJ, Chandler RA, Grow ML: Facial fractures in children. *Plast Reconstr Surg* 1966; 37:209.

Myer CM, Grobello P, Bolton RT, et al: Blunt laryngeal trauma in children. *Laryngoscope* 1987; 97:1243.

Ousterhout DK, Vargervik K: Maxillary hypoplasia secondary to midface trauma in childhood. *Plast Reconstr Surg* 1987; 80:491.

Rowe NL: Fractures of the jaws in children. *J Oral Maxillofac Surg* 1969; 27:497.

Tate RJ: Facial injuries associated with the battered child syndrome. *Br J Oral Maxillofac Surg* 1971; 9:41.

Wheat PM, Evaskus DS, Laskin DM: Effects of temporomandibular joint meniscectomy on adult and juvenile primates. *J Dent Res* 1977; 58:139.

52 Eye Trauma

William V. Good

Anatomy ■

Evaluating an eye injury requires an understanding of normal eye anatomy. The *cornea* is a transparent shield covering the front part of the eye. It provides most of the refracting of light and helps maintain the integrity of the eye. Behind the cornea is the *anterior chamber,* an area filled with *aqueous fluid.* The *iris* separates the anterior chamber from the *posterior chamber.* The *ocular lens* rests behind the iris and is supported by *lens zonules. Vitreous gel* fills the posterior cavity of the eye. The *eye wall* has three layers: the inner retinal layer, middle choroidal layer, and the outer scleral layer. This outer sclera is white, and is lined by fascia, referred to as *conjunctiva* and Tenon's fascia.

The *orbit* consists of the bones that encase the eye. The orbit contents include the globe, extraocular muscles, fascia, and adipose tissue. The anterior orbit is divided from the posterior orbit by an extension of peri-orbita called the *orbital septum.* This natural barrier is responsible for the characteristic clinical picture in preseptal versus orbital cellulitis (see Chapter 117).

The *cavernous sinus* transmits the third, fourth, fifth, and sixth nerves to the orbit. Oculosympathetics and the internal carotid artery also course through the cavernous sinus. Injury to this region can cause any combination of cranial neuropathies.

Mechanisms of Injury and Pathophysiology ■

Eye trauma may be blunt or penetrating (i.e., from sharp objects); there is some overlap. A second category of eye injury is accidental versus nonaccidental.

BLUNT INJURIES

The globe is protected by an important bony encasement. This bony encasement surrounds the eye and consists of a frontal bone superiorly; lacrimal and ethmoid bones medially; maxillary, palatine, and zygomatic bones inferiorly; and sphenoid and zygomatic bones laterally. There is considerable variation in anatomy: some eyes are deeply set in the orbit and others are relatively proptosed. Obviously, blunt trauma is more likely to injure a globe that protrudes beyond the anterior limits of the bony orbit.

When a blunt force such as a kick or a blow by a fist strikes the globe, the globe expands, transmitting pressure to the orbital bones. The maxillary and ethmoid bones are vulnerable to fracture, but the superior and lateral walls of the orbit are rarely fractured due to blunt trauma of the globe.

Blunt injury causes contusions of the lids and ocular surface. Eyelid ecchymosis is common. The subcutaneous tissue surrounding the eye is distensible, allowing bruising to spread circumferentially around the eye and across the bridge of the nose. Corneal abrasions and subconjunctival hemorrhages are also quite frequent. The conjunctiva surrounds the globe and inserts at the corneal scleral limbus, the junction between the cornea and the sclera. When a bruise develops underneath the conjunctiva, the surface of the conjunctiva is elevated but clearly demarcated from the cornea. Therefore, a subconjunctival hemorrhage presents as an elevated red mass up to but not including the cornea.

Rarely, blunt injury to the eye will cause a rupture of the globe, most often beneath the rectus muscles and medial to the superior oblique muscle or occasionally at the corneal scleral limbus where the cornea and sclera meet.

PENETRATING OR SHARP INJURIES

Sharp injuries are much more likely to cause a rupture. The speed and direction with which the object strikes the eye are important; high-velocity projectiles are more likely to penetrate the eye. The bones of the orbit tend to protect the eye from posterior penetrating injuries, but the anterior segment of the eye remains especially vulnerable.

The shape of the projectile is relevant. A BB or shotgun pellet may glance off the globe and embed in orbital tissue. Sharper objects are much more likely to actually penetrate the eye.

ACCIDENTAL AND NONACCIDENTAL TRAUMA

An eye injury can be the result of child abuse (see Chapter 128). One inflicted injury of special importance is the so-called "shaken-baby" syndrome, which causes a fairly characteristic constellation of eye findings. The crying baby has increased intravenous pressure. Simultaneous shearing forces of shaking put added pressure on intraretinal vessels. This may result in a hemorrhage into the retina and vitreous. When intraocular hemorrhage occurs, subarachnoid hemorrhage and retinal hemorrhages appear on fundoscopic examination. The syndrome is called Tersen's syndrome and is virtually pathognomonic for child abuse in infancy.

Clinical Findings ■

Accurate diagnosis and treatment of eye trauma is premised on careful, methodical history and physical exam. Important *history* includes:

1. Time of injury
2. Mechanism
3. Velocities
4. Direction of impact
5. Characteristics of penetrating object
6. History of visual or other eye problems
7. Immunization and allergy histories
8. Symptoms of vision loss, double vision, blurriness, or discharge
9. Quality and location of pain

Physical examination must include the eye as well as the surrounding bones and soft-tissue structures. Compare the injured side to the uninjured side, when clinical findings are ambiguous. Ensure that all the following structures are evaluated and that physical findings are documented on an anatomic map of the face and eye:

1. Eyelids
2. Lacrimal passages
3. Conjunctiva and sclera
4. Cornea (including fluorescein staining)
5. Anterior chamber
6. Pupil (shape, responsiveness, consensual response)
7. Iris, lens, vitreous humor
8. Retina
9. Extraocular movement
10. Orbit and surrounding soft tissues
11. Vision (use Snellen chart or pediatric version)

Specific Conditions ■

BLOW-OUT FRACTURES

Clinical Findings

Blow-out fractures result from blunt trauma to the globe and orbit. Fractures of the inferior and medial walls of the orbit cause intra-orbital tissue to collapse into maxillary and ethmoid sinuses, respectively. The cardinal signs and symptoms of blow-out fractures are enophthalmos, double vision, and loss of sensation in the distribution of the infra-orbital nerve (see Table 52-1). The enophthalmos is caused by loss of orbital volume, with orbit tissue displaced into surrounding cavities (e.g., maxillary sinus). Double vision is caused by herniation of extraocular muscles into the maxillary or ethmoid sinus. The usual ocular motility disturbance involves double vision in straight and upgaze due to entrapment of the inferior rectus muscle. The infra-orbital nerve, which courses along the floor of the orbit, is particularly vulnerable to injury of the maxillary bone.

Treatment

The optimal time for surgical treatment is 5–10 days after the injury. This allows traumatic edema to subside. Indications for treatment are double vision and cosmetically unacceptable enophthalmos. Treatment consists of repositioning prolapsed orbit contents in the orbit and repairing bony defects. The mere presence of a fractured orbital bone is seldom an indication for surgical repair.

CORNEAL ABRASIONS

Clinical Findings

Corneal abrasions result from sharp or blunt trauma. A corneal abrasion is diagnosed by the presence of a positive fluorescein test. Instillation of fluorescein into the inferior cul-de-sac is followed by an exam-

---

TABLE 52–1. *Clinical Findings in Blow-Out Fracture*

Enophthalmos
Anesthesia of infraorbital nerve
Double vision

ination with a blue cobalt light. In areas where corneal epithelium is abraded, there is increased fluorescence.

Treatment

There are three aspects to the treatment of a corneal abrasion:

1. Treat the extreme pain. A cycloplegic agent (Cyclogyl 1%, scopolamine 0.25%) will dilate the pupil and reduce the amount of reflex ciliary spasm. This spasm is responsible for much of the discomfort.
2. Prevent secondary infection. The corneal epithelium is an important antimicrobial barrier. Use prophylactic antibiotic ointment.
3. Patch the eye with the eyelid closed in order to improve the pain and facilitate more rapid healing of the corneal epithelium.

Examine corneal abrasions daily or refer the patient to an ophthalmologist to ensure that the corneal epithelium has healed. Most corneal abrasions will heal in 1–2 days, but occasionally a corneal abrasions takes a week or longer to heal. In such cases, the use of therapeutic contact lenses may be indicated.

SUBCONJUNCTIVAL HEMORRHAGES

Clinical Findings

Subconjunctival hemorrhages occur spontaneously or as the result of trauma (Figure 52-1). The hemorrhage

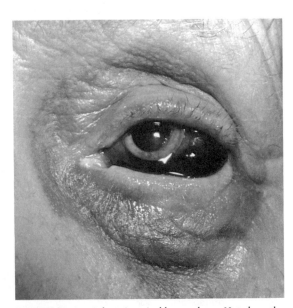

FIGURE 52–1. Subconjunctival hemorrhage. Note how the hemorrhage is elevated and spares the cornea.

is striking and elicits concern on the part of parents and physicians. The hemorrhage itself is seldom of any visual consequence, but it may indicate an occult rupture of the globe. When a subconjunctival hemorrhage is noted, perform a very careful inspection of the globe to confirm that the ocular structures are normal, and that there is no laceration of cornea or sclera.

Treatment

Subconjunctival hemorrhages may occur spontaneously or with Valsalva's maneuver. Bleeding diatheses will occasionally cause subconjunctival hemorrhages. No treatment is usually required.

LENS SUBLUXATION

Clinical Findings

Lens subluxation results from blunt or sharp trauma to the eye. The diagnosis is made by the characteristic finding of a lens edge in the pupil space. Occasionally, it is necessary to dilate the pupil to see the edge of the lens. Normally with dilation, it should be impossible to identify the lens equator.

Treatment

Refer the patient to an ophthalmologist. If the lens edge is not on the visual axis, it may be possible to correct the reduced vision with glasses or a contact lens. Occasionally, lensectomy is indicated.

IRIS INJURIES

Abnormal Pupil Shape

After eye trauma, the pupil and iris may appear abnormal. If the pupil appears nonreactive to light, and if the patient has normal mental status, the differential diagnosis includes traumatic rupture or paralysis of the iris sphincter, and traumatic third-nerve palsy. The latter is diagnosed by the co-existence of paralysis of the inferior, medial, and superior rectus muscles. If the child has depressed mental status and an unreactive pupil, consider intracranial third-nerve compression from bleeding and increased pressure (see Chapter 50).

Traumatic Iritis

Blunt eye trauma interferes with the blood-aqueous barrier. Inflammatory cells spill into the anterior chamber, resulting in the characteristic triad of pain, redness, and photophobia. Traumatic iritis usually resolves spontaneously. Topical steroids will expedite resolution, but their use may be complicated by cataract and glaucoma.

Hyphema

Trauma at the root of the iris may cause a hyphema. A hyphema occurs when there is bleeding inside the eye in the anterior chamber. The so-called "eight-ball" hyphema occurs when the entire anterior chamber fills with blood.

The management of hyphemas requires special considerations. Recommend strict bed rest. Cycloplegia may also be helpful. Do not use steroid eye drops. Although epsilon aminocaproic acid is occasionally used in adults, its use in children causes nausea and vomiting, which may exacerbate the hyphema. The black patient with a hyphema may have sickle-cell disease; such patients have more trouble clearing the hyphema and are more likely to develop complications.

The most dreaded complication of hyphema is corneal blood staining, which occurs when the corneal endothelium is compromised and intraocular pressure is elevated. Glaucoma is an occasional complication of a hyphema.

GLAUCOMA

Damage to the trabecular meshwork from trauma may cause glaucoma 10 or 20 years after the injury. Therefore, refer any patient with a history of blunt trauma or a hyphema for a yearly eye exam.

RETINAL INJURIES

Clinical Findings

The retinal sequelae of blunt and sharp trauma include hemorrhage, choroidal rupture, and detachment.

Retinal hemorrhage may be diffuse or feather-edged, depending on the particular layer of retina involved. Feather-edged hemorrhages occur in the nerve fiber layer. When the retinal hemorrhage occurs outside the area of the macula, resorption without vision damage is the rule. On the other hand, macular retinal hemorrhage may cause fibrosis and scarring, resulting in decreased vision.

Choroidal ruptures, which result from forceful blunt trauma, are concentric ruptures most common in the macula. Although visual acuity is seldom dramatically reduced, a choroidal rupture renders an eye more susceptible to delayed scarring (subretinal neovascularization). Occasionally a retinal hemorrhage will break into the vitreous.

Detachment results from blunt or penetrating injury, especially in a myopic patient. Fundoscopic exam reveals a bullous, wrinkled, elevated, pale retina with visual loss.

Treatment

The management of retinal and vitreous injuries is expectant. Consult an ophthalmologist. Seldom is it appropriate to intervene surgically. Apply a protective eye shield to all such patients.

OPTIC NERVE INJURIES

Clinical Findings

Indirect injury to the optic nerve occurs when there is blunt trauma to the face, particularly the frontal bone. Diagnostic findings include decreased vision in the presence of an otherwise normal eye exam. The examiner will always find a Marcus-Gunn pupil, which is diagnosed with the so-called swinging flashlight test. The involved pupil constricts poorly to direct visual stimulation and strongly to consensual stimulation. When the light is moved from the uninvolved eye to the involved eye, the involved pupil dilates.

There is no confirmed acceptable treatment for indirect injury to the optic nerve. Early ophthalmologist consultation is imperative. A trial of high-dose intravenous steroids may be indicated with the hope that intracanalicular inflammation will subside and reduce compression on the optic nerve. There is no convincing evidence that surgical decompression of the optic nerve improves visual acuity.

RUPTURED GLOBE

Clinical Findings

Perhaps the most feared injury is the ruptured globe, *a surgical emergency* that requires immediate ophthalmologist consultation.

Any eye injury should raise the suspicion of a rupture. Loss of normal anterior segment anatomy usually indicates that uvea has prolapsed through a wound. A soft eye usually indicates a ruptured globe, but measuring intraocular pressure may be dangerous because any pressure applied to a ruptured globe can result in extrusion of intraocular contents. Finding dark tissue on the surface of the eye suggests prolapsed uvea (see Figure 52-2). A localized subconjunctival hemorrhage or chemosis occasionally masks an occult scleral rupture.

If there is any suspicion of an intraocular foreign body, obtain appropriate films. A metallic foreign body can usually be seen with routine X-rays (Figure

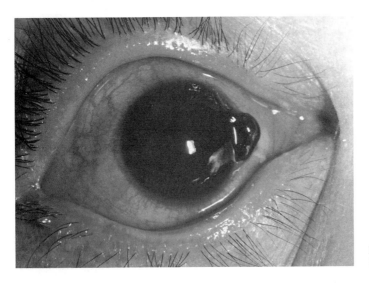

FIGURE 52-2. Corneoscleral laceration. Note prolapsed uveal tissue at nasal limbus.

52-3). Orbit CT scans are also very helpful in localizing an intra-orbital or intra-ocular foreign body. Ultrasound is seldom of value.

Treatment

When a ruptured globe is suspected, first protect the globe. Tape a metal shield across the orbit to protect the patient and others from inadvertently pushing on the eye. The use of ocular lubricants is contraindicated; in fact, do not apply eye drops or medicine of any kind to the eye, because of probable intraocular toxicity. Obtain an ophthalmology consultation immediately.

Complications

Complications of ruptured globes are listed in Table 52-2. The most dreaded complication is *sympathetic ophthalmia,* in which the immune system is sensitized to uveal tissue and causes a panuveitis in the normal fellow eye. Sympathetic ophthalmia can result in bilateral blindness. Fortunately, this complication is rare.

Siderosis bulbi occurs when there is retained intraocular iron. Iron stains epithelial cells, resulting in a progressive deterioration of visual acuity.

Amblyopia occurs in young children when an eye is not being used. It is divided into three categories.

Occlusion amblyopia causes profound unilateral visual loss in the presence of significant media opac-

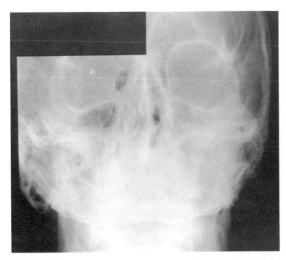

FIGURE 52-3. Intraocular foreign body, circled in right globe.

TABLE 52-2. *Complications of Ruptured Globe*

Sympathetic ophthalmia
Retained foreign body
Amblyopia
Strabismus
Endophthalmitis
Cosmetic deformity

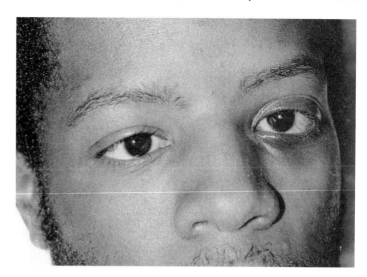

FIGURE 52–4. Carotid-cavernous fistula. Note left eye proptosis, redness, and left sixth nerve palsy.

ity. Obviously, a significant cataract or corneal laceration from an injury could result in this type of amblyopia.

Strabismic amblyopia occurs when the eyes are not aligned and the patient uses one eye preferentially.

Endophthalmitis occurs in 3–7% of cases of rupture or laceration of the globe. Signs and symptoms of endophthalmitis include increased intraocular inflammation, eyelid swelling, pain, and decreased vision. Any one of these symptoms should prompt an immediate ophthalmologist evaluation. Delays of even a few hours can result in total loss of vision.

CAVERNOUS SINUS FISTULA

Clinical Findings

Cavernous sinus fistula is a rare complication of blunt eye and orbit trauma. Signs and symptoms include redness, proptosis, dilated conjunctival vessels, iritis, a bruit, and decreased vision (Figure 52-4). A sixth-nerve palsy will occasionally be present. Treatment is based on the degree of discomfort and reduced vision. The fistula can be embolized, and some fistulae resolve spontaneously.

INJURIES TO OCULAR ADNEXAE

Lid Margin Laceration

Close lid margin lacerations carefully to avoid scarring and deformity. First, close the tarsus with deep, interrupted vicryl sutures. Then use 6-0 or 7-0 nylon sutures to approximate the lid margin.

Canalicular Injury

If the lid margin laceration is located nasally, the canaliculi (upper and lower) must be explored to ensure their integrity. Injury requires ophthalmology consultation for intubation and closure under the operating microscope. Failure to recognize this problem will result in epiphora and the need for more extensive surgery at a later date.

For cellulitis, see Chapter 117.

Bibliography ■

Feist RM, Farber MD: Ocular trauma epidemiology. *Arch Ophthalmol* 1989; 107:503–505.

Good WV, Hoyt CS: Behavioral correlates of poor vision in children. *Int Ophthalmol Clin* 1989; 29:57–60.

Lambert SL, Johnson TE, Hoyt CS: Optic nerve sheath and retinal hemorrhages associated with the shaken-baby syndrome. *Arch Ophthalmol* 1986; 104:1509–1517.

Lessell S: Indirect optic nerve trauma. *Arch Ophthalmol* 1989; 107:382–387.

Sanders M, Hoyt WF: Hypoxic ocular sequelae of carotid-cavernous fistulae. *Br J Ophthalmol* 1969; 53:82–97.

Schein OD, Hibberd PL, Shingleton BJ: The spectrum and burden of ocular injury. *Ophthalmology* 1988; 95:300–305.

53 Dental Trauma

Raymond L. Braham and Merle E. Morris

Few dental emergencies exert as great a psychological impact on children and parents as a traumatic injury to a child's mouth with disfigurement of the anterior teeth. Traumatic injuries to the teeth occur most frequently when children learn to walk, start school, ride bicycles or skateboards, or engage in contact sports such as football or hockey. The maxillary incisors are most commonly affected. Treatment is determined by the child's age, the severity of damage to the oral structures, and the elapsed time since the injury. The initial objective of the emergency physician or dentist is to relieve the anxiety of both parent and child, then to treat pain and establish a specific diagnosis.

Clinical Findings and Ancillary Data ■

Examine every patient who has suffered an injury to the head or face for the possibility of a mandibular or maxillary fracture. While leg fractures and facial lacerations are often readily detected, several days or even weeks may pass before a fracture of the jaw is discovered. Obviously, at this later date the fracture is very much more difficult to treat. Depressed fractures sometimes are masked by severe edema. A contusion of the jaw suggests a fracture and often provides information as to the direction, type, and force of trauma.

Carefully examine all the teeth. Displaced fractures in dentulous areas are revealed by a depressed or raised segment and a break in continuity of the occlusal plane, especially in the mandible. In the absence of visible displacement, palpate the area. Place the forefingers of each hand on the mandibular teeth, thumbs below the jaw. Beginning with the right forefinger in the retromolar area of the left side, and with the left forefinger on the left bicuspid teeth, alternate each hand in an up-and-down movement. If a fracture is present there will be movement between the fingers and an audible grating sound (crepitus). Minimize such movements to prevent further trauma to

the area, ingress of infection, and pain. After examining the teeth, do an evaluation of maxillofacial structures, as outlined in Chapter 51.

Obtain a dental radiograph of the injured area. If only a single tooth is involved, a simple intra-oral periapical radiograph will suffice, but if the injured area is a wider one it is better to arrange for an extra-oral panoramic radiograph. This serves not only to detect fractures and possible foreign bodies, but also as a baseline for subsequent therapy. When a jaw fracture is suspected, refer the patient immediately to an oral surgeon.

Soft-Tissue Injuries ■

It is not uncommon, especially in children, to encounter trauma as a result of post-anesthesia lip, tongue, or cheek-biting. This invariably happens when a posterior inferior alveolar nerve block is administered unilaterally. After leaving the dental office, and despite warnings, the patient finds that the anesthetized lip and associated half of the tongue feel strange. The child often will bite through the lip or tongue because no sensation is present, creating some very dramatic lesions. The parent will commonly bring the child to an emergency department (ED) clinician who did not carry out the dental treatment; the key history of the recent dental visit is not given. The lesion can be confused with those associated with acute primary herpetic stomatitis (Figure 53-1), but the absence of a fever and the presence of an associated newly placed dental restoration (Figure 53-2) will enable the physician to make the correct diagnosis.

Treatment is symptomatic and palliative. Keep the wound clean with warm dilute saline and recommend acetaminophen. In very severe cases, antibiotics may be necessary.

Another lesion, fortunately less common, in the differential diagnosis of traumatic lip-biting is the "serpiginous" ulcer associated with secondary syphilis.

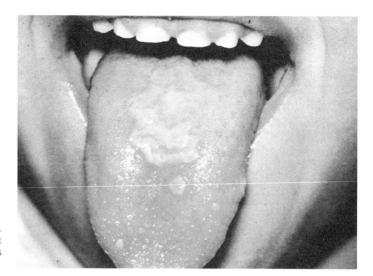

FIGURE 53–1. Postanesthesia bite of tongue. The differential diagnosis of this lesion must exclude primary herpetic gingivo-stomatitis and secondary syphilis.

A soft-tissue injury that has become more prevalent in recent times is the electrical burn caused when an infant or toddler chews on a live electrical wire, such as that attached to a television set (Figure 53-3). Treatment of these injuries is discussed in Chapter 61. Avoid suturing, and refer the patient to a pediatric dentist who can make an acrylic appliance that will control the healing of the lip so as to leave a minimal scar.

Soft-tissue lacerations are relatively common as a result of traumatic injuries, since the intra-oral mucous membranes are relatively fragile. Although lac-erations are sometimes due to direct contact with foreign objects, most result when tissue comes in direct contact with the teeth, resulting in wound edges that are often jagged and irregular in depth. Clean and debride all soft-tissue lesions. In the case of shallow abrasions, it is usually sufficient to advise the parent have the child rinse with a warm saline mouth-bath several times a day after the wound has been debrided.

Deep wounds must be closed after debridement. Infiltrate the general area with a local anesthetic containing a vasoconstrictor (epinephrine), which also

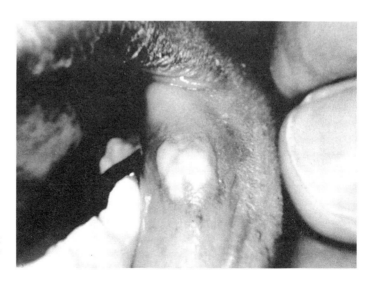

FIGURE 53–2. Postanesthesia bite of lip. Note the stainless-steel crown, which had just been placed on the primary molar close to the lesion.

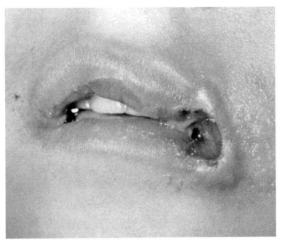

FIGURE 53–3. Electrical burn at commissure of lip, caused by chewing on a television cord.

helps control local hemorrhage. Remove devascularized tissue but save viable tissue. Before suturing soft tissues, palpate the area carefully to ensure that no tooth or other fragment is buried in the tissues. Since the intra-oral vascular bed is very extensive, carefully prevent hemorrhage and cicatrization when suturing wounds in the oral mucosa.

Suture deep tissues with 4-0 or 5-0 plain gut or an

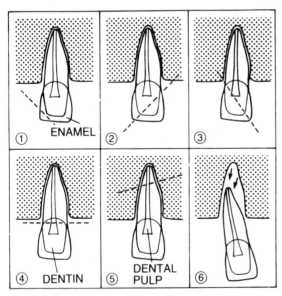

FIGURE 53–4. Classification of dental fractures; see Table 53–1.

absorbable suture; mucosal edges may be sutured with 4-0 silk, plain gut, or polyglycolic acid sutures. When suturing the mucocutaneous junction of the lip, meticulously approximate the edges. A step in the vermilion border of the lip, as a result of suturing, eventuates in a significant cosmetic defect (and could easily bring about a lawsuit!).

Because of their vascularity, the oral tissues are usually resistant to infection. However, assess each case individually according to the nature of the wound and mechanism of injury. If there is no great damage to the actual teeth or maxilla or mandible, it is amazing what Mother Nature can do by herself in a week or two, with only general debridement and regular checks by the physician or dentist.

Hard-Tissue Injuries ■

The nature of injuries to the teeth themselves differs between the primary and permanent dentitions. Because the child's alveolar process has more cellular and fibrous elements than the adult's, it is more plastic and more easily deformed. Hence, a blow on the teeth of the child will cause deformation and yielding of the alveolar process, which explains the higher frequency of displaced primary incisors when they are subjected to trauma. In children past the age of 9 or 10 years, the stronger alveolar bone does not yield so readily and the force of the blow, transmitted to the rigidly held tooth, is more likely to result in a fracture. In addition, the longer and thicker roots of the permanent teeth have a broader area for periodontal attachment and offer greater resistance to displacement.

TREATMENT OF ALIGNMENT DISRUPTIONS

If a primary incisor is totally *avulsed,* tidy up the debris, ensure that the whole tooth is out, and refer the patient to a dentist as soon as possible. Reimplantation of primary incisors rarely works.

Much more common is the *straight intrusion.* If the tooth is just pushed straight in vertically, it may re-erupt on its own, especially if the child is under 2 years of age; however, if the labial plate is broken the tooth should be extracted. So it is "wait and see."

If the tooth is *partially luxated* but otherwise intact, it may be irrigated with warm saline, pushed gently into place with finger pressure, and left alone.

TOOTH FRACTURES

Assessing and treating trauma to the permanent dentition is more complex. The classification system, il-

TABLE 53–1. *Classification of Dental Fractures*

Class 1. Crown fracture involving enamel only. The injury may result in enamel loss or simply a craze line or crack
Class 2. A crown fracture involving enamel and dentin, but not the dental pulp
Class 3. A crown fracture involving enamel, dentin, and dental pulp, but with considerable tooth structure remaining
Class 4. A crown fracture in which most of the crown of the tooth is lost. Involves the same tissues as Class 3 injury but much more extensive
Class 5. A root fracture that may be horizontal, vertical, or diagonal
Class 6. A displacement of the tooth, either total or partial, from the bony socket

lustrated in Figure 53-4 and outlined in Table 53-1, is based on the widely accepted classification of incisor injuries by Ellis and Davey and the World Health Organization.

Treatment

Class 1 injury may or may not involve enamel structure. If the tooth remains intact and asymptomatic, no emergency treatment is necessary. If enamel loss results, three options are available:

1. Do not treat. Recommended for cases of minimal enamel loss and no roughness
2. Smooth the fracture area with a dental stone. Recommended when there is minimal enamel loss and a sharp edge
3. Restore the area. This should be done by a dentist but is not a major emergency.

Class 2, 3, and 4 injuries require specialized dental equipment and training. Once the initial diagnosis has been made, refer the patient to a dentist without delay. Class 2 injuries are likely to cause mild to moderate discomfort, but appropriate pain medication will usually suffice until morning. *Since Class 3*

TABLE 53–2. *Protocol for ED Care of the Avulsed Tooth*

1. Clean the tooth gently in TEPID running water. Do NOT scrub it.
2. Administer local anesthetic.
3. Remove the blood clot from the socket with a moistened cotton applicator or fine surgical suction, and examine the alveolus for fracture.
4. Using finger pressure, replant the tooth firmly in the socket.
5. Verify the position of the tooth, preferably with an intra-oral radiograph.
6. Stabilize the tooth with a temporary split as previously described.
7. Refer to a dentist for follow-up without delay.

and 4 injuries involve the dental pulp, the tooth's vitality is at stake and a dentist must be consulted immediately.

The location of the root fracture is the single most important factor in deciding the future of teeth with *Class 5 injuries.* The closer the fracture is to the apex of the root, the more favorable the prognosis. Stabilize the tooth and refer the patient to a dentist without delay. The simplest way to stabilize a tooth is to mold some lead foil (such as that from a dental X-ray packet) around the tooth and two adjacent teeth and cover the whole with surgical cement (zinc oxide and eugenol).

Class 6 injuries involve partial or total avulsion of the tooth from the alveolus. The simplest treatment for the various forms of partial avulsion is to administer an infiltration-type local anesthetic and gently manipulate the tooth or teeth as close to normal position as possible. Then refer the patient to a dentist without delay. *For the totally avulsed tooth, time is of the essence in regard to the prognosis.* Good results have been obtained if the tooth is replanted within half an hour of the accident. Once the tooth has been out of the mouth for two hours, the chances of a favorable prognosis are greatly decreased.

If the parent or child calls the ED or office before presenting, ensure that appropriate advice is given for immediate action. Stress the urgency of coming in immediately. If the tooth has fallen to the ground, gently rinse it under *tepid* water and replace it in the socket without pressure. The tooth should *not* be scrubbed. If the tooth cannot be replaced, milk has been shown to be the best transporting medium in which to bring it to the ED. Once in the ED, use the clinical protocol outlined in Table 53-2.

Caveats and Disposition ■

The management of dental trauma is one of the most difficult areas of dental care. A successful prognosis depends totally on the rapid availability of emergency care, a skillful diagnosis, and appropriate treatment. It is imperative that every ED establish an emergency call relationship with the local dental society so that expert care is always close at hand.

Bibliography ■

Braham RL, Roberts MW, Morris ME: Management of dental trauma in children and adolescents. *J Trauma* 1977; 17: 11;857–865.

Ellis RW, Davey KW: *The classification and treatment of injuries to the teeth of children,* 5th ed. Chicago: Yearbook Medical Publishers, 1970.

World Health Organization: *International classification of disease - Application to dentistry and stomatology, ICD-DA,* 2nd ed. Geneva: World Health Organization, 1978.

Wright GZ, Friedman CM: Management of dental trauma. In: Braham RL, Morris ME, eds: *Textbook of pediatric dentistry,* 2nd ed. revised reprint. Toronto and Philadelphia: BC Decker, 1988, pp. 565–592.

54 Spinal Trauma

Michael S. Edwards and Philip H. Cogen

About 7,000–8,000 spinal-cord injuries occur each year in the United States; more than half of these injuries are suffered by people younger than 25 years old. From 2–10% occur in infants (0 to 3 years), children (3 to 12 years), and young adolescents (12–15 years). Spinal-cord injuries are twice as common in boys as in girls and have a peak incidence during the summer. Most result from motor-vehicle accidents, but in infants and young children falls account for a significant number. The mortality rate from spinal-cord injuries among children ranges from 10–59%.

Many spinal-cord injuries in children can be prevented by proper use of safety equipment (e.g., infant car seats) and with educational programs that encourage recreational safety.

Anatomy and Pathophysiology ■

Significant differences in anatomy and biomechanics between the adult and pediatric spine account for the characteristic patterns of spinal injury seen in children. Forces of injury capable of distracting the spine are not well checked because of several factors, which also allow subluxation or other injuries to occur with surprisingly little force:

1. The supple ligamentous structures of the child's spine permit a markedly high degree of spinal mobility. The spine does not obtain the ligamentous characteristics of the adult spine until 8 to 10 years of age. Cervical musculature, which plays an important role in the stability and alignment of the adult spine, is poorly developed in the child. The articular facets of the child's spine are more horizontally positioned than those of the adult spine: in infancy, they may be as low as 30 degrees, increasing to 70 degrees by 10 years of age.
2. An infant's spine is primarily cartilaginous; it ossifies progressively throughout childhood. Injuries in infants and young children tend to be avulsions or epiphyseal separations rather than true fractures.
3. Odontoid injuries in children usually produce a separation through the basilar synchondrosis and into the body of C2. Injuries in this age group are essentially splits in the cartilaginous endplates. They routinely heal well with spontaneous fusion.
4. The fulcrum for flexion-extension in children is different from that in adults. The greatest amount of motion is at the C2-C3 level, and the fulcrum gradually moves caudally with the child's increasing age. The anatomic and biomechanical features of the immature spine make the upper cervical spinal segments from C1 to C3 particularly vulnerable to injury.
5. Little other than prevention can significantly reduce the effects of the primary injury on the spinal cord. The primary event produces immediate disruption of the spinal gray and white matter. The subsequent progression of neurologic dysfunction develops over a period of hours or days and is the result of a series of mechanisms (secondary injury) that are set into motion by the primary injury.
6. Secondary injury from reduction of spinal cord blood flow following trauma may produce extracellular ion fluxes, decreased oxygen and glucose utilization, production of toxic free radicals, lipid peroxidation, and possibly the release of neuropeptides. Pharmacologic management is targeted to treat the secondary injury.

Mechanisms of Injury and Clinical Presentations ■

INFANTS AND CHILDREN

In infants and children, 70% of fractures and dislocations in the cervical region occur above the C3 level. Locked facets, which are commonly found in adults, do not occur in children. *Rotatory subluxation,* an injury rare in adults, is relatively common in the infant and young child. It is usually the result of minor trauma associated with the sudden rotation and twisting of the neck beyond its normal range.

267

The child presents with painful torticollis and local tenderness to palpation in the posterior neck region over the C1-C2 spinous processes. The diagnosis is confirmed by radiographs made with the child's mouth open to show the odontoid processes asymmetrically placed between the lateral articular masses of the atlas. Reduction is usually achieved by light cervical traction using 3 to 5 pounds of weight. If reduction cannot be achieved using traction or if subluxation recurs after traction has been discontinued, an atlantoaxial fusion may be required.

Atlanto-occipital dislocation is rarely recognized clinically because it usually produces cervical medullary compression, resulting in respiratory arrest and death. Nine of thirteen reported cases have been in children younger than 18 years old. The shallow articular surfaces of the atlas and the small size of the occipital condyles in children make the stability of this region almost entirely dependent on ligamentous integrity. The relatively large head and weakness of the cervical musculature in infants make them especially vulnerable to this type of injury.

The mechanism that produces this injury is extreme hyperextension in association with lateral flexion. The diagnosis is made on the basis of plain radiographs when there is malalignment of the odontoid with respect to the anterior aspect of the foramen magnum and of the posterior arch of the atlas with respect to the posterior edge of the foramen magnum. MRI demonstrates the severity of cord injury. The initial treatment is supportive care and mechanical ventilation. Achieve spinal stability and realignment under neurosurgical guidance in the emergency department (ED) with a halo apparatus. Occipital-cervical fusion is necessary later.

The frequency of *odontoid fracture* in children is unknown. It is controversial whether os odontoideum is an anatomic abnormality or is the result of trauma. In the infant and young child, the transverse ligament is stronger than the incompletely ossified dens and with traumatic subluxation the atlanto-dental interval (ADI) is usually maintained. Most odontoid fractures in children are similar to epiphyseal separations that occur in the long bones and they readily heal if their position is re-established and immobilization is maintained.

Neurologic signs are insidious in almost 50% of infants and children, while the other 50% present with the acute onset of neurologic dysfunction. Neck pain is a major feature in 66% of patients. Treatment depends on whether cord compromise occurs on flexion or extension. If the lesion is reducible with positioning or traction under neurosurgical guidance, then stabilization is important. If it is nonreducible, then an anterior or posterior operative decompression followed by a stabilization procedure is necessary. Fractures of the pedicles of C2 (hangman's fracture), lower cervical spine fractures, thoracic and lumbar fractures are rare in children.

OLDER CHILDREN AND ADOLESCENTS

Spinal motion characteristics of the adult are usually attained by 8 years of age but may be delayed until age 12. Then the spine is ossified, the ligaments and joint capsules have lost their laxity, the facets have assumed a vertical orientation, and the cervical paraspinal musculature is much stronger. Spinal injuries assume an adult pattern and most occur in the lower cervical segments. The injuries that occur are predominately *wedge compression fractures* and *anterior subluxation and dislocation* caused by axial loading and hyperextension.

Thoracic lumbar fractures become relatively more common because of flexion-rotation injuries caused by motor-vehicle accidents. Fractures of the vertebral column are divided into *stable* and *unstable* types (Figure 54-1).

Stable fractures are those that produce wedging of the vertebral bodies and are rarely associated with neurologic injury. However, burst fractures may produce impaction of disc and/or bone fragments into the spinal canal and are frequently associated with neurologic deficits.

Unstable fractures are associated with disruption of the posterior ligamentous structures, which produces dislocation of the vertebral bodies and may be associated with unilateral or bilateral locked facets. *Rotational dislocation fractures are the most unstable of all vertebral fractures.* Shear fractures occur in the thoracic and lumbar regions and are a burst fracture in conjunction with fracture of the neural arches. Compression fractures producing more than a 50% reduction in the height of the vertebral body are chronically unstable.

SCIWORA

Spinal-cord injury without associated radiographic abnormality (SCIWORA) may occur in 16–66% of children younger than 8 years of age who have severe spinal injuries. The most common cause is motor-vehicle accidents. The pathophysiology has not been established but may be related to severe flexion or hyperextension injuries with subsequent ischemic damage to the spinal cord. An extreme degree of ligamentous suppleness may predispose the pediatric spine to severe subluxation at the time of injury that then spontaneously reduces itself. This subluxation may produce mechanical damage to the cord and severe neurologic deficits.

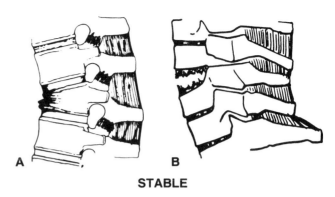

STABLE

FIGURE 54–1. (**A**) Wedge compression fracture in which the posterior ligamentous structures are preserved. (**B**) Dislocation resulting from a hyperextension injury; preservation of the posterior supporting structures makes this a stable injury. (**C**) Fracture dislocations occurring when the posterior ligamentous structures are disrupted, producing instability; if the facet joints become locked, complete reduction with traction may be impossible, requiring surgical intervention to realign the spine. (**D**) Rotation dislocation occurring when the posterior ligamentous structures and the articular capsules are disrupted along with a slice fracture of the lower vertebral body. (Reprinted with permission from Holdsworth F: Fractures, dislocations and fracture–dislocations of the spine. *J Bone Joint Surg* 1963;45(B):7–9)

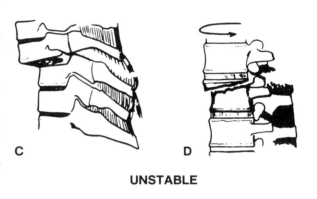

UNSTABLE

The diagnosis of SCIWORA requires a complete radiographic series including flexion-extension views. CT, often with intrathecally administered contrast agent, and/or MRI are usually necessary to exclude spinal-cord compression. In most cases these diagnostic tests show either no abnormality or a partial block soon after the initial injury. MRI performed 1–3 months after the injury may reveal atrophy of the spinal cord if there is neurologic residual. About half the children with SCIWORA have a late onset of neurologic deterioration 30 minutes to 4 days (mean 1.2 days) after the injury. The paralysis usually develops rapidly once it begins and most frequently culminates in a complete cord lesion. The pathophysiology of delayed cord injury is undetermined.

Traumatic infarction may account for as many as 8% of spinal-cord injuries in children. An injury to the chest or abdomen is usually the initiating event. The children are typically neurologically intact at presentation but develop a profound and usually complete paraplegia within hours or days thereafter and rarely have any neurologic recovery. Plain radiographs and myelograms show a normal spine but spi-

nal angiography may reveal occlusion of the anterior spinal artery.

The long-term prognosis of SCIWORA is poor. Children with complete lesions and those with severe incomplete lesions do not recover. The initial neurologic status is the major predictor of the extent of recovery.

SPINAL INJURIES IN ATHLETES

The "burning hands" syndrome occurs in football players who suffer neck trauma. It is characterized by burning dysesthesias in the hands and fingertips and occasionally in the feet. The pathophysiology is thought to be a central cord contusion (central spinothalamic tract) secondary to hyperextension of the cervical spine. Treat any athlete with spinal trauma and complaints of paresthesias or dysesthesias in the extremities, even without neck pain, as if a fracture or dislocation were present. A careful radiologic evaluation is necessary because more than half the children with these symptoms have a cervical fracture or dislocation.

Treatment ∎

PREHOSPITAL CARE

At the site of injury, immobilize the neck. If a helmet (e.g., motorcycle or football helmet) is in place, leave it alone if breathing is adequate. Assess the level of consciousness, perfusion, and ventilation. If ventilation is inadequate, institute airway protection, preferably by endotracheal intubation accomplished with manual in-line cervical traction. If there is no perfusion, begin cardiopulmonary resuscitation (see Chapter 6). Place the child on a spinal board and sandbag and tape the head during transport to an appropriate facility.

EMERGENCY DEPARTMENT

In the ED, maintain the child in the supine position and support the head if necessary to maintain a neutral cervical spine configuration. For suspected cervical injuries, ensure neck immobilization with sandbags and tape over the forehead or a semirigid plastic collar and tape; alternatively, hold the head and neck manually to minimize spinal movement. Use a long spineboard if a thoracic or lumbar fracture is suspected. If movement of the body is necessary to clear the airway, to prevent aspiration, or to complete mandatory physical or radiographic evaluation, log-roll the patient with manual spinal traction.

Assess the ventilatory status. *Adequate tissue oxygenation is critical to avert secondary injury to the spinal cord.* Do not move the neck to establish an airway. When airway obstruction, apnea, or ineffective breathing is present, perform either endotracheal intubation with strict in-line manual cervical traction, blind nasotracheal intubation, or needle cricothyrotomy, as outlined in Chapters 48 and 49. *Do not delay definitive airway management in patients with suspected spine injuries; treatment of hypoxia and respiratory acidosis always has first priority.*

Ensure adequate perfusion. Ischemia causes shock and multiple system failure, including secondary injury to the brain and spinal cord. Chapter 48 outlines the ED treatment of hypoperfusion. Hypotension and bradycardia may indicate spinal shock, or loss of sympathetic tone (i.e., venous pooling in the lower extremities) from a high cervical spinal-cord injury. Volume replacement or vasopressor drugs usually resolve the hypotension. Corticosteroids, although used routinely in many centers, have shown no evidence of clinical efficacy.

Assessment of spinal-cord injury is frequently complicated by head trauma and a reduced level of consciousness. Evaluate the severity of a child's head injury on the Glasgow Coma Scale or with a pediatric

modified version (Table 16-1). Management of head injury, respiratory depression, hypotension, or severe hemorrhage always precedes treatment of the spinal-cord injury.

In infants, young children, and uncooperative patients, define a motor and/or sensory level if possible (Figure 54-2). A level to pinprick sensation may be the only useful modality. A change in skin temperature with warmth below the level of injury owing to vasodilatation or an absence of sweating (warm dry skin) below the level of injury may help localize the lesion. In cooperative patients, perform and fully document a complete sensory and motor examination including evaluation of the superficial and deep tendon reflexes. Assess rectal sphincter tone and perianal sensation, then evaluate the bulbocavernosus reflex. *The findings of complete motor and sensory paralysis with persistence of the bulbocavernosus reflex is a bad prognostic finding, indicating that spinal shock cannot account for the paralysis.*

In all children with neurologic dysfunction, insert an indwelling bladder catheter to prevent severe bladder distention and to evaluate fluid balance and renal function. Children with cervical or upper thoracic spinal-cord injuries usually develop an ileus. Therefore, place a nasogastric tube to prevent abdominal distention, regurgitation, and possible aspiration.

Cervical and upper thoracic injuries producing paralysis and sensory loss may mask an intraabdominal process (e.g., perforated viscus or ruptured spleen). Evaluate all hemodynamically stable patients with abdominal trauma with abdominal CT and/or peritoneal lavage (see Chapter 56).

If an acutely unstable spinal fracture is identified, apply skeletal traction early in the child's ED management. In older children, Gardner-Wells tongs or a halo device may be applied in minutes. In infants, especially those younger than 18 months, the cranium is too thin and soft to safely place an external fixation device; in these patients, apply traction safely by placing two 1-cm trephinations in both parietal bones, through which wires can be passed and connected to skeletal traction. These procedures require neurosurgical consultation.

In adolescents and older children, reduction of the cervical spine is accomplished by placing about 5 lb of weight on the traction apparatus for each spinal level involved (i.e., C4-C5 subluxation, 20 lb; C5-C6 subluxation, 25 lb; and so on). For the young child and infant, this amount of weight is inappropriate, and 1–3 lb per segment added slowly is a more rational plan considering the ligamentous suppleness in this age group. Because locked facets rarely if ever occur in children, reduction is usually successful in the acute phase of the injury.

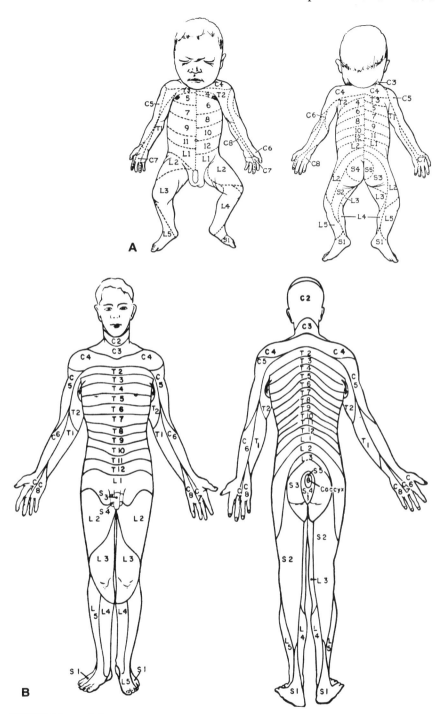

FIGURE 54–2. (**A**) Dermatomal chart of an infant. Reproduced by permission from Brann AW Jr, Schwartz J. Central nervous system disturbances, Part one: Assessment of neonatal neurologic function. (In: Fanaroff AA, Martin RJ, eds. *Neonatal-perinatal medicine,* 4th ed. St. Louis: CV Mosby, 1987) (**B**) Dermatomal chart of an adolescent. (Reprinted with permission from Barr ML, Kiernan JA: The human nervous system, 5th ed. Philadelphia: Harper & Row, 1988)

When neurosurgical assistance is not immediately available, consult the nearest general trauma center, pediatric trauma center, or pediatric critical care center, and arrange transport as soon as the patient is stable, with the patient's spine carefully immobilized en route.

Ancillary Data ■

The initial radiologic evaluation depends on the site of suspected spinal injury. The following are initial studies. However, if static radiographs do not reveal subluxation or dislocation and an injury to the cervical, thoracic, or lumbosacral spine is still suspected, get flexion and extension views of the spine with a qualified physician in attendance. These films must be obtained with caution, especially in the infant and young child in whom passive motion of the spine is necessary. If muscle spasm limits neck motion, repeat the dynamic studies when spasm has resolved and full flexion and extension is possible.

CERVICAL SPINE

Evaluate cervical vertebral trauma first with a plain cross-table lateral radiograph. All seven cervical vertebrae must be visualized; in order to do so, it may be necessary to pull the patient's shoulders down or to obtain a lateral swimmer's view. If the lateral radiograph shows no abnormalities, obtain a plain anterior-posterior (AP) radiograph and a third with the child's mouth open to evaluate the odontoid.

THORACIC SPINE

Suspected thoracic spine injuries require plain AP and lateral radiographs. All 12 thoracic vertebrae must be visualized.

LUMBAR AND SACRAL SPINE

Obtain plain AP and lateral radiographs of all five lumbar vertebrae and the sacrum to adequately evaluate the lumbosacral spine.

STANDARD CHEST, ABDOMINAL, AND LONG-BONE RADIOGRAPHS

Order these radiographs as indicated from the history and physical examination. The child with significant spinal trauma almost always has other associated major injuries.

PLAIN CT WITH BONE WINDOW SETTINGS

This study is frequently useful in defining a suspected abnormality visualized by plain radiographs, by determining the location and extent of bone injury, especially in the upper cervical spine where neural arch fractures may not be detected by plain radiographs. CT may be particularly helpful in differentiating synchondrosis from fracture.

MYELOGRAPHY

This is essential if there is evidence of neurologic dysfunction. The sensitivity is increased by using intrathecal water-soluble contrast agent in conjunction with CT (i.e., CT myelography). If a block to the flow of intrathecal contrast agent is identified, the upper and lower extent of the block must be determined by placing contrast agent in the subarachnoid space through a C1-C2 puncture by a neurosurgeon.

MAGNETIC RESONANCE IMAGING

MRI is replacing CT with and without intrathecal contrast administration. For the present, however, the child requiring physiologic monitoring or ventilatory support is more safely evaluated using CT techniques.

Caveats ■

The radiographic appearance of the pediatric spine is complicated by the normal occurrence of multiple epiphyseal plates, incomplete ossification, and hypermobility because of the supple ligamentous structures. Epiphyseal plates are ubiquitous in infants and children, and a complete knowledge of their appearance and time of resolution is not essential to the evaluation of the pediatric spine. However, there are important anatomic points:

1. At birth, the atlas (C1) has three ossification centers, one for the body of the vertebra and one for each of the neural arches. Therefore, in 80% of neonates the anterior arch of C1 appears to be discontinuous. The neural arches usually close by the third year of life to form a complete ring and subsequently fuse to the body of C1 by age 7 years.
2. The axis (C2) has four centers of ossification, one for the odontoid process, one for the vertebral body, and one for each neural arch. In all children younger than 3 years and in 50% of children under 5 years of age, the dens is separated on plain radiographs from the body of C2 by a broad cartilaginous band that corresponds to an intervertebral disk. This radiolucent line may be visualized until a child is 11 years old and should not be misinterpreted as a fracture.

3. Ligamentous laxity and the horizontal position of the facet joints allows for excessive mobility in the pediatric spine. In the infant, the normal distance on plain radiographs from the anterior arch of C1 to the odontoid process is ≤ 5 mm.
4. Of all plain lateral radiographs in normal children under the age of 8 years, 40% show C2 shifted forward and tilted downward in relation to C3. More than 50% of these children have a 3-mm or greater degree of forward displacement. This "pseudo-subluxation" can be differentiated from true subluxation by forced hyperextension. In true subluxation, the anterior displacement cannot be reduced, but with pseudosubluxation, the displacement is always easily reduced.
5. Immature vertebral bodies are wedged anteriorly; this appearance should not be mistaken for a compression fracture. By age 10 years, the pediatric spine has taken on the attributes of the adult spine anatomically and radiographically and should be assessed and treated as an adult spine.

Disposition ■

SURGICAL MANAGEMENT

The decision to operate in acute spinal injuries is more often based on orthopedic than neurosurgical considerations. Immediate neurosurgical intervention is seldom necessary, except in the following circumstances:

1. Complete neurologic loss below the level of injury in children for whom there is a possibility of preserving or recovering an important nerve root
2. Children with an anterior cord syndrome on neurologic examination in whom CT and/or myelography, or MRI, shows anterior cord compression

IN-HOSPITAL CARE

Neurosurgical management includes reduction and traction immobilization, usually in the ED, then inpatient care. Immediate transfer to a facility properly qualified to manage pediatric spinal trauma is imperative in all cases.

REHABILITATION

Spinal-cord injury with severe residual neurologic dysfunction does not often occur in children but its consequences are devastating, particularly in view of a child's long life expectancy. Children with spinal-cord injury have special needs because of their potential for continued physical, intellectual, psychological, and social growth. The goals of rehabilitation are to provide for the child's optimal neurologic recovery, to provide skills that compensate for lost or impaired functions, and to permit the fullest functional development. This is best accomplished in a pediatric rehabilitation center that has adopted a multidisciplinary approach.

Bibliography ■

Bailey DK: The normal cervical spine in infants and children. *Radiology* 1952; 59:487–500.

Choi U, Hoffman H, Hendrick EB, et al: Traumatic infarction of the spinal cord in children. *Neurosurgery* 1986; 65: 608–610.

Faden AI: Pharmacologic therapy in acute spinal-cord injury: Experimental strategies and future directions. In: Becker DP, Povlishok T, eds: *Central nervous system trauma status report 1985.* Bethesda, Md.: NINCDS 1985;481–485.

Hadley MN, Zabramski M, Browner CM, et al: Pediatric spinal trauma: Review of 122 cases of spinal cord and vertebral column injuries. *Neurosurgery* 1988; 68:18–24.

Kewalramani LS, Kraus F, Sterling HM: Acute spinal cord lesions in a pediatric population: epidemiological and clinical features. *Paraplegia* 1980; 18:206–219.

Kewalramani LS, Tori A. Spinal cord trauma in children. Neurologic patterns, radiologic features, and pathomechanics of injury. *Spine* 1980; 5:11–18.

Maroon C: "Burning hands" in football spinal cord injuries. *JAMA* 1977; 238:2049–2051.

Mayfield K, Erkkila C, Winter RB: Spine deformity subsequent to acquired spinal-cord injury. *Bone Surg* 1981; 63A:1401–1411.

Menezes AH. Os odontoideum: Pathogenesis, dynamics and management. *Concepts Pediatric Neurosurg* 1988; 8: 133–145.

Pang D, Wilberger E: Spinal-cord injury without radiographic abnormalities in children. *Neurosurgery* 1982; 57:114–129.

Pueschel SM, Scola FH: Atlantoaxial instability in individuals with Down syndrome: Epidemiologic, radiographic, and clinical studies. *Pediatrics* 1987; 80:555–560.

Ruge R, Sinson GP, McLone DG, et al: Pediatric spinal injury: The very young. *Neurosurgery* 1988; 68:25–30.

Wilberger E: *Spinal cord injuries in children.* Mount Kisco: Futura, 1986.

55 Chest Trauma

Frank R. Lewis

Thoracic trauma is a major cause of mortality, accounting for 25% of traumatic deaths, yet effective therapy for 85–90% of victims (tracheal intubation and tube thoracostomy) is readily available in almost every emergency department (ED). Moreover, intubation of children is possible in most prehospital settings. About 50% of traumatic thoracic deaths occur after patients reach the ED; most are preventable. This leads to two conclusions: injuries are not appropriately suspected and recognized, or necessary therapy is not implemented in a timely, effective manner.

Mechanisms of Injury and Pathophysiology ■

Thoracic injuries in children differ markedly from those in adults. These differences result from several factors: the type and mechanism of injuries, and the anatomic differences between children and adults. In children, blunt trauma occurs far more often than penetrating trauma, although the latter is increasing significantly in urban areas and among teenagers. Motor vehicles are the primary mechanism of injury. However, in contrast to adults, who usually sustain injury as automobile occupants, children are also injured as pedestrians and are therefore unprotected in the impact.

Flexibility of the child's thorax is another factor. In adults, thoracic deformability is limited, and rib fractures compose the most common sequelae of blunt trauma. The ribs absorb some of the impact energy, preventing transmission to structures beneath, and the number and severity of the fractures provides a rough guide as to the trauma severity. In children, the flexible chest wall absorbs relatively little energy, transmitting it instead to underlying structures. The flexibility of the ribs allows them to bend and deform to extreme degrees without fracturing. *Therefore, young children rarely experience rib fractures; older children and teenagers do so more commonly.*

The principles of assessment and treatment of acute pediatric thoracic injuries are similar to those followed for adults; however, appropriate adjustments in tube sizes and drug dosages for the smaller body size are imperative. This chapter first addresses general principles of diagnosis and treatment, then describes specific conditions.

Clinical Findings and Initial Treatment ■

PRIMARY ASSESSMENT: AIRWAY AND BREATHING

The ABCs—*A*irway, *B*reathing, and *C*irculation—require immediate evaluation upon the child's arrival in the ED. In the first 30 seconds, the physician can assess the respiratory status and determine appropriate therapy (see Chapters 48 and 49).

A brief observation conveys an enormous amount of information:

1. Is the patient awake or unconscious? If unconscious, the child may need tracheal intubation for airway protection.
2. Is the patient apneic or making respiratory efforts? If apneic, the patient may require immediate clearing of the pharynx and ventilation with a bag-valve-mask device using 100% oxygen. Rapid intubation may also be indicated.
3. Are respiratory efforts slow or rapid, shallow or deep, labored or easy? Is the patient displaying normal chest and abdominal expansion with inspiration or a "rocking" pattern typical of diaphragmatic breathing? Are the accessory muscles being used? Are both sides of the chest moving equally, or is one side splinted or moving paradoxically?
4. If respiratory effort is present, is air actually being exchanged?
5. Are airway noises present (stridor, rhonchi, or wheezing) or is breathing quiet? If noise is present,

is it primarily inspiratory or expiratory? Is inspiration or expiration unduly prolonged? Inspiratory noise and prolonged inspiration usually indicate extrathoracic airway (upper airway) obstruction. Expiratory noise and prolonged expiration indicate intrathoracic (lower airway) obstruction.

After making these observations, the physician can implement the appropriate level of airway management.

Following airway stabilization, evaluate the chest wall, lungs, and pleural spaces:

1. On palpation, is any crepitus in the subcutaneous fat? Mild to moderate crepitus is often seen with pneumothoraces. Marked crepitus over the whole thorax, head, and neck typifies tracheal or major bronchial disruption.
2. On palpation of the chest wall, does the patient experience any tenderness or exhibit any obvious deformities or unstable portions of chest wall? Does inspiration yield a paradoxical motion? Rib fractures cause uniform pain upon palpation to awake patients, and a careful exam can usually define which ribs are broken. With multiple fractures, particularly of the middle ribs (4–8), chest wall instability is more likely, and paradoxical movement can be very subtle, especially in the young child.
3. Are the breath sounds equal and the trachea midline? Unequal breath sounds classically signify pneumothorax, but the difference is often subtle and difficult to distinguish in a noisy ED. For that reason, pneumothoraces are rarely diagnosed on clinical grounds alone. The trachea is rarely shifted enough to detect unless a tension pneumothorax exists and cardiopulmonary effects are present.

When intubation and assisted ventilation do not relieve respiratory distress, presume a pneumothorax and insert a chest tube before obtaining a chest X-ray. The clinical findings will usually dictate the side for insertion, but if this cannot be determined, establish bilateral intubation. The trivial morbidity of unneeded chest tubes far outweighs the potentially lethal consequence of not inserting a needed chest tube.

CIRCULATION

The final area of assessment is circulation. The physician must determine two things: (1) the patient's intravascular volume status and (2) the adequacy of cardiac pump function. The signs of shock include hypotension and tachycardia, but in children these often appear ambiguous (see Chapters 8 and 48).

A clinical sign of great value in hypotensive patients with chest trauma is distention of the external jugular neck veins. Even in obese patients, these are easily visible, and the clinician can determine an approximate venous pressure from direct observation. Flat neck veins that do not distend during expiration, even with the patient flat, indicate a venous pressure near zero and probable hypovolemia. On the other hand, *neck veins tautly distended during all phases of respiration signify cardiac tamponade or tension pneumothorax.* This single sign is the only clinical finding that distinguishes these two causes of shock from hypovolemia. Inspect the cardiac monitor or electrocardiogram for disturbances of rate and rhythm that may interfere with pump function.

Treatment for hypotension is outlined in Chapter 48, and the child should receive treatment with multiple lines, isotonic fluid, and blood products as indicated.

Ancillary Data ■

Following stabilization, a chest X-ray will usually define the intrathoracic pathology. An upright posterior-anterior film is best because it allows clearest visualization of air-fluid levels. *Most intrathoracic conditions can be clearly identified or at least suspected based on chest X-ray findings.* Obtain blood specimens for serial hematocrits and arterial blood gas measurements. Pulse oximetry provides excellent ongoing monitoring of oxygen saturation. During all ancillary testing, the patient should be closely monitoring, with respiratory status, vital signs, intake and output, and mental status re-evaluated every 5–10 minutes during the first hour. The clinical course is initially unpredictable, and failing to follow the patient closely may result in late detection of hypovolemia and respiratory distress.

If the patient requires transport to radiology for CT scanning, angiography, or other contrast studies, a nurse and physician must remain at the bedside to provide intensive monitoring.

Disposition ■

Rather than observing a child with respiratory distress and hemodynamic instability in the ED, it is better to obtain immediate surgical consultation and to establish an appropriate disposition, either to the operating room, the pediatric ward, or the intensive care unit.

An unstable patient must not leave the ED until definitive treatment is instituted or he or she is taken directly to the operating room.

Specific Conditions ∎

PNEUMOTHORAX

Pneumothoraces fall into three classes: *simple, open,* and *tension*. Penetrating trauma injuries, such as stabbings or gunshot wounds, often cause direct lung injury. In blunt trauma, lung lacerations usually result from the jagged ends of fractured ribs.

Simple Pneumothorax

A simple pneumothorax, by far the most common, is a partial or total collapse of the lung as a result of air leakage into the pleural space. This most commonly occurs from a laceration or penetration of the lung parenchyma with air leakage from the small airways or alveoli.

A simple pneumothorax may cause shortness of breath or no symptoms at all. Chest wall pain usually occurs from the injury itself. Rarely does a simple pneumothorax pose a major threat to life, as patients can survive quite well with the function of a single lung. When a pneumothorax occurs, blood flow through the collapsed lung is markedly reduced, thereby averting hypoxemia from shunting of blood through the nonventilated lung.

All traumatic pneumothoraces, even small ones, warrant re-expansion via chest tubes (see Chapter 139 for procedure). The danger of not inserting a chest tube in a clinically insignificant pneumothorax is deterioration when the patient is not fully monitored. Normally the air leak will decrease and stop within a three-day period, and the tube can be removed. The patient should remain on suction for 12–24 hours after the leak stops, with the tube then placed on water seal without suction for 24 hours. If the lung remains fully expanded, the tube can be removed.

A large air leak may necessitate an additional chest tube, but this is uncommon and raises the suspicion of a major bronchial or tracheal disruption. When the size of the leak makes lung re-expansion impossible, the patient requires surgery either to repair or resect the source of the leak. If the size of the leak is unusual, the patient should undergo bronchoscopy to rule out a major airway injury.

Open Pneumothorax

An open pneumothorax is one in which there is a communication from the pleural space to the outside air. This is a life-threatening condition because the air movement through the chest wall prevents the development of negative intrathoracic pressure with inspiration and therefore prevents effective ventilation. Fortunately, this injury is extremely rare in civilian practice. Treatment requires closing the chest wall opening, initially with temporary material such as petrolatum-impregnated gauze or even plastic wrap and a sterile dressing, then surgically reconstructing the area. Chest tube usage for lung re-expansion is identical to that of the previous situation.

Tension Pneumothorax

A tension pneumothorax, created by positive pleural pressure, commonly results when a patient with a simple pneumothorax receives positive-pressure ventilation. In some situations, it can occur with spontaneous breathing and a flap valve mechanism, but these are uncommon. The treatment is the same as for a simple pneumothorax but is more urgent. When tube thoracostomy cannot be performed immediately, needle thoracostomy (Chapter 139) may be a temporizing measure.

A tension pneumothorax may severely compromise the patient. The principal danger results from displacement of the mediastinum to the opposite side, such that the vena cava is partially occluded at the diaphragm and thoracic inlet, thereby reducing venous return to the heart. Compression of the opposite lung also occurs, preventing it from expanding effectively and compromising even the "good" lung. Hemodynamic collapse develops rapidly without effective treatment.

HEMOTHORAX

Hemothoraces commonly co-exist with pneumothoraces and result from the same mechanisms. Injuries that disrupt the airways and cause air leakage from the lungs also usually cause bleeding. A chest radiograph diagnoses this condition and approximates the volume of the hemothorax. *The rate and amount of bleeding from lung injuries is normally small because the central portions of the lung and the pulmonary arteries are rarely injured and pulmonary circulation operates at low pressure, only slightly higher than venous pressure.* The exceptions include injuries to the intercostal and internal mammary arteries, which are at systemic pressure and can bleed massively.

A hemothorax is generally harmful only because of the blood loss. The degree of compression of lung parenchyma is normally not significant enough to compromise ventilation since the thoracic volume is large in comparison to the blood volume, and the patient will exsanguinate before lung compression becomes limiting.

Hemothorax treatment is the same as for pneumothorax: insertion of a chest tube. Do not remove the chest tube until only serous drainage is present and the total amount is less than 1 ml/kg/day.

Surgical evaluation is imperative in every case requiring chest tube insertion. When bleeding is massive or continues at an unacceptable hourly rate, thoracotomy may be necessary for control. Only 5–15% of patients experience this complication. In such cases, a systemic artery generally accounts for the bleeding. Adults require thoracotomy if total drainage exceeds 1,500 ml or continues for more than 3–4 hours at 300 ml/hr; specific standards have not been defined for children, but about the same amounts in proportion to weight seem reasonable (20–25 ml/kg total, or 4–5 ml/kg/hr).

FLAIL CHEST

Children rarely develop flail chest because of rib flexibility and the infrequency of rib fracture. It becomes more common in teenagers. The condition results from the fracture of multiple adjacent ribs, usually at two sites, so that a portion of the chest wall becomes unstable and moves paradoxically with respiration. If a slight amount of paradox is observed but the patient can breathe effectively, the child should be observed in an intensive care unit. A patient experiencing respiratory distress or marked hypoxemia requires immediate intubation and mechanical ventilation to "splint" the chest wall pneumatically. Intubation should usually continue for 12–14 days to allow fibrous adhesions to develop around the rib ends and stabilize the fracture sites.

PERICARDIAL TAMPONADE

Rupture of the heart from blunt trauma is quite rare and almost uniformly fatal. This injury generally occurs with penetrating trauma, most often stab wounds. When the trauma directly injures a coronary artery, immediate myocardial dysfunction develops and the patient rarely reaches the hospital alive. Those who do rarely have coronary artery injuries and can be managed without heart-lung bypass.

The signs of pericardial tamponade include shock and distended neck veins. The heart tones are also usually muffled, but a noisy environment makes these difficult to detect. Definitive diagnosis can be made by ultrasound; however, a patient in distress cannot wait for this, and the diagnosis must be made clinically.

The preferred treatment is emergent surgery for thoracotomy and operative decompression of the pericardium. If this is impossible, attempt pericardial aspiration (see Chapter 139). However, technical success with this procedure in cardiac wounds has proven problematic. If the patient arrests in the ED while being observed, appropriate treatment consists of performing open thoracotomy in the left fourth interspace with the pericardium opened longitudinally. After pericardial decompression, these patients typically resuscitate easily.

WOUNDS TRAVERSING THE MEDIASTINUM

Gunshot wounds crossing one thorax to the other are a subset of penetrating trauma that requires special evaluation. The bullet tract is usually not very clear. The major vascular structures generally necessitate evaluation by angiography and the esophagus by Hypaque swallow. An air leak or subcutaneous crepitus indicates the need for a bronchoscopy. Failure to detect an intrathoracic esophageal perforation promptly often becomes a fatal mistake and at best creates prolonged septic complications.

Bibliography ∎

Baker SP, O'Neill B, Karpf RS: *Injury fact book.* Lexington, Mass.: Lexington Books, 1984.

Eichelberger MR, Randolph JG: Thoracic trauma in children. *Surg Clin North Am* 1981; 61:1181.

Eichelberger MR, Randolph JG: Pediatric trauma: An algorithm for diagnosis and therapy. *J Trauma* 1983; 23:91.

Haller JA Jr: Thoracic injuries. In: Welch KJ, Randolph JG, Ravitch MM, et al, eds: *Pediatric surgery.* Chicago: Yearbook Medical Publishers, 1986, pp. 143–154.

Smyth BT: Chest trauma in children. *J Pediatr Surg* 1979; 14:41.

Velcek FT, Weiss A, Dimaio D, Klotz DH, Kottmeier TK: Traumatic death in urban children. *J Pediatr Surg* 1977; 12:375.

56 Abdominal Trauma

Mark A. Schiffman and James Betts

Undiagnosed or inadequately treated abdominal injuries are the most common cause of unexpected death following trauma in children. Severe abdominal trauma may not be clinically apparent in a pediatric trauma victim, who may have more obvious injuries elsewhere, such as a concussion or long-bone fracture, or who may be unable to assist the examiner because of young age or altered mental status.

Mechanisms of Injury and Pathophysiology ■

Severe blunt trauma to the abdomen in pediatrics is usually caused by motor-vehicle accidents ("auto versus child" is more common, but sometimes the child is a passenger), falls, bicycle accidents, and child abuse. Penetrating injuries, once rare in children, are becoming more common, particularly in urban areas, largely due to a rising frequency of nonaccidental trauma. Nevertheless, *blunt injuries still constitute 90% of serious abdominal trauma in childhood.*

Blunt injury to the abdomen has several mechanisms and produces several types of injury to various solid and hollow organs. The most common problem is *compression* of a solid organ, such as the spleen or liver, causing contusion, laceration, or burst injury. Immediate blood loss occurs, of variable degree, usually into the peritoneum.

A second possibility is injury to a hollow viscus or mesenteric vessel, usually from a *deceleration* mechanism and shearing of vascular attachments. The intestine is also subject to compression injury (e.g., between the abdominal wall and vertebral bodies) and burst injury (requiring a closed loop). Peritonitis is the usual sequela, secondary to seepage of blood and/or potent digestive enzymes. Peritonitis usually manifests within 6–24 hours, rarely later. Also, blunt injury to the small bowel, particularly the duodenum, can cause an intramural hematoma that results in bowel obstruction.

Abdominal injury may also involve structures in the retroperitoneal region, specifically the pancreas, third and fourth parts of the duodenum, kidneys, urinary bladder, and rarely the colon. The resulting irritation by blood or digestive enzymes occurs in the retroperitoneal space; anterior abdominal examination may be completely normal, despite severe but occult pathophysiology. Retroperitoneal injury presents special difficulties to early diagnosis.

Clinical Findings ■

Abdominal trauma must be suspected based on the mechanism or physical examination. Therefore, a detailed history of the event is imperative. In blunt trauma, key features are the speed of the automobile, the use of restraints, the time since the event, the distance of the fall, and the type of surface struck. Important features in penetrating injury are the type and caliber of weapon, the distance from the gun, the length of the knife blade, and the trajectory of penetration.

Consider injury to the abdomen in anatomic injuries from the nipple line to the pelvis. Often, abdominal and thoracic, or abdominal and pelvic, injury occurs concurrently; occasionally diaphragmatic disruption is present, usually from penetration between two body cavities, which poses further compromise to vital function.

Clinical findings that may point to a diagnosis of intraabdominal injury are summarized in Table 56-1. However, these signs and symptoms are neither sensitive nor specific. *Fully 50% of significant abdominal injuries may present without positive findings on anterior abdominal examination.* Ensure that children are fully exposed for examination. All patients require a thorough physical assessment, including genital exam and rectal exam with stool testing for blood, as well as careful evaluation of long bones for associated fractures. Serial examination of the abdomen is key to early detection of serious injury.

TABLE 56–1. *Physical Signs and Symptoms Suggestive of Abdominal Trauma*

Pain
Tenderness
Distention
Peritoneal signs (may be late in uncomplicated
    hemoperitoneum)
    Absent or diminished bowel sounds
    Rebound tenderness
Ecchymoses
Tire tracks
Seat-belt marks
Heme-positive nasogastric aspirate
Heme-positive urine
Heme-positive stool
Kehr's sign: pain in left shoulder induced by palpation of
    LUQ
Turner's sign: ecchymotic discoloration of the flank
Cullen's sign: ecchymotic discoloration of the umbilicus
Unexplained hypotension or other signs of hypovolemic
    shock

(Source: Schiffman MA: Nonoperative management of blunt abdominal trauma in pediatrics. *Emerg Med Clin North Am* 1989; 7)

The most common seriously injured intraabdominal organ is the spleen, followed by the liver; injuries to the kidneys and renal collecting system are quite common but are typically minor and do not require sophisticated diagnostic or therapeutic interventions. Injuries can also occur to the pancreas, stomach, small and large bowel, and mesentery; these may present nonspecifically in the immediate post-injury period, or with abdominal pain, guarding, and signs of shock.

Trauma to the spleen is almost always due to blunt injury to the abdomen, usually from motor-vehicle accidents, bicycle accidents, or falls. Physical findings may be masked by trauma elsewhere, particularly closed head injury. The patient may complain of left upper quadrant (LUQ) pain, sometimes radiating to the left shoulder; LUQ tenderness and rebound tenderness may be elicited on examination. *If the patient is unconscious, an apparently normal abdominal examination is meaningless.* Suspect splenic trauma in the setting of early or late stages of hemorrhagic shock, or with a rapidly distending abdomen.

Liver injuries are the leading cause of death following blunt abdominal trauma; often, disruption of the inferior vena cava is present. Patients with liver trauma present similarly to those with trauma to the spleen (few clinical findings except shock or dropping hematocrit, but a suspicious history of blunt abdominal injury). Patients may complain of right upper quadrant (RUQ) pain, with RUQ tenderness, rebound tenderness, and abdominal distention.

Trauma to the small bowel also may be difficult to diagnose clinically. Usually, the erosion of digestive juices into surrounding structures, rather than blood, causes important pathophysiology, and pain. Sometimes, intramural hematomas are responsible for blood loss and bowel obstruction. Although most patients with small bowel injuries do have some abdominal tenderness in the ED, hours to days may elapse before the diagnosis is made. A high index of suspicion, serial examinations, and early use of ancillary diagnostic modalities is imperative.

The large bowel is infrequently injured in children. Penetrating injury is invariably present, with entry commonly between the anterior axillary line and flank. Signs and symptoms are similar to those of small bowel injury.

The pancreas is likewise an infrequent source of pediatric abdominal injury. Because detection by physical exam is exceedingly difficult, ancillary testing is necessary in almost every case. Turner's sign (ecchymotic flank discoloration) and Cullen's sign (ecchymotic periumbilical discoloration) suggest retroperitoneal injury and should prompt an aggressive search for pancreatic trauma.

Injury to the kidneys, ureters, or bladder usually presents with hematuria. These injuries are typically minor (see Chapter 57), but may involve severe vascular injury and occur together with other significant abdominal injury. Penetrating injuries, especially from gunshots, are often the mechanism in severe genitourinary tract trauma.

Ancillary Data ■

CLINICAL LABORATORY

All patients with potentially serious abdominal injuries require laboratory analysis for complete blood count, electrolytes, BUN, creatinine, coagulation studies, platelet count, amylase, hepatic transaminases, and urinalysis. *The most important test is blood type and crossmatch.* Hematocrit may be difficult to evaluate. Early hemorrhage may be associated with a normal value, since equilibration may not have occurred. Serial hematocrits every 30–60 minutes are far more sensitive, but must be evaluated in light of the dilutional effects of intravenous hydration. Preexisting anemia may further complicate hematocrit interpretation.

The serum amylase correlates moderately well with injury to the pancreas or duodenum, and serum transaminases correlate very well with injuries to the liver. Urinalysis is the best screen for injury to the kidneys and collecting system, but may be normal in the face of massive injury, if disruption of the collecting system is present.

ROENTGENOGRAMS

Radiology offers only limited assistance in assessing abdominal trauma. Chest roentgenography may identify abdominal free air in cases of perforation of a hollow viscus, or the splenic shadow may be enlarged or the gastric bubble displaced medially in cases of splenic injury and hemorrhage. In a patient with shock or rapidly dropping hematocrit, a one-shot intravenous pyelogram can immediately assess the vascular integrity of the kidneys.

PERITONEAL LAVAGE

Diagnostic peritoneal lavage (DPL) may be of major value in early identification of abdominal injury in the hemodynamically stable patient. For the child with refractory shock and clinical findings suggestive of abdominal injury, immediate exploratory laparotomy is indicated. However, many major trauma victims respond to aggressive resuscitative measures, so that further diagnostic studies are possible in the ED before commitment to operative intervention.

TABLE 56–2. *Diagnostic Peritoneal Lavage: Pros and Cons*

Pros

Extremely sensitive to presence of intraperitoneal blood

Can detect intraperitoneal white blood cells and enzymes, providing diagnostic clue to the presence of small bowel or pancreatic injury

Can be performed rapidly without moving the patient from the ED

Relatively inexpensive

Cons

Technically difficult in small child

Too sensitive to hemoperitoneum, resulting in unnecessary laparotomies

Cannot define the specific organ damaged or the extent of the damage

Cannot reliably detect retroperitoneal injury

Potential false positive resulting from diapedesis of retroperitoneal blood

Potential false positive from traumatic tap

Can miss small bowel injuries if performed too early

Potential injury to intra-abdominal organs resulting from introduction of the catheter or trochar

Renders subsequent physical examination unreliable

(Source: Schiffman MA: Nonoperative management of blunt abdominal trauma in pediatrics. *Emerg Med Clin North Am* 1989; 7)

TABLE 56–3. *Abdominal CT Scanning: Pros and Cons*

Pros

Detects injury to all intraperitoneal and retroperitoneal organs simultaneously

Accurately detects as little as 25 mL of free intraperitoneal blood

Bony structures are well visualized

Excellent for renal injuries

Cons

Radiation exposure (approximately equal to fluoroscopy)

Patient exposed to IV and GI contrast for optimal results

Patient motion must be controlled

Patient must leave ED for an area not well suited to resuscitation

Expert radiologic interpretation is required at all hours

Accuracy in diagnosing trauma to pancreas and bowel is questioned

(Source: Schiffman MA: Nonoperative management of blunt abdominal trauma in pediatrics. *Emerg Med Clin North Am* 1989; 7)

In DPL, after bladder catheterization, a large-bore catheter is introduced into the peritoneal cavity in the midline, at or just below the umbilicus; normal saline is instilled and re-collected to examine for obvious blood, bile, or fecal material, and laboratory analysis of red and white blood cell counts. Ordinarily, this procedure is carried out by the consulting surgeon or by the ED physician or pediatrician in close cooperation with the surgeon. Any positive finding requires careful consideration for laparotomy. Table 56-2 summarizes the advantages and disadvantages of DPL in evaluating abdominal injury. Technical difficulties with young children are frequently the limiting factors.

COMPUTERIZED AXIAL TOMOGRAPHY (CT)

CT is the mainstay of current diagnostic modalities for abdominal trauma. It is sensitive and specific. Its advantages and disadvantages are presented in Table 56-3; Table 56-4 compares DPL to CT.

Treatment ∎

Treatment of abdominal trauma follows the guidelines for resuscitation and stabilization presented in Chapter 48. *Delay in providing blood products is the*

TABLE 56-4. *CT versus Peritoneal Lavage in the Diagnosis of Pediatric Intra-abdominal Injuries*

	Peritoneal Lavage	CT
Sensitivity to hemoperitoneum	++++	++++
Noninvasive	+	++++
Allows specific diagnosis	0	++++
Sensitivity to ruptured hollow viscus	++++	++
Speed of exam	+++	+
Retroperitoneal injury	0 (some false +)	++++
Requires sedation	Usually	Yes
Requires movement of patient from ED	No	Yes
Sensitivity for renal injury	0	++++
Ruins subsequent physical exam	Yes	No
Leads to unnecessary laparotomy	++	No

most common preventable cause of mortality in major abdominal trauma.

Empty the stomach with a nasogastric tube. This permits evaluation of gastric contents for blood; decompresses the stomach of air and gastric contents; avoids distention from ileus; and facilitates physical examination of the abdomen. Use an orogastric tube when significant facial trauma or cerebrospinal fluid rhinorrhea is present.

Next, place an indwelling Foley catheter if there are no contraindications (see Chapter 57).

PENETRATING TRAUMA

Knife and bullet wounds account for about 5–10% of abdominal injuries in children. Evaluate stab wounds in stable, cooperative patients first by local exploration of the wound to exclude peritoneal penetration. In case of minimal peritoneal penetration by a knife, many patients can be managed expectantly, after thorough surgical consultation without immediate exploratory surgery. In these cases, DPL or CT may further clarify the depth of penetration.

All bullet wounds to the abdomen that penetrate the peritoneum must be explored in the operating room due to the massive dissipation of kinetic energy and resultant likelihood of serious injury.

OPERATIVE MANAGEMENT

Several advances in the diagnosis and treatment of abdominal injuries have decreased the need for operative treatment of abdominal injuries in children:

1. Newer imaging technology that allows accurate, noninvasive diagnosis of splenic, hepatic, and renal injuries
2. An increased awareness of the immunologic role of the spleen and the need for maximal splenic preservation
3. Evidence that most splenic and many hepatic injuries heal spontaneously without operative intervention

Thus, the patient can be spared the morbidity of laparotomy in many cases. Patients meeting the criteria in Table 56-5 may be candidates for nonoperative management. The pediatric surgeon is best prepared to determine the therapeutic options.

Disposition ■

The least seriously injured patients can be closely observed over a period of hours with serial examinations and repeated hematocrits to monitor for deterioration or development of significant findings.

Stable patients in whom intraabdominal injury is seriously suspected should undergo noninvasive testing (such as CT, ^{99}Tc scintigraphy, intravenous pyelography, or ultrasound), depending on the likely problem and the available expertise.

Unstable patients may be candidates for immediate abdominal exploration.

Surgical consultation should be obtained immediately in all but the most trivial of abdominal injuries. Patients initially evaluated in a poorly equipped facility must be considered for early transfer to a pediatric trauma center, general trauma center, or pediatric critical care unit.

TABLE 56-5. *Requirement for Nonoperative Management of Abdominal Trauma*

Patient physiologically stable
Less than ½ blood volume transfused
Pediatric ICU or equivalent observation capabilities
Surgical back-up immediately available in case of deterioration
Absence of obvious indication for immediate laparotomy, such as pneumoperitoneum or peritonitis

Bibliography ■

Bass BL, Eichelberger MR, Schisgall R, et al: Hazards of nonoperative therapy in hepatic injury in children. *J Trauma* 1984; 24:978–982.

Berger P, Kuhn J: CT of blunt abdominal trauma in childhood. *AJR* 1981; 136:105–110.

Chaikof E, McCabe C: Fatal overwhelming postsplenectomy infection. *Am J Surg* 1985; 149:534–539.

Cobb LM, Vinocur CD, Wagner CW, et al: Intestinal perforation due to blunt trauma in children in an era of increased nonoperative treatment. *J Trauma* 1986; 26:461–463.

Federle M, Maull K: Proper use of computed tomography with abdominal trauma. *Emerg Med Reports* 1988; 9(20): 153–160.

Haftel AJ: Evaluation of blunt abdominal trauma in childhood. In: Barkin RM, ed: *The emergently ill child: Dilemmas in assessment and management.* Rockville, Md.: Aspen, 1987.

Hoelzer DJ, Brian MB, Balsara VJ, et al: Selection and non-operative management of pediatric blunt trauma patients: The role of quantitative crystalloid resuscitation and abdominal ultrasonography. *J Trauma* 1986; 26:57–62.

Karp MP, Cooney DR, Pros GA, et al: Non-operative management of pediatric hepatic trauma. *J Pediatr Surg* 1983; 18:512–518.

Kuhn JP: Diagnostic imaging for the evaluation of abdominal trauma in children. *Pediatr Clin North Am* 1985; 32:1427–1447.

Power R, Green J, Ochsner M, et al: Peritoneal lavage in pediatric patients sustaining blunt abdominal trauma: A reappraisal. *J Trauma* 1987; 27:6–10.

Ruffing RP, Marx JA: Blunt abdominal trauma: Diagnostic triage and management. In: Barkin RM, ed: *The emergently ill child: Dilemmas in assessment and management.* Rockville, Md.: Aspen, 1987.

57 Genitourinary Tract Trauma

Jack W. McAninch

Traumatic injuries are the leading cause of death in children, and genitourinary injury occurs in about 10–15% of all abdominal trauma. Since injuries to other organ systems are often more obvious, the emergency department (ED) physician must be mindful of the potential for urologic injury and must perform the appropriate diagnostic evaluation early.

Renal Injuries ■

ETIOLOGY AND PATHOPHYSIOLOGY

Renal injuries are the most common injuries of the urinary system. Although well protected by heavy lumbar muscles, ribs, vertebral bodies, and viscera, the kidneys have unusual mobility. Consequently, parenchymal damage and vascular injuries due to stretch on the vessels occur easily. Additionally, minimal trauma may cause renal injury in kidneys with a pre-existing pathologic condition such as tumor or hydronephrosis.

Blunt traumatic injuries caused by automobile accidents, falls, or blows to the abdomen account for most renal injuries in children. Rapid deceleration injuries sustained in high-speed vehicular collisions or falls can result in major renal vascular injury. Penetrating injuries, usually from gunshot or stab wounds, occur rarely in children. The extent of injury cannot be judged on the basis of hematuria or the appearance of the entrance or exit wound.

Microscopic or gross hematuria after abdominal trauma indicates urologic injury. *However, gross hematuria may occur in minor renal trauma and microhematuria in major trauma.* Moreover, 30% of renal vascular injuries are reportedly not associated with hematuria. Thus, the presence of hematuria demands urologic evaluation. Rapid deceleration blunt trauma and penetrating flank injuries, even without associated hematuria, are also indications for assessment of the upper urinary tract (Figure 57-1).

CLINICAL FINDINGS

History

Pain may be localized to one flank or over the abdomen, but the presence of visceral injury or pelvic fracture may obscure symptoms of renal injury. Nausea, vomiting, and abdominal pain may be present. Extensive blood loss and symptoms of shock may result from retroperitoneal bleeding.

Physical Examination

A systematic physical examination provides necessary information to direct urologic evaluation. Fractures of the lower ribs are associated with renal injuries, pelvic fractures with bladder and urethral injuries. Diffuse abdominal pain may indicate intraperitoneal bladder rupture or retroperitoneal hematoma. An abdominal bruit may suggest a renal vascular injury. Perineal hematoma, a dislocated prostate on rectal examination, and blood at the urethral meatus are associated with urethral injury. Scrotal contusions and hematomas require evaluation for possible testicular rupture.

Concurrent abdominal trauma is usually evident. Flank ecchymosis or lower rib fractures may be present. Extensive blood loss and shock may result from retroperitoneal bleeding. A palpable mass may indicate a retroperitoneal hematoma or urinoma. If the retroperitoneum has been torn, hemoperitoneum will cause diffuse abdominal tenderness and ileus.

Ancillary Data

Radiographic imaging begins with excretory urography. Patients with gross or microscopic hematuria (more than 5 RBC/HPF or positive dipstick testing) and those suspected of having renal injury should receive 2 ml/kg of intravenous contrast medium with the resuscitation fluids (more hemodynamically sta-

283

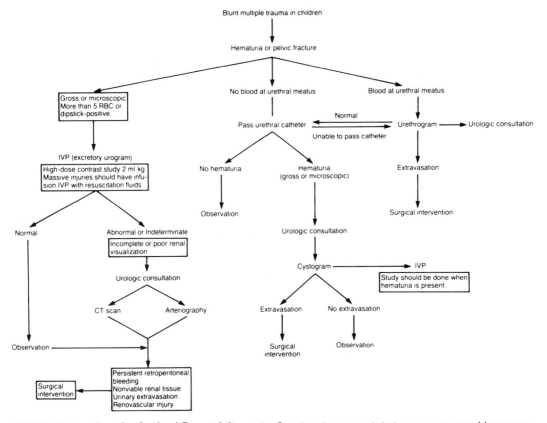

FIGURE 57–1. Algorithm for the differential diagnosis of genitourinary-tract injuries consequent to blunt trauma in children.

ble patients can undergo a routine study). The initial film after injection will not only identify bony fractures, free intraperitoneal air and displaced bowel, but will also establish the presence or absence of both kidneys and define the renal outlines, the collecting systems, and the ureters. Nephrotomography is indicated when the urogram does not fully define the extent of injury. Excretory urography combined with tomography can adequately define 85% of renal injuries.

Computed tomography (CT) provides excellent information regarding renal injuries: it defines the depth and extent of lacerations; sensitively demonstrates extravasation; clearly depicts the size and extent of retroperitoneal hematoma; and detects arterial injury. Arteriography, which defines arterial injuries and renal lacerations, can be used when CT is unavailable or not definitive. Radionuclide renal scanning is used in defining renal trauma, but is not readily available in the emergency setting and is not as sensitive as either CT or arteriography. Sonography

in its current stage of development is nonspecific and does not provide sufficient diagnostic information.

MINOR RENAL TRAUMA

Renal trauma is minor in 85% of cases; renal contusions, subcapsular hematomas, and superficial cortical lacerations are considered minor. These injuries usually cause diminution or delay in excretion of contrast dye in the affected kidney.

MAJOR RENAL TRAUMA

Deep corticomedullary lacerations may extend into the collecting system, resulting in perirenal urinary extravasation. Large retroperitoneal and perinephric hematomas may accompany these deep lacerations. Extravasation of contrast dye, an obscured renal outline, and a shift in the normal position and axis of the affected kidney are associated radiographic signs.

VASCULAR INJURIES

Of all patients with blunt trauma, 1% suffer vascular injuries to the renal system. These include total avulsion of the renal artery and vein, partial avulsion of the segmental branches of these vessels, and main renal artery or segmental artery thrombosis without avulsion.

No excretion of contrast on intravenous urography suggests a main renal artery injury, severe contusion causing vascular spasm, or absence of the kidney and requires further evaluation with CT or arteriography. Likewise, abnormal or indeterminate results of urography necessitate additional studies in the stable patient.

TREATMENT AND DISPOSITION

Treat conservatively (with careful follow-up) patients with microscopic hematuria and minor injuries (contusions and superficial parenchymal lacerations) defined by appropriate staging. Patients with gross hematuria and minor injuries require urologic consultation and hospitalization; place them on strict bed rest until their gross hematuria resolves. Obtain immediate urologic consultation for possible surgical intervention for vascular injuries and for major renal parenchymal injuries associated with extensive extravasation or an expanding or pulsatile hematoma. Penetrating injuries from gunshot and stab wounds require surgical exploration unless thorough diagnostic testing (CT or arteriography) demonstrates only a minor parenchymal injury without extravasation.

COMPLICATIONS

Complications of recurrent bleeding, persistent urinary extravasation, retroperitoneal urinoma, and perirenal abscess can occur within a few days of injury. Late complications include hypertension and hydronephrosis. Follow all patients who have major renal injuries with imaging studies and renal radionucleotide scans.

Ureteral Injuries ■

The ureter is rarely injured. Gunshot and stab wounds are the most common causes of ureteral injury from external trauma. In children, blunt trauma can avulse the ureter from the ureteropelvic junction. The complications that arise from failure to recognize ureteral injury include urinoma, abscess, fistula formation, and hydronephrosis.

CLINICAL FINDINGS

Diagnosis of ureteral injury is primarily based on suspicion. Physical findings are nonspecific and usually relate to the associated intraabdominal injuries; microhematuria is present in 90% of cases. Gunshot wounds to the abdomen and stab wounds to the lumbar or flank area can cause ureteral injury and require diagnostic evaluation.

ANCILLARY DATA

Perform excretory urography for all penetrating injuries over the course of the ureter or in suspected injury from blunt trauma. The urogram may reveal only faint extravasation of contrast, mild ureteral dilation proximal to the injury, or mild hydronephrosis. When the results are equivocal, obtain a retrograde ureterogram in the stable patient.

TREATMENT AND COMPLICATIONS

All patients with suspected or documented ureteral injuries require urologic consultation. Prompt surgical exploration with ureteral repair is necessary. Complications consist of abscess and retroperitoneal urinoma in delayed diagnosis. Ureteral obstruction can occur postoperatively.

Bladder Injuries ■

Bladder ruptures most commonly occur in association with blunt trauma and pelvic fracture (Figure 57-1). Indeed, the bladder or urethra is ruptured in about 15% of pelvic fractures, usually from automobile/pedestrian accidents. Extraperitoneal rupture (75%) is often due to perforation from bony fragments; however, intraperitoneal rupture (25%) may occur in the absence of pelvic fracture if the bladder is distended during a direct blow to the lower abdomen. *Suspect bladder rupture in children even if presenting symptoms are minimal.*

CLINICAL FINDINGS

Pelvic fracture and gross hematuria will be present in over 90% of cases. Hemodynamic instability is commonly due to the extensive blood loss from disruption of pelvic vessels and associated injuries. Signs of an acute abdomen indicate intraperitoneal rupture. Evidence of lower abdominal injury from gunshot or stab wounds should lead one to suspect bladder injury.

ANCILLARY DATA

Obtain urine by urethral catheterization unless there is blood at the urethral meatus. Bloody urethral discharge indicates urethral injury and urethrography must be done promptly. When catheterization is possible, examine the urine for blood. Gross hematuria is common, microscopic hematuria less so. Obtain urine cultures for the presence of infection.

A plain abdominal film demonstrates the associated pelvic fractures. Obtain retrograde cystograms in the presence of gross hematuria or microscopic hematuria associated with pelvic fracture or penetrating lower abdominal injury. Contrast material should completely distend the bladder (a handy rule-of-thumb for bladder capacity in children is 60 ml plus 30 ml for each year of life: e.g., a 2-year-old would be expected to have a 120-ml capacity). Obtain a film of the lower abdomen. After complete emptying, obtain a drainage film to demonstrate areas of extraperitoneal extravasation, which, in 15% of cases, may have been obscured on the filling film. This technique, properly performed, is nearly 100% sensitive for bladder rupture.

An intravenous pyelogram is indicated for all patients with trauma-induced hematuria, as abdominal trauma may injure the kidneys and ureters as well.

TREATMENT AND COMPLICATIONS

Treat shock and hemorrhage and obtain urologic consultation when bladder rupture is suspected. Early operative repair with suprapubic drainage is successful and associated with minimal complications. Nonoperative management has been successful in extraperitoneal injuries.

Urethral Injuries ■

Urethral injuries are uncommon and occur most often in boys secondary to blunt trauma. Injuries to the posterior urethra are associated with pelvic fracture in 95% of cases; those to the anterior urethra commonly occur with straddle injuries. Stricture, impotence, incontinence, and chronic urinary tract infection are potential severe complications.

ETIOLOGY AND PATHOPHYSIOLOGY

The posterior urethra, consisting of the prostatic and membranous portions, is most commonly injured during blunt trauma associated with pelvic fractures. The urethra is usually first sheared off proximal to the urogenital diaphragm. The prostate is displaced superiorly by the developing hematoma. The anterior urethra, consisting of the portion distal to the urogenital diaphragm, can be lacerated and bruised from straddle injuries or instrumentation.

CLINICAL FINDINGS

The patient usually complains of abdominal pain and inability to urinate. Blood at the meatus is the most important sign of urethral injury. Retrograde urethrography is indicated before catheter passage. *Attempts to pass a urethral catheter may result in conversion of a partial disruption to a complete disruption or in infection of the periprostatic hematoma.*

Physical examination will reveal suprapubic tenderness and pelvic fracture. Rectal examination may demonstrate superior displacement of the prostate and a large pelvic hematoma. However, superior prostatic displacement will not occur if the puboprostatic ligaments remain intact or if the disruption is complete.

ANCILLARY DATA

Extravasation of contrast material on retrograde urethrography superior to the urogenital diaphragm confirms the diagnosis of posterior urethral laceration.

TREATMENT AND COMPLICATIONS

Urologic consultation is mandatory (Figure 57-1). Initial management should consist of a suprapubic cystostomy to provide urinary drainage; complications are rare. Plan for subsequent stricture repair within three months.

Testicular Trauma ■

Blunt trauma to the scrotum can result in testicular rupture and in large hematoceles.

CLINICAL FINDINGS

Pain, nausea, and vomiting often accompany testicular injury. Scrotal ecchymosis and large hematomas may make testicular examination difficult.

ANCILLARY DATA

Sonography is highly sensitive in diagnosing testicular rupture. Testicular scanning can also suggest rupture, but it is more time-consuming and appears to be less reliable.

TREATMENT AND COMPLICATIONS

Obtain urologic consultation when testicular rupture is suspected. Exploration and repair of testicular rupture and penetrating testicular injuries is imperative. When rupture is excluded, conservative treatment with scrotal elevation and sitz baths should be adequate. Very large hematomas may require surgical drainage to reduce morbidity. *Testicular atrophy secondary to necrosis can follow major testicular injury.*

Genital Skin Loss ■

Avulsion injuries, burns, and gunshot and stab wounds can result in major penile and scrotal skin loss. Obstructive rings at the base of the penis can cause gangrene and urethral injury. Investigate possible associated urethral damage by urethrography. Debride and repair superficial lacerations in the ED. For avulsion injuries and gangrene, however, debride immediately but delay reconstruction.

Bibliography ■

Ahmed S, Morris LL: Renal parenchymal injuries secondary to blunt abdominal trauma in childhood: A 10-year review. *Br J Urol* 1982; 54:470.

Berger PE, Munschauer RW, Kuhn JP: Computed tomography and ultrasound of renal and perirenal diseases in infants and children. *Pediatr Radiol* 1980; 9:91.

Bretan PN Jr, McAninch JW, Federle MP, et al: Computerized tomographic staging of renal trauma: 85 consecutive cases. *J Urol* 1986; 136:561.

Bright TC, White K, Peters PC: Significance of hematuria after trauma. *J Urol* 1978; 120:455.

Carroll PR, McAninch JW: Major bladder trauma: The accuracy of cystography. *J Urol* 1983; 130:887.

Cass AS: Blunt renal trauma in children. *J Trauma* 1983; 23:123.

Corriere JN Jr, Sandler CM: Mechanisms of injury, patterns of extravasation and management of extraperitoneal bladder rupture due to blunt trauma. *J Urol* 1988; 139:43.

Drago JR, Wisnia LG, Palmer JM, et al: Bilateral ureteropelvic junction avulsion after blunt abdominal trauma. *Urology* 1981; 17:169.

Fournier GR Jr, Laing FC, Jeffrey RB Jr, et al: High-resolution scrotal ultrasonography: A highly sensitive but nonspecific diagnostic technique. *J Urol* 1985; 134:490.

Kuzmarov IW, Morehouse DD, Gibson S: Blunt renal trauma in the pediatric population: A retrospective study. *J Urol* 1981; 126:648.

McAninch JW, Kahn RI, Jeffrey RB Jr, et al: Major traumatic and septic genital injuries. *J Trauma* 1984; 24:291.

58 Skeletal Trauma

John A. Ogden

Because skeletal trauma accounts for 10–15% of all childhood injuries, the evaluating physician should be familiar with the probable mechanism of injury, the short-term biologic responses of the injured part, and the appropriate guidelines for initial diagnosis and treatment of the specific injury. Relying on principles of diagnosis applicable to injuries of the adult skeleton may cause errors in judgment and early treatment that may result in permanent defects.

In the emergency department (ED), diagnosis and treatment are initiated and potential acute and long-term problems identified. The ED or primary physician must be aware of indications for referral and discuss with parents the need for consultation and specialized treatment. The ED physician must also warn the family about potential complications.

A *fracture* is the disruption of the normal continuity of the bone, cartilage, or both. The disruption may or may not cause a break in the continuity of the bone; sometimes in children the developing cortical bone bends or buckles rather than breaking completely.

Sprains (ligament injuries) are unusual in children, but become more common in adolescents. Most sprains prior to skeletal maturity are avulsions of cartilage and bone from the epiphysis; the ligament is generally intact.

Because the chondro-osseous epiphyses of children are variably radiolucent, evaluation and radiologic diagnosis may be difficult. Sometimes a fracture must be inferred on the basis of clinical judgment when roentgenographic substantiation is not immediately possible. However, subsequent reactive bone formation days to weeks later makes the diagnosis certain. Always splint the injured part before sending the patient for radiologic tests.

Each fracture must be described adequately, because proper description allows better communication between the primary physician and the consulting physicians.

Anatomic Location ■

The fracture's location may have a major impact on acute treatment and potential long-term problems (Figure 58-1).

Diaphyseal: Involvement of the central shaft, which is progressively composed of mature, lamellar bone

Metaphyseal: Involvement of the flaring ends of the bone, which are composed of endosteal trabecular bone and cortical immature fiber bone, both of which predispose to the torus (buckle) fracture

Physeal: Involvement of the endochondral growth mechanism

Epiphyseal: Involvement of the chondro-osseous end of a bone. The epiphysis may be injured *only* in the cartilaginous portion, which may make diagnosis extremely difficult if not impossible with normal radiographic methods.

Articular: Involvement of the joint surface. The injury may be part of a more extensive epiphyseal injury, or it may be localized only to the articular cartilage.

Epicondylar: Involvement of regions around the elbow that serve as major muscle attachments

Subcapital: Involvement just below the epiphyses of certain bones, such as the proximal femur or radius

Cervical: Involvement along the neck of a specific bone, such as the proximal humerus or femur

Supracondylar: Involvement above the level of the condyles and epicondyles (e.g., distal humerus)

Transcondylar: Located transversely across the condyles. This is usually a physeal fracture of the distal humerus or femur.

Intercondylar: Involvement of the epiphysis; the fracture splits the normal condylar anatomic relationships.

Malleolar: Involvement of the distal regions of the fibula and tibia

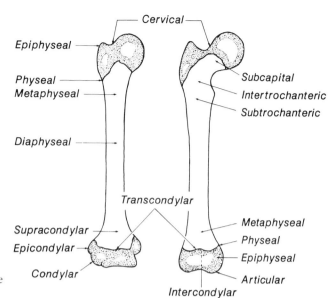

FIGURE 58–1. Common anatomic areas of fracture in the immature skeleton.

Types of Fractures ■

The basic fracture patterns are as follows (see Figure 58-2:

Longitudinal (A): The fracture line follows the longitudinal axis of the diaphysis.

Transverse (B): The fracture line is at a right angle to the longitudinal axis.

Oblique (C): The fracture line is variably angled relative to the longitudinal axis.

Spiral (D): The fracture line encircles a portion of the shaft.

Impacted (E): This is a compression injury in which the cortical and trabecular bone tissues are crushed.

Comminuted (F): The fracture has multiple, variable-sized fragments.

Bowing (G): The bone is deformed beyond its capacity for full elastic recoil into *permanent* plastic deformation. The younger the child, the more likely this may occur. It is common in the fibula and the ulna, both of which may bow, while the paired bone (i.e., tibia or radius) fractures. Such permanent deformation may limit the reducibility of the fractured bone of the pair.

Greenstick (H): The bone is completely fractured, with a portion of the cortex and periosteum remaining intact on the compression side. Since the intact cortical bone is usually plastically deformed (bowed), an angular deformity is common, which may necessitate conversion to a complete fracture by reversal of the deformity.

Torus (I): This is an impaction injury in which the bone buckles, rather than fracturing completely. A relatively stable injury is created.

Treatment ■

Before satisfactory treatment, the child's apprehensions must be dispelled and appropriate pain relief given. If reduction is necessary, proper levels of sedation or anesthesia are essential. Local anesthetic infiltration of the fracture site may be used, but only under rigidly sterile conditions. Intravenous regional block or selective nerve block may be accomplished in older, cooperative children. The use of intravenous agents (e.g., diazepam) must be undertaken with caution. Remember that diazepam is basically an amnesic, not an analgesic agent. The child will feel and react to pain, but will not remember doing so. The drug response may be delayed. Any child being sent to another area for post-reduction films must be appropriately alert, lest respiratory arrest occur in an area where observation and resuscitation are difficult.

If a fracture requires muscle relaxation for reduction, general anesthesia is more useful. This is particularly true for supracondylar humeral and dorsally displaced distal radial fractures. When general anesthesia is used, admit the child to the hospital for overnight observation of the neurovascular response to both the injury and the manipulation.

The basic principle of fracture reduction is to reverse the mechanism of injury. Reduction by this

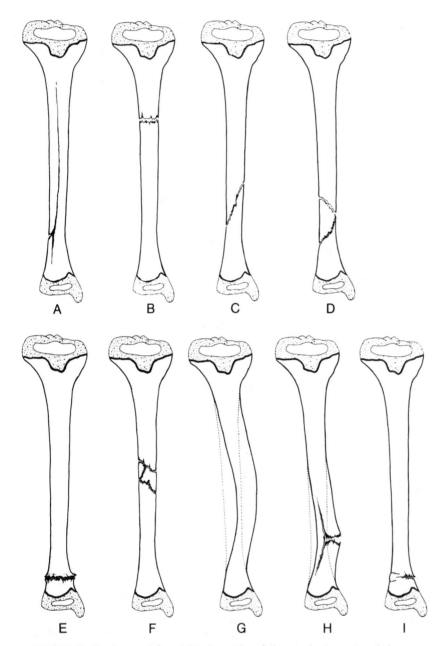

FIGURE 58–2. Patterns of partial and complete failure in the immature skeleton.

method depends on the presence of the partially in-tact soft-tissue linkage (i.e., the periosteum). Another step in fracture treatment is to align the fragment that can be more easily controlled. Usually the distal fragment is controlled more easily, and should be aligned longitudinally with the proximal fragment. The proximal fragment adopts a position caused by the pull of the muscles attached to it.

Closed reduction is adequate to maintain normal alignment of most fractures in children, because the remodeling of their bones engenders good anatomic and functional results. Rotational deformities must be corrected. Except in fractures involving joints and epiphyses, absolute anatomic reduction of the bone fragments is not always necessary, and sometimes should be purposely avoided. Angulation in the middle third of long bones is unacceptable, and should be corrected as close to normal as possible. Some angulation in the metaphyses may be acceptable if enough remodeling potential is present. Direct apposition of bone ends is less important. Side-to-side apposition, especially in the midfemur, is desirable and usually leads to prompt, strong osseous union. The younger the child, the greater the amount of anticipated remodeling.

The thoughtless use of internal fixation should be strongly discouraged in treating fractures in children, but it is incorrect to deny such application altogether. Operative treatment should be used whenever closed reduction does not achieve an acceptable result. Many types of fractures of the physis and epiphysis are best treated by immediate open reduction and internal fixation. However, open reduction may be dangerous if performed several days or weeks after the epiphyseal injury because the danger of damage to the growth plate increases.

Children devise ingenious methods for destroying immobilization devices, so casts or splints must be applied securely. As a general rule, one or more joints on either side of the fracture should be immobilized. Follow-up radiographs should be obtained about five to ten days after reduction. During this time, the reactive swelling and pain are subsiding and the child's activity level is increasing, so the cast may loosen and cause the reduction to be lost. This is also the period during which a loss of reduction or a less acceptable angulation is easiest to correct.

Growth Mechanism Injuries ■

About 15% of fractures in children involve the physis, or growth plate. Boys sustain physeal injuries more often than girls. The physes are open longer in boys than in girls, extending the duration of exposure to potential injury. The distal physes are injured more often than the proximal physes.

In any injury to a growth mechanism, no matter how minor it may appear, it is imperative to discuss with the parents the risk of growth slowdown or arrest, shortening, and angular deformity.

Most epiphyseal injuries are associated with displacement of the shaft relative to the secondary ossification center. The greater the displacement, the more evident the injury. At times, displacement or widening of the plate may be minimal. Epiphyseal injuries occasionally may be seen only in non-standard projections (e.g., oblique views).

Because of the elastic capacity of developing bone and contiguous soft tissues, the injured part may spring back into anatomic position after the deforming force is removed. This is particularly common in epiphyseal fractures around the knee. These fractures are the childhood and adolescent analogue of ligamentous injuries in the adult. Stress application may "open" a fracture sufficiently to document the injury.

The basic growth mechanism injuries are shown in Figure 58-3.

TYPE 1

The fracture extends transversely across the hypertrophic and calcified zones of the physis. Displacement may be minimal, making this pattern hard to diagnose radiographically. The most common injury pattern in infants and young children, it must be strongly considered in an infant instead of a dislocation, which is anatomically less likely. This pattern is frequent in child abuse and patients with myelomeningocele.

Closed reduction is indicated for most Type 1 injuries. In certain injuries, such as the distal humerus, temporary pin fixation may be necessary.

TYPE 2

The fracture extends partially along the physeal-metaphyseal interface and then propagates into the metaphysis, creating the characteristic triangular metaphyseal fragment (Thurstan Holland sign). This is the most common physeal injury pattern and becomes increasingly prevalent after age 4 years.

Closed reduction is usually indicated. The periosteum is intact along the metaphyseal fragment and diaphysis, creating a stable hinge to work against during reduction. Infrequently, open reduction may be necessary, especially to remove soft tissues displaced into the fracture gap.

TYPE 3

The fracture propagates transversely along the physeal-metaphyseal interface and then turns to cross the entire physis, epiphysis, ossification center, and articular cartilage. This creates an unstable epiphyseal fragment with disruption of all zones of the growth plate and loss of continuity of the articular surface.

These injuries usually require open reduction and internal fixation. Direct particular attention toward restoring the articular surfaces. Discuss growth arrest potential with parents.

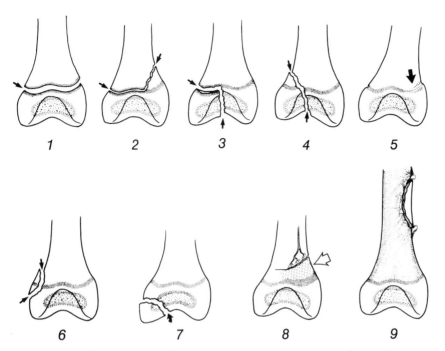

FIGURE 58–3. Patterns of growth mechanism injuries. See text for details.

TYPE 4

The fracture extends from the articular surface to the metaphyseal cortex, traversing epiphysis (and its ossification center), physis, and metaphyseal bone. The metaphyseal fragments of Type 2 and Type 4 injuries may be confusing; the physician must distinguish between them to institute proper treatment.

Treatment requires open reduction and internal fixation. Both the physis and articular surface must be anatomically restored. Discuss growth arrest potential with parents.

TYPE 5

Originally this fracture was thought to be due to a crushing of the physis, but microscopic splitting, linear disruption, and microvascular compromise of the physis are more likely mechanisms. Diagnosis cannot be made at the time of injury and usually is made retrospectively.

TYPE 6

This fracture involves the peripheral growth plate. It usually results from a localized contusion or avulsion of the peripheral portion of the growth mechanism,

as might occur from a lawn-mower accident or if the ankle is caught in a spoked wheel.

Treatment involves local care of soft-tissue injury and reduction of large fragments. Do *not* replace small avulsion fragments. Discuss the possibility of a peripheral osseous bridge.

TYPE 7

This fracture is within the epiphysis, propagating from the articular surface through the epiphyseal cartilage into the secondary ossification center. It is common at the malleoli, within the distal humerus (capitellum) or distal femur as an osteochondral fracture, and in the tibial tuberosity (Osgood-Schlatter's lesion).

Treatment involves immobilization when undisplaced, and open reduction and fixation when displaced.

TYPE 8

This type of fracture involves the metaphyseal growth and remodeling mechanisms. It represents a temporary phenomenon related to vascular alterations.

Treatment includes appropriate reduction and immobilization for the area involved. Warn parents that hypervascularity may lead to angular growth (e.g., valgus angulation complicating proximal tibial metaphyseal fracture)

TYPE 9

This category includes any direct injury causing permanent damage to the periosteum and affecting the bone's ability to grow circumferentially. Wringer and degloving injuries may be associated with significant avulsion of the periosteum. Damage to the interosseous area in paired bones also may cause contiguity of damaged periosteal elements, leading to synostosis.

Treatment includes evaluating muscle compartment pressures, appropriate care of soft tissues, and stabilization of fracture fragments by either open or closed methods.

STRESS FRACTURES

Stress fractures may be confused with neoplasms if seen early. They are often present when a new sport is attempted or there is too much activity in a regular sport. The fibula and tibia are the most common sites; the medial proximal tibia may be affected, as in adult. Many osteochondroses (e.g., Panner's, Sever's and Osgood-Schlatter's lesions) are chronic overuse injuries from childhood sports.

CHILD ABUSE

Signs of child abuse are a characteristic metaphyseal "corner fracture" and multiple fractures in different stages of healing. Coordination with pediatric staff and state regulatory agencies (see Chapter 128) is necessary.

Specific Conditions ■

PROXIMAL CLAVICLE

True sternoclavicular dislocation is very unlikely. A physis and epiphysis are present, along with a meniscus; a physeal injury occurs.

Diagnosis: Pain is felt over the sternoclavicular joint. If anteriorly displaced, the proximal end is palpable. If posteriorly displaced, a "hollow" is evident. There may be difficulty swallowing or breathing. Take oblique sternoclavicular joint views and cross-sectional images.

Treatment: Attempt closed reduction for anterior displacement. The fracture may require pin fixation to ensure stability. Posterior displacement usually requires open reduction.

Concern: Protrusion into mediastinal structures may cause tracheal or esophageal pressure.

CLAVICLE-DIAPHYSIS

This is the most common fracture in the preschool child. Do not confuse it with congenital pseudoarthrosis.

Diagnosis: Deformity is palpable. The greenstick pattern is common in young children. Angulation also is common; watch for skin injury. Comminution is more likely in older children.

Treatment: Accurate anatomic reduction is rarely necessary. Apply a figure-eight clavicle strap; it may require readjusting during the first seven to ten days.

Concern: Children under age 3 often get a large callus, but this remodels, usually within a year.

DISTAL CLAVICLE

This is usually a physeal injury. It is *not* usually a joint dislocation prior to skeletal maturity. The periosteal sleeve is partially intact and attached to an *intact* acromioclavicular joint.

Diagnosis: Pain is felt over the acromioclavicular joint. This injury is easy to confuse with acromioclavicular separation and may require a stress view (have the patient hold a weight).

Treatment: Closed reduction or internal fixation (percutaneous) if unstable.

Concern: Excessive subperiosteal bone.

SHOULDER DISLOCATION

Neonates do not suffer dislocations, but instead physeal fractures of the proximal humerus. This is an unusual injury prior to skeletal maturity

Diagnosis: Loss of motion, palpable gap under the acromion, displacement of humerus from glenoid.

Treatment: Closed reduction.

Concerns: Recurrent dislocation; the child may habitually duplicate the dislocation.

HUMERUS-PROXIMAL EPIPHYSIS

The Type 1 pattern is common in children under age 10; the Type 2 pattern is common in children over age 10.

Diagnosis: Painful shoulder; shortening (overriding) in younger child. A laterally displaced metaphysis may be palpable. This is often misinterpreted as shoulder dislocation in a neonate following a difficult delivery.

Treatment: Closed reduction followed by appropriate immobilization (sling and swathe or cast). Avoid a "Statue of Liberty" cast. Bed rest with arm in abduction, if unstable. Internal fixation is rarely indicated. Overriding is acceptable, except in a patient approaching skeletal maturity.

Concerns: Herniation through periosteal sleeve; entrapment of biceps tendon; longitudinal growth slowing.

HUMERUS-DIAPHYSIS

The cortex is progressively rigid, leading to changing patterns of fracture.

Diagnosis: Angular deformity, swelling; a greenstick injury is common. A spiral fracture may occur in adolescents. The fracture may displace when complete.

Treatment: Closed reduction.

Concerns: Radial nerve injury, angulation.

HUMERUS-SUPRACONDYLAR

Double column, due to olecranon and coronoid fossae, makes reduction unstable.

Diagnosis: Swollen elbow. A detailed neurovascular assessment is essential. There is usually posterior displacement with extensive periosteal stripping.

Treatment: Initial closed reduction, with or without percutaneous pinning; skeletal traction; open reduction.

Concerns: An impacted fracture may be in varus even when "undisplaced." Watch for nerve injury, vascular injury, compartment syndrome (Volkmann's ischemia), and cubitus varus.

HUMERUS-TRANSCONDYLAR

This is usually a Type 1 physeal injury.

Diagnosis: Must be distinguished from elbow dislocation; frequent as birth injury; usually medially displaced, whereas a dislocation is usually laterally displaced.

Treatment: Closed reduction or open reduction and fixation.

Concern: Angular deformity (cubitus varus).

HUMERUS-LATERAL CONDYLE

This is a Type 3 or 4 physeal injury.

Diagnosis: Pain and swelling; may also have soft tissue damage medially. Assess displacement. A stress film may be indicated.

Treatment: Pin fixation, with open reduction in most cases. Beware the undisplaced or minimally displaced injury: reassess within a few days, and alter treatment as necessary.

Concerns: Loss of reduction after a few days when swelling subsides; relative instability of "undisplaced" lesion; delayed union or nonunion; avascular necrosis; premature physeal closure.

HUMERUS-MEDIAL CONDYLE

This is a Type 3 or 4 physeal injury.

Diagnosis: Swollen, painful elbow; usually displaced; may be confused with medial epicondylar fracture.

Treatment: Open reduction, internal fixation.

Concerns: Delayed union or nonunion.

HUMERUS-MEDIAL EPICONDYLE

This involves a major muscular attachment. It may displace *progressively* due to isometric contractures.

Diagnosis: May be part of elbow dislocation (the epicondyle may be within the joint). The displacement varies and may worsen over several days as the soft tissue swelling decreases. Stress films may be necessary to assess the real extent of displacement.

Treatment: Closed if separation is less than 2 mm; otherwise pin fixation and open reduction. Neurolysis of cubital tunnel and ulnar nerve.

Concerns: Ulnar nerve injury (acute or chronic); delayed union or nonunion; chronic pain; elbow instability.

"LITTLE LEAGUE ELBOW"

Osteochondritis of the capitellum; this is sometimes called Panner's disease.

Diagnosis: Pain in the elbow, especially when throwing; sclerotic and lytic regions.

Treatment: Discontinue the sport, switch to a different position, or reduce the amount of time playing. Immobilization may be indicated.

Concerns: Joint incongruency; loss of motion.

ELBOW DISLOCATION

This is usually posterolateral.

Diagnosis: Swollen, often hyperextended. Look for associated chondro-osseous damage (especially radial head or medial epicondyle).

Treatment: Closed reduction; May require open reduction and fixation of associated injuries.

Concerns: Neurovascular damage; entrapment of medial epicondyle in joint; myositis ossificans; recurrent dislocation.

"NURSEMAID'S ELBOW"

This hyperpronation injury involves partial displacement of the annular ligament.

Diagnosis: The child holds the arm in pronation. Radiology is not useful, other than to rule out other injuries.

Treatment: Gentle quick supination with your thumb on the child's radial head.

Concern: Recurrence.

PROXIMAL ULNA

Diagnosis: Painful olecranon; inability to extend arm. Do not misinterpret a small secondary ossification center as a metaphyseal fracture fragment. Similarly, do not interpret a displaced metaphyseal fragment as a secondary ossification center.

Treatment: Usually open reduction, tension band fixation.

Concerns: Refracture; nonunion.

PROXIMAL RADIUS

Metaphyseal compression injury is the most common pattern.

Diagnosis: Pain; swelling over radial head; loss of forearm rotation. Assess the degree of angular displacement.

Treatment: If it is a metaphyseal injury, attempt closed manipulation with pressure over radial head. Epiphyseal injuries usually require open reduction.

Concerns: Avascular necrosis (susceptible intracapsular blood supply) and joint incongruency; malunion may cause loss of supination/pronation.

MONTEGGIA INJURY

The biomechanical interrelationships of the radius and ulna "necessitate" some type of injury of both bones. The usual pattern is a radial head dislocation with proximal or middle third ulnar fracture.

Diagnosis: Obtain appropriate views of the elbow to assess radio-humeral relationships when only an ulnar fracture (or even plastic bowing) occurs *anywhere* along the course of the ulna. This may occur even when both bones are fractured.

Treatment: Adequate closed or open reduction of radial dislocation (the ulna is usually stable when the radius is reduced).

Concerns: Annular ligament disruption or displacement, leading to unstable proximal radioulnar joint; incomplete reduction of radius. Be careful to initially recognize the injury.

RADIUS AND ULNA-DIAPHYSIS (BOWING)

The changing microstructure of the radius and ulna make plastic deformation of one or both likely in the younger child.

Diagnosis: Pain in forearm. This injury is often difficult to assess radiographically since both bones have a normal curvature.

Treatment: Cast or splint for 10 to 14 days.

RADIUS AND ULNA-DIAPHYSIS (GREENSTICK)

This is the typical pattern in a young child with relatively porous diaphysis.

Diagnosis: Swelling, pain. Sometimes the deformity is palpable or visually evident. Some of the cortex remains intact.

Treatment: Three-point pressure in cast necessary; may require completion of fracture.

Concern: Angular change as swelling subsides and incomplete greenstick springs into an increasing deformity.

RADIUS AND ULNA-DIAPHYSIS (BOTH BONES)

Fracture patterns change as the cortices mature. The greenstick pattern is more common in children under age 10; a complete fracture is more common after age 10.

Diagnosis: Angular deformity is common. Assess fracture patterns, degree of displacement, and any overriding.

Treatment: Closed reduction under age 10; open reduction, internal fixation more likely in child older than 10.

Concerns: Malunion; nonunion of one or both bones; decreased pronation/supination.

RADIUS AND ULNA (DISTAL METAPHYSIS)

This is one of the most frequently injured areas. A torus injury is common. The periosteum is intact dorsally and disrupted on the volar surface.

Diagnosis: "Silver spoon" deformity when displaced; painful, variably swollen wrist. Assess median nerve carefully.

Treatment: Torus: splint for about two weeks; angulated: correct the deformity; dorsally displaced: closed reduction by "walking" the distal fragment. Reassess after a few days to ensure angulation does not recur.

Concerns: Failure to reduce displacement (may require open reduction); angulation; acute carpal tunnel syndrome.

RADIUS (DISTAL PHYSIS)

This is one of the most common physeal injuries.

Diagnosis: Pain, swelling over distal radius; variably displaced. Look at the ulnar styloid.

Treatment: Gentle closed reduction.

Concerns: Growth slowing or arrest; ulnar styloid nonunion.

PELVIC RAMI

The rami should be considered analogous to a long bone, with an epiphysis at either end. Displacement of the rami should be considered a growth mechanism injury. The periosteal sleeve may be intact and eventually will fill in the apparent radiologic defect. Evaluate the sacroiliac region (dislocation versus chondro-osseous separation), as the entire hemipelvis may be involved.

Diagnosis: Assess possible visceral injury (bladder, urethra). A CT scan is important. Apparent widening of the symphysis pubis is usually a physeal separation.

Treatment: Bed rest; progressive weight bearing (fractures heal rapidly). External fixation may be necessary. Embolization for excessive hemorrhage.

ILIAC SPINES

Traction "apophysis" at origin of major thigh and leg musculature This is often termed "hip pointer" and usually occurs during athletic activity.

Diagnosis: Look for radiographic displacement of osseous fragment. Impossible to diagnose if only the cartilaginous portion is avulsed; however, subsequent callus makes the fracture evident.

Treatment: Discontinue the sport. Crutches with progressive weight bearing for three to six weeks; reconditioning for muscles involved in the sport.

Concerns: Exostosis; chronic pain.

ISCHIUM

This "apophyseal" injury is the major origin of hamstring muscles.

Diagnosis: Pain over tuberosity, following either chronic exertion or acute injury; may have irregular bone formation. This must be distinguished from a tumor or osteomyelitis.

Treatment: Discontinue sports until asymptomatic. Significant displacement may require surgical fixation.

HIP DISLOCATION

Normal laxity in children may contribute to dislocation with minimal trauma. The injury is usually posterior; anterior is much less common.

Diagnosis: Shortened, adducted leg with posterior dislocation; shortened, abducted leg with anterior dislocation Displacement of femoral head. Look for peripheral acetabular fracture (posteriorly), but do *not* confuse with normal secondary ossification centers appearing during adolescence.

Treatment: Closed reduction; open reduction when necessary.

Concern: Avascular necrosis.

FEMUR (PROXIMAL PHYSIS)

The capital femur and greater trochanter have variable cartilaginous continuity, causing differing morphologic lesions. In the neonate, both regions are injured together, whereas the older child sustains injury only to the capital femoral physis.

Diagnosis: Painful hip motion. May only have slight widening of the capital femoral physis. In the neonate, do not confuse with congenital dysplasia of the hip.

Treatment: Aspiration of hip joint; may require capsulotomy to decrease pressure. Closed reduction in infant; older child may require internal fixation (use smooth pins to allow for growth).

Concerns: Ischemic necrosis; premature closure of physis.

FEMUR (SLIPPED CAPITAL FEMORAL EPIPHYSIS)

This is usually a chronic injury in the adolescent, but it may occur acutely following a fall or contact in athletics. Infrequently, it may occur during attempted reduction of hip dislocation.

Diagnosis: Beware when there is pain *anywhere* between the groin and knee. Lateral is the most diagnostic view; anteroposterior may appear normal.

Treatment: Traction for relief of joint irritation and gradual spontaneous reduction; possible gentle manipulative reduction of acute injury; internal fixation.

FEMORAL NECK

Diagnosis: Painful hip motion. The leg is externally rotated when fracture is complete. Assess the degree of displacement.

Treatment: Traction; internal fixation.

Concerns: Nonunion, delayed union, coxa vara, and ischemic necrosis (beware of vascular injury to femoral head).

LESSER TROCHANTER

This is an avulsion injury of attachment of iliopsoas tendon. It is often seen in adolescent athletes, especially sprinters.

Diagnosis: Pain in groin or inner thigh. This injury cannot be diagnosed if only cartilage is avulsed (look for callus at two to three weeks).

Treatment: Crutches, progressive weight bearing; discontinue athletic activity until healed (three to six weeks); must have progressive muscular rehabilitation.

FEMUR (DIAPHYSIS)

There is minimal displacement in the infant and young child, but a greater tendency to overriding after age 2 years. The femur normally has mild anterolateral bowing.

Diagnosis: Swollen, painful thigh. Carefully assess for neurovascular injury and monitor blood loss into thigh. Assess the extent of overriding and angulation and assess the hip for concomitant dislocation.

Treatment: Allow overriding of 1 to 2 cm; traction with emphasis on longitudinal and rotational alignment; early cast, especially in younger children.

Concern: Overgrowth is very common in children ages 2 to 10 years.

FEMUR (DISTAL PHYSIS)

This region is a major contributor to leg length (40%).

Diagnosis: Pain, swelling above knee; possible hemarthrosis or knee effusion. May require a stress view.

Treatment: Closed reduction of Types 1 and 2; internal fixation of Type 2 may be indicated if unstable. Types 3 and 4 require open reduction, internal fixation.

Concern: Growth arrest.

KNEE DISLOCATION

The medial and lateral ligaments are not usually disrupted; cruciate ligament injury is more likely. Neurovascular structures are relatively fixed just above femoral condyles, increasing susceptibility to injury.

Diagnosis: Carefully examine neurovascular status and look for accompanying fractures.

Treatment: Closed reduction; immobilization for four to six weeks.

Concerns: Vascular disruption; compartment syndrome; ligamentous laxity.

PATELLAR DISLOCATION

There is usually lateral displacement, with disruption of medial soft tissues.

Diagnosis: Patella located along lateral condyle. Look for associated fractures from condyles or patellar margins.

Treatment: Closed reduction (reassess for fractures after reduction); three to four weeks of extension immobilization; progressive rehabilitation. Accompanying fracture may require fixation.

PATELLAR SUBLUXATION

The movement of the patella varies from longitudinal axis.

Diagnosis: Apprehension when the examiner attempts to lateralize the patella; decreased height of lateral condyle and asymmetric shape of patella in "sunrise" views.

Treatment: Quadriceps rehabilitation; infrequently requires surgery prior to skeletal maturation.

KNEE LIGAMENTS

Prior to skeletal maturity this is usually a chondro-osseous disruption, rather than a ligament injury.

Diagnosis: Pain and tenderness over ligament, especially over chondro-osseous attachment; joint effusion, bleeding; small avulsion fracture.

Treatment: Closed, with three to four weeks of immobilization until the fracture heals.

PATELLAR FRACTURE

Variable amount of cartilage is present, depending on age. Most frequent fractures are in the mid-portion.

Diagnosis: Painful patella; knee effusion. Bipartite patella, while normally considered a radiologic variant, may also be an acute injury.

Treatment: Closed, if not displaced; open reduction, tension band wiring.

DISTAL PATELLA

Chronic failure is usually referred to as Sinding-Larsen-Johansson injury (analogous to Osgood-Schlatter's lesion at the other end of the patellar tendon).

Diagnosis: Pain at lower (inferior) part of patella; there may be a very thin piece of bone at the distal chondro-osseous junction ("sleeve" fracture). May be a retrospective diagnosis, especially in chronic injury.

Treatment: Immobilization in cylinder cast for at least three weeks; progressive rehabilitation.

TIBIAL SPINES

This is the analogue of cruciate ligament injury in the adult.

Diagnosis: Swollen knee; motion restriction; hemarthrosis. A lateral view is essential to show anteroposterior extent of the injury and the degree of displacement.

Treatment: Closed, if undisplaced; open, if displaced.

Concerns: Chronic cruciate ligament insufficiency; nonunion with or without pain.

OSGOOD-SCHLATTER'S LESION

This is a chronic stress injury.

Diagnosis: Painful tibial tuberosity; irregular ossification within the tuberosity. Late stage may be associated with ossicle formation.

Treatment: Immobilization for one to three weeks until the pain is gone; temporary discontinuation of sports; progressive quadriceps strengthening; rarely, lateral retinacular release or resection of ossicle(s) indicated. Do not inject steroids.

Concern: Enlargement of the tuberosity.

PROXIMAL TIBIOFIBULAR JOINT

Diagnosis: Painful anterolateral mass. May require oblique views.

Treatment: Closed reduction.

Concerns: Peroneal nerve dysfunction; chronic pain and instability.

PROXIMAL TIBIAL METAPHYSIS

Diagnosis: Pain, swelling distal to knee; usually an incomplete tibial fracture (fibula may not appear injured).

Treatment: Closed, with three-point pressure to maintain alignment.

Concern: Progressive valgus deformity.

TIBIA/FIBULA (DIAPHYSIS)

Increased thickening of the cortex is a factor in changing fracture patterns.

Diagnosis: Painful, swollen lower leg. Assess compartment pressure, neurovascular status, fracture pattern, degree of overriding, shortening.

Treatment: Closed reduction. Maintain length as much as possible.

Concern: Increased possibility of delayed union or nonunion as child matures into adolescence.

TODDLER'S FRACTURE

This injury, which may involve the tibia or the fibula, occurs as the child is first walking, when the diaphysis still has considerable woven rather than osteon bone.

Diagnosis: Pain in leg, limping. Look for bowing of the fibula.

Treatment: Cast immobilization.

TIBIA/FIBULA (DISTAL EPIPHYSIS, TYPES 1 AND 2)

This fracture may displace with rotation only.

Diagnosis: Painful, swollen ankle. Normal irregularity of physis just above malleolus should not be misinterpreted as a fracture. Must distinguish Type 2 from more complex injuries. Be wary of pure rotational displacement.

Treatment: Closed reduction.

Concern: Growth arrest.

TIBIA/FIBULA (TRIPLANE)

This is a combination of Type 3 and 4 injuries.

Diagnosis: Swollen, painful ankle. Anteroposterior/lateral views will not reveal morphology of injury; may require CT imaging for complete delineation.

Treatment: Open reduction.

Concern: Growth arrest.

TIBIA/FIBULA (FRACTURE OF TILLAUX)

This injury relates to the pattern of the closure of the physis: the medial side closes before the lateral side.

Diagnosis: Painful, swollen ankle. May require oblique or mortise view to delineate extent of injury; CT scan may delineate degree of separation.

Treatment: Closed when fracture is undisplaced; open, with fixation, if displacement interrupts joint congruity.

TALUS

Vascularity changes with chondro-osseous maturation.

Diagnosis: Pain with ankle motion; swollen in ankle region; neck fracture; os trigonum: acute versus chronic.

Treatment: Neck fracture: closed versus open depends upon displacement; osteochondritis: immobilization; os trigonum: immobilization.

Concerns: Ischemic necrosis; chronic joint pain.

CALCANEUS

There is variability of secondary ossification in apophysis.

Diagnosis: Pain in heel. Variable sclerosis of apophysis difficult to diagnose (possibility of Sever's disease).

Treatment: Closed whenever possible.

TARSAL NAVICULAR

There is variability in ossification.

Diagnosis: Pain in dorsum of midfoot; irregularity of ossification (osteochondritis); presence of accessory navicular. A bone scan is useful.

Treatment: Immobilization, excision of accessory navicular if chronically painful.

METATARSALS

Shaft fractures are more common than physeal.

Diagnosis: Painful, swollen; especially on dorsum of the foot. Variable displacement of metatarsals in shaft fracture. Angulation of distal physeal fractures.

Treatment: Closed reduction.

FIFTH METATARSAL

This is an apophyseal injury.

Peroneal musculature attaches here.

Diagnosis: Point tenderness, swelling over proximal end of metatarsal. Do not confuse with secondary ossification center.

Treatment: Closed reduction, immobilization.

FOOT PHALANGES

Injuries are most common in the great toe; small bones minimize injury in the other four toes.

Diagnosis: Painful, swollen toe. Assess physeal injury, especially in stubbing injury.

Treatment: Closed reduction when necessary. Antibiotics if open nail or pulp space injury.

Concerns: Nail injury, infection.

PUNCTURE WOUNDS TO THE FOOT

Such injuries may extend to skeletal components or joints.

Diagnosis: Small puncture wound may be all that is readily evident. Look for foreign material (e.g., wood, metal) and for osseous cortical injury.

Treatment: Antibiotic coverage; debridement when indicated.

Concerns: Osteomyelitis, septic arthritis, abscess.

Bibliography ■

Borden S: Roentgen recognition of acute plastic bowing of the forearm in children. *Am J Roent* 1975; 123:524.

Ogden JA: Injury to the immature skeleton. In: Touloukian RJ, ed: *Pediatric Trauma,* 2nd ed. St. Louis: CV Mosby, 1989.

Ogden JA: Injury to the growth mechanism of the immature skeleton. *Skel Radiol* 1981; 6:237.

Ogden JA: Skeletal growth mechanism injury patterns. *J Ped Orthop* 1982; 2:371.

Ogden JA: *Skeletal injury in the child,* 2nd ed. Philadelphia: WB Saunders, 1989 (in press, est. Oct.)

Ogden JA: The uniqueness of growing bones. In: Rockwood CA Jr, Wilkins KE, King RE, eds: *Fractures: Children,* Vol. 3, 2nd ed. Philadelphia: JB Lippincott, 1984.

Rang M: *Children's fractures,* 2nd ed. Philadelphia: JB Lippincott, 1981.

Salter RB, Harris WR: Injuries involving epiphyseal plates. *J Bone Joint Surg* 1963; 45A:587.

59 Hand Trauma

Ronald A. Dieckmann and Robert E. Markison

Injuries to the hand and wrist are common emergencies of childhood. Most cases involve minor trauma to the skin or soft tissues and require only routine wound care. Occasionally, however, vital underlying structures are affected by blunt or penetrating injuries, crushes, burns, envenomations, infections, or amputations. These injuries require meticulous initial clinical assessment, appropriate ancillary tests, and precise early treatment. A major diagnostic challenge to the examining physician is establishing trust and cooperation with panicky parents and a frightened child, in order to accomplish accurate evaluation.

Anatomy and Function ■

The hand is a complex structure, with multiple functional units:

1. The skin and soft-tissue cover
2. The circulation
3. The motor and sensory nerves
4. The musculotendinous structures
5. The skeleton, including joints and ligaments

Figure 59-1 illustrates the functional anatomy of the hand, in a superficial-to-deep plane dissection. Figure 59-2 presents the sensory innervation of the hand. Figure 59-3 shows the arrangement of carpal bones at the wrist.

The hand's functions are diverse and delicate. It is the functional end of a cantilevered musculoskeletal system reaching from the shoulder to the fingertips. Coordinated movement and sensation depend on dynamic and balanced interrelationships of intrinsic and extrinsic motor structures that drive a sensate glove of soft-tissue cover. Figure 59-4 shows the "position of function" of the hand. This position includes 20–30 degrees of wrist extension, 50–60 degrees of metacarpophalangeal (MCP) flexion, with the thumb in line with the radius. Injury to the functional units of the hand causes disruption in this posture.

Treatment techniques must ensure maintenance of the functional position during repair and healing,

whenever possible. Flexor tendon injuries are an exception, since proper splinting of these injuries requires wrist flexion to minimize stress on divided tendons.

Clinical Findings ■

Hand emergencies involve one or several symptoms and signs:

Pain
Swelling
Stiffness
Loss of soft tissue
Specific structural unit failure (e.g., loss of sensation, loss of movement, or deformity)

HISTORY

A focused history includes the exact mechanism of injury, the time of the injury, the relative cleanliness of the penetrating object, depth and direction of penetration, amount of soft-tissue loss, blood loss, and prior hand problems. Inquire about the specific symptoms noted above. Sometimes loss of sensation or movement is not easily elicited in the very young child, and instead requires clinical detection. Establish the child's tetanus immunization and allergy status.

PHYSICAL EXAMINATION

Physical assessment must be gentle and methodical. Always spend the first moments of the encounter establishing rapport, enlisting parental assistance when necessary, and providing explanation. Disrobe and expose the neck, shoulders, and bilateral arms and remove bracelets, rings, and other clothing. *Analgesia is imperative* (see Chapter 39) and must *never* be withheld in the child with severe pain who is hemodynamically stable. Occasionally, chemical sedation may be necessary to accomplish the examination; morphine sulfate, 0.1–0.2 mg/kg subcutaneously or intravenously, with hydroxyzine, 1 mg/

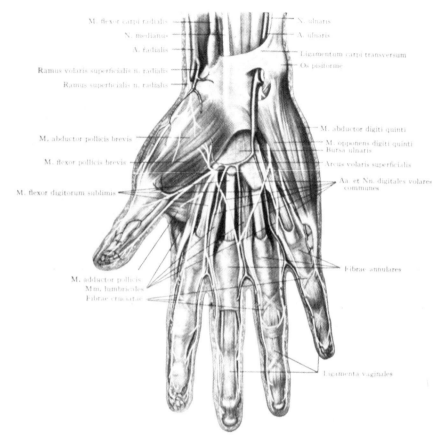

FIGURE 59–1. Functional anatomy of the hand. (From Markison RE, Kilgore ES: Hand. In Davis JH (ed): *Clinical Surgery.* St Louis: CV Mosby, 1987; p. 2292.)

kg intravenously or intramuscularly, provides excellent sedation. To elicit maximum information, inspect the hand and instruct the patient on appropriate independent maneuvers prior to palpation, whenever possible.

Ensure that all functional units of the hand and wrist are individually evaluated. Begin with simple inspection of the hand and wrist, then test sensation, motor function, circulation, and skeletal integrity. Finally, after the clinical exam, exploration may be necessary to determine the extent of the hand injury.

Inspection

First, look at the functional position and contour of the hand. Bony deformity, edema, and musculotendon disruption may be immediately obvious. Then, observe the skin and soft-tissue cover for color and

for external trauma such as lacerations, abrasions, contusions, puncture wounds, crush or degloving injuries, or burns. Assess which areas are painful.

Sensation

Determine if sweating is present by inspecting the involved part with an otoscope or by dragging a smooth plastic pen across the anatomic area; sweat will cause the pen to drag from friction, while dry denervated skin allows the pen to glide smoothly. Since peripheral autonomic fibers travel within nerve sheaths, absence of sweating suggests nerve disruption in the corresponding sensory distribution. Soaking the hand for 5 minutes in warm water will further assist in identifying insensate areas: denervated skin will not wrinkle.

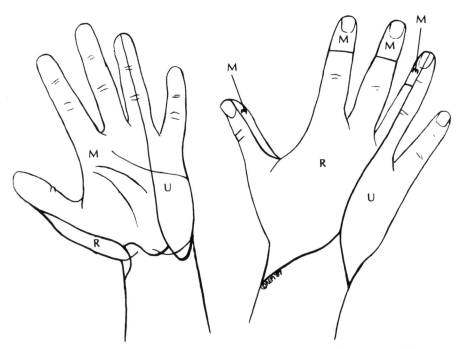

FIGURE 59-2. Sensory innervation of the hand: median (*M*), ulnar (*U*), and radial (*R*) nerves. From Markison RE, Kilgore ES: Hand. In Davis JH (ed): *Clinical Surgery.* St. Louis: CV Mosby, 1987; p. 2292.)

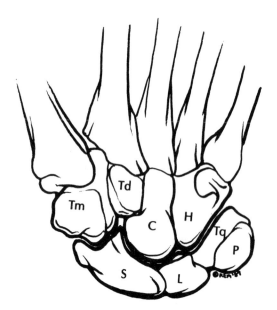

FIGURE 59-3. Arrangement of carpal bones at the wrist: *Tm,* Trapezium; *Td,* Trapezoid; *C,* Capitate; *H,* Hamate; *L,* Lunate; *Tq,* Triquethrum; *P,* Pisiform. (From Markison RE, Kilgore ES: Hand. In Davis JH (ed): *Clinical Surgery.* St. Louis: CV Mosby, 1987; p. 2292.

Test all three nerves—radial, median, and ulnar. Sensory distribution is shown in Figure 59-2. Use a blunt paper clip with ends 1 cm apart to establish two-point discrimination. The finger pads normally distinguish two points 2–5 mm apart, the palm and dorsum 5–10 mm. *Never use "sharp and dull" testing*

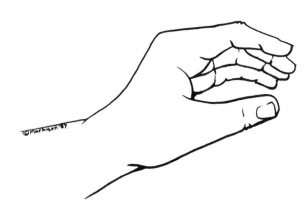

FIGURE 59-4. Position of function of the hand. (From Markison RE, Kilgore ES: Hand. In Davis JH (ed): *Clinical Surgery.* St. Louis: CV Mosby, 1987; p. 2292.)

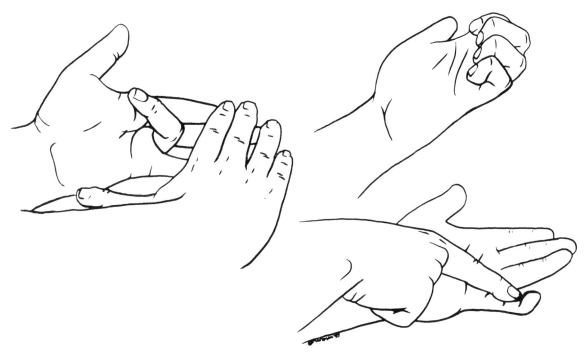

FIGURE 59–5. Above, testing for flexor digitorum sublimis; **right** and **below,** testing for flexor digitorum profundus. (From Markison RE, Kilgore ES: Hand. In Davis JH (ed): *Clinical Surgery.* St. Louis: CV Mosby, 1987; p. 2292.)

in children, as it provides no worthwhile information and is abusive. Always evaluate sensation distal to the injury, and before local anesthesia is administered. Isolated digital nerve injuries are the most commonly missed nerve disruption.

Motor Function

Evaluate every individual musculotendinous unit. First, have the patient perform a series of movements *bilaterally:*

1. Hold hands over head, palms forward (observe for symmetry).
2. Open and close hands, slowly then quickly (check symmetric extrinsic muscle function).
3. Spread, then adduct fingers (establishes ulnar nerve innervation).
4. Oppose thumbs individually to each digit (establishes median nerve innervation).
5. Press the palms together, then the dorsums, with maximum wrist flexion (median nerve function) and extension (radial nerve function).

These maneuvers will provide a good idea of neuromotor function. Then, do specific testing of the following tendons:

1. Flexor longus pollicis: touch thumb tip to base of little finger.
2. Flexor profundus digitorum: see Figure 59-5.
3. Flexor sublimis digitorum: see Figure 59-5.
4. Extensor tendons: extend each finger against resistance.

Circulation

Inspect for cyanosis or pallor. Feel for coolness. Then, determine capillary refill to measure perfusion, particularly with wounds of the flexor surfaces. In children, refill occurs normally in less than 2 seconds. The Allen test evaluates the balance of inflow (radial and ulnar arteries) circulation into the hand. With the child clenching and elevating the hand, compress both arteries at the wrist. Then have the patient lower and open the hand; release one vessel and observe for refill. Repeat to test the other artery. Normal filling of the entire hand from either artery takes 2–3 seconds.

Skeleton

Evaluate bony and ligamentous injuries through careful inspection for deformity, then by palpation of areas of pain. Usually, radiographic studies are necessary to fully assess the location and severity of fractures and dislocations. Test joint stability by applying gentle stress in every plane, then comparing to the normal side.

WOUND EXPLORATION

When the clinical exam does not disclose deep structure injury, proceed to proper wound care after local anesthesia and sterile preparation, as presented in Chapter 62. Wound exploration may disclose injuries to deep structures that are not apparent clinically. Proper wound care technique includes copious pressure irrigation, meticulous removal of clots and foreign bodies, and minimal debridement of devitalized tissue.

Often, a pneumatic tourniquet is necessary to achieve adequate visualization for optimal repair. First, paint the involved area with povidone-iodine solution and drape sterilely; then, inflate the properly sized blood pressure cuff to 100 mm Hg above systolic pressure after 1 minute of extremity elevation. Do not inflate longer than 30 minutes.

Ancillary Data ■

Radiographic studies are of great value in assessing hand and wrist injuries. Bilateral radiographs provide a normal comparative film and are helpful in distinguishing growth plates from fractures. Radiographs may detect fractures, dislocations, osteomyelitis, foreign bodies, or air in the joints and soft tissues. Xeroradiography is especially helpful in locating soft-tissue foreign bodies. Ultrasound is sensitive for assessing infections, especially tenosynovitis, and deep abscesses. *Do not put needles into infected areas of the child's hand.*

When hand infections are diagnosed, other important ancillary data includes gram stain and culture of available tissue, complete blood count, glucose, and electrolytes. Tissue biopsy may be helpful in ambiguous cases.

Treatment and Disposition ■

If the hand injury involves only superficial skin and soft-tissue cover, use the wound care techniques outlined in Chapter 62. Splinting is necessary if the wound requires sutures and crosses the joint (see below). If a fracture is diagnosed, consult a hand specialist to determine immediate treatment and disposition. *Beware of diagnosing sprains of the wrist*

or hand in the ED, since an occult fracture may be present. Instead, splint and refer.

If deeper structures are involved, consult a hand surgeon immediately. These injuries are not well suited for ED management, and instead require better lighting, sterility, and instrumentation available in the operating room. When deep involvement of musculotendinous units, nerves, arteries, or bones is diagnosed, provide initial ED measures as outlined in Table 59-1 to anticipate operative treatment.

SPLINTING TECHNIQUES

Many hand and wrist injuries require splinting after repair or while awaiting operative treatment. Splinting minimizes pain and swelling and provides an anatomic position for healing. Infants may need circumferential plaster rather than a splint to maintain adequate positioning.

For distal finger injuries, aluminum and foam splints with tape are usually adequate. When one whole finger needs splinting, usually include the adjacent fingers as well. Other premade splints are available commercially, but they are often not sized correctly for children with injuries proximal to the interphalangeal joint. An easy method for constructing a custom splint for more severe injuries is to first measure the distance over the involved area from

---

TABLE 59-1. *Emergency Department Approach to Hand Injuries Requiring Operative Repair*

---

1. *Stop bleeding.* Usually pressure alone will suffice, with a compression bandage. If bleeding persists, examine carefully for foreign body. Never ligate or cauterize hand vessels. Rarely, a pneumatic tourniquet is necessary.
2. *Avoid probing the wound.* Once an operative intervention is deemed necessary by clinical assessment, minimize wound manipulation in the ED. Occasionally, wound exploration is necessary to determine the extent of the injury, if clinical assessment is inconclusive. Once deep involvement is determined, close the wound, using temporary sutures if necessary to preclude bacterial contamination.
3. *Elevate to minimize swelling and pain.*
4. *Splint the extremity*
5. *Provide analgesia,* as outlined.
6. *Provide antimicrobial coverage,* usually with a cephalosporin.
7. *Update tetanus immunization.*
8. *Obtain appropriate radiographs.*
9. *Document findings and treatment* on the chart, using an anatomic map.

one joint proximal to one joint distal. Wrap with soft cotton. Take one or two rolls of appropriate-width plaster roll and create 10–12 layers of measured length. Wet and wring out the plaster, then apply and mold to the anatomic area. Wrap with cut bias or stockinette. After drying, the splint will be hard and durable. A shoulder sling will provide further support; elevate the hand above the heart.

Specific Conditions ■

INJURIES TO THE SKIN AND SOFT-TISSUE COVER

For lacerations, punctures, and foreign bodies, see Chapter 62. For animal bites, see Chapter 93. For arthropod envenomations, see Chapter 101. For burns, see Chapter 61.

DEEP SPACE INFECTIONS

Tenosynovitis, palmar space infections, necrotizing fasciitis, and osteomyelitis occasionally occur in childhood. Flexor tenosynovitis, the most common, usually begins with a puncture wound to the proximal or middle phalanx, which develops into an abscess and erodes into the flexor sheath. The infection proliferates rapidly proximally and destroys tendons if not aggressively managed. Clinical findings are fusiform swelling and slight finger flexion, erythema and tenderness of the flexor sheath, and pain with passive finger extension. Ultrasound may be helpful in ambiguous cases. Treatment requires operative drainage in most cases. Early consultation with a hand surgeon is imperative.

Palmar space infections and necrotizing fasciitis present with systemic toxicity and diffuse hand swelling, rapidly advancing erythema and induration, pain, and heat. These conditions require immediate surgical debridement and drainage (see Chapter 118). Osteomyelitis is discussed in Chapter 119.

FELON

This condition presents as a pulp space infection of the distal phalanx, with erythema, pain, and swelling. Minor trauma or a puncture wound is often the cause. Treatment is incision and drainage to avoid progression to osteomyelitis or flexor tenosynovitis. Make a longitudinal incision on the mid-palmar aspect of the pad of the finger and open widely. Elevation and warm soaks are helpful; soaks can start one day after drainage.

INJECTION INJURIES

High-pressure injection of paint or grease into the hand is often devastating to delicate structures, since the substance jets into paths of least resistance, such as the flexor sheaths and deep spaces of the hand. External clinical findings may be minimal. Immediate consultation with a hand surgeon, and appropriate decompression and wide debridement are essential.

PARONYCHIA

This staphylococcal infection of the nail fold is a relatively common hand disorder. Improper nail trimming is often responsible. The condition presents as a fluctuant, erythematous tender mass along the nail. Treatment consists of digital block with 1% lidocaine and elevation of the nail fold to evacuate pus. Longitudinal incisions are occasionally necessary. After incision and drainage, pack the wound open with petrolatum-impregnated gauze. Sometimes, removal of all or part of the nail is necessary for extensive or chronic infections. Elevation and soaks are helpful.

RING ON A SWOLLEN FINGER

Treatment consists of either removal with a ring-cutter or with the string method. The latter technique involves wrapping a string circumferentially around the edematous finger from distal to proximal to force edema out of the finger. Next, apply petrolatum or Lubrifax generously to the coil of the string. Then, pull the proximal end of the string, inserted under the ring, to slowly advance the ring over the compressed soft tissues.

SUBUNGUAL HEMATOMA

Blood under the nail is usually secondary to blunt injury. A distal phalangeal fracture may or may not be present. Treat by decompression, either with an electric cautery device or with a red-hot paper clip. The nail must be decompressed distal to the lunula to avoid injury to the germinal matrix. Usually, digital nerve block is unnecessary, if the physician exercises appropriate finesse. Ensure that the pressure exerted on the decompression device is steady, gentle, and then deliberately reduced as the nail is penetrated to avoid painful contact of the hot end of the instrument with the nail bed.

SUBUNGUAL SPLINTER

This painful condition is treated by trimming the nail with scissors or a scalpel until the end of the splinter is visualized. It can usually be extracted with a splinter forceps.

TIP AMPUTATION

Treat soft-tissue loss from the distal pulp conservatively, if bone is not exposed. Usually, only debridement, copious irrigation, and hemostasis is indicated, along with careful dressing, splinting, and elevation. Skin grafts are usually unnecessary, and granulation occurs within 4–8 weeks. When bone is exposed, consult a hand surgeon for consideration of operative repair.

WHITLOW

Herpes simplex type 1 is the pathogen causing this painful lesion of the distal phalanx. Usually, the virus originates from oral lesions. Extreme burning pain is often present, with serous exudate and clusters of tiny vesicles. Staining may reveal the virus; gram stains show no organisms. Do not incise this lesion. Treatment includes analgesics, splinting, warm soaks, and topical acyclovir 5% ointment. Sometimes, decompression of the nail is necessary for subungual lesions or for secondary bacterial infections. Prescribe a penicillin or cephalosporin when secondary infection is present.

INJURIES TO THE CIRCULATION

Vascular injuries are uncommon but easily overlooked. Pulses are palpable distally in 20% of cases. In 50% of cases, nerve injuries co-exist. When arterial bleeding is observed, stop hemorrhage by direct pressure and compressive bandages, or rarely with a tourniquet. *Never clamp vessels, since nerve injury may result.* Such cases require immediate operative repair.

More subtle presentations occur. The Allen test (see above in "Clinical Findings") may disclose major arterial interruption or other signs of circulatory impairment. Obtain surgical consultation and arrange an immediate arteriogram in such patients.

Compartment syndromes from expanding hematomas can occur in any of the four fascial forearm compartments. Swelling and the five "P's" (*p*allor, *p*ain on passive movement, *p*aresthesias, *p*aresis, and *p*ulselessness) are cardinal features. Immediate surgical consultation is imperative. Therapeutic options include immediate exploration with fasciotomy, arteriogram, or conservative management with ice, compression, and elevation.

MUSCULOTENDINOUS INJURIES

When clinical evaluation or wound exploration discloses musculotendinous disruption, treatment is best accomplished in the operating room after surgical consultation. Follow guidelines for anticipatory

ED management of operative hand injuries in Table 59-1.

Tendinitis of forearm or flexor or extensor tendons crossing the wrist may present as forearm or wrist pain. Repetitive actions, usually in sports activities, are typically responsible (see Chapter 60 for diagnosis and treatment).

NERVE INJURIES

Nerve injuries heal less predictably than traumatic disruptions of other deep structural units of the hand. With prompt, capable management, however, children have good likelihood for recovery of neuronal continuity. Nerve injuries have a spectrum of severity and prognosis. Diagnosis and treatment are based on clinical findings, never on ancillary tests such as nerve conduction studies. If a nerve disruption is suspected clinically, immediately consult a hand surgeon. Usually, initial management consists of primary wound closure in the ED, then operative repair timed for optimal outcome to nerve regeneration.

SKELETAL INJURIES

The hand skeleton has a fixed unit for stability and mobile units for precise movement and force. The eight carpal bones (Figure 59-3) and the second and third metacarpals form the fixed unit; the remaining hand bones form three other distinct motor units: the thumb and first metacarpal; the index finger; and the long, ring, and little fingers with the fourth and fifth metacarpals. Multiple and varied joint types, numerous collateral ligaments, and a balanced extrinsic and intrinsic musculotendinous system provide advanced dexterity and stability to the hand.

Hand fractures, dislocations, and sprains may occur; they can be simple, comminuted, open, or closed (see Chapter 58). Treatment must restore skeletal alignment within hours to safeguard optimal healing. The most frequent conditions in childhood are described below.

Phalangeal Fractures

This is the most common fracture of childhood. Examination reveals pain, swelling, and point tenderness. A subungual hematoma may be present. *Deformity is established when fingernails of the flexed hand are deviated from their normal orientation directly toward the scaphoid tubercle.* Radiographic studies usually disclose the fracture; obtain both anterior-posterior and lateral projections.

Treatment of closed, nondisplaced fractures of the middle and distal phalanges consists of splint immobilization of the involved and adjacent fingers. A proximal phalangeal fracture requires a dorsal splint with 30 degrees of wrist extension, 50–60 degrees of MCP joint flexion, and 10–15 degrees of intraphalangeal (IP) joint flexion. Open, epiphyseal, angulated, and rotational fractures usually require consultation for appropriate reduction and immobilization.

Mallet Finger

This occurs as a hyperextension injury, from a blow to the fingertip by a ball. The extensor tendon is avulsed from the base of the distal phalanx. Salter fractures may accompany this injury. Examination reveals tenderness and swelling at the distal, dorsal phalanx, which is held in flexion, with loss of distal extension. Standard radiographs may demonstrate the avulsion of the dorsal, proximal lip of the distal phalanx. Treatment includes splinting the distal IP joint (Figure 59-6) for 6 weeks, and referral. When the fracture involves the joint surface, consult a hand specialist for consideration of operative reduction.

Metacarpal Fractures

These fractures are the result of direct blunt force. The commonest is the boxer's fracture of the head

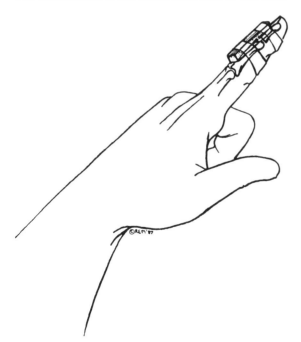

FIGURE 59–6. Splinting the mallet finger. (From Markison RE, Kilgore ES: Hand. In Davis JH (ed): *Clinical Surgery.* St. Louis: CV Mosby, 1987; p. 2292.)

TABLE 59–2. *Management of an Amputated Part*

1. Retrieve the distal part.
2. Rinse with a balanced saline solution.
3. Wrap in a gauze moistened with isotonic solution.
4. Place in a dry, sterile container.
5. Place the container on crushed (never dry) ice.

of the little finger metacarpal. Clinical findings are local tenderness, swelling, and angulation and rotation. Radiographs easily reveal the fracture. Treatment consists of careful reduction and 3–4 weeks of splint immobilization (casting is necessary in younger children). Apply plaster from the mid-forearm to the distal phalanges, with the wrist in 20–30 degrees of extension and the MCP joint at 50–60 degrees flexion. Consult a hand specialist for advice and follow-up.

Carpal Fractures and Dislocations

Falling on an outstretched hand causes the most frequent carpal fracture of the scaphoid bone. Clinical findings include snuffbox tenderness and grip weakness. Obtain both wrist and navicular radiographs. Since circulation is tenuous to the navicular, when clinical signs are present, even in the absence of positive radiographs, treat presumptively for fracture and refer for repeat radiographs and orthopedic follow-up in 10 days. Management of the nondisplaced fracture requires a long arm cast with thumb spica. Some hand specialists also immobilize the digits. Consultation from the ED is indicated prior to patient discharge.

A second childhood injury associated with falling on the outstretched hand is the perilunate dislocation. Tenderness, swelling, and wrist pain occur. The inexperienced physician may attribute the clinical findings to a wrist sprain; significant disability may result if the injury remains untreated. Radiographs may reveal disruption of carpal alignment on the lateral projection. Consultation is imperative to accomplish adequate reduction.

JOINT INJURIES

Ligamentous disruptions of the hand in children are unusual, because ligament is stronger than bone. Tear of the ulnar collateral ligament of the thumb is the most common; this injury is called the skier's or gamekeeper's thumb. Examination reveals local tenderness, swelling, and ligamentous laxity with stress of the joint toward the radial side. Radiographs with stress may reveal opening of the joint and/or an associated fracture. Acute treatment often involves surgical repair. Consult a hand specialist when the diagnosis is established.

AMPUTATIONS

Amputations through hand structures can involve any component. The distal phalanx is most common, although more proximal amputations, sometimes involving the entire hand, occur infrequently. Follow the steps in Table 59-2 for management of the amputated part. Consult a hand surgeon for consideration of replantation. Reattachment is usually impossible when amputation is beyond the distal joint. In the ED, follow anticipatory guidelines for operative repair (Table 59-1).

Bibliography ■

Kilgore ES: *The hand: Surgical and non-surgical management.* Philadelphia: Lea & Febiger, 1977.

Markison RE, Kilgore ES: Hand. In: Davis JH, ed: *Clinical surgery.* St. Louis: CV Mosby, 1987.

Newmeyer WL: *Primary care of hand injuries.* Philadelphia: Lea & Febiger, 1979.

60 Sports Trauma

Dee Hodge

About 6 million children participate in high-school sports; 20 million more are involved in out-of-school recreational and competitive sports. With this increased participation, sports-related injuries are common. The exact incidence is unknown, but about 1 million children sustain sports injuries annually. The incidence of injury increases as the athlete gets older and larger.

Etiology and Pathophysiology ■

Sports-related injuries are largely determined by the sport. Football accounts for the greatest total and the most serious injuries. Gymnastics has the greatest percentage of injuries compared to the number of participants, but most are minor. Basketball accounts for frequent sprains and strains, most involving the leg or foot. Hockey and soccer are associated with contusions.

Sports injuries are due to either repeated microtrauma (overuse syndromes) or macrotrauma (fractures, strains, sprains, and contusions). Ninety-five percent of sport injuries are soft-tissue injuries. About two-thirds of these injuries are sprains or strains. Ten to fifteen percent are contusions and 2–3% are lacerations. Only 5–6% of sport injuries are fractures. In children and adolescents, the ligaments around major joints are stronger and more resistant to tensile forces than the adjacent epiphyseal plate. Injuries that result in musculotendinous or ligamentous failure in adults frequently will produce apophyseal avulsion in children. Therefore, always consider the possibility of bony injuries following mechanisms that would cause only soft-tissue injuries in the adult athlete.

This chapter deals with the more common soft tissue macro- and microtrauma seen in the pediatric athlete. Emphasis is on immediate diagnosis and treatment. Fractures, dislocations, and wound management are dealt with in Chapters 58 and 62.

Sprains, Strains, and Contusions ■

A *sprain* is an injury to a ligamentous structure. Sprains are graded according to severity (see Table 60-1). Sprained ligaments are painful with limitation of motion. There is swelling and localized tenderness over the anatomic course of the injured structure. Laxity of ligaments is best appreciated immediately after injury before appreciable swelling has occurred, using varus and valgus and anterioposterior stress in several positions of flexion and extension. X-rays with stress views may be necessary to evaluate for possible epiphyseal fractures. Sometimes initial X-rays are negative, yet follow-up films in 7–10 days reveal periosteal reaction indicative of bony fracture.

A *strain* is an injury to a muscle-tendon unit. These injuries are also graded I–III (see Table 60-2). These injuries are most commonly seen as hamstring or rectus femoris "pulls." Strains associated with large hematomas are more severe.

A *contusion* is a soft-tissue trauma caused by a direct blow. Bleeding occurs within the fascial compartment, resulting in pain, spasm, and limitation of motion. In general, these injuries have little long-term consequence. They are staged as mild, moderate, or severe depending on the amount of swelling and tenderness and the decrease in function.

Contusions to the lower leg can result in vascular compromise in the form of *acute compartment syndrome*. This is most often seen with blows to the anterolateral leg. Symptoms of compartment syndrome include five Ps: increasingly severe *P*ain and *P*aresthesias; on physical exam, progressive *P*aresis or weakness of the foot and toe dorsiflexors; then late development of *P*ulselessness and *P*allor, when compartment pressures are quite high. Therefore, *the presence of distal pulses does not rule out the diagnosis.* Compartment syndromes are a true orthopedic emergency and, if suspected, require immediate referral for possible surgical decompression and fasciotomy.

TABLE 60-1. *Classification of Sprains*

Grade 1   There is stretching or microscopic tearing of the ligament. There is normal joint stability and the patient can move the joint with minimal discomfort.

Grade 2   There is partial overt tearing of ligament but at least some ligamentous continuity remains. There is an increase in joint instability, pain, and disability.

Grade 3   There is a total loss of ligament continuity. Ecchymosis is present. The joint is unstable, extremely painful, and unusable.

TREATMENT

In general, the treatment for sprains, strains, and contusions is the same:

1. For the first 6–12 hours, minimize the initial swelling. This will expedite diagnosis and rehabilitation. Apply ice immediately using a wet elastic wrap both to hold the ice pack in place and to protect the skin. Do not apply ice directly to the skin. Leave ice in place at least 30 minutes and repeat every 4 hours until bleeding and swelling have stabilized.
2. In most cases, compress and elevate the injury site for the first 24 hours. A mnemonic to recall this therapeutic routine is *ICE,* for *Ice, Compression,* and *Elevation*).

TABLE 60-2. *Classification of Strains*

Grade I or first degree	There is minimal disruption and no deficit in the muscle tendon unit. Mild local tenderness is present.
Grade II or second degree	There is partial tearing with bleeding and spasm. There is no deficit in the muscle tendon unit.
Grade III or third degree	There is complete disruption of the muscle-tendon unit. Marked bleeding occurs with spasm, and pain in the affected limb. The exam may be difficult because of hematoma, but a palpable defect is evident. Grade III strains are rare in young children, but tendon avulsion with an attached piece of bone is not uncommon.

3. Immobilization may be necessary for some injuries, with a preformed splint, a formed plaster splint, or occasionally a plaster or fiberglass cast. Surgical repair is occasionally necessary.

Rehabilitation consists of techniques to improve muscle strength and endurance. This can be accomplished with exercise techniques alone or in combination with isometrics, isotonics, and isokinetics. The patient's complaints of pain should guide the rehabilitation program.

Overuse Syndromes ■

Overuse syndromes consist of stress fractures, tendonitis, apophysitis, and other inflammatory syndromes. In the rapidly growing child, muscle and tendon growth lags behind bone growth, causing decreased flexibility. This inflexibility, when combined with inadequate pre-exercise stretching, leads to great stress on the apophysis. Factors that contribute to overuse injuries include training errors, hard and/or canted surfaces, improper shoes and equipment, bone alignment abnormalities, leg length discrepancy, muscle imbalance, muscle weakness, and poor flexibility. The history is critical in making the diagnosis: a recent increase in work-out time or intensity or beginning a new sport is a frequent historical factor.

Prevention depends on pre-exercise stretching, strengthening, and proper technique. Rest, ice, compression, and elevation are the treatment for most of these problems. For the athlete, cryotherapy, an alternate exercise program aimed at correcting muscle weakness, stretching, splints, or braces may be used. Medications include only nonsteroidal anti-inflammatory medicines; steroids and strong analgesics should be used with caution. Physical therapy is invaluable in management. Most athletes require individualized rehabilitation programs and frequent follow-up with a sports specialist, orthopedist, or primary physician.

Specific Injuries ■

ACROMIOCLAVICULAR SPRAINS OR SEPARATIONS

These ligamentous disruptions are common and often are seen in football players, secondary to falls onto the shoulder. Clinical diagnosis may be difficult. Swelling and tenderness occur directly over the AC joint. The diagnosis and treatment are based on bilateral shoulder stress X-rays. Grade I sprains have normal X-rays and are managed symptomatically with rest, analgesics, and a shoulder strap. Grade II sprains have minor AC widening on X-rays; treatment consists of immobilization and referral. Grade III sprains have both AC and coracoacromial widening on X-ray. Pain is usually severe and joint mobility is limited. Grade III injuries require immobilization and early referral to the orthopedist.

Acromioclavicular contusion is seen in football players who were not wearing shoulder pads. The "shoulder pointer" is a common site for contusion. Treatment is symptomatic.

UPPER EXTREMITY OVERUSE SYNDROMES

Rotator cuff impingement syndrome is being seen more frequently in children participating in swimming, pitching, and racquet sports. Pain is located anteriorly and superiorly at the site of the coracoacromial ligament. *"Little League elbow"* is a catch-all diagnosis that encompasses several clinical entities, including medial epicondylitis, lateral impingement, posterior impingement from muscular imbalance, and ulnar nerve impingement. Osteochondritis dessicans and avulsion fracture must be excluded. *Wrist capsulitis* is often seen in the gymnast from weight-bearing on dorsiflexed hands. Pain is on the dorsum of the wrist. On physical examination, there is diffuse tenderness over the dorsum of the wrist with mild swelling. Obtain hand and wrist X-rays to rule out occult fractures. Management of these entities is the same as for other overuse injuries.

"WRIST SPRAINS"

Ligamentous injuries of the wrist are rare in children. Hence, even with negative X-rays, the maxim in children is "a sprained wrist is a fractured wrist until proven otherwise." Splint all wrist injuries, and refer to an orthopedist for repeat X-rays and follow-up evaluation.

BACK STRAIN

Back strain most commonly involves the lumbosacral or the upper thoracic areas. This is an injury of older adolescents. Pain is usually bilateral; on physical exam there is usually spasm and tenderness of the paraspinous muscles, and positive back pain with straight leg-raising. The neurologic exam is normal. X-rays are usually unnecessary except with acute trauma. Treatment includes anti-inflammatory medications, muscle relaxants, and heat. All back strains should respond within 10 days. Rehabilitation includes working on increased flexibility and correcting underlying muscle imbalance.

ACUTE LOWER EXTREMITY INJURY

The quadriceps are the most common sites for muscle contusions and hematomas. These usually present as warm, swollen, painful masses. Myositis ossificans (calcification at the site of the hematoma) can be a sequela. Treatment equals "ICE" immediately. Rehabilitation involves pain-free stretching and strengthening exercises.

"Hip pointer" is another common contusion site, especially among football players who were not wearing hip pads. Treatment of such iliac crest contusions is symptomatic.

KNEE SPRAINS

Knee sprains are frequently serious sports injuries; they usually involve the medial collateral or anterior cruciate ligament. Occasionally epiphyseal fractures are present. The patient will complain of a sense of instability, a feeling of the knee "going out," a sensation or sound of a pop or tear at the time of injury, and an inability or unwillingness to bear weight. Joint instability may be present on physical exam (see Figures 60-1A and 60-1B). A modified Lachman drawer test (anterior-posterior glide) is positive in most anterior cruciate ligament tears, but is also seen in avulsion fractures of the tibial insertion of the ligament. Varus and valgus stress testing of the medial and lateral collateral ligaments will reveal laxity if there is tearing of these structures. With ligamentous knee injuries, swelling of the joint and hemarthrosis occur within 12 hours of injury. X-rays are necessary to rule out fracture. Immobilization, ICE, analgesics, and early orthopedic evaluation is imperative. Occasionally, needle aspiration of tense hemarthrosis is necessary in the ED to relieve pain.

ANKLE SPRAINS

Most ankle injuries occur when the ankle is inverted and plantar flexed. Most of these injuries are sprains involving the anterior talofibular, calcaneofibular, and posterior talofibular ligaments. Salter fractures must also be considered and excluded in the child and younger adolescent. With inversion and external rotation injury, there is damage to the medial deltoid ligaments and possible "push-off" fracture of the fibula. Grading of ankle sprains is described earlier. Tenderness over the bony prominence of the tibia, fibula, and/or the fifth metatarsus is suspicious of a fracture. Check ligamentous stability by stress-testing the injured ankle and comparing it to the uninjured ankle (see Figure 60-2). This is best done immediately at the time of injury or after the swelling has decreased. X-rays (AP, lateral, and Mortise views)

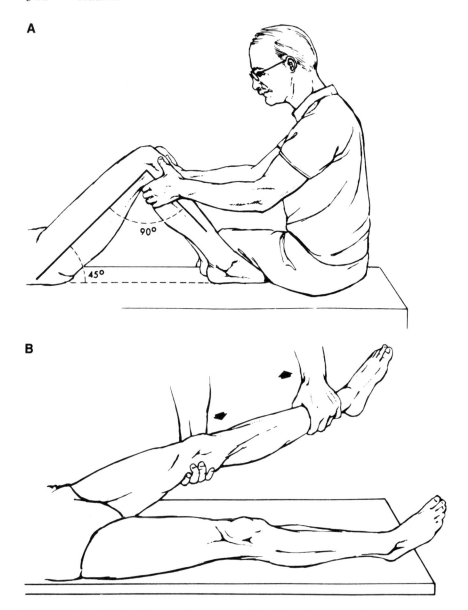

FIGURE 60–1. **(A)** Anterior-posterior stress test. The athlete lies on the table with his injured knee flexed to 90 degrees and his hip flexed to 45 degrees. The examiner sits on the toes of the injured leg with the foot in neutral position, faces the athlete, and places both hands on the portion of the calf immediately below the knee joint with his fingers in the popliteal space and his thumbs over the tibia. To test the anterior cruciate ligament, the examiner pulls the lower leg toward himself and then pushes it back; he repeats the maneuver in the uninjured leg and compares the results. If the injured leg moves forward and/or backward more than the uninjured leg, this is a positive anterior drawer sign and implies a torn ligament. The same procedure is repeated, except that the examiner pushes the lower leg back away from himself and then pulls it forward, to test the integrity of the posterior cruciate. **(B)** The knee in stress. Collateral stress test. With the athlete lying on his back with both knees extended, the examiner holds the injured leg firmly with one hand placed slightly above the ankle and places his other hand on the lower lateral aspect of the thigh and around under the knee. To

(*continued*)

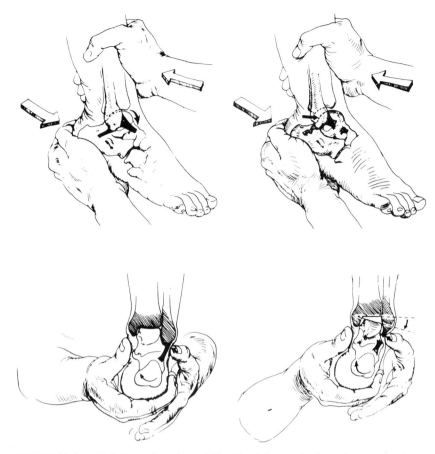

FIGURE 60-2. Clinical tests for ankle stability. **Top left,** anterior draw sign test to evaluate the intactness of the anterior talofibular ligament; **top right,** positive anterior draw sign; **bottom left,** test to evaluate the stability of the anterior talofibular and the calcaneofibular ligaments; **bottom right,** ankle is unstable if the anterior talofibular and calcaneofibular ligaments are torn. (Reproduced with permission from Hoppenfeld S: *Physical Examination of the Spine and Extremities.* New York: Appleton-Century-Crofts, 1976:222.)

are usually indicated. Management follows the general treatment guidelines. In addition, grade II injuries are best treated with immobilization and crutches for one week. Grade III injuries require full casting and may need surgical repair.

LOWER EXTREMITY OVERUSE SYNDROMES

Osgood-Schlatter Syndrome

This is commonly seen in adolescents and is due to traction of the patellar tendon on the apophysis of

---

FIGURE 60-1. (continued).
test the medial collateral ligament, he gently pushes inward on the thigh while gently pulling the lower leg away from the midline of the body at the same time. The same maneuver is repeated with the injured knee at 30 degrees of flexion. Both maneuvers are then repeated in the uninjured knee and the results in the two knees are compared. The lateral collateral ligament can be tested in the same manner, except that this time the examiner pulls outward on the thigh while pushing inward on the lower leg. (From Grossman M, Pascoe D: *Quick Reference to Pediatric Emergencies.* Philadelphia: JB Lippincott, 1984:78, 79.)

the tibia. Sports involving repeated flexion and forced extension are precipitating factors. There is pain over the tibial tubercle, which is often very prominent. X-rays are negative but may rule out other diagnoses. Treatment includes rest, immobilization, and analgesics. Changing sports is usually indicated.

Patellofemoral Syndrome

This overuse syndrome is frequently associated with anatomic problems and other risk factors. Pain is varied: it may be a dull ache behind the knee cap or joint, or it may be along the medial or lateral aspect of the knee. Pain is present after exercise, especially running, during forced extension from a fully flexed position, or after sitting with the leg acutely flexed. Physical exam shows normal range of motion. Tenderness and crepitus may be elicited while pressing on the patella during flexion and extension of the knee. Anatomic abnormalities may be noted, including vastus medialis atrophy, high-riding patellae, genu valgum and tibia vara, and tight hamstring muscles. Other syndromes to exclude are chondromalacia patella and osteochondritis dessicans; the latter diagnosis can be made by X-ray evaluation. Treatment is conservative and consists of nonsteroidal anti-inflammatory medications and decreased activity.

Anterior Leg Pain

Pain along the anterior aspect of the tibia after exercise is often called "shin splints." This entity may be one of three different processes: a stress fracture of the tibia, inflammation of the tendons attaching to the tibia, or acute compartment syndrome. Tendonitis presents with linear tenderness along the anterior or medial edge of mid-shaft distal tibia. Compartment syndromes are less frequent but pose a true emergency caused by increased pressure in the muscle fascial compartment due to overuse and impairment of venous outflow.

Achilles Tendonitis

This usually occurs in children with short Achilles tendons or tight calf muscles, in circumstances of repeated forcible traction. Pain usually occurs after exercise and may occur in the morning on awakening. Tenderness is present around the tendon itself at the level of the malleoli, when palpating between the thumb and forefinger. Achilles tendon rupture is excluded on physical exam if quadriceps compression results in plantar flexion of the foot. Treatment is symptomatic. Heel risers may be helpful.

Plantar Fascitis

Inflammation of the plantar fascia is an incapacitating syndrome due to increase in duration or frequency of exercise, frequently involving hill-running. Pain is felt in the arch or heel. Physical exam usually reveals pain along the medial aspect of the plantar fascia, exaggerated by dorsiflexion of the foot. The patient usually limps, favoring the lateral aspect of the foot. Diagnosis is by history and physical exam. X-rays are not helpful. Differential diagnosis includes stress fractures of the metatarsals or calcaneus or apophysitis of the calcaneal growth plate.

Apophysitis of the Calcaneal Growth Plate

Also known as Sever's disease, this overuse syndrome is commonly seen in children between ages 8 and 13 and is associated with an increase in running activity. The condition is manifested by a limp. On physical exam the heel is sore to lateral compression. There is swelling and induration of the heel and the heel cord is tight. Treatment consists of a heel riser to raise the height of the affected heel ½"–¾" higher than the front of the foot. Anti-inflammatory agents are helpful. The patient should be re-evaluated in 1–2 weeks, usually by a pediatric orthopedist or sports specialist.

Bibliography ■

Committee on School Health, American Academy of Pediatrics: School health: A guide for health professionals. Elk Grove Village, Illinois: American Academy of Pediatrics, 1987.

Garrick JG: Sports medicine. Pediatr Clin North Am 1986; 33:1541–1550.

Herring SA, Nilson KL: Introduction to overuse injuries. Clin Sports Med 1987; 6:225–239.

Ireland ML, Andrews JR: Shoulder and elbow injuries in the young athlete. Clin Sports Med 1988; 7:473–494.

Jones DC, James SL: Overuse injuries of the lower extremity. Clin Sports Med 1987; 6:273–290.

Kellett J: Acute soft tissue injuries: A review of the literature. Med Sci Sports Exerc 1986; 18:489–500.

McManama GB: Ankle injuries in the young athlete. Clin Sports Med 1988; 7:547–562.

Mosher JF: Current concepts in the diagnosis and treatment of hand and wrist injuries in sports. Med Sci Sports Exerc 1985; 17:48–55.

Simmons BP, Lovallo JL: Hand and wrist injuries in children. Clin Sports Med 1988; 7:495–526.

Smith RW, Reischl SF: Treatment of ankle sprains in young athletes. Am J Sports Med 1986; 14:465–471.

Steiner ME, Grana WA: The young athlete's knee: Recent advances. Clin Sports Med 1988; 7:527–546.

Tursz A, Crost M: Sports-related injuries in children. Am J Sports Med 1986; 14:294–299.

Webber A: Acute soft-tissue injuries in the young athlete. Clin Sports Med 1988; 7:611–624.

61 Thermal Injury

Val Selivanov

Children represent a large segment of the estimated annual 2 million burn victims in the United States. Scald thermal injury is the most common type of thermal injury, and children are the largest group of scald victims. Thermal burns are common pediatric emergencies; inhalation and electrical burns occur less often.

Society is increasingly recognizing that intentional thermal injury is a major form of child abuse. In fact, 39% of pediatric burn unit admissions may result from intentional injury. All burned children seen in emergency departments (EDs) must be considered potential abuse victims.

Etiology and Pathophysiology ■

THERMAL

The basic mechanism of thermal injury, like that of all trauma, is abnormal energy transfer to and through tissue. The temperature (kinetic energy delivered to the tissue), duration of exposure, total surface area exposed, association of other injuries such as fractures, hemorrhage and smoke inhalation, and physiologic age of the victim determine the clinical problem and prognosis.

The uncomplicated natural history of burns is simply that of normal wound healing. All burns risk complications. Major burns carry the immediate risk of hypovolemic shock. All burns carry a late risk (days later) of infection and metabolic exhaustion leading to sepsis. All moderate burns potentiate a far-late (after months or years) risk of cosmetic and functional impairment due to excess collagen deposits forming hypertrophic scars and contractures. Emotional scar sequelae may be severe.

INHALATION

Inhalation injuries occur when burns are sustained in a closed-space environment. Injury is caused by inhaling microscopic smoke particles (noxious compounds, chemical irritants, and reactants) into the distal bronchial/alveolar tree. The combustion of plastics and synthetic construction materials releases polyvinyl chloride, hydrocyanic acid, and acetaldehyde, which combine with lung water to produce corrosive acids and alkalis. Cyanide and carbon monoxide poisoning may occur concurrently. The composite pathophysiology is that of severe chemical pneumonitis with increased capillary permeability and destruction of normal alveolar architecture. Clinically, this presents within 24 hours as hypoxemia with permeability edema.

Fluid requirements exceeding initial estimates based on body surface area (BSA) burned should raise the suspicion of occult injury and/or superimposed inhalation injury.

ELECTRICAL

Children rarely experience electrical injuries except for home outlet and electric-cord injuries in infants and toddlers. These injuries result from low-amperage alternating current, which causes both deep thermal injury and direct tissue destruction. High-voltage electrical injuries are more devastating and may cause ventricular fibrillation and tetanic-like clonic contractions of skeletal muscle. Hypoxia and renal failure secondary to myoglobinuria often complicate these injuries. Lightning causes direct current, massive energy level injuries with a different pathophysiology (see Chapter 97).

Higher voltage/amperage, industrial electrical burns injure small surface areas but exhibit dramatic entry and exit sites that resemble high-velocity bullet wounds. The total volume of tissue injured is variable and not readily evident. The current travels along neurovascular bundles and can cause direct heat damage to muscles and viscera as well as vessel thrombosis. Signs of muscle ischemia and necrosis may not become evident for hours.

Clinical Findings ■

Most pediatric burns seen in non—burn-center EDs do not carry a significant risk for later systemic sepsis, as most "small burns" re-epithelialize in 10–14 days without complication. Nevertheless, the key lies in distinguishing small, simple wounds from potentially serious ones based on accurate estimation of burn depth and size.

BURN DEPTH

Most initial burn assessments overestimate area and underestimate depth. An initial lack of blistering may cause erythematous regions of dermal burns to appear as first-degree or partial-thickness burns. These may prove within hours to be dermal or full-thickness injuries with raised epithelium. Burn wounds are dynamic; some blistered areas, especially those immediately adjacent, may rapidly convert to full thickness. Initial distinction in the ED between second- and third-degree burns is often impossible. Therefore, burn depth may be best estimated initially as either *partial* or *full thickness*. Nomenclature using first-, second-, and third-degree categories for depth is probably accurate retrospectively but not in the ED setting. Table 61-1 lists histologic and clinical characteristics of full-thickness, partial-thickness (including deep dermal and shallow), and indeterminant-depth burns.

BURN SIZE

Rapidly estimating the size of a small burn is imperative for effective treatment. To estimate burn size, the clinician should visually superimpose the patient's palm over the burned area, counting the number of "palms" it takes to cover the injury; the palmar area of any given patient is usually 1% of total skin surface. To estimate larger burn areas (>12%), a pediatric modified Lund-Browder chart (Figure 61-1) is useful.

Chart documentation on burn victims must include anatomic mapping of injured areas with estimation of depth and size of BSA burned.

TABLE 61–1. *Initial Characterization of Burn Depth*

Full Thickness

Involves epidermis and entire dermis into fat

Insensate

May appear charred or pale

Partial Thickness

Deep Dermal
Dermal appendages spared on histologic evaluation. Cannot be determined clinically.

Pale with some erythematous spots

May be insensate or very painful

Shallow
Epidermis and only superficial layers of dermis involved.

Epidermis, although burned, may be partly retained, not exposing dermis.

Dermis where exposed is erythematous and painful.

Most epidermis will be gone within 36 hours.

Indeterminate

This category acknowledges that it is not always possible in the emergency department to determine the depth of all areas of a burn topography. Depth may be more accurately assessed in the following 24–36 hours.

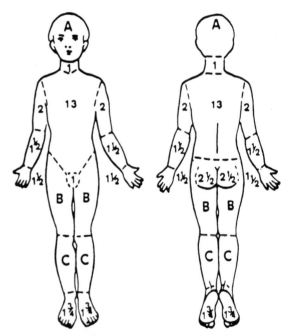

Percentage of surface area of head and legs at various ages.

Area in Diagram	Age in Years				
	0	1	5	10	15
A = ½ of head	9½	8½	6½	5½	4½
B = ½ of one thigh	2¾	3¼	4	4¼	4½
C = ½ of one lower leg	2½	2½	2¾	3	3¼

FIGURE 61–1. Modified Lund-Browder chart. Estimations of burn size must take patient age into account.

INHALATION INJURY

The clinician should suspect smoke inhalation and carbon monoxide poisoning (see Chapter 71) when a burn occurs in a closed space. Cyanide poisoning may also be present (see Chapter 76). Carbonaceous sputum is a *sine qua non* finding for smoke inhalation. Singed nasal hairs, circumoral burns, hoarseness, and wheezing breath sounds are all suggestive but notoriously variable physical findings. Erythema of visible oral pharynx, dyspnea, and secretions with sputum flecked with black carbon provide the strongest physical evidence. These findings should prompt consideration of prophylactic intubation.

All patients with inhalation history should receive 100% oxygen for presumptive carbon monoxide poisoning until carboxyhemoglobin concentrations exclude this diagnosis. Other ED studies include arterial blood gas measurements and chest X-rays.

ELECTRICAL INJURY

Clinical findings in electrical injury vary widely, ranging from mild local injury to life-threatening multisystem destruction. The infant who sucks on an electric plug in a home outlet usually exhibits a burn to the corner of the mouth involving full-thickness lip (see Chapter 53 and Figure 53-3).

Most electrical injuries display small entry and exit wounds. Extensive internal injury may initially be occult. Assessment includes evaluation of cardiac rhythm, neurologic status, and musculoskeletal integrity. Underlying muscle and visceral damage, including long-bone fractures from clonic contractions, must be excluded, as must also be thrombosis and extremity and intestinal ischemia. Additionally, distal neurovascular status should be checked.

Laboratory evaluation for electrical injury includes complete blood count (CBC), electrolytes, BUN, creatinine, creatinine phosphokinase (CPK) with MB and BB fractions, urinalysis (to check for myoglobin), and ECG. Arterial blood gases may disclose an early base deficit and alert the clinician to extensive internal injury.

Treatment ■

PREHOSPITAL MANAGEMENT

Immediately after a small thermal injury, cool-water application is appropriate; however, such treatment 10 to 20 minutes post-injury increases the risk of vasoconstriction and may increase the zone of necrosis. Therefore, running cool tap water over a burn is rational only in the first minutes after the burn.

Initially apply a dry, sterile dressing or a clean, dry, preferably warm sheet. Air currents moving across denuded areas of dermis cause pain in partial-thickness injuries. Transporting the patient with a wet saline dressing causes increased heat loss and may contribute to dangerous hypothermia.

Field personnel should leave all blisters intact and apply no topical ointments. Provide 100% oxygen by nonrebreather mask if inhalation injury is suspected.

EMERGENCY DEPARTMENT MANAGEMENT

The Major Burn: Resuscitation

A burn exceeding 10% to 12% BSA in the pediatric patient is a "major burn" and should be managed aggressively (Table 61-2).

Airway and breathing adequacy are the first priorities. Signs of airway injury necessitate early prophylactic intubation before hypoxia, hypercapnea, and respiratory failure develop. Airway edema may render late intubation impossible. Patients not intubated should receive 100% high-flow oxygen by nonrebreather mask to increase carbon monoxide elimination. Carboxyhemoglobin levels, arterial blood gas measurements, and bedside pulse oximetry, combined with careful clinical evaluation and constant monitoring for respiratory distress, are the most important ED guides to the level of intervention required. Steroids are contraindicated.

Fluid resuscitation is indicated to treat hypovolemia and prevent florid burn shock. After burn depth and size have been estimated in the ED, initial IV rates must be established based on total area of second- and third-degree burns (Table 61-2). *The initial estimated fluid requirement for the first 24 hours are 3–4 ml/percent of total BSA involved/kg.* This formula serves only as a guide for calculating the initial hourly IV rate; actual infusion rates are adjusted based on measures of perfusion.

Half-hourly and hourly monitoring of urine output provides the best method for evaluating fluid needs. An indwelling Foley catheter is mandatory for titrating total IV rate to achieve 1–2 ml urine output/kg/hour.

TABLE 61–2. *Resuscitation for Burned Children*

1. Intubate early.
2. Administer 100% oxygen by nonrebreather mask or endotracheal tube.
3. Initiate fluid bolus: 10–20 ml/kg crystalloid.
4. Maintain fluid requirements: 3–4 ml/kg/day/ percentage body surface area burned.
5. Titrate fluids to urine output:
   2–2.5 ml/kg/hr infants
   1 ml/kg/hr children

Urine output in this range ensures adequate tissue perfusion. The IV rate must be titrated to physiologic parameters and may vary in children.

Once burn size approaches 30–40% BSA, at least two secure, large-bore, indwelling IV catheters must be started.

The fluid of choice for major ED resuscitations is Ringer's lactate, Plasmalyte, or any isotonic fluid; these closely resemble what is lost in burn blisters. Although capillaries lose some protein, exogenous protein from colloid solutions cannot be expected to stay in the vascular space. Morbidity and mortality rates for comparable burn injuries are equal when treated with either crystalloid or colloid.

Escharotomy is rarely required, but a burn surgeon must evaluate the need for it in all major burns. When consultation is not promptly available and an extremity or thorax burn is full-thickness circumferential, the emergency physician may be forced to perform escharotomy. This should be done in the volar-dorsal plane down into subcutaneous tissue.

Burns in Dangerous Locations ■

The overwhelming majority of pediatric burns are small (less than 1% BSA). Their seriousness, however, depends upon *location* in addition to BSA and depth. Pediatric facial burns tend to swell later. Neck burns tend to macerate and carry significant contracture potential. Burns to the feet, perineum, and hands and circumferential extremity burns are difficult to clean, debride, and dress. These require burn surgeon consultation, inpatient care, and early physical therapy.

BURNS SUITABLE FOR OUTPATIENT MANAGEMENT

Most burns seen in the ED can be cared for safely and properly on an outpatient basis, using the approach outlined in Table 61-3.

Outpatient Dressings

Burn injuries suitable for outpatient management may be dressed in an "open" or "closed" method. In the "open" method, apply silver sulfadiazine to a fine-mesh gauze; the gauze holds the topical antimicrobial in apposition to the wound surface. A dry, bulky dressing is optional. Silver sulfadiazine is effective for eight hours. For outpatient care, dressing changes every eight hours are optimal, but 12–24-hour changes are acceptable.

Table 61–3. *Outpatient Burn Therapy*

1. Wash the wound, debride larger blisters, and cover with a dry, sterile Kerlex wrap and bulky dressing. Splint or immobilize extremities.
2. Leave most blisters intact. They will burst spontaneously under an occlusive dressing. Blister fluid is rich in immunoglobulins and does not become an infection risk for days. The pain caused by unnecessary debridement, especially in children, does not warrant immediate, mandatory blister removal.
3. Administer any necessary tetanus toxoid boosters for all burns. Determine completeness of the initial immunization series and time since last booster (Chapter 138). Systemic oral or parenteral antibiotics are *not* indicated at initial presentation. During the first post-injury hours, the wound may be lightly colonized but is certainly not infected when seen fresh. Only a gentle cleansing with warm saline solutions or light soaps such as dilute Ivory and a clean dressing are necessary.
4. The burn need not necessarily be treated with silver sulfadiazine.
5. A surgical consultant should assess all electrical injuries. Electrical injuries destroy more tissue than first appearances suggest, and patients should generally be admitted to monitor for late sequelae.
6. Schedule follow-up for the next day, preferably with a physician with burn interest and experience.

The "closed" method is based upon the recognition that outpatient burns heal most efficiently if simply kept clean and protected. Small burns do not require topical antibiotics. Apply a lightly impregnated petrolatum gauze or fine-mesh gauze moistened in saline to small intact blisters or unroofed blisters. Wrap the wound in dry, bulky, but comfortable sterile gauze dressings. The gauze should be thick enough to allow drainage into but not through the dressing. Elastic webbing may be applied over the bulky dressing. The dressing may be left intact for 48 hours, at which time the patient must return for follow-up care.

If the patient exhibits no fever, no pain by history, no adjacent erythema, and no proximal lymphadenopathy, the bulky dressing may be left intact for another five days. Schedule a return visit for that time, and inspect the wound during that visit.

By the fifth day, small burn wounds carry little risk of infection or conversion to deeper injury. At this time, evidence of healing should be visible. A similar occlusive dressing may be applied for another five days. Healthy individuals should experience complete healing within two weeks.

LATE-PRESENTING BURN WOUNDS: COMPLICATIONS AND CAVEATS

Many burn wounds present initially to the ED four to seven days post-injury. At four to seven days, many burns become soupy and develop yellow-green drainage. This drainage is merely a mixture of burn transudate and topical antimicrobial compound. The wound edges reveal slight hyperemia measured in millimeters. Concerns regarding these wounds include the potential for deeper tissue loss and the presence of incipient sepsis.

Infected, deteriorating, late-presenting burn wounds manifest with systemic symptoms that accompany the ugly local wound. Fever, anorexia, depressed mental status, listlessness, and signs of dehydration indicate a serious, complicated wound. Low-grade fevers (less than 100°F) occur commonly in uncomplicated wounds.

Fortunately, most questionable wounds that present on the fourth to seventh day are usually still good healing wounds. Often they have not been dressed with enough absorbent cotton, or the dressings have not been changed often enough with silver sulfadi-

azine. The transudate-antimicrobial combination may appear as pus. Also, silver sulfadiazine may fade exposed dermis to a white shade, making it appear suspiciously pale and avascular and mimicking a full-thickness wound.

A child with a four- to seven-day-old wound who appears alert and healthy without systemic signs of toxicity should receive mild analgesia/sedation. The physician may then gently wash the wound with warm saline and perform a gauze-like warm washcloth debridement of the pus-like fluid over the burn. A thin layer of soft yellow eschar may also be gently rubbed off in this manner. Following removal of the soupy material, pink re-epithelialization is usually evident. If no exposed fat, no bleeding granulation, and no extended erythema of the wound margins are evident, then the wound is probably healing naturally. It should be rewrapped with absorbent cotton gauze or Telfa with enough outer absorbing layers to contain potentially forming transudate and move it away from the wound surface. Consultation is advisable, and patient follow-up with a burn surgeon within 24–48 hours is indicated.

If any symptoms or indications of systemic toxicity are present, initiate an IV line and arrange transfer or admission to a burn center. A child's ability to take liquids and nutrition after sustaining a thermal injury is a critical parameter for suspecting early systemic toxicity. Again, if in doubt, it is wiser to admit.

Treatment of early superficial infection and prompt excision of necrotic tissue, with autografting when possible, are the current mainstays of serious burn wound management, decreasing morbidity and mortality and improving late functional and cosmetic results.

TABLE 61–4. *Admission Guidelines for Burned Children*

More than 10% body surface area
More than 5% full-thickness burns
Location
  Face
  Neck
  Both hands
  Both feet
  Perineum
Burn types
  Inhalation
  Electrical
  Chemical
  Circumferential
Associated injuries
  Disabling soft-tissue trauma
  Fractures
  Head injury
Complicating medical conditions
  Diabetes
  Heart disease
  Pulmonary disease
Social problems
  Child abuse
  Neglect
  Homelessness

Disposition ■

As a general rule, pediatric burns exceeding 10% BSA, smaller burns involving the face, neck, hands, feet, or perineum, circumferential burns, electrical burns, inhalation injuries, and any suspected intentional burns require admission or transfer to the care of a burn surgeon, preferably within a burn center.

If criteria for admission, as listed in Table 61-4, are not met, the patient may receive outpatient management as described.

No burn treatment is as effective as prevention. Water at 136°F, not uncommon in household water heaters, causes full-thickness skin loss within 10 seconds of constant exposure. Simply lowering water heater temperatures prevents many burn injuries.

Other prevention measures include installing outlet covers, placing electrical units away from water sources, and turning pan handles away from the edge of the stove.

Bibliography ■

Burke JF, Quinby WC Jr, Bondoc CC: Primary excision and prompt grafting as routine therapy for the treatment of thermal burns in children. *Surg Clin North Am* 1976; 56(2):477–494.

Durtschi MB, Kohler TR, Finley A, et al: Burn injury in infants and young children. *Surg Gynecol Obstet* 1980; 150:651–656.

Feldman KW, Schaller RT, Feldman JA, et al: Tap water scald burns in children. *Pediatrics* 1978; 62:1–7.

Graves TA, Cioffi WG, McManus WF, et al: Fluid resuscitation of infants and children with massive thermal injury. *J Trauma* 1988; 28:1656–1659.

Heimbach DM, Engrav LH: *Surgical management of the burn wound.* New York: Raven Press, 1984.

Showers J, Garrison KM: Burn abuse: A four-year study. *J Trauma* 1988; 28:1581–1583.

Shuck JM: Outpatient management of the burned patient. *Surg Clin North Am* 1978; 58(6):1107–1117.

Solomon JR: Pediatric burns. *Critical Care Clinics* 1985; 1(Mar):159–173.

62 Wound Care

D. Demetrios Zukin and Jonathan Grisham

Wounds are common pediatric emergencies. Lacerations, punctures, abrasions, and embedded foreign bodies are universal problems in childhood. Simple wound care requires both functional and cosmetic considerations.

Mechanisms of Injury and Pathophysiology ■

CLASSIFICATION OF LACERATIONS

There are three types of lacerations. The first type is a *shear* laceration and is caused when the skin is cut by a sharp object, such as glass or a knife. Shear lacerations are generally clean, with straight edges and little damage to the surrounding tissues. The second type is a *tension* laceration, caused by a blow to the skin, without a bone immediately below the surface. Tension lacerations tend to have irregular edges as well as increased damage to the tissue immediately adjacent to the wound edge. The third type is a *compression* laceration, which occurs when the skin is crushed between a bone and a hard surface, as occurs when a child falls and strikes the forehead against the floor. Compression lacerations have increased infection potential and tend to heal with more scarring than shear or tension wounds.

FACTORS AFFECTING WOUND INFECTION RATES

Several factors affect the wound infection rate. Highly vascular regions, such as the face and scalp, are more resistant to infection. Extremities are most frequently infected. Shear lacerations have a lower infection rate than compression injuries. Extremity wounds repaired within six hours of the time of injury and facial wounds repaired within 12 hours have a lower infection rate than when wound repair is delayed. Suturing technique also influences the infection rate: wounds with tight sutures and wounds with inverted edges are more prone to infection. Wounds that are grossly contaminated, such as those resulting from animal or human bites, have higher infection rates than clean wounds.

Clinical Findings ■

The assessment of a child with an open wound must first exclude more serious, sometimes occult pathophysiology from injury to vital structures, as outlined in Chapter 48.

The history should include allergies, medications, medical illnesses, last meal, and the time and mechanism of the injury. Document the patient's tetanus status, and provide tetanus prophylaxis as recommended by the Centers for Disease Control (Table 62-1). In an unimmunized patient, give both tetanus immune globulin (250 IU given IM) and tetanus toxoid (0.5 ml IM) for tetanus-prone wounds such as puncture wounds and suturable lacerations.

Physical assessment of wounds must evaluate the status of the circulation, motor function, and sensation of the injured area. *The sensory-motor examination must precede the administration of local anesthesia.* Patients with major or complicated injuries (i.e., those involving nerves, tendons, or arteries) and uncooperative young children should be made NPO upon presentation to the ED because sedation or general anesthesia may be required.

Further evaluation of the extent of the wound occurs during cleaning, irrigation, and debridement. When obvious sensory-motor deficits or musculotendinous disruptions are found during the exploration of deep lacerations, it is unnecessary and unwise to proceed in the ED, since these cases will usually require operative repair; manipulation in the ED may introduce further infection risk. Once the need for further consultation for operative closure is established, close the wound with sterile dressings and do not disturb it further.

Table 62-2 outlines the basic steps in wound evaluation and treatment.

TABLE 62–1. *Tetanus Prophylaxis*

	Tetanus Toxoid Immunizations	Requires Tetanus Toxoid	Requires Tetanus Immune Globulin
Clean Wounds *(Clean, superficial abrasions and lacerations)*	Three or more, last within 10 yr	No	No
	Three or more, last within >10 yr	Yes	No
	Fewer than three or unknown	Yes	No
Tetanus-Prone Wounds *(Contaminated deep punctures, tenuous blood supply, sutured lacerations)*	Three or more, last within 5 yr	No	No
	Three or more, last within >5 yr	Yes	No
	Fewer than three or unknown	Yes	Yes

Techniques for Wound Repair ■

MATERIALS

Sutures

Table 62-3 summarizes the properties of various suture materials. Table 62-4 lists recommended sutures for various anatomic wound sites.

Needles

Manufacturers place a life-size picture of the needle on the suture package. For most lacerations, choose a ⅜-circle needle. The half-circle is useful for the web spaces between fingers and toes.

Needles come with various cross-sectional configurations. The type most commonly used for wound repair is the cutting needle, which has a triangular configuration with the apex of the triangle honed to a sharp edge. Taper needles, with a circular configuration, have difficulty passing through the epidermis.

Forceps

The design may be smooth or rat-toothed. Toothed forceps cause less crushing of skin because less pressure is required to secure the skin edge.

Skin Hooks

Skin hooks cause less tissue damage than forceps, but hooks also afford less control of the wound edge than forceps.

Needle Holders

Hold the suture needle with the needle holder at the junction of the middle and proximal thirds, near to where the suture attaches to the needle. Needle holders have either smooth or corrugated surfaces. Smooth is best for use with small needles. Learn to "palm" the needle holder, aiming the index finger toward the needle, rather than placing the fingers in the finger holes, for better accuracy and control.

Scissors

Iris scissors are best for minor excisions and debridement along the wound edges.

Scalpel Blades

#10: large, cutting surface on belly, for making deep incisions.

#11: pointed tip. Cutting surface on the tip, for lancing abscesses, or for marking out a region for debridement.

#15: small, curved blade, with the cutting surface on the distal portion of the curve.

SEDATION

Any agent that will adequately sedate a child for laceration repair may cause apnea. Therefore, withhold sedation when possible. Instead, gain the patient's cooperation by carefully explaining what is going to take place, enlisting the assistance of the parent or caretaker when possible, ensuring complete local anesthesia, and using a gentle approach. Patients who fight during local anesthesia administration often fall asleep during the actual suturing. A papoose board is useful, especially with uncooperative toddlers.

In the patient who is too uncooperative to permit wound repair despite the above steps, chemical sedation may be needed. Useful agents include meperidine 1–2 mg/kg IM; midazolam 0.1 mg IM; or fentanyl 2 micrograms/kg IV. Fentanyl has the ad-

TABLE 62–2. *Steps in Wound Care*

Step	Hints and Cautions
Examine the patient	Include sensory, motor, and perfusion exam.
	Consider child abuse if physical findings are not consistent with history.
Sedation/papoose	Usually not necessary; local anesthesia and immobilization usually suffice.
	All parenteral sedatives have the potential for causing apnea.
Local anesthesia	It is less painful to inject through the wound edge than through intact skin.
	The usual dose is 0.4 ml/kg of 1% lidocaine (4 mg/kg).
	Raise a wheal at the wound edges.
Irrigation	Normal saline is the irrigation solution of choice.
	Use a 20-ml syringe, and an 18 g angiocath.
	Always wear protective mask and goggles.
Topical antisepsis	Apply dilute Betadine solution (*not* the cytotoxic detergent scrub) directly into the open wound, and then paint surrounding intact skin.
Trim the wound edges	Use either a sharp iris scissors or a #15 scalpel.
	Never shave the eyebrows.
Close the wound	Use nylon (Ethicon, Dermalon) or prolene for the skin.
	Use Dexon or Vycril for the deep layer.
	Perform a layered closure on the face whenever possible. Never put deep sutures into the hand.
Bandage the wound	Keep the wound clean and covered.
	Splint areas of motion, such as knees, elbows, and hands.
Wound check	For infection-prone wounds, have the patient return for a wound check in 2 days (1 day for bites).
Suture removal	Remove sutures relatively early (4 days for facial lacerations) and then reinforce the wound for an additional 1–2 weeks with skin tape.

vantage of being short-acting and reversible with naloxone. Ideally, patients should be NPO prior to sedation, should have both cardiac and respiratory monitors during sedation, and should be discharged only after they can sit without support, talk, and walk with minimal assistance (or, for infants, once they have returned to their presedation level of consciousness). Sedation should only be deep enough to make suturing possible, in conjunction with physical immobilization.

LOCAL ANESTHESIA

Local Infiltration

Whenever possible, use local anesthesia before irrigation, for the sake of the patient's comfort. There is no greater infection rate injecting through the open wound edge as compared to through the intact skin,

and it is much less painful to the patient. For soiled wounds it is necessary, however, to irrigate prior to anesthetic administration.

Choose an appropriate anesthetic agent, as outlined in Table 62-5. Raise a wheal in the dermis. An anesthetic instilled into the subcutaneous fat will drip out of the wound and will not give adequate anesthesia.

For most purposes, 1% lidocaine is adequate. A 2% solution is useful for regional blocks where a diffusion gradient is needed. Ensure there is no history of allergy to local anesthetics.

TAC

TAC is a mixture of tetracaine, adrenaline, and cocaine that serves as an effective topical anesthetic for minor skin wounds. A common formulation is 0.5% tetracaine, 1:2,000 topical epinephrine, and 11.8%

TABLE 62–3. *Suture Materials*

	Material	Properties
Absorbable Sutures	Vicryl and Dexon (polyglycolic acid)	Lowest infection rates of absorbables, because breakdown products inhibit bacterial growth. Lowest tissue reactivity of absorbables. Good tensile strength. Braided, so hold knots well, but makes gradual cinching down of ties more difficult. Can take 40 or more days to absorb, but usually lose tensile strength within 14 days. Come both dyed and undyed. For emergency-department use, *choose undyed.*
	Plain gut	Most tissue reactivity of the absorbables. Higher infection potential than Vicryl or Dexon. Absorbs in 4–8 days, so useful where rapid absorption required, such as inside the mouth.
	Chromic gut	Greater tensile strength and lower infection potential than plain gut. Slower absorption than plain gut.
	Fast-absorbing gut (Ethicon)	Specifically made for skin sutures in children where suture removal may be difficult. Fast-absorbing gut loses most of its strength by day 5, and can be plucked from the wound without the use of scissors or scalpel.
Nonabsorbable Sutures	Silk	The standard for all sutures in terms of ease of use and conformity to tissue contours. Unfortunately, silk, being a foreign protein, induces more tissue reaction and has a higher infection potential than nylon or Prolene.
	Nylon (Ethylon and Dermalon)	Monofilament. Low tissue reactivity, low infection rate. Suitable for most emergency-department wounds. Knots tend to unravel; use 4–5 throws per knot.
	Polypropylene (Prolene)	Monofilament. Similar tissue reactivity and infection potential to nylon, but slightly easier to handle.

cocaine. Usually 4–10 ml applied with pressure over ten minutes with a soaked 2"×2" gauze will achieve adequate anesthesia. It works best on face and scalp.

Use TAC with caution for small skin lacerations. *It must never be applied to mucosal surfaces* because of high absorption rates and the possibility of serious untoward consequences, including seizures and death from cocaine toxicity.

TABLE 62–4. *Suture Chart*

Region	Suture[1]	Suture Removal[2]
Face	**Skin:** 6-0 nylon or prolene	4 days
	Deep: 5-0 Vycril or dexon	
Scalp	3-0, 4-0, or 5-0 nylon or prolene	5–7 days
	Galea: 2-0 Vycril or Dexon	
Hand	5-0 or 6-0 nylon or Prolene; **No deep sutures**	Joint, 10–14 days; other, 7–10 days
Extremities	**Skin:** 4-0 or 5-0 nylon or Prolene	Joint, 10–14 days; other, 7–10 days
	Deep: 4-0 Vycril or Dexon	
Trunk	**Skin:** 4-0 or 5-0 nylon or Prolene	7 days
	Deep: 4-0 Vycril or Dexon	
Oral mucosa and tongue	6-0 Vycril or Dexon or 4-0 or 5-0 plain gut	Absorbable

[1] Skin sutures: those selected to close the upper layer of a two-layer closure; deep sutures: those selected to close the lower layer of a two-layer closure.
[2] Because of the low tensile strength of the wound during the first 10–20 days, lacerations on the face and over joints should be reinforced with skin tape following suture removal.

TABLE 62–5. *Local Anesthetic Chart*

Lidocaine (without epi) 4 mg/kg (0.4 ml/kg 1% solution)

Lidocaine (with epi)[1] 7 mg/kg (0.7 ml/kg 1% solution)

Marcaine (bupivacaine)[2] (1.25 mg/kg (0.5 ml/kg) 0.25%)

---

[1] *Do Not* use anesthetic *with epinephrine* for the hands, feet, penis, tip or bridge of nose, or tip of ears.

[2] Longer acting than lidocaine, but not yet approved for use in infants and young children. Cardiotoxic in overdosage; avoid inadvertent IV push.

REGIONAL BLOCK

Regional block consists of anesthetizing the nerve that supplies the larger anatomic area. A commonly used block is the digital nerve block for finger lacerations. Regional blocks are an ideal means of providing local anesthesia because there is no edema or deformity in the area to be sutured.

Wound Preparation ■

HAIR REMOVAL

Most lacerations require no hair removal. For scalp wounds some hair removal is sometimes needed if the hair cannot be kept out of the surgical field. Hair can also be kept out of the field by taping it with paper tape, or by applying Lubrifax. There is no difference in the infection rates in scalp lacerations treated with or without hair removal. *Never shave the eyebrows:* they are slow to grow back, and serve as valuable landmarks during suturing.

IRRIGATION

Forceful (7 psi of pressure) irrigation of wounds effectively washes away both bacteria and foreign material from soiled wounds. Use protective goggles and masks during irrigation to protect against body substance exposures (e.g., hepatitis virus or HIV). *Proper wound irrigation is the best way to prevent infection.* The best method for irrigating soiled lacerations is to fit a 20- or 30-ml syringe with a 16- or 18-gauge catheter and press firmly on the plunger to direct the flow of solution directly into the wound. Use 100–250 ml of irrigating volume for most suturable wounds. Clean wounds, such as those caused by sharp metal or glass, are generally not as highly soiled and may require less volume. Sterile saline is the irrigating solution of choice because fluids instilled into a wound under pressure are absorbed systemically.

TOPICAL ANTISEPTICS

See Table 62-6. The topical antiseptic of choice for use in the ED is 1% povidone-iodine solution (a 1:10 dilution of the stock 10% Betadine prep solution with aqueous base). Dilute povidone-iodine solution applied for one minute directly into the open wound significantly lowers the wound infection rate without harming the healing process. Unlike the normal saline used for irrigation, the Betadine prep solution is dabbed on with a sterile pledget, not irrigated into the wound under pressure. Then paint the Betadine prep solution on the surrounding intact skin just prior to draping.

Unlike the mild aqueous solution, Betadine Surgical Scrub (povidone-iodine in a harsh detergent base) is highly cytotoxic, as are all detergents, and should *never* be applied to subcutaneous tissues.

DEBRIDEMENT

All foreign material must be removed. In addition, carefully trimming irregular wound edges will result in a finer result. Remove grossly devitalized tissue. Debridement can be carried out with either a scalpel or scissors.

HEMOSTASIS

The following steps are useful for obtaining hemostasis:

1. *Apply direct pressure* for 10 to 20 minutes (remove all clots and foreign bodies).

TABLE 62–6. *Antiseptic Agents*

Agent	Antibacterial Efficacy	Tissue Toxicity
Alcohol (70%)	10	10
Betadine surgical scrub[1]	9	8
pHisoHex[1]	8	8
Hydrogen peroxide	3	5
Quaternary ammonia	6	3
Hexachlorophene solution[2]	8	2
Betadine prep solution[2]	9	1
Shur-Clens (plurionic F-68)	1	0.5
Sterile water	0	0.5
Sterile saline	0	0

[1] A detergent preparation

[2] An aqueous solution

2. *Epinephrine 1:1,000,* 1 ml diluted with 4–5 ml of saline on a 4″ × 4″ gauze, held over the bleeding region for 5 minutes will stop small dermal bleeders. Larger vessels must be ligated, however, because the vasoconstriction is temporary.

3. *Suture the wound.* Very effective in wounds such as scalp lacerations that continue to bleed slowly even after local pressure. The wound must be observed for several minutes for hematoma formation, prior to bandaging.

4. *Locate, clamp, and ligate arterial bleeders.* Pressure over a main artery (such as with a BP cuff inflated proximal to an extremity laceration) may facilitate the ligation of arterial bleeders. Do not inflate the BP cuff more than 20–30 minutes. If more time is required, repair is usually best accomplished in the operating room. Do not ligate arterial bleeders in the hand (or major arteries elsewhere in the body) without first obtaining consultation regarding the possibility of microsurgical repair.

Suturing Technique ■

SKIN SUTURES

Simple Interrupted Sutures

Use monofilament nylon or polypropylene. A key to cosmetic skin closure is to have the edges either lie flat or evert slightly, as opposed to having them fold in. Edge eversion can be obtained by entering the skin at a 90-degree angle rather than at a tangent, as shown in Figure 62-1. In situations where the edges tend to invert despite proper technique, use a vertical mattress suture (see below).

Running Sutures

The running suture is ideal for pediatric wound repair, because it is much quicker than multiple interrupted sutures. In addition, subsequent removal of the sutures is easier with the running stitch. The first loop is made in the same way as the interrupted suture, but then one continues down the wound without cutting and tying until the wound is closed. Figure 62-2 illustrates the technique of tying the final knot.

Vertical Mattress Suture

See Figure 62-3. Because it ensures wound edge eversion, the vertical mattress suture is useful in regions such as the web space between the thumb and index finger, where inversion is often a problem.

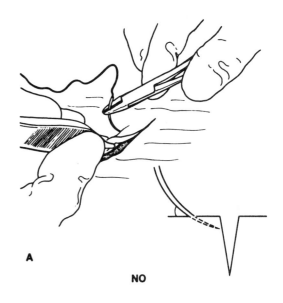

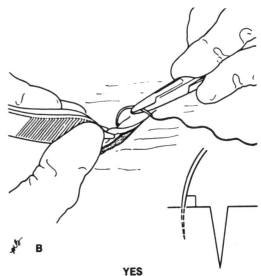

FIGURE 62–1. The simple interrupted suture. (**A**) Do not enter the skin with the needle at a tangent, as this will yield too little tissue at the base of the suture loop. (**B**) The skin should be entered at a 90 degree angle. See text for details. (Reprinted with permission from Zukin DD, Simon RR: Emergency wound care. Rockville, MD: Aspen Publishers, 1987:43.)

Corner Stitch

See Figure 62-4. The corner stitch, or half-buried horizontal mattress, goes through the tips of the skin flaps of stellate lacerations. The suture is placed just below the epidermis, at the dermal-epidermal junc-

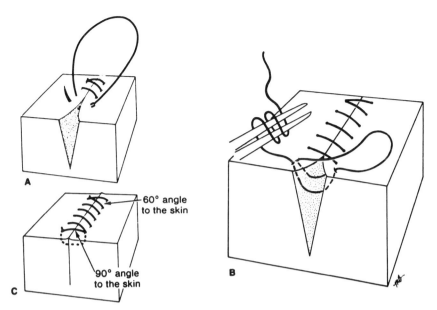

FIGURE 62–2. The running suture. (**A**) Begin with a simple suture at one end of the wound, and then run down the length of the laceration. (**B**) and (**C**) To complete the repair, knot the suture to itself. By using this technique the suture lies diagonally above the skin. (Reprinted with permission from Simon RR, Brenner BE: *Procedures and techniques in emergency medicine.* Baltimore: Williams & Wilkins, 1982:302.)

tion. The half-buried horizontal mattress is a superior means of repairing small flaps because the stitch does not retard the blood flow to the flap (remember that the skin vessels run deep to the dermal-epidermal junction).

Deep or Buried Sutures

A layered closure (i.e., a deep layer and a skin layer) improves the cosmetic outcome in facial lacerations in children. The deep suture serves three vital functions. First, it provides two to three weeks of additional support to the wound after the skin sutures are out. Thus the scar is less likely to widen with time. Second, the deep layer avoids the development of unsightly pitting in the injured region caused by lack of healing of the deep portions of the wound. Third, the deep layer serves to preserve the normal functioning of the muscles of facial expression.

The opposite rule holds true for other parts of the body. In the extremities, and the hand in particular, the deep sutures increase the risk of infection and have the potential of damaging vital nerves, arteries, and tendons.

The most common deep suture for laceration repair is the *buried knot stitch* illustrated in Figure 62-5.

Begin and end at the base of the wound, so as to bury the final knot. In some cases the deep sutures along a wound must all be placed prior to tying, because the tying of one suture can make the placement of the subsequent deep sutures more difficult.

SKIN TAPES (STERI-STRIPS)

Skin tapes are useful for shallow, non-gaping wounds. Tapes are not practical for use in toddlers and young children, who tend to pull them off. Never use Steri-Strips for extensor surface lacerations.

Before applying skin tapes, wait for full hemostasis; tapes will not adhere to moist areas. Next, prepare adjacent skin with tincture of benzoin to enhance sticking. Allow the benzoin to dry and become tacky, then apply the strips.

SKIN STAPLES

Disposable skin staplers are significantly faster for repairing lacerations than conventional sutures because knot-tying is not needed. Staples are ideal for small scalp lacerations. Since the staples are quite thick, if more than one or two are to be placed, use a local anesthetic prior to closure. Disposable staple removers are required.

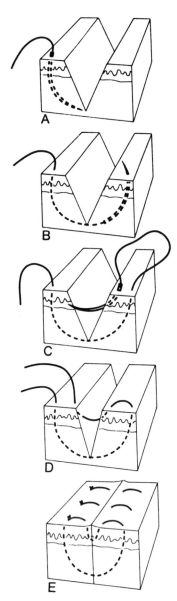

FIGURE 62-3. The vertical mattress suture. (Reprinted with permission from Simon RR, Brenner BE: *Procedures and techniques in emergency medicine.* Baltimore: Williams & Wilkins, 1982:303.)

Aftercare ■

CLEAN DRESSING

Use a three-layered bandage on most wounds. The first layer consists of fine mesh placed directly over the wound. Xeroform gauze is excellent because it does not adhere to the wound as does plain gauze. The second layer consists of 2"×2" or 4"×4" gauze to absorb exudate. The third layer consists of a wrap-around dressing such as Conform® to secure the bandage in place. Slight pressure will aid in hemostasis and decrease local edema.

For small abrasions and lacerations, a conventional Band-Aid will suffice.

ELEVATION

Instruct patients to keep the wounded region elevated when possible, to prevent edema. Use a sling for significant upper extremity wounds.

SPLINTS

Splint lacerations over joints for 7–10 days. Crutches are helpful for lower extremity wounds.

ANTIBIOTICS

Prophylactic antibiotics have not been proved effective in decreasing the incidence of wound infections in simple lacerations. Antibiotics may have a place in certain animal and human bites (see Chapter 93).

WOUND CHECK

In any case with a high potential for infection, the patient should return in 48 hours to be checked for signs of infection. In the case of sutured dog or cat bites, the check should be at 24–36 hours.

SUTURE REMOVAL

See Table 62-4. Unsightly suture marks occur when epithelial cells grow down the tracks of skin sutures. Because these tracks can form on a child's face in as little as five days, prompt removal of facial sutures is needed. Most suture marks regress and disappear with time.

Other Soft-Tissue Injuries ■

ABRASIONS

Anesthetize the surface with topical lidocaine (4%). Be careful about the quantity of lidocaine applied

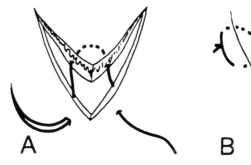

FIGURE 62–4. The corner stitch. Either a half-buried horizontal-mattress suture (**A**) or three simple interrupted sutures (**B**). In both examples, half of the suture lies beneath the skin, in the subcuticular plane (dashed lines). (Reprinted with permission from Simon RR, Brenner BE: *Procedures and techniques in emergency medicine.* Baltimore: Williams & Wilkins, 1982:306.)

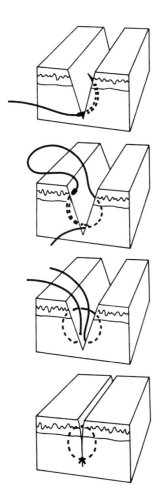

FIGURE 62–5. The buried knot suture. (Reprinted with permission from Simon RR, Brenner BE: *Procedures and techniques in emergency medicine.* Baltimore: Williams & Wilkins, 1982:308.)

because some systemic absorption can occur. Hold the gauze in place for 10 minutes (parents can be helpful in this regard). If there are no contraindications, such as abdominal trauma or head trauma, a dose of Demerol (1–2 mg/kg, IM) may be given 10–20 minutes prior to cleaning a large, painful region (but beware of possible respiratory depression). *Ground-in foreign matter must be removed or else an unsightly "road tattoo" will result.*

Dress abrasions either with a topical antibiotic salve such as Neosporin or Silvadene, or with a semi-occlusive dressing such as Duoderm, Tegaderm, or Xeroform.

FOREIGN BODIES

Embedded glass fragments show up on soft-tissue radiographs of injured regions more than 75% of the time; hence X-rays are indicated to screen for both glass and metallic foreign bodies. Taping a metallic marker (such as a bent paper clip) to the skin before taking the X-ray can aid in locating the object beneath the skin. Ensure there is adequate local anesthesia before probing for the foreign body. Special instruments, such as foreign-body forceps, with tapered blades facilitate foreign-body removal.

PUNCTURE WOUNDS

Puncture wounds may contain foreign material. For example, bits of fabric and plastic may become embedded in the foot when a patient steps on a nail while wearing running shoes. Puncture wounds of the foot deep enough to reach the bone can result in osteomyelitis, often with Pseudomonas as the causative organism.

Bibliography ∎

American Academy of Pediatrics, Committee on Drugs, Section on Anesthesiology: Guidelines for the elective use of conscious sedation, deep sedation, and general anesthesia in pediatric patients. *Pediatrics* 1985; 76:317–321.

Bennett RG: Selection of wound closure materials. *J Am Acad Derm* 1988; 18:619–637.

Dushoff IM: A stitch in time. *Emerg Med* 1988; 20:23:57.

Edlich RF, Rodeheaver GT, Morgan RF, et al: Principles of emergency wound management. *Ann Emerg Med* 1988; 17:1284–1302.

Gravett A, Sterner S, Clinton JE, et al: A trial of povidone-iodine in the prevention of infection in sutured lacerations. *Ann Emerg Med* 1987; 16:167–171.

Zukin DD, Simon RR: *Emergency wound care.* Rockville, Md.: Aspen, 1987.

VIII
Toxicology

63 Emergency Management of Childhood Poisoning

Kent R. Olson and William Banner, Jr.

Drug overdose and poisoning are important problems in pediatrics, accounting for many emergency department visits and hospitalizations. In 1987, of approximately 1.2 million calls to 63 poison control centers participating in a national data collection program, 731,954 (60%) involved children under age 5; 22 of these children died, and 107,844 others became ill. Of 4,740 unintentional poisoning deaths in 1986 reported by the Centers for Disease Control, 93 were in children under five, 24 were in children 5–9 years old, and 249 were in the age group 10–19.

The next several chapters provide practical advice on the rapid assessment and treatment of acute childhood poisoning or drug overdose.

The Asymptomatic Patient ■

The asymptomatic patient may have been exposed to or ingested a lethal dose of a poison and not yet have any manifestations of toxicity. Therefore, it is always important to:

Quickly assess the potential danger
Perform decontamination to prevent absorption
Observe the patient for an appropriate interval.

If the toxin is known, the potential danger can be assessed by consulting a text or computerized information resource (e.g., Poisindex) or by calling a regional poison control center (Table 63-1). Risk assessment will generally take into account the dose ingested (in mg/kg), the time interval since ingestion, and the presence of any clinical signs or elevated serum levels of the toxin. Be aware that the history given by the patient or family may be unreliable.

The choice of gastric decontamination procedure depends on the toxin (see Chapter 64 for more discussion of methods). Generally, if the ingestion occurred within 15–20 minutes, and if there are no contraindications, induce emesis with ipecac syrup.

The Symptomatic Patient ■

The following complications may occur, depending on the type of poisoning.

COMA

The most common cause of death in comatose patients is respiratory failure (hypoventilation or apnea), which may occur abruptly. Pulmonary aspiration of gastric contents may also occur, especially in victims who are comatose or convulsing. Respiratory failure may cause or aggravate other complications such as arrhythmias, hypotension, and seizures. Protection of the airway and assisted ventilation are the most important interventions in any poisoned patient.

Airway

Establish a patent airway by proper positioning, suction, and an artificial nasal or oropharyngeal airway. If the patient is deeply comatose, or if there is no gag or cough reflex, perform endotracheal intubation. These airway interventions may be unnecessary if the patient is intoxicated by an opioid and responds rapidly to IV naloxone (see below).

Breathing

Clinically assess the quality and depth of respiration, and provide assistance if necessary with a bag-valve-mask device or mechanical ventilator. Administer supplemental oxygen. The arterial carbon dioxide tension measured by blood gases is useful in determining the adequacy of ventilation. The arterial oxygen tension may reveal hypoxemia, which may be caused by respiratory arrest, bronchospasm, pulmonary aspiration, or non-cardiogenic pulmonary edema.

TABLE 63–1. *AAPCC Certified Regional Poison Control Centers*

The American Association of Poison Control Centers (AAPCC) is a nationally recognized body that has certified 36 regional poison centers as meeting their minimum operating criteria. Regional poison control centers operate 24 hours a day using specially trained and dedicated staff with access to a variety of texts, files, and computerized poison information resources. They can also provide immediate telephone consultation with a physician specializing in medical toxicology. The following is a list of certified regional poison control centers in the USA by state:

State	Poison Center	Phone Number	State	Poison Center	Phone Number
Alabama	Children's Hospital of Alabama Regional Poison Control Center, Birmingham	(800) 292-6678 (205) 933-4050	Minnesota	Hennepin Regional Poison Center, Minneapolis	(612) 347-3141
				Minnesota Regional Poison Center, St. Paul	(800) 222-1222 (612) 221-2113
Arizona	Arizona Poison and Drug Information Center, Tucson	(800) 362-0101 (602) 626-6016	Missouri	Cardinal Glennon Children's Hospital Regional Poison Center, St. Louis	(800) 392-9111 (314) 772-5200
	Samaritan Regional Poison Center, Phoenix	(602) 253-3334			
			Montana	Rocky Mountain Poison and Drug Center, Denver, CO	(800) 525-5042
California	Fresno Regional Poison Control Center, Fresno	(800) 346-5922 (209) 445-1222			
	Los Angeles County Medical Association Regional Poison Control Center, Los Angeles	(800) 82-LAPCC (213) 664-2121	Nebraska	Mid-Plains Poison Center, Omaha	(800) 642-9999 (402) 390-5400
			New Jersey	New Jersey Poison Information and Education System, Newark	(800) 962-1253 (201) 923-0764
	San Diego Regional Poison Center, UCSD Medical Center, San Diego	(800) 876-4766 (619) 543-6000	New Mexico	New Mexico Poison and Drug Information Center, Albuquerque	(800) 432-6866 (505) 843-2551
	San Francisco Bay Area Regional Poison Center, San Francisco	(800) 523-2222 (415) 476-6600	New York	Long Island Regional Poison Control Center, East Meadow	(516) 542-2323
	UC-Davis Medical Center Regional Poison Center, Sacramento	(800) 342-9293 (916) 734-3692		New York City Poison Control Center, New York City	(212) 340-4494 (212) 764-7667
Colorado	Rocky Mountain Poison and Drug Center, Denver	(800) 332-3073 (303) 629-1123	Ohio	Central Ohio Poison Center, Columbus	(800) 682-7625 (614) 228-1323
Florida	Florida Poison Information Center, Tampa	(800) 282-3171 (813) 253-4444		Regional Poison Control System and Drug and Poison Information Center, Cincinnati	(800) 872-5111 (513) 558-5111
Georgia	Georgia Poison Control Center, Altanta	(800) 282-5846 (404) 589-4400			
Kentucky	Kentucky Regional Poison Center, Louisville	(800) 722-5725 (502) 589-8222	Oregon	Oregon Poison Center, Portland	(800) 452-7165 (503) 279-8968
Maryland	Maryland Poison Center, Baltimore	(800) 492-2414 (301) 528-7701	Pennsylvania	Delaware Valley Regional Poison Center, Philadelphia	(215) 386-2100
Massachusetts	Massachusetts Poison Control System, Boston	(800) 682-9211 (617) 232-2120		Pittsburgh Poison Center, Pittsburgh	(412) 681-6669
Michigan	Blodgett Regional Poison Center, Grand Rapids	(800) 632-2727 (616) 774-7851			
	Poison Control Center, Children's Hospital of Michigan, Detroit	(800) 462-6642 (313) 745-5711	Rhode Island	Rhode Island Poison Center, Rhode Island Hospital, Providence	(401) 277-5727

(From American Association of Poison Control Centers. March 1990)

(*continued*)

TABLE 63–1. *AAPCC Certified Regional Poison Control Centers* (*continued*)

The American Association of Poison Control Centers (AAPCC) is a nationally recognized body that has certified 36 regional poison centers as meeting their minimum operating criteria. Regional poison control centers operate 24 hours a day using specially trained and dedicated staff with access to a variety of texts, files, and computerized poison information resources. They can also provide immediate telephone consultation with a physician specializing in medical toxicology. The following is a list of certified regional poison control centers in the USA by state:

State	Poison Center	Phone Number	State	Poison Center	Phone Number
Texas	North Texas Poison Center, Dallas	(800) 441-0040 (214) 590-5000	Washington, D.C.	National Capitol Poison Center, Washington, D.C.	(202) 625-3333
	Texas State Poison Center, Galveston Houston Austin	(800) 392-8548 (409) 765-9728 (713) 654-1701 (512) 478-4490	West Virginia	West Virginia Poison Center, Charleston	(800) 642-3625 (304) 348-4211
Utah	Intermountain Regional Poison Center, Salt Lake City	(800) 456-7707 (801) 581-2151	Wyoming	Rocky Mountain Poison and Drug Center, Denver, CO	(800) 442-2702

Circulation

Measure the pulse and blood pressure, and estimate tissue perfusion (e.g., measurement of urinary output, skin signs, blood pH). Insert an IV line and draw blood for routine (blood count, glucose, electrolytes) and toxicologic testing.

Dextrose, Thiamine, and Naloxone

Unless promptly treated, severe hypoglycemia causes irreversible brain damage. In all comatose or convulsing children, give 25% dextrose 2 ml/kg IV, unless a rapid bedside blood sugar test rules out hypoglycemia. In poorly nourished patients who may have marginal thiamine stores, give thiamine 50 mg IM or IV.

Naloxone, 0.4–2 mg IV, may reverse opioid-induced respiratory depression and coma (note that these are much higher doses than previously recommended). If opioid overdose is strongly suspected, give additional doses of naloxone (up to 5–10 mg may be required). Caution: Naloxone has a short duration of action (2–3 hours); repeated doses may be required and continuous observation for several hours is mandatory.

See Tables 63-2, 63-3, 63-4, and Chapter 20.

HYPOTENSION

Hypotension may be caused by venodilation, arteriolar vasodilation, depressed cardiac contractility, or a combination of these effects. Most patients respond to empiric treatment with IV fluid boluses (normal saline or other isotonic crystalloid, or colloids, 20 ml/kg once or twice). Caution: Do not give hypotonic fluids such as 0.25 NS or 5% dextrose, as these may cause severe hyponatremia. If fluid therapy is unsuccessful, infuse dopamine IV 5–15 mcg/kg/min.

For hypotension caused by a cyclic antidepressant overdose, administer sodium bicarbonate 1–2 mEq/kg IV bolus (see Chapter 77). For beta-blocker over-

TABLE 63–2. *Initial Management of Coma*

A   Airway Control

B   Breathing

C   Circulation

D   Dextrose 25%, 2 ml/kg IV

    Thiamine, 50–100 mg IM or IV

    Naloxone, 0.4–2 mg IV

TABLE 63–3. *Common Drugs/Poisons Causing Coma*

Ethanol
Cyclic antidepressants
Phenothiazines
Opioids
Barbiturates
Benzodiazepines
Clonidine
Antihistamines

TABLE 63–4. *Important "Rule-Outs" in Coma*

Head trauma or other intracranial mass lesion
Hyperglycemia, hypoglycemia
Hypernatremia, hyponatremia
Hyperthermia, hypothermia
Hypoxemia
Shock
Infection (encephalitis, meningitis)

TABLE 63–6. *Common Drugs/Poisons Causing Hypertension*

Phenylpropanolamine
Ephedrine and pseudoephedrine
MAO inhibitor interactions
Cocaine and amphetamines
Phencyclidine (PCP)

dose, administer glucagon 0.1 mg/kg IV bolus (see Chapter 69). For calcium antagonist overdose, administer calcium chloride 25 mg/kg IV (maximum 1 gram) (see Chapter 70).

See Table 63-5.

HYPERTENSION

Severe hypertension (e.g., after phenylpropanolamine overdose) can produce acute intracranial hemorrhage. Treat hypertension if the diastolic pressure is greater than 100–105 mm Hg or the systolic pressure is greater than 160–170 mm Hg, or if the child has a systolic blood pressure above the 95th percentile for age and manifests end-organ injury from hypertension (see Chapter 11). Administer phentolamine 0.01–0.05 mg/kg IV or nitroprusside 0.5–5 ug/kg/min IV. If excessive tachycardia is present, add propranolol 0.01–0.05 mg/kg IV or esmolol 25–50 μg/kg/min IV. Do *not* give beta blockers alone, as this may paradoxically worsen hypertension.

See Table 63-6 and Chapter 11.

ARRHYTHMIAS

Arrhythmias are often caused by hypoxemia or electrolyte imbalance, and these problems should be treated. If ventricular arrhythmias persist, lidocaine or phenytoin are usually effective. Caution: avoid Type Ia (quinidine, procainamide, disopyramide)

TABLE 63–5. *Common Drugs/Poisons Causing Hypotension*

Opioids
Clonidine
Antihypertensives
Phenothiazines
Cyclic antidepressants
Calcium antagonists
Beta blockers
Iron

agents, as these may aggravate arrhythmias caused by cyclic antidepressants, calcium antagonists, or beta blockers. For tachyarrhythmias induced by sympathomimetic agents, use propranolol or esmolol (25–50 μg/kg/min IV). Treat wide QRS complex tachycardia caused by cyclic antidepressant overdose with sodium bicarbonate, 1–2 mEq/kg IV bolus.

See Table 63-7 and Chapter 12.

CONVULSIONS

Convulsions are usually effectively controlled with common anticonvulsants. A few drugs and toxins may require antidotes or other specific therapies (Table 63-9). Rule out other causes of convulsions, such as hypoxia, hypoglycemia, hypocalcemia, hyponatremia, and central nervous system infections.

Administer diazepam 0.1–0.2 mg/kg IV or, if IV access is not immediately available, midazolam 0.1–0.2 mg/kg IM. If the patient continues to convulse, administer phenobarbital 15 mg/kg IV over no less than 30 minutes and/or phenytoin 15 mg/kg IV over no less than 30 minutes.

See Table 63-8 and Chapter 26.

HYPERTHERMIA

Hyperthermia may result from prolonged seizures or other causes of muscular hyperactivity (Table 63-10). Severe hyperthermia (temperature above 40–41°C) may rapidly cause brain damage. Treat hyperthermia aggressively by removing clothing, spraying with tepid water, and fanning. If this is not rapidly effective, induce neuromuscular paralysis with pancuronium 0.1 mg/kg IV. Once paralyzed, the patient must be intubated and mechanically ventilated. In addition, absence of visible seizure activity may give the false impression that brain convulsions have ceased; however, this must be confirmed with EEG.

HYPOTHERMIA

Hypothermia commonly accompanies sedative-hypnotic, phenothiazine, and other depressant drug ov-

TABLE 63–7. *Common Drugs/Poisons Causing Arrhythmias*

Arrhythmia	Common Causes
Sinus bradycardia	Beta blockers, organophosphates, digitalis, opioids, clonidine, barbiturates, sedative-hypnotics
AV block	Beta blockers, digitalis glycosides, calcium antagonists, cyclic antidepressants, lithium
Sinus tachycardia	Theophylline, caffeine, cocaine, amphetamines, phencyclidine, beta agonists, iron, anticholinergics (including cyclic antidepressants), antihistamines, salicylates, MAO inhibitors
Wide QRS complex	Cyclic antidepressants, Type Ia and Ic antiarrhythmics, some phenothiazines, hyperkalemia

erdoses (Table 63-11). Hypothermic patients may have a barely perceptible pulse and blood pressure and often appear dead. Hypothermia may cause or aggravate hypotension.

Hypothermia treatment is discussed in Chapter 95; gradual rewarming is preferred unless the patient is in cardiac arrest. Because undressed infants and small children rapidly lose body heat, warming lamps are recommended for routine use in comatose children.

Diagnosis of Unknown Poisoning ■

Most commonly, the identity of the ingested substance is known, but occasionally the child is found with an unlabeled container or the suicidal adolescent refuses to cooperate. Often, a tentative clinical diagnosis can be made by performing a directed physical examination and obtaining common clinical laboratory tests. This may allow empiric interventions or indicate specific toxicologic tests.

PHYSICAL EXAMINATION

Important diagnostic variables in the physical exam include *blood pressure, pulse rate, temperature, pu-pil size, sweating, and the presence or absence of peristaltic activity.* Many drugs fit into one of four common syndromes:

1. *Sympathomimetic syndrome* (Table 63-12): Blood pressure and pulse rate are elevated, although with severe hypertension reflex bradycardia may occur. The temperature is often elevated, pupils are dilated, and the skin is sweaty. Patients are agitated, anxious, or even psychotic.
2. *Sympatholytic syndrome* (Table 63-13): Blood pressure and pulse rate are both decreased. The temperature is low. The pupils are small. Peristalsis is usually decreased. Patients are usually obtunded or comatose.
3. *Cholinergic syndrome* (Table 63-14): Stimulation of muscarinic receptors causes bradycardia, miosis, sweating, hyperperistalsis, bronchorrhea, wheezing, salivation, and urinary incontinence. Nicotinic receptor stimulation may produce initial hyper-

TABLE 63–8. *Common Drugs/Poisons Causing Convulsions*

Cyclic antidepressants
Cocaine and amphetamines
Phencyclidine (PCP)
Theophylline
Isoniazid
Lindane
Camphor
Antihistamines
Phenothiazines

TABLE 63–9. *Convulsions Requiring Special Consideration*

Toxin/Drug	Comments
Isoniazid (INH)	Give pyridoxine, 5–10 g IV
Lithium	May require hemodialysis
Organophosphates	May respond to pralidoxime (2-PAM) or atropine
Strychnine	"Convulsions" are actually spinally mediated muscle spasms; usually require neuromuscular paralysis.
Theophylline	Convulsions are indication for charcoal hemoperfusion.
Cyclic antidepressants	Hyperthermia and cardiotoxicity are common complications. Consider neuromuscular paralysis.

TABLE 63–10. *Common Drugs/Poisons Causing Hyperthermia*

Cocaine and amphetamines
Phencyclidine (PCP)
Cyclic antidepressants
MAO inhibitors
Anticholinergics
Salicylates
Pentachlorophenol
Antipsychotics

tension and tachycardia, as well as fasciculations and muscle weakness.

4. *Anticholinergic syndrome* (Table 63-15): Tachycardia with mild hypertension is common. The temperature is often elevated. Pupils are widely dilated. The skin is flushed, hot, and dry. Peristalsis is decreased, and urinary retention is common. Patients may have myoclonic jerking or choreoathetoid movements. Agitated delirium is frequently seen.

ANCILLARY DATA

The following laboratory tests are recommended for routine screening of the overdose patient:

Serum osmolality and osmolar gap
Electrolytes
Serum glucose
Blood urea nitrogen (BUN) and creatinine
Urinalysis

In addition, obtain a stat serum acetaminophen level and a serum ethanol level in all patients, regardless of the history of ingestion.

Osmolar Gap

Under normal circumstances, the serum osmolality is estimated by the following calculation:

TABLE 63–11. *Common Drugs/Poisons Causing Hypothermia*

Opioids
Ethanol
Phenothiazines
Barbiturates
Sedative-hypnotics
Hypoglycemic agents

TABLE 63–12. *Some Causes of Sympathomimetic Syndrome*

Cocaine
Amphetamines
Phencyclidine (pupils usually normal or small)
Phenylpropanolamine (bradycardia common)

$$Osm = 2(Na)[mEq/L] + Glucose[mg/dL]/18 + BUN[mg/dL]/2.8$$

The normal osmolality is 290 mOsm/L. The osmolality may be directly measured using the freezing point depression osmometer or vaporization method. The difference between the calculated and the measured osmolality is known as the osmolar gap.

$$Osm\ gap = Measured\ Osm - Calculated\ Osm$$

The gap may be increased by large quantities of small-molecular-weight substances (Table 63-16). An elevated gap is most commonly caused by ethanol. The presence of a combined osmolar and elevated anion gap should suggest poisoning by methanol or ethylene glycol. Caution: If the vaporization osmometry method is used, alcohols may be vaporized, resulting in a falsely normal measured osmolality.

Anion Gap

Metabolic acidosis associated with an elevated anion gap is usually due to accumulation of lactic acid or other organic acids (Table 63-17). The calculation of the anion gap is:

$$Anion\ gap = Na - Cl - HCO_3 = 8-12\ mEq/L$$

Always also check the osmolar gap; combined anion and osmolar gap suggests poisoning by methanol or ethylene glycol.

TABLE 63–13. *Some Causes of Sympatholytic Syndrome*

Ethanol
Barbiturates
Sedative-hypnotics
Clonidine
Opioids

TABLE 63–14. *Some Causes of Cholinergic Syndrome*

Organophosphates
Carbamates
Physostigmine
Nicotine

TABLE 63–16. *Common Drugs/Poisons Causing Elevated Osmolar Gap*

Ethanol
Isopropyl alcohol
Methanol
Ethylene glycol
Propylene glycol
Acetone

Toxicology Laboratory

The routine toxicology screen is of minimal value in the initial care of the poisoned patient because it is time-consuming, expensive, and frequently erroneous. Routine laboratory values may provide a clue to the diagnosis (Table 63-18). On the other hand, specific quantitative levels may be extremely helpful (Table 63-19), especially if specific antidotes or interventions would be indicated based upon the results.

If a toxicology screen is ordered, urine is the best specimen for broad qualitative screening. Blood is poorly sensitive for psychotropic agents, opioids, and stimulants.

Abdominal X-Rays

Abdominal X-rays may reveal radiopaque iron tablets, drug-filled condoms, or other toxic material. Recent studies suggest that few tablets are predictably visible. The X-ray is useful only if positive.

DECONTAMINATION OF SKIN AND EYES

Skin

Corrosive agents rapidly injure the skin and must be removed immediately. In addition, many toxins are readily absorbed through the skin, and systemic absorption can only be prevented by rapid action. Wash affected areas with copious lukewarm water or saline. Wash behind ears, under nails, and in skin folds. For oily substances (e.g., pesticides), wash with soap and shampoo hair.

Eyes

Act quickly to prevent serious damage. Flush with copious lukewarm water or saline. If available, instill local anesthetic drops before beginning irrigation. Place the victim under a tap or stream of water, and direct the flow across the nasal bridge. Lift the tarsal conjunctiva to look for undissolved particles and to enhance irrigation. Continue irrigation for 10 minutes (or at least 1 liter to each eye). If the toxin is an acid or a base, check the pH of the tears after irrigation.

After irrigation, perform a fluorescein exam of the eye using a Wood's lamp to identify any corneal injury. Patients with serious corneal injury should be immediately referred to an ophthalmologist.

For *gastrointestinal decontamination* see Chapter 64; for *enhanced elimination of toxins* see Chapter 65.

Disposition ■

Observe asymptomatic or mildly symptomatic patients for at least 4–6 hours, unless the assessment is a nontoxic ingestion, in which case the patient might

TABLE 63–15. *Some Causes of Anticholinergic Syndrome*

Cyclic antidepressants
Atropine and scopolamine
Antihistamines
Phenothiazines (hypotension; pupils usually small)

TABLE 63–17. *Common Drugs/Poisons Causing Elevated Anion Gap Acidosis*

Salicylates
Methanol
Ethylene glycol
Isoniazid
Iron
Phenformin
Cyanide
Carbon monoxide

TABLE 63–18. *Common Causes of Other Laboratory Findings*

Lab Finding	Causes
Hypokalemia	Theophylline, caffeine, barium, beta agonists
Hyperkalemia	Fluoride, digitalis glycosides, beta blockers, rhabdomyolysis
Hypoglycemia	Insulin, oral hypoglycemics, beta blockers, liver failure
Hyperglycemia	Theophylline, caffeine, iron
Leukocytosis	Lithium, iron, theophylline

TABLE 63–19. *Specific Quantitative Levels and Potential Interventions*

Toxin/Drug	Potential Intervention
Acetaminophen	N-acetylcysteine
Carboxyhemoglobin	100% oxygen
Digoxin	Digitalis antibodies
Ethylene glycol	Ethanol, dialysis
Iron	Deferoxamine
Lithium	Dialysis
Methanol	Ethanol, dialysis
Methemoglobin	Methylene blue
Salicylate	Dialysis
Theophylline	Hemoperfusion

be discharged immediately. After this interval, the patient may be discharged if asymptomatic and after having received adequate gastric decontamination.

Before discharge, perform a psychosocial evaluation. Children less than 14–16 months and older than 4–5 years do not usually experiment with drugs found around the house, and an ingestion in these age groups should raise the possibility that they were given to the child, perhaps by a psychotic parent or a sibling. Intentional ingestions in adolescents, especially girls, should raise the possibility of unwanted pregnancy or sexual or physical abuse in the home. *Evaluate all intentional ingestions for suicidal risk.*

Bibliography ■

Ellenhorn M, Barceloux D: *Medical toxicology: Diagnosis and treatment of human poisoning.* New York: Elsevier, 1988.

Goldfrank LR et al, eds: *Goldfrank's toxicologic emergencies.* New York: Appleton-Century-Crofts, 1985.

Haddad LM, Winchester JF: *Clinical management of poisoning and drug overdose.* Philadelphia: WB Saunders, 1983.

Olson KR et al: Physical assessment and differential diagnosis of the poisoned patient. *Med Toxicol* 1987; 2:52–81.

64 Gastrointestinal Decontamination

Milton Tenenbein

The intent of gastrointestinal decontamination is to remove the poison from the GI tract, or to bind it to a nonabsorbable agent, preventing its absorption. Traditional interventions include *ipecac-induced emesis, gastric lavage,* and *activated charcoal administration.* Although all of these interventions have been widely used for decades, there is little documented proof of benefit. Recent studies suggest that activated charcoal may be the single most important procedure for patients with acute poisoning.

Syrup of Ipecac ■

Syrup of ipecac, which acts both on the gastric mucosa and on the chemoreceptor trigger zone, is effective within 15–20 minutes in more than 90% of patients. Its safety is well established.

Give 15 ml to children less than 2 years old and 30 ml to those who are older, along with no more than 250 ml of water. If vomiting does not occur within 20 minutes, administer a second dose.

Ipecac should not be given to any patient with an unprotected airway (obtunded, comatose, or convulsing) because of the risk of aspiration of gastric contents. It should also be avoided if the ingestant is likely to produce coma or seizures in a short period of time (e.g., camphor, strychnine, clonidine). Ipecac is also contraindicated for caustic or corrosive ingestions (Table 64-1). Hydrocarbon ingestion is not a specific contraindication, but since most hydrocarbons lack systemic toxicity, emesis is usually not indicated (see Chapter 79).

Whether or not ipecac improves clinical outcome is questionable. Extensive review of animal and human literature indicates that it removes only about one-third of the ingestant from the stomach. In addition, emesis delays the administration of activated charcoal.

Gastric Lavage ■

Gastric lavage is generally used when ipecac is unsafe or after ipecac has failed. Patients who are obtunded, comatose, or convulsing require endotracheal intubation prior to passage of the gastric tube. The largest possible tube should be passed (at least a 30 French gauge) to facilitate removal of tablet particles. Ingestion of a caustic or corrosive agent is a relative contraindication, as there is a risk of aggravating esophageal injury. Gastric lavage is not specifically contraindicated for hydrocarbon ingestions; it is usually simply not indicated.

After passage of the tube, confirm its position by auscultation over the stomach during air injection. During lavage, place the patient on the left side. This lessens the risk of irrigation of the toxicant into the small intestine.

Lavage the stomach with 10 ml/kg (maximum 200 ml) aliquots plus the volume of the lavage tube, which can be measured just before its insertion. Use warmed saline in small patients to prevent hypothermia and water intoxication.

The effectiveness of gastric lavage, like that of ipecac, is questionable. In teenagers, about one-third of the toxin is removed from the stomach. However, in small children, the volume removed is less because of the smaller tube size. Gastric lavage complications (esophageal trauma, aspiration pneumonia) are more worrisome and occur at a greater frequency (3% in one study).

Activated Charcoal ■

Activated charcoal is now the primary GI decontamination procedure for many acute poisonings. Charcoal adsorbs most ingestant, preventing their absorption into the bloodstream. It is easier to remem-

TABLE 64–1. *Contraindications to Gastric Emptying Procedures*

Ipecac:

Presence of (or threat of rapid onset of) coma, convulsions, or obtundation

Ipecac or Gastric Lavage:

Ingestion of a caustic or corrosive substance

Nontoxic ingestion

TABLE 64–2. *Agents Poorly Adsorbed by Activated Charcoal*

Simple ions (e.g., iron, lithium, cyanide)
Simple alcohols (e.g., ethanol, methanol)
Strong acids or bases

ber what it doesn't adsorb than what it does (Table 64-2).

To prevent desorption of toxin from charcoal in the gut, give large amounts of charcoal (25–50 g for toddlers and preschoolers and 50–100 g for teenagers, as a slurry in water). Charcoal usually must be given by a nasogastric tube, since most small children will not drink it voluntarily.

There are no absolute contraindications for charcoal administration. It must be used with caution in patients who are obtunded, comatose, or convulsing.

Administration of a cathartic is frequently recommended along with activated charcoal. The presumed benefits are prevention of charcoal-induced constipation and the clearance of the charcoal drug mass before drug desorption can occur. However, there are no data supporting these contentions. Do not use potent cathartics such as sorbitol in preschoolers, since fluid depletion or electrolyte imbalance may result. The general use of cathartics at any age is questionable.

Multiple-dose charcoal administration (10–20 g every few hours) is a relatively new intervention. It enhances the removal of already absorbed toxin from the blood, probably because the repeated charcoal administration keeps the concentration of free drug within the GI tract near zero, maintaining a gradient from blood to bowel. Hence, it is also referred to as *GI dialysis.* The best data demonstrating effectiveness are for phenobarbital and theophylline. The treatment should probably not be used in depressed patients with absent bowel sounds, as they are at risk for charcoal obstruction (see also Chapter 65).

Whole-Bowel Irrigation ■

Whole-bowel irrigation recently has been described as a GI decontamination procedure for acute poison-

ing. It consists of giving large volumes of polyethylene glycol electrolyte solution to irrigate out GI tract contents. This fluid produces no net absorption or secretion of water or electrolytes. For poisoning, it is given by nasogastric tube at 2 L/hr for adolescents and adults and 500 ml/hr for preschoolers. The irrigation is continued until the rectal effluent is clear; this usually takes several hours.

The indications for whole-bowel irrigation include: the ingestion of a very large amount of a toxic substance; ingestion of sustained-release or enteric-coated pharmaceuticals; ingestion of substances not adsorbed by activated charcoal, such as iron or lithium. Contraindications include obstruction or perforation of the bowel, ileus, or significant GI hemorrhage. Use a nasogastric tube, since patients will not drink the required amount. Avoid ipecac, because after its administration patients often cannot tolerate the large volumes required. A dose of charcoal can be given before initiating whole-bowel irrigation. IV metoclopramide can be given to control vomiting.

Whole-bowel irrigation is not a panacea. Because it is both labor-intensive and time-consuming, it is generally unsuitable as a primary GI decontamination procedure.

Bibliography ■

Kulig K, Bar-Or D, Cantrill SV, et al: Management of acutely poisoned patients without gastric emptying. *Ann Emerg Med* 1985; 14:562–567.

Rodgers GC Jr, Matyunas NJ: Gastrointestinal decontamination for acute poisoning. *Pediatr Clin North Am* 1986; 33:261–285.

Tenenbein M, Cohen S, Sitar DS: Efficacy of ipecac-induced emesis, orogastric lavage and activated charcoal for acute drug overdose. *Ann Emerg Med* 1987; 16:838–841.

Tenenbein M: Whole-bowel irrigation as a gastrointestinal decontamination procedure after acute poisoning. *Med Toxicol* 1988; 3:77–84.

65 Enhancing the Elimination of Toxins

William Banner, Jr.

Dialysis and other extracorporeal removal procedures have long been considered part of the glamorous side of toxicology, but gastric decontamination and supportive care are more likely to improve outcome. For those rare circumstances where these techniques are necessary, a basic understanding of these methods is essential.

The decision to implement an extracorporeal removal technique is based on several factors:

1. Has supportive care been unsuccessful, or is it likely to be?
2. Are the risks of the procedure worth the potential benefit?
3. Is the drug removed effectively by extracorporeal procedures?

HAS SUPPORTIVE CARE FAILED? ARE THE RISKS WORTH IT?

Consulting a medical toxicologist or a regional poison center is advised (see Table 63-1). Table 65-1 lists specific drugs and serum concentrations at which extracorporeal removal must be considered. At high concentrations of some long half-life drugs such as phenobarbital, it is predictable that a long duration of advanced life support will be necessary. In such cases, the relative risks of maintaining a patient in the intensive care unit on mechanical ventilation have to be weighed against the risks of extracorporeal removal.

WILL THE METHOD WORK?

Drugs and toxins have intrinsic pharmacokinetic properties that influence their ability to be removed by these procedures. A drug with a volume of distribution greater than 1 liter/kg has more tissue stores outside plasma than within the plasma. Extracorporeal removal techniques are most successful for drugs with small volumes of distribution. Unfortunately, many toxic drugs such as tricyclic antidepressants, digoxin, and benzodiazepines have a large volume of distribution and are not effectively removed.

An additional consideration is the *intrinsic clearance*. Drugs with a high intrinsic clearance may be removed by the body so rapidly that an extracorporeal technique may only marginally decrease the duration of the toxic exposure.

Repeated Dose Charcoal ■

Filling the small bowel with charcoal to adsorb drugs which back-diffuse across the richly vascular, high-surface-area bowel is a new concept (see also Chapter 64). Generally, 10–20 gm activated charcoal is given every 3–4 hours with a dose of cathartic every third to fourth dose. Avoid excessive use of cathartics, since massive charcoal diarrhea may lead to serious fluid and electrolyte disturbances. This technique will enhance the elimination of drugs such as carbamazepine, theophylline, and phenobarbital.

Renal Elimination ■

An overrated method of enhancing elimination is vigorous diuresis. This approach, with urinary alkalinization, has been advocated for acidic drug ingestions such as salicylate and phenobarbital. However, the creation of excessive amounts of urine often results in dilute drug concentrations in urine instead of dramatic increases in elimination. Also, aggressive administration of fluids may cause electrolyte imbalance and pulmonary edema. Acidification of the urine has been advocated in the management of ingestions of weak bases such as amphetamine, but acidification may aggravate systemic acidosis as well as promote deposition of myoglobin in the kidney in patients with rhabdomyolysis.

TABLE 65–1. *Serum Concentrations that May Indicate Need for Dialysis or Hemoperfusion*

Drug or Poison	Serum Concentration	Preferred Procedure
Carbamazepine	>80 mg/L	HP
Ethylene glycol	>50 mg/dL	HD
Methanol	>50 mg/dL	HD
Phenobarbital	>150 mg/L	HP
Salicylate	>120 mg/dL	HD
Theophylline	>100 mg/L	HP

HD = hemodialysis
HP = hemoperfusion

Dialysis and Hemoperfusion ■

Reports of dialysis techniques to remove toxins have vastly overrated their effectiveness by focusing on clearance calculations instead of the impact on total body burden of drug. Peritoneal dialysis can be instituted easily but provides extremely poor drug removal rates. Generally, a drug that can be renally eliminated will achieve higher clearances through the kidneys than through peritoneal dialysis. Hemodialysis will remove water-soluble toxins with low molecular weight and a low volume of distribution (Table 65-2). Even if a drug has a small volume of distribution, other factors are also important. Drugs with large size (>600 daltons), low water solubility, or high protein binding are generally not well-removed by hemodialysis, although they may be by charcoal hemoperfusion.

Charcoal hemoperfusion is generally more efficient than dialysis. However, alcohols and glycols, lithium, sodium, and potassium are not well-bound to charcoal and require hemodialysis for removal. Although salicylate can be removed more efficiently by charcoal hemoperfusion, it is preferable to use hemodialysis to correct the metabolic acidosis and electrolyte abnormalities.

TABLE 65–2. *Toxins Commonly Removed by Dialysis*

Methanol
Ethylene glycol
Lithium
Sodium
Potassium
Bromide
Salicylate
Bromates

Bibliography ■

Hampson ECGM, Pond SM: Failure of haemoperfusion and haemodialysis to prevent death in paraquat poisoning: A retrospective review of 42 patients. *Med Toxicol Adverse Drug Exp* 1988; 3:64–71.

Heath A, Knudsen K: Role of extracorporeal drug removal in acute theophylline poisoning: A review. *Med Toxicol Adverse Drug Exp* 1987; 2:294–308.

Neuvonen PJ, Olkkola KT: Oral activated charcoal in the treatment of intoxications: Role of single and repeated doses. *Med Toxicol Adverse Drug Exp* 1988; 3:33–58.

66 Acetaminophen

Michael McGuigan

Acetaminophen is widely used in a variety of over-the-counter and prescription products. Accidental and intentional ingestions are common and may go unrecognized because initial symptoms are nonspecific and because patients and physicians may not recognize that the ingested product contains acetaminophen.

Toxicity results from the metabolism of acetaminophen. Normally, when a small portion of acetaminophen is metabolized by the hepatic (and renal) cytochrome p-450 pathway, a toxic intermediate is formed that is immediately detoxified by combining with cellular glutathione. In an acute overdose, the quantity of toxic intermediate is sufficient to deplete glutathione stores, and the toxic metabolite attacks cellular macromolecules. Hepatic (and sometimes renal) damage occurs.

The amount of acetaminophen required to deplete glutathione stores is about 140 mg/kg. It is difficult to predict a particular child's toxic dose because of variability in glutathione stores and in the relative contribution of p-450 to overall acetaminophen metabolism. Children under 12 years appear to be more resistant to toxicity because of less active p-450 metabolism of acetaminophen.

Clinical Findings ■

Early after ingestion, there are no specific symptoms or signs of acetaminophen toxicity. Nausea, vomiting, and abdominal discomfort may be the only symptoms during the first 12–24 hours after a large ingestion. Clinical and biochemical evidence of hepatic and renal damage are usually not apparent for 24–48 hours. Acute liver damage is characterized by jaundice, enlarged tender liver, elevated serum transaminases, prolonged prothrombin time, and rarely, encephalopathy and death. Acute renal tubular necrosis occasionally occurs.

The only reliable indicator of acute serious ingestion is the serum acetaminophen concentration. The level should be plotted against time since ingestion on the Rumack-Matthew nomogram (Figure 66-1) to predict the likelihood of hepatic damage and the need for antidotal therapy.

Prior to development of overt hepatic damage, the symptoms and signs of acetaminophen overdose are nonspecific. Because of this, suspect acetaminophen overdose routinely in any case of drug ingestion.

The toxicologic differential diagnosis of acute hepatic damage includes arsenic, iron, mushrooms (some species of amanita, galerina, and lepiota), carbon tetrachloride, and other halogenated hydrocarbon solvents. Hepatic damage may also occur as an allergic or idiosyncratic reaction to chronic use of anticonvulsant medications (phenytoin, phenobarbital, or valproate). The medical differential diagnosis includes Reye's syndrome, viral hepatitis, and Wilson's disease.

Treatment ■

SUPPORTIVE CARE

Early after ingestion, there should be no serious respiratory, cardiovascular, or central nervous system complications, unless other drugs have been ingested. Vomiting may be treated with any antiemetic.

Once hepatic damage is evident, supportive care includes careful monitoring of mental status (including signs of encephalopathy and increased intracranial pressure), vital signs, fluid balance, blood glucose, and prothrombin time. Fresh-frozen plasma may be required to correct coagulopathy. Standard therapy for encephalopathy may include oral neomycin and/or lactulose and medical therapy to reduce intracranial pressure. If massive hepatic failure occurs, with intractable encephalopathy, consider liver transplantation.

Decontamination

Empty the stomach with induced emesis or gastric lavage (see Chapter 64). Lavage is the preferred method if it is readily available. Do not induce emesis

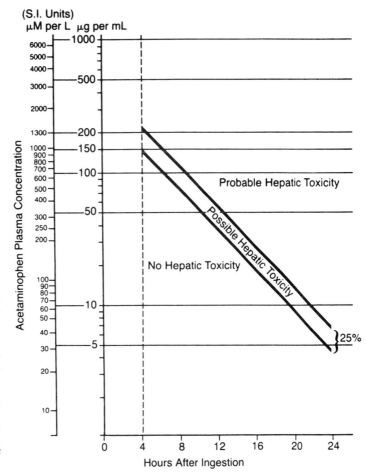

FIGURE 66–1. Nomogram for acute acetaminophen poisoning. Note: (1) Time refers to time of ingestion. (2) Serum levels drawn before 4 hours may not represent peak levels. (3) The graph is useful only for single acute ingestions. (4) The lower solid line 25% below the standard nomogram is included to allow for possible errors in acetaminophen plasma assays and estimated time from ingestion of an overdose. (5) If the acetaminophen level at least 4 hours following an overdose falls above the lower solid line, administer the entire course of acetylcysteine treatment. (Reproduced with permission from Rumack B and Matthew: *Pediatrics* 1975;55:871)

if the patient presents more than 4 hours after ingestion, because continued vomiting may delay use of oral n-acetylcysteine. Administer activated charcoal and a cathartic (because of concerns about the ability of charcoal to adsorb some of the antidote n-acetylcysteine, some toxicologists recommend an increased loading dose (190 mg/kg) of n-acetylcysteine).

TABLE 66–1. *N-acetylcysteine Treatment Protocols*

	Loading Dose	Maintenance Dose
Protocol 1	140 mg/kg PO	70 mg/kg PO every 4 hours for 14 doses
Protocol 2*	140 mg/kg IV	70 mg/kg IV every 4 hours for 12 doses
Protocol 3*	150–170 mg/kg IV	50–60 mg/kg IV over 4 hours, followed by 110–115 mg/kg IV over 16 hours

* Caution: The IV route is NOT approved in the United States; the U.S. preparation of n-acetylcysteine is not formulated for parenteral use. Also, any formulation of n-acetylcysteine can cause hypotension and flushing if given rapidly IV.

SPECIFIC TREATMENT

The antidote of choice is n-acetylcysteine, which serves as a glutathione substitute and scavenges toxic metabolite as it is produced. N-acetylcysteine is most effective if given within the first 8–10 hours after ingestion, and is of questionable value if given later than 16–24 hours after ingestion. If a serum level of acetaminophen is not immediately available, or if the patient presents at 7–8 hours after ingestion, start therapy empirically.

Of the three available treatment protocols (Table 66-1), only the oral route is approved for use in the United States. The commercially available U.S. oral preparation should not be given IV. If IV therapy is considered, contact a regional poison center (Table 63-1) for assistance.

DISPOSITION

All patients with suspected acetaminophen overdose involving more than 140 mg/kg should have a serum acetaminophen level drawn at least 4 hours after ingestion to determine the need for antidotal therapy. Admit all patients requiring n-acetylcysteine.

Bibliography ■

Rumack BH: Acetaminophen overdose in young children. *Am J Dis Child* 1984; 138:428–433.

Rumack BH: Acetaminophen overdose in children and adolescents. *Pediatr Clin North Am* 1986; 33:691–701.

67 Alcohols and Ethylene Glycol

Mary Ellen Mortensen

Alcohols (isopropanol, ethanol, methanol) and ethylene glycol are small, membrane-permeable molecules metabolized by alcohol dehydrogenase and other hepatic enzymes. Alcohols are well absorbed by oral, dermal, and inhalation routes; ethylene glycol is well absorbed only by the oral route. Intoxication with all agents produces CNS depression and interferes with hepatic (especially glucose) metabolism. Metabolites of methanol (formic acid) and ethylene glycol (oxalic and hippuric acids) cause metabolic acidosis and serious systemic toxicity.

All of these agents increase the measured serum osmolality and the *osmolar gap* (see Chapter 63) in proportion to blood alcohol or glycol concentration. Metabolic acidosis with an elevated *anion gap* (see Chapter 63) may be present with methanol and ethylene glycol poisoning.

Mild symptoms can occur with 0.3 gm/kg of isopropyl alcohol (0.5 mL/kg of 70%) and intoxication is likely with 1 mL/kg of 70%; blood levels greater than 340 mg/dL are usually fatal. Intoxication with ethanol occurs with ingestion of 1 gm/kg. Fatalities may occur with ingestion of more than 3 g/kg, corresponding to less than 2–3 ounces of strong liquor in a small child. Methanol is toxic at doses of 0.4 mL/kg; 30 mL is considered potentially fatal. Ethylene glycol at 1.5 mL/kg can be fatal if untreated.

Clinical Findings ■

Initial gastric irritation, especially after isopropyl alcohol ingestion, may lead to nausea, vomiting, and hematemesis. Generalized CNS intoxication usually occurs within 30–60 minutes of ingestion of any of the agents: elation, then confusion, ataxia, nystagmus, progressing to stupor, coma, and respiratory depression. Direct myocardial depression and vasodilation may lead to hypotension. Hypoglycemia may result from alcohol inhibition of gluconeogenesis, especially in young children.

Methanol metabolism causes metabolic acidosis, which may be delayed up to 72 hours as formic acid accumulates. Ocular findings include decreased acuity, scotomata ("being in a snowstorm"), dilated pupils, decreased pupillary light response, retinal edema, and hyperemic optic disks.

Ethylene glycol intoxication is also characterized by metabolic acidosis that develops after a delay of several hours, with the accumulation of oxalic, glycolic, and hippuric acids. Progressive signs of intoxication include tachycardia, mild hypertension, congestive heart failure, and shock. Renal toxicity is characterized by calcium oxalate crystalluria, oliguria, and acute tubular necrosis.

The differential diagnosis includes overdose with narcotics, barbiturates, sedatives, and salicylates. Other causes of coma include head trauma, sepsis or CNS infection, and metabolic disturbance. Table 63-17 summarizes toxic causes of anion gap metabolic acidosis.

Treatment ■

SUPPORTIVE CARE

Maintain a patent airway and provide assisted ventilation if needed. Correct metabolic acidosis with IV bicarbonate 1–2 mEq/kg per dose, and replace fluid and electrolyte losses with IV crystalloid solutions. Restore euglycemia with IV or PO dextrose and reassess frequently. Correct hypotension with IV fluids and Trendelenberg position. Passive rewarming is sufficient for mild hypothermia (see Chapter 95).

Decontamination

Induced emesis is not recommended if more than 30 minutes have passed since ingestion. Gastric lavage is the preferred method of stomach emptying. Alcohols and glycols do not efficiently adsorb to activated charcoal (see also Chapter 64).

Wash with soap and water to decontaminate heavily exposed skin. Dermal application of alcohols, es-

TABLE 67–1. *Indications for Ethanol Administration for Methanol or Ethylene Glycol Intoxication*

Methanol
Blood methanol >20 mg/dL

Ethylene Glycol
Blood ethylene glycol >25 mg/dL

Either
Metabolic acidosis and markedly elevated osmolar gap

Severely symptomatic patient

Patient considered for or awaiting hemodialysis

TABLE 67–3. *Guidelines for Initiating Hemodialysis in Methanol or Ethylene Glycol Poisoning*

Compound	Indication
Methanol	Refractory metabolic acidosis
	Deep coma
	Visual impairment
	Blood level > 50 mg/dL
Ethylene glycol	Refractory metabolic acidosis
	Deep coma
	Oxalate crystalluria
	Blood level > 50 mg/dL
	Renal failure

pecially in a small room, can produce significant inhalation exposure.

SPECIFIC TREATMENT

Indications for ethanol administration to block methanol or ethylene glycol metabolism, and recommended ethanol doses, are presented in Tables 67-1 and 67-2. Table 67-3 summarizes the indications for hemodialysis. Hemodialysis is rarely necessary for ethanol or isopropyl alcohol intoxication, unless

TABLE 67–2. *Ethanol Doses to Achieve and Maintain Blood Ethanol of 100 MG/dL*

Loading Dose
0.7 g/kg (1 mL/kg) of 100% (v/v) ethanol (Dilute to 20–30% for PO or NG) (Dilute to 5–10% in D_5W for IV)

Maintenance Dose
Immediately after loading, administer 130 mg/kg/hr (0.16 mL/kg/hr of 100% ethanol, diluted to 5–10% as above)

Hemodialysis Dose
Increase maintenance dose to 250–350 mg/kg/hr.

Measure blood ethanol frequently and adjust dose to achieve 100–150 mg/dL. Monitor blood glucose during prolonged ethanol administration.
(Adapted from Goldfrank LR, Flomenbaum NE, Lewin NA, et al, eds. *Goldfrank's toxicologic emergencies,* 3rd ed, Appleton-Century-Crofts, E. Norwalk, Conn., 1986.)

progressive clinical deterioration occurs despite aggressive supportive therapy.

Folate and thiamine have been recommended for methanol and ethylene glycol intoxication but remain unproven, although harmless, therapies. A specific alcohol dehydrogenase inhibitor, 4-methylpyrazole, is under investigation for treatment of methanol and ethylene glycol intoxication.

DISPOSITION

Patients who remain asymptomatic 2–3 hours after suspected ethanol or isopropyl alcohol ingestion can be discharged. Blood levels of methanol or ethylene glycol help to determine the need for admission and aggressive care, but are often not readily available. When these levels are unavailable, patients should be observed at least 8 hours for symptoms and biochemical abnormalities (anion gap, osmolar gap). Empiric ethanol administration and hospital admission may be warranted if a potentially lethal ingestion of methanol or ethylene glycol is suspected.

Bibliography ■

Jacobsen D, McMartin KE: Methanol and ethylene glycol poisonings. Mechanism of toxicity, clinical course, diagnosis and treatment. *Med Toxicol Adverse Drug Exp* 1986; 1:309–334.

Litovitz T: The alcohols: Ethanol, methanol, isopropanol, ethylene glycol. *Pediatr Clin North Am* 1986; 33:311–324.

68 Anticoagulant Rodenticides

S. Alan Tani

Anticoagulant rodenticides are commonly of the short-acting type (warfarin) or the long-acting type. The two classes of long-acting anticoagulants are indandiones (including diphacinone, chlorophacinone, and pindone) and 4-hydroxycoumarins (including difenacoum, brodifacoum, and bromodialone). All of these oral anticoagulants block the synthesis of vitamin K-dependent clotting factors.

Single ingestions of the short-acting type of anticoagulant rodenticides are generally nontoxic. However, large single ingestions (greater than 1 oz) of long-acting anticoagulant rodenticides may result in anticoagulation persisting for weeks to months.

Clinical Findings ■

Patients presenting within 24 hours of ingestion are generally asymptomatic. Hemorrhage and its complications are the most common clinical findings after that period of time. Prolongation of the prothrombin time is maximal at 24 hours following ingestion of short-acting anticoagulants, and 36 to 72 hours following long-acting anticoagulants. Serum levels for anticoagulants are not generally available.

Trauma must be considered in patients presenting with hemorrhage. Ingestion of other types of rodenticides must be considered in patients presenting with symptoms other than prolongation of prothrombin time or hemorrhage.

Treatment ■

SUPPORTIVE CARE

Actively bleeding patients may require transfusions of crystalloid, whole blood, packed red blood cells, or fresh-frozen plasma.

Decontamination

Induce vomiting with syrup of ipecac or perform gastric lavage, then follow with activated charcoal and sorbitol (see Chapter 64).

SPECIFIC TREATMENT

Patients with markedly elevated prothrombin times should receive SC (or slowly IV) vitamin K_1, 0.6 mg/kg in children and up to 25 mg in adults. Give smaller PO or SC doses (1–5 mg in children and 10 mg in adults) in cases of suspected toxicity with normal or slightly elevated prothrombin times. Do *not* use vitamin K_3 (menadione); it is ineffective.

DISPOSITION

Single ingestions of warfarin-containing rodenticides rarely produce toxicity and require treatment only if symptoms of bleeding develop. On the other hand, ingestions of long-acting anticoagulants require baseline and repeat prothrombin times at 24 and 48 hours. Patients with severely elevated prothrombin times or clinical hemorrhage require hospital admission.

Bibliography ■

Kumer K, Nwangu PV: Clinical toxicology of warfarin from commercial rodenticides: Symptoms, diagnosis and management. *Clinical Toxicology Consultant* 1981; 3: 23–27.

Lipton RA, Klass EM: Human ingestion of a "super-warfarin" rodenticide resulting in a prolonged anticoagulant effect. *JAMA* 1984; 252:3004–3007.

69 Beta-Adrenergic Blocker Intoxication

Pierre Gaudreault

Beta-blocking agents are used in a variety of conditions such as angina, cardiac arrhythmias, hypertension, migraine, thyrotoxicosis, and glaucoma.

Toxic manifestations result from accentuation of their pharmacologic properties. In overdose, beta blockers lose their specificity and both beta$_1$ and beta$_2$ receptors are blocked, resulting in decreases in heart rate, myocardial contractility, cardiac output, and conduction velocity. In addition, the membrane-stabilizing activity of drugs like propranolol, oxprenolol, and alprenolol will contribute to myocardial contractility. The partial sympathomimetic action of acebutolol, alprenolol, oxprenolol, pindolol, and practolol is responsible for tachycardia and hypertension encountered occasionally with these agents.

The exact mechanism responsible for neurologic manifestations is unknown. Lipophilic drugs with membrane-stabilizing activity such as propranolol and oxprenolol are more likely to induce seizures and rapid loss of consciousness than agents lacking these properties. However, sotalol (an hydrophilic drug devoid of membrane-stabilizing activity) can also induce seizures.

Toxic doses and patient susceptibility vary greatly: for example, one patient died after taking 3.2 g of sotalol, while another survived after taking 8 g. Patients with myocardial disease may develop signs of serious toxicity at lower blood concentrations than patients with a normal heart. A prudent approach would be to consider that any patient who has ingested more than three to five times the recommended daily dose is at risk for toxicity.

Clinical Findings ■

Following an acute overdose, signs and symptoms usually occur within 1–2 hours after ingestion. Signs of toxicity have lasted for more than 72 hours in some cases.

In general, beta blockers affect primarily the cardiovascular and central nervous systems. Patients with severe intoxications will present with bradycardia and hypotension. The neurologic effects most commonly encountered are seizures and alteration of the level of consciousness. Other symptoms include nausea, vomiting, and rarely bronchospasm or respiratory arrest. Toxic manifestations depend on the individual drug (Table 69-1).

Laboratory abnormalities include hypoglycemia, hyperkalemia, and ECG changes such as first-degree atrioventricular block and sinus bradycardia. Massive intoxications induce disappearance of P waves, intraventricular conduction defects, and asystole. Drugs with membrane-stabilizing activity, such as propranolol, may induce a widening of the QRS complex.

Serum drug levels do not correlate reliably with severity of intoxication. In addition, treatment decisions rely on the patient's clinical status regardless of plasma concentrations.

Treatment ■

SUPPORTIVE CARE

As for all emergency situations, maintain a patent airway and assist ventilation if needed. Give atropine (0.01–0.02 mg/kg IV) to patients with hemodynamically significant bradycardia. Treat hypotension with IV fluids and dopamine (see Chapter 63). Control seizures with diazepam. If necessary, add phenytoin (15 mg/kg IV over 30 minutes) and phenobarbital (15 mg/kg IV over 30 minutes). Hypoglycemia can be treated with glucose and glucagon. If there is evidence of bronchoconstriction, give beta$_2$-agonist agents and aminophylline.

TABLE 69–1. *Toxic Manifestations of Beta Blockers*

Drugs	Beta Receptor	Pulse	Blood Pressure	Coma	Seizure	Respiratory Arrest	Death
Acebutolol	$\beta 1$	↓	↓				+
Alprenolol	$\beta 1$–$\beta 2$	↓	↓				+
Atenolol	$\beta 1$	↓	↓				
Metoprolol	$\beta 1$	↓		+			+
Oxprenolol	$\beta 1$–$\beta 2$	↓	↓	+	+	+	+
Pindolol	$\beta 1$–$\beta 2$	↑[1]	↑				
Practolol	$\beta 1$	↑[1]					
Propranolol	$\beta 1$–$\beta 2$	↓[2]	↓	+	+	+	+
Sotalol	$\beta 1$–$\beta 2$	↑[3]	↓		+		+

[1] Sinus tachycardia, hypertension
[2] Rarely ventricular fibrillation, QRS widening
[3] Ventricular tachyarrhythmias more frequent, QT prolongation.

Decontamination

In children, ipecac-induced emesis is the most convenient technique of emptying the stomach. Alternately, perform gastric lavage with the largest orogastric tube possible in patients with coma, seizures, or cardiotoxicity (see Chapter 64).

Administer activated charcoal orally or by gastric tube. Give 1 g/kg body weight every 4 to 6 hours until the patient evacuates a stool containing charcoal.

Forced diuresis is not indicated in beta-blocker intoxication. The efficacy of dialysis and hemoperfusion have never been evaluated, but based on their pharmacokinetic data these techniques would not be effective and they are not recommended.

SPECIFIC TREATMENT

Glucagon, with its inotropic effect independent of the beta receptors, has been the most effective drug in the treatment of beta-blocker-induced hypotension and bradycardia. The ideal dose has not been established, but begin with 1–2 bolus doses of 0.1 mg/kg IV (maximum: 10 mg/dose) followed by infusion of 0.05–0.1 mg/kg/hr. Ventricular tachycardia and fibrillation following sotalol intoxication may benefit from infusion of lidocaine.

DISPOSITION

Discharge patients who remain asymptomatic 6 to 8 hours after the time of ingestion and who have evacuated a stool containing activated charcoal. Admit any patient with cardiovascular or neurologic signs of toxicity.

Bibliography ■

Prichard BNC, Battersby LA, Cruickshank JM: Overdosage with β-adrenergic blocking agents. *Adv Drug React Ac Pois Rev* 1984; 3:91–111.

Weinstein RS: Recognition and management of poisoning with beta-adrenergic blocking agents. *Ann Emerg Med* 1984; 13:1123–1131.

70 Calcium Antagonists

Michael D. Reed

Calcium antagonists (diltiazem, nifedipine, and verapamil; Table 70-1) are primarily used as antiarrhythmic and antianginal agents, as well as in the treatment of hypertension. Chemically and pharmacologically, each drug is slightly different. Both diltiazem and verapamil decrease AV nodal conduction to a greater extent but produce less vasodilatation than nifedipine.

The calcium antagonists interfere with the entry of calcium into cells through voltage-dependent channels. They also possess limited affinity for α-adrenergic receptors, and competitive α-antagonism may occur in the presence of high drug concentrations. In contrast, calcium channel antagonists have little effect on skeletal muscle.

Clinical Findings ■

The signs and symptoms seen in overdoses result from an exaggeration of cardiovascular effects, including vasodilatation, negative inotropism, and depression of cardiac automaticity and conduction. Changes in mental status (lethargy, mental confusion, seizures, coma) depend on the degree of cerebral hypoperfusion resulting from systemic hypotension.

There are no specific laboratory findings. Serum calcium is not affected. Toxicology screening does not test for calcium antagonists, and serum concentrations of these drugs are not useful clinically.

Other drug intoxications that may result in bradycardia and hypotension include digitalis glycosides, beta blockers, clonidine, and possibly large intoxications with a narcotic analgesic.

Treatment ■

SUPPORTIVE CARE

Maintain a patent airway, and assist ventilation if needed. Give repeated fluid boluses (10–20 ml/kg) and vasopressors (i.e., norepinephrine/dopamine) as needed to support cardiac output and blood pressure. Avoid digitalis glycosides. Treat bradycardia with atropine (0.02 mg/kg; minimum dose 0.1 mg). Cardiac pacing is often necessary for severe myocardial depression, advanced heart block, or asystole.

TABLE 70–1. *Comparative Cardiovascular Effects of Therapeutic Doses of Calcium Antagonists*

Parameter	Diltiazem	Verapamil	Nifedipine
Sinus rate	↓	unchanged	↑
AV node conduction	↑↑	↑↑↑	unchanged
Peripheral arteriolar dilatation	+	++	+++
Hypotension	+	++	+++
Coronary arterial dilatation	++	++	+++
Myocardial contractility	↓	↓↓↓	↓↓
Cardiac output	↑	unchanged	↑↑

(Adapted from Conti CR, et al, *Emerg Med Reports* 1984; 5:29–36.)

Decontamination

Empty the stomach with emesis or gastric lavage, and administer activated charcoal (see Chapter 64). Considering these drugs' high degree of protein binding, large volumes of distribution, and extensive hepatic metabolism, diuresis, forced diuresis, hemodialysis, and hemoperfusion are of limited clinical utility.

SPECIFIC TREATMENT

Intravenous calcium may antagonize negative inotropic effects, but has little influence on vasodilation and AV block. Administer IV calcium chloride 25 mg/kg (maximum 1 gm) over 3–5 minutes; this dose may be repeated one or two times. Exercise caution with calcium administration by maintaining ionized calcium ≤6.5 mg/dl.

DISPOSITION

Admit all symptomatic children to the intensive care unit or arrange immediate transfer to a pediatric critical care center. Monitor asymptomatic children for at least 4–6 hours. Admit for cardiac monitoring children who are asymptomatic but have ingested a time-release preparation (e.g., Calan SR).

Bibliography ■

Snover SW, Bocchino V: Massive diltiazem overdose. *Ann Emerg Med* 1986; 15:1221–1224.

Weiner DA: Calcium channel blockers. *Med Clin North Am* 1988; 72:83–115.

71 Carbon Monoxide

Kent R. Olson

Carbon monoxide (CO) is a colorless, odorless gas produced by incomplete combustion of carbon-containing material. Common sources are automobile exhaust fumes, poorly ventilated kerosene or gas stoves, and smoke inhalation from fires. Fetal exposure may occur from maternal inhalation.

CO binds to hemoglobin with an affinity 250 times that of oxygen. This results in reduced oxyhemoglobin saturation and decreased oxygen-carrying capacity. In addition, the oxygen dissociation curve shifts to the left, impairing oxygen delivery to the tissues. CO may also directly inhibit cellular cytochrome oxidase, and it binds to myoglobin, contributing to impaired myocardial contractility.

The level considered immediately dangerous to life or health is 1,500 ppm (0.15%). Several minutes of exposure to 1,000 ppm (0.1%) may result in 50% saturation of carboxyhemoglobin (COHgb) and fatal poisoning. *Because fetal hemoglobin has an even greater affinity for CO than mature hemoglobin, infants are at greater risk from exposure to the same levels as older children and adults.*

Clinical Findings ■

The presentation may be quite variable, depending on the degree and duration of exposure. Symptoms and signs are nonspecific and the diagnosis may be overlooked. Most patients will have headache, nausea, and dizziness, and many will present with vomiting and diarrhea. With more severe exposures, impaired thinking, syncope, coma, convulsions, cardiac arrhythmias, hypotension, and death may occur. Survivors of serious poisoning may suffer neurologic sequelae such as parkinsonism and personality and memory disorders.

There are no reliable specific clinical findings; cherry-red skin coloration may be apparent at autopsy but is not commonly noted in the emergency department. Venous blood may be bright red due to the red color of the COHgb complex. The routine arterial blood gas measurement is falsely normal, because it measures oxygen dissolved in plasma but does not directly measure oxygen saturation or oxygen content. Pulse oximetry is also falsely normal. Metabolic acidosis due to cellular hypoxia may be noted.

Accurate diagnosis depends on measurement of the COHgb concentration. Table 71-1 correlates symptoms and signs with COHgb concentration.

Other gases that may cause altered mental status, coma, and metabolic acidosis include hydrogen cyanide and hydrogen sulfide. Any victim of smoke inhalation from a fire should be suspected of co-intoxication by cyanide (see Chapter 76) or methemoglobinemia (see Chapter 83).

Treatment ■

SUPPORTIVE CARE

Maintain the airway, and assist ventilation if needed. If smoke inhalation also occurred, consider early intubation for airway protection. Do not treat mild or moderate metabolic acidosis with bicarbonate or hyperventilation, since acidosis facilitates oxygen delivery to the tissues.

TABLE 71–1. *Symptoms and Signs of Carbon Monoxide Poisoning*

COHgb Level (%)	Signs and Symptoms
0–15	Usually none, or mild headache
15–30	Headache, nausea, dizziness
30–45	Severe headache, vomiting, confusion
45–60	Syncope, seizures, coma
>60	Coma, hypotension, death

Decontamination

Remove the victim from exposure immediately and administer the highest available concentration of supplemental oxygen. Rescuers should wear protective self-contained breathing apparatus.

SPECIFIC TREATMENT

Immediately administer 100% oxygen by tight-fitting facial mask or endotracheal tube. Breathing 100% oxygen reduces the half-time of the COHgb complex from 6 hours (in room air) to about 1 hour.

Hyperbaric oxygen (HBO) provides 100% oxygen under 2–3 atmospheres of pressure and can further enhance the elimination of CO (half-time reduced to 20–30 minutes). However, it remains controversial whether HBO is more effective than 100% oxygen alone, and transport of an unstable patient long distances for HBO treatment may be risky. Consult a medical toxicologist or a regional poison center for advice and information about HBO chambers (see Table 63-1).

DISPOSITION

Admit all symptomatic patients and those with COHgb levels greater than 25%.

Bibliography ∎

Olson KR: Carbon monoxide poisoning: Mechanisms, presentation, and controversies in management. *J Emerg Med* 1984; 1:233–243.

72 Cardiac Glycoside Intoxication

William Banner, Jr., and Garth S. Orsmond

The cardiac glycosides are naturally occurring compounds found in foxglove, lily of the valley, oleander, and other plants. These glycosides inhibit the sodium-potassium ATP-ase pump in the myocardium. Intoxication may result from acute overdose or chronic therapeutic use. When single acute doses exceed 25 μg/kg, toxicity is possible. When toxicity resulting from a cardiac glycoside occurs in the therapeutic setting, predisposing factors should be considered (Table 72-1).

Clinical Findings ■

Non-cardiac manifestations of toxicity include nausea, vomiting, and changes in vision in children old enough to describe them. Hyperkalemia is common with severe, acute overdose, but is not usually present with chronic intoxication, where hypokalemia is more common because of diuretic therapy. The first cardiac effect is increased vagal tone, resulting in decreased heart rate and delayed conduction through the AV node and the bundle of His. Cardiac glycosides also decrease the rate of spontaneous depolarization in Purkinje and ventricular muscle fibers; sudden ventricular arrhythmias may occur (Table 72-2). *Elevated serum potassium correlates with tissue effect and may be a more reliable indicator of toxicity than serum digoxin concentrations in acute overdose.*

The ECG manifestations of digoxin intoxication are nonspecific and may also be caused by congenital heart disease, cardiac surgical interventions, severe electrolyte disturbances, and other drugs affecting cardiac conduction. In the neonate, falsely high concentrations of digoxin may be measured because of the presence of digoxinlike substances in the serum. The volume of distribution of digoxin is very large (6–7 L/kg) and distribution to tissues takes several hours. Since toxicity is related to tissue concentrations and not serum levels, high serum digoxin concentrations during the early pre-distribution phase may not be associated with signs of toxicity.

Treatment ■

SUPPORTIVE CARE

Many common antiarrhythmic agents may predispose to lethal rhythm disturbances and should generally be avoided (Table 72-3). Useful antiarrhythmics include atropine (to increase heart rate and improve conduction) and phenytoin (to activate the sodium/potassium ATP-ase pump). Lidocaine may be useful for ventricular arrhythmias (Table 72-4).

Because hypokalemia associated with chronic diuretic therapy may aggravate cardiac arrhythmias in patients with chronic intoxication, potassium replacement should be undertaken cautiously in such patients. However, with acute ingestion and with very severe chronic intoxication, paralysis of the sodium-potassium ATP-ase pumping mechanism may occur and severe hyperkalemia may result. In these situations, treatment of *hyperkalemia* is indicated instead of replacement of potassium. Hyperkalemia may be corrected with Kayexalate, glucose, and insulin, and correction of acidosis with sodium bicarbonate (see Chapter 102). Calcium should *not* be used, as it may aggravate digitalis-induced tachyarrythmias. *Under no circumstances* should empiric potassium therapy be

---

TABLE 72–1. *Factors Increasing Cardiac Glycoside Toxicity*

Hypokalemia or hypercalcemia
Low glomerular filtration rate
Myocarditis
Cardiac surgery
Quinidine, amiodarone, or verapamil kinetic interactions

TABLE 72–2. *Cardiac Glycoside-Induced Arrhythmias*

Heart block (all degrees)
Premature ventricular contractions (may be coupled)
Supraventricular tachyarrhythmias
Ventricular tachycardia
Ventricular fibrillation

TABLE 72–4. *Useful Therapies in Cardiac Glycoside Intoxication*

Atropine
Lidocaine
Phenytoin
Pacing
Fab fragments

started without knowledge of the serum concentration of potassium.

Decontamination

After acute ingestion, induce emesis with ipecac syrup or perform gastric lavage (see Chapter 64). Caution: These procedures may increase vagal tone and enhance AV block and bradycardia induced by cardiac glycosides. Administer activated charcoal and cathartic.

Enhancing Elimination

Measures such as hemodialysis and charcoal hemoperfusion have no value to enhance the removal of *digoxin* because of its high degree of tissue binding. However, the volume of distribution of *digitoxin* is small, and hemoperfusion and repeated-dose charcoal have been effective.

SPECIFIC TREATMENT

Rapid and effective reversal of cardiac glycoside poisoning can be achieved with digoxin-specific Fab antibody fragments (Digibind®). The Fab-digoxin complex is rapidly excreted by simple glomerular filtration. In the presence of renal failure, dissociation

of the complex and clinical relapse probably does *not* occur. While specifically manufactured against digoxin, the Fab fragments have documented efficacy against all the cardiac glycosides, although dosing may be somewhat more empiric.

The dose of digoxin Fab fragments is calculated from the estimated total body burden of digoxin. The formula shown below can be used to estimate Fab fragment doses based on the serum digoxin concentration (SDC).

$$\text{Body Burden} = \frac{\text{SDC (ng/mL)} \times 5.6 \times \text{Wt (kg)}}{1000}$$

This formula is not reliable after acute overdose because transiently elevated serum concentrations may occur before complete tissue distribution. An alternative method of estimating body burden, especially useful in acute ingestions, is based on the ingested dose (for oral ingestions, it can be assumed that about 80% of an oral dose will be absorbed). After an estimate of the total body burden of digoxin has been made, 40 mg of Fab fragments can be used per 0.6 mg of digoxin in the body. Table 72-5 shows

TABLE 72–3. *Relatively Contraindicated Therapies in Cardiac Glycoside Intoxication*

Beta-receptor blockers
Calcium
Verapamil
Quinidine
Procainamide
Disopyramide
DC cardioversion

TABLE 72–5. *Estimated Fab Dose From Digoxin Level or Acute Oral Dose*

Chronic* Digoxin Level (ng/ml)	Acute Oral Digoxin Dose (µg/kg)	Digibind Dose (mg/kg)
5.0	33	1.8
7.5	50	2.8
10.0	66	3.7
12.5	75	4.6
15.0	100	5.6

* Post-distributional or equilibrium level. Cannot be used early after acute overdose.

estimated Fab doses in mg/kg based on serum concentrations or oral ingested dose.

Fab fragments are normally reconstituted at a concentration of 10 mg/ml. They should be filtered before use and should be given as a slow infusion (i.e., over 3–4 minutes). The incidence of true hypersensitivity reaction appears extremely low. Serum digoxin concentrations measured after the administration of Fab fragments may be misleadingly high because of translocation of digoxin from tissue to serum. Repeated doses of Fab fragments are usually unnecessary if the body burden was properly calculated, but may be given if manifestations of toxicity (particularly hyperkalemia and arrhythmias) do not resolve in 20–30 minutes.

DISPOSITION

Because of the prolonged absorption of these compounds, all except the most trivial of ingestions warrant close observation for at least 12 hours. Asymptomatic patients seen more than 12 hours after an acute ingestion with very low serum digoxin concentrations and no elevation of serum potassium may be presumed to have ingested minimal amounts and do not need inpatient therapy. Admit symptomatic patients to an intensive care unit or arrange immediate transfer to a pediatric critical care center.

Bibliography ∎

Leikin J, Vogel S, Graff J, et al: Use of Fab fragments of digoxin-specific antibodies in the therapy of massive digoxin poisoning. *Ann Emerg Med* 1985; 14:175–178.

Smith TW, Butler VP, Haber E, et al: Treatment of life-threatening digitalis intoxication with digoxin-specific Fab antibody fragments. *New Engl J Med* 1982; 307:1357–1362.

73 Caustics

Mary Ellen Mortensen

Caustics include acids (hydrochloric, hydrofluoric, sulfuric, phosphoric) and alkalis (lye, ammonia, sodium hydroxide, sodium hypochlorite), as well as a variety of other corrosive agents such as phenols, chlorates, metals (e.g., mercuric chloride) and cationic detergents. Acids produce a self-limiting coagulation necrosis. Hydrofluoric acid is unique in producing a severe deep penetrating injury, due to the highly electronegative fluoride ion. Corrosive alkalis cause penetrating and progressive liquefaction necrosis. Gastric injury is more common after ingestion of acids, which are usually in a liquid form; in contrast, esophageal injury is more common with granular alkaline drain openers.

The toxicity of caustics depends upon concentration, duration of contact, and the exposed tissue. One or two swallows of lye may be fatal, but several ounces of ingested household bleach (3–5% hypochlorite) may not.

Clinical Findings ■

ACIDS

Ingestion may cause hematemesis and epigastric pain, or no symptoms prior to gastric perforation. The oropharynx may appear normal or reddened. Dermal exposure produces severe pain; concentrated acid burns are well demarcated. Ocular exposure may cause conjunctivitis, edema, and corneal injury; secondary corneal infection and scarring may lead to permanent visual impairment. Inhalation of acid gas, mists, or vapors may precipitate bronchospasm and chemical pneumonitis, which may progress to noncardiogenic pulmonary edema after 6–8 hours (or as long as 24–36 hours after inhalation of fuming nitric acid).

ALKALIS

Ingestion causes oropharyngeal pain, drooling, and dysphagia; the mucous membranes appear white and soapy. The absence of oral burns does not exclude esophageal injury. Hoarseness and stridorous breathing suggest upper airway compromise; complete airway obstruction may occur suddenly. Findings after ocular and inhalation exposures are similar to those for acids.

MIXTURES

Chlorine bleach mixed with strong acid releases chlorine gas. Chlorine bleach and ammonia produce chloramine gas. Inhalation effects are described above under "Acids."

OTHERS

Ingestion of phenols produces caustic effects as well as CNS excitation, seizures, methemoglobinemia, and hepatic and renal dysfunction. Dermal contact can cause painless, full-thickness burns. Chlorates can cause hemolysis and methemoglobinemia. Paraquat can cause caustic injury to the mouth, esophagus, and stomach, and respiratory fibrosis. Mercuric chloride produces caustic burns and acute renal failure.

ANCILLARY DATA

Laboratory abnormalities depend upon symptomatology. Hemorrhage may lower hemoglobin. Dehydration and electrolyte abnormalities are common. Oxidizing agents such as phenols and chlorates may produce methemoglobinemia and hemolysis. Radiographic signs of gastric or esophageal perforation include intramural air, subdiaphragmatic free air, and mediastinal emphysema.

ENDOSCOPY

Endoscopy is indicated after caustic ingestion in symptomatic patients without perforation (oral burns, nausea, vomiting, abdominal pain, etc.) and in some asymptomatic patients, depending on the time since ingestion, the agent, and the amount ingested. Consider barium swallow if patients present more than 48 hours after ingestion.

DIFFERENTIAL DIAGNOSIS

Other causes of acute upper airway obstruction include foreign body aspiration and infection (e.g., epiglottitis, peritonsillar abscess, tonsillar cellulitis). Acute abdomen may result from perforated viscus secondary to infection, obstruction, ulceration, and trauma; medical causes include pancreatitis, tumor, lymphadenitis, ulcer disease, and, in post-pubertal females, ectopic pregnancy and gynecologic disorders. Thermal injury can produce mucosal or dermal burns.

Treatment ■

SUPPORTIVE CARE

Airway obstruction requires rapid oral (not blind nasotracheal) intubation, or cricothyroidotomy if orotracheal visualization is impossible. Assisted ventilation may be needed, with positive end-expiratory pressure for severe pulmonary edema. Treat hypotension and shock with IV fluid replacement, and transfuse to replace blood loss. Vasopressors may be needed for unresponsive shock.

Decontamination

Ingestion: If able to swallow, the patient should drink 1–2 glasses of milk or water to dilute the material. Do *not* induce emesis. Do not give activated charcoal (except after paraquat ingestion). Cautious gastric lavage may be indicated for a large liquid caustic ingestion, providing signs of perforation are not present.

Ocular: Flush with copious amounts of water or saline for 15–30 minutes, checking the pH of tears at regular intervals. Refer to an ophthalmologist if there is evidence of corneal injury on fluorescein examination.

Dermal: Flush with copious amounts of water; castor oil or vegetable oil application may decrease phenol absorption. Remove contaminated clothing.

Inhalation: Remove from exposure.

SPECIFIC TREATMENT

The use of steroids to prevent esophageal strictures after corrosive alkali ingestion is controversial. Ste-

TABLE 73–1. *Classification of Endoscopic Findings in Alkali Ingestion*

Superficial (First Degree)
Mild, nonulcerative esophagitis, hyperemic mucosa without loss of tissue

Transmucosal (Second Degree)
Ulcerative lesions, mild transmucosal involvement with shallow ulcers. Moderately severe: deep craters with muscle-layer involvement

Transmural (Third Degree)
Ulcerative, severe: few areas of intact mucosa, transmural involvement. Very severe: widespread tissue destruction, mediastinitis, abscess formation

(Adapted from Friedman EM, Lovejoy FH Jr: The emergency management of caustic ingestions. *Emerg Med Clin North Am* 1984; 2:81)

roid therapy is based on endoscopic findings (Table 73-1) and is recommended only for second-degree burns. Give methylprednisolone 20 mg IV every 8 hours (<2 years old) or 40 mg IV every 8 hours (>2 years old); when oral intake tolerated, prednisone 2 mg/kg/day for 3–4 weeks. Start broad-spectrum antibiotic therapy only if there is evidence of perforation, infection, or sepsis. Follow-up esophagoscopy or barium swallow should be done 3–4 weeks after the injury or if signs of obstruction (dysphagia) occur.

For hydrofluoric acid burns, injections of calcium gluconate may be required; consult a regional poison control center immediately for advice (Table 63-1).

Disposition ■

Admit all symptomatic patients. Observe asymptomatic patients for at least 6 hours in the emergency department if earlier admission is unnecessary.

Bibliography ■

Friedman EM, Lovejoy FH: The emergency management of caustic ingestions. *Emerg Med Clin North Am* 1984; 2: 77–86.

Moore WR: Caustic ingestions: Pathophysiology, diagnosis, and treatment. *Clin Pediatr* 1986; 25:192–196.

74 Clonidine and Antihypertensives

Olga F. Woo

CLONIDINE AND RELATED AGENTS

Clonidine, guanabenz, and methyldopa all act centrally to decrease sympathetic outflow by stimulating alpha-2 adrenergic (inhibitory) receptors. In addition, guanabenz has ganglionic blocking properties, and methyldopa is metabolized to a false neurotransmitter (alpha-methylnorepinephrine). As little as one tablet of 0.1-mg clonidine will produce toxic symptoms, but 10 mg shared by twin 34-month-old girls was not fatal. Ingestion of or skin absorption from transdermal clonidine patches has also caused toxicity. No pediatric overdoses have been reported with methyldopa, but ingestion of more than the maximum daily dose (65 mg/kg) is expected to cause symptoms.

PRAZOSIN AND RELATED AGENTS

Prazosin and phenoxybenzamine are selective oral alpha-1 receptor adrenergic blocking agents, but the latter is seldom prescribed for the treatment of hypertension. Terazosin and trimazosin are new oral agents that will be available in the future. These drugs cause vasodilation by decreasing alpha-1-mediated vasoconstrictor tone. Serious acute overdoses seldom occur.

CAPTOPRIL AND RELATED AGENTS

Captopril, enalapril, and lisinopril block the enzyme peptidyldipeptide carboxyhydrolase from converting angiotensin I to angiotensin II, thereby inhibiting vasoconstriction. Enalapril requires metabolism to enalaprilat to be active.

RESERPINE AND RELATED AGENTS

Reserpine, guanethidine, and guanadrel are ganglionic blocking agents that produce sympatholysis by depleting catecholamines and neurotransmitters at presynaptic ganglionic nerve terminals centrally and peripherally. Acute overdosages of these agents have not resulted in serious poisonings; survival of reserpine overdoses ranging from 25 mg to 1 g have been reported. The duration of effect may be 3 days or more.

HYDRALAZINE AND RELATED VASODILATORS

Hydralazine and minoxidil are vasodilators that directly dilate peripheral arterioles to lower blood pressure.

Clinical Findings ■

The primary presentation of antihypertensive drug overdoses is hypotension. Other manifestations depend on the agent's specific pharmacologic properties (see Table 74-1). Centrally acting agents such as clonidine produce bradycardia and CNS depression; peripheral vasodilators typically produce hypotension with orthostatic dizziness or syncope and tachycardia. Clonidine may also demonstrate biphasic effects: initially there may be transient hypertension due to peripheral alpha stimulation.

An acute ingestion should be suspected when a child appears lethargic. Progression to various levels of consciousness may result in coma and/or apnea. Hypoxic ischemia to the brain may also produce seizure activity.

Diagnosis depends on a reliable history for exposure and evidence of cardiotoxic effects. Other signs and symptoms, such as miosis and hypothermia, may also provide helpful clues. Immediate toxicologic analysis to detect these agents in blood or urine is generally unavailable.

The differential diagnosis includes beta blockers, calcium channel blockers, sedative-hypnotic agents, barbiturates, antidepressants, phenothiazines, and opiates.

TABLE 74–1. *Antihypertensive Agents*

Agent Group	Reported Toxic Dose (mg)	Onset (min)	Signs and Symptoms
Central Alpha-2 Agonist			
Clonidine	0.1–10	30	Miosis, apnea, coma, bradycardia, hypotension, hypothermia, hyporeflexic
Guanabenz	12–480	60	Same as clonidine
Methyldopa	No reported cases		
Peripheral Alpha-1 Antagonist			
Prazosin	No reported cases		
Angiotensin Inhibitor (Peripheral)			
Captopril	No reported cases		Stupor
Enalapril	No reported cases		
Lisinophil	No reported cases		
Ganglionic Blocker (Central and Peripheral)			
Reserpine	25–1,000	As late as 12 hr	Miosis, apnea, coma, bradycardia, hypotension, hyperthermia, vomiting, diarrhea, flushing, nasal congestion
Guanethidine	No reported cases		
Guanadrel	No reported cases		
Vasodilators			
Hydralazine		30–45	Lethargy, hypotension, tachycardia
Minoxidil	100	30–60	Hypotension, tachycardia

Treatment ■

SUPPORTIVE CARE

Protect the airway and assist ventilation if necessary. Transient hypertension after clonidine overdose does not require treatment, but close observation and monitoring are important. Hypotension usually responds to supine position and IV fluid bolus therapy (10–20 ml/kg saline). Atropine may be used to treat symptomatic bradycardia. If the hypotension is unresponsive to fluid therapy and the supine position, administer dopamine and/or norepinephrine. Use a warming blanket to correct hypothermia. Recovery is usually complete within 24 hours with supportive care.

Decontamination

Empty the stomach with ipecac-induced emesis (if the ingestion occurred within 30 minutes) or gastric lavage, and administer activated charcoal (see Chapter 64). There is no evidence that repeated doses of activated charcoal will hasten the elimination of these drugs.

SPECIFIC TREATMENT

There are no specific antidotes for these agents. Giving naloxone in clonidine poisoning may produce an equivocal or transient clinical response. Tolazoline has been recommended to treat clonidine-induced hypertension, but the response is unreliable and can paradoxically worsen the hypertension.

Extracorporeal drug removal (e.g., dialysis or hemoperfusion) is unnecessary and ineffective.

Disposition ■

Observe asymptomatic patients for at least 6 hours before discharge from the emergency department. Admit all symptomatic patients for a 24-hour observation period.

Bibliography ■

Loggies JMH, Saito H, Kah I, et al: Accidental reserpine poisoning: Clinical and metabolic effects. *Clin Pharmacol Ther* 1967; 8:692–695.

Olsson JM, Pruitt AW: Management of clonidine ingestion in children. *J Pediatr* 1983; 103:646–650.

75 Cocaine and Amphetamines

S. Alan Tani

Cocaine, amphetamines, and related drugs are widely abused for their stimulant effects. They may be ingested, snorted, injected, or smoked. Cocaine is commonly sold as the hydrochloride salt or the free base ("freebase" or "crack"). The free base form of cocaine is preferred for smoking because it is readily volatized, whereas the salt form decomposes with heating. Amphetamines are synthetic stimulants with similar properties to cocaine. A new smokable form of methamphetamine, known as "ice," has recently become popular.

These drugs produce intoxication by directly stimulating the central nervous system and peripheral adrenergic neurons and inhibiting catecholamine reuptake. In addition, cocaine has local anesthetic effects which may produce membrane depression in very high doses. The toxic dose is highly variable depending on individual tolerance. Acute absorption of more than 1 mg/kg of any of these drugs should be considered potentially harmful.

Clinical Findings ■

Smoking and intravenous injection of these drugs produces nearly immediate onset of effects, whereas the time to onset of effects after oral or mucosal absorption may be delayed 20–30 minutes or longer. Infants have developed toxicity (including seizures) following passive inhalation of cocaine-laden smoke or breast-feeding. Occasionally toxicity occurs up to several hours after a bag, vial, balloon, or condom containing one of these drugs is ingested. Initial effects of mild central nervous stimulation include euphoria, talkativeness, dilated pupils, paranoia, and tachycardia. With larger doses diaphoresis, agitation, hypertension, and psychosis may occur. Severe hypertension may cause intracranial hemorrhage or myocardial necrosis. Severely overdosed patients may develop seizures, muscle rigidity, agitated delirium, hyperthermia, and cardiovascular collapse. Secondary damage from hyperthermia and seizures includes rhabdomyolysis and renal failure (Table 75-1). Neonates born to cocaine-abusing mothers ("crack babies") may have poor muscle tone and feeding, weak cry, and lethargy.

The diagnosis of stimulant intoxication should be suspected in any child or adolescent presenting with hypertension, tachycardia, diaphoresis, and agitation. These drugs and their metabolites can be detected in the urine on toxicologic screening. Blood levels are neither available nor reliable measures of toxicity. The differential diagnosis includes other illicit stimulants and hallucinogens (*e.g.,* phencyclidine [PCP], LSD), nonprescription decongestants and diet pills, antihistamines, anticholinergics, and withdrawal from alcohol or other sedative-hypnotic drugs. Also consider other life-threatening medical conditions such as sepsis, meningitis, or exertional heat stroke.

Treatment ■

Maintain a patent airway and provide intensive supportive care as described in Chapter 63. Patients with mild intoxication can often be managed with calm reassurance and mild sedation. On the other hand, those with severe agitation or major medical complications require aggressive intensive care. Manage hyperthermia with external cooling (tepid sponging, fanning) and, if necessary, neuromuscular paralysis. If rhabdomyolysis is suspected, check the urine for myoglobin (positive hemoglobin dipstick test) and measure the serum CPK. Rhabdomyolysis is treated by alkalinizing the urine and administration of intravenous fluids to prevent myoglobin deposition in the kidney. Obtain a CT brain scan in patients with focal neurologic deficits or other evidence of intracranial hemorrhage.

DECONTAMINATION

After ingestion of cocaine or amphetamines, empty the stomach with gastric lavage and administer activated charcoal and a cathartic. If the patient is cooperative, activated charcoal may be given orally

TABLE 75–1. *Clinical Features of Cocaine and Amphetamine Intoxication*

Central Nervous System
    Talkativeness, euphoria
    Agitation, psychosis
    Seizures
    Intracranial hemorrhage
Cardiovascular
    Tachycardia
    Hypertension
Renal
    Renal tubular necrosis from myoglobinuria
Metabolic/other
    Hyperthermia
    Rhabdomyolysis

without prior gut emptying. Do not induce emesis because of the risk of aggravating agitation and hypertension and because of the risk of abrupt onset of seizures. Patients who have ingested a bag, condom, or other container should be admitted for observation until the bag is passed in the stool. Radiographic contrast procedures, whole bowel irrigation, and endoscopic retrieval have all been used to manage such ingestions, although most patients have been treated successfully with repeated doses of activated charcoal and cathartics and hospital observation.

There is no role for enhanced extracorporeal elimination procedures such as dialysis or hemoperfusion because these drugs are highly tissue bound. Although urinary acidification may enhance renal excretion of amphetamines, the marginal benefit does not justify the risk of aggravating myoglobinuric renal toxicity.

SPECIFIC TREATMENT

There are no specific antidotes. Several therapeutic drugs are useful for management of specific complications (see Chapter 63). Treat agitation or seizures with sedatives such as diazepam, lorazepam, or midazolam. Prolonged seizures may require general anesthesia with pentobarbital. Hypertension should be treated with phentolamine or nitroprusside; mild hypertension in an awake and cooperative patient may be treated with oral or sublingual nifedipine if it does not resolve with sedation. Tachyarrhythmias are treated with esmolol or propranolol rather than usual antiarrhythmic drugs.

Disposition ■

All children with a history of exposure to these drugs should be evaluated in an emergency department. Asymptomatic or mildly symptomatic children may be discharged after 6–8 hours of observation unless they have ingested a bag, vial or other container. All children should be evaluated for possible child abuse. Patients with significant symptoms, and those with suspected ingestion of a drug-filled container, should be admitted to the intensive care unit or transferred to a pediatric critical care center.

Bibliography ■

Garland JS, Smith DS, Rice TB et al: Accidental cocaine intoxication in a nine-month-old infant: presentation and treatment. *Pediatr Emerg Care* 1989; 5:245–247.

Ernst AA, Sanders WM: Unexpected cocaine intoxication presenting as seizures in children. *Ann Emerg Med* 1989; 18:774–777.

Chasnoff IJ, Lewis DE, Squires L: Cocaine intoxication in a breast-fed infant. *Pediatrics* 1987; 80:836–838.

76 Cyanide

Kent R. Olson

Cyanide is a rapidly acting lethal poison, which may exist as a gas or liquid or as a salt with sodium, potassium, and other cations. Cyanide gas is released when acid comes in contact with cyanide salts or with cyanogenic compounds such as nitriles and cyanogenic glycosides found in a variety of plants (pulverized pits of apricots, plums, peaches, etc). Cyanide gas is also produced by combustion of a variety of synthetic and natural materials, and is an important contributor to death in smoke inhalation victims. Cyanide is also released from sodium nitroprusside.

Cyanide binds to intracellular cytochrome oxidase, inhibiting aerobic metabolism. The victim experiences "chemical asphyxia" because of the inability to utilize oxygen. The potentially lethal dose by inhalation of cyanide gas is approximately 100–300 ppm. The estimated lethal adult oral dose of hydrogen cyanide liquid is 50 mg. The estimated lethal oral dose of cyanide salts (e.g., potassium cyanide) is 200–300 mg for an adult and 1.2–5 mg/kg in a child. The lethal oral dose of cyanogenic glycosides and other compounds is unpredictable owing to variations in content of cyanogenic material and rate of conversion to cyanide. Very rapid rates of nitroprusside infusion (i.e., greater than 10–20 ug/kg/min) may induce signs of cyanide toxicity, although deaths have not been reported.

Clinical Findings ■

Symptoms occur almost immediately after inhalation but may be delayed for several minutes after ingestion or skin exposure. Initial manifestations include headache, dyspnea, dizziness, confusion, restlessness, nausea, vomiting, and tachypnea. With a lethal exposure, shock, convulsions, coma, respiratory arrest, and death may occur within 5–10 minutes. The skin is usually clammy and diaphoretic, although cyanosis may be absent because of the higher venous content of oxygen. Breath or gastric contents may have a distinct almond-like odor (discernible by only about 50% of the population). Arterial blood gases will usually reveal severe metabolic acidosis. The venous oxygen content (or oxyhemoglobin saturation) may be elevated because tissue oxygen uptake is reduced. There is no rapid bedside laboratory test for cyanide. Blood cyanide levels are useful in confirming toxicity but are not readily available to be useful in the emergency department. Blood levels greater than 2–2.5 mg/L are considered potentially lethal.

Suspect cyanide poisoning in any patient with sudden onset of coma, shock, and metabolic acidosis. Other toxins producing similar manifestations include hydrogen sulfide and carbon monoxide. Suspect combined cyanide and carbon monoxide poisoning in any patient with smoke inhalation.

Treatment ■

SUPPORTIVE CARE

Establish a patent airway and assist ventilation if needed. High-flow supplemental oxygen is of questionable value for cyanide but is useful for co-existing carbon monoxide poisoning.

For patients in shock, give boluses of IV crystalloid (normal saline or lactated Ringer's solution) 10–20 ml/kg once or twice. Reverse acidosis with sodium bicarbonate boluses 1–2 mEq/kg.

Decontamination

Inhalation: Remove the victim from exposure, while protecting the rescuer with a self-contained breathing apparatus.

Ingestion: If ingestion occurred within the previous 5–10 minutes, and hospital care or activated charcoal therapy is not immediately available, promptly induce emesis with digital oropharyngeal stimulation or with ipecac syrup. If charcoal is available, immediately administer at least 60–100 g orally or by gastric tube, if possible (see Chapter 64). Although charcoal has a relatively low affinity for cyanide, it has been shown to effectively bind it at a ratio of approximately 50:1.

TABLE 76–1. *Antidotal Treatment of Cyanide Poisoning*

Available Agents in Cyanide Antidote Kit

Amyl nitrite 0.3 ml ampules: break and inhale

Sodium nitrite 3% solution: 0.2–0.4 ml/kg, based on Hgb

Sodium thiosulfate 25% solution: 1.6 ml/kg

Sodium Nitrite Dose Based Upon Hemoglobin

Hgb (mg/dL)	Sodium Nitrite (mg/kg)	Sodium Nitrite 3% Solution (ml/kg)
7.0	5.8	0.19
8.0	6.6	0.22
9.0	7.5	0.25
10.0	8.3	0.27
11.0	9.0	0.30
12.0	10.0	0.33
13.0	10.8	0.36
14.0	11.6	0.39

SPECIFIC TREATMENT

For patients with signs of cyanide poisoning, administer the cyanide antidote kit (see Table 76-1). Break an ampule of amyl nitrite (0.2 ml) under the nose or over the endotracheal tube while starting an IV line.

Then give sodium nitrite 3% solution IV, about 0.3 ml/kg (exact dose is based on hemoglobin; see Table 76-1). Caution: Excessive administration of nitrites can produce severe hypotension and methemoglobinemia. Also give sodium thiosulfate 25% solution IV, 1.6 mL/kg. Sodium thiosulfate is essentially harmless and may be given empirically when the diagnosis is in doubt. Nitrites and thiosulfate may be repeated once at one-half the original dose, if needed.

Disposition ■

Patients who inhaled hydrogen cyanide gas will experience maximal absorption and onset of symptoms immediately after exposure. If they are improving or asymptomatic upon arrival in the emergency department, further toxicity is unlikely. On the other hand, patients who ingested cyanide salts or cyanogenic compounds may have a delayed inset of poisoning (from minutes to several hours). Thus, observe any patient with a potential cyanide ingestion for at least 6 hours (12 hours if a cyanogenic glycoside or nitrile is involved). Admit all symptomatic patients to an intensive care unit or transfer to a pediatric critical care center.

Bibliography ■

Lambert RJ et al: The efficacy of superactivated charcoal in treating rats exposed to a lethal oral dose of potassium cyanide. *Ann Emerg Med* 1988; 17:595–598.

77 Cyclic Antidepressant Overdose

William Banner, Jr.

Cyclic antidepressants (also known as tricyclic antidepressants) continue to be a serious source of lethal overdose in both children and adults. These drugs produce toxicity by various mechanisms. The mechanism of antidepressant effects appears to be inhibition of re-uptake of catecholamines and serotonin at the presynaptic nerve terminal. In overdose, there may be an early elevation of circulating catecholamines and sympathomimetic effects. As the nerve terminals are depleted, there may be a relative lack of catecholamines, resulting in bradycardia and hypotension. The most lethal effect of cyclic antidepressants is a quinidine-like membrane-depressant effect on cardiac conduction. Other mechanisms include alpha-adrenergic blockade and antimuscarinic (atropine-like) effects. *One misconception is that the lethality of these compounds is caused by an anticholinergic-like syndrome that can be reversed with drugs that increase cholinergic tone.*

The minimum toxic dose of tricyclic antidepressants is variable, but consider ingestions of greater than 10–20 mg/kg life-threatening.

Clinical Findings ■

Clinical manifestations of cyclic antidepressant poisoning are shown in Table 77-1. Serious effects can be quite abrupt in onset, and it is not unusual for an ambulatory patient to suffer sudden seizures, coma, and cardiac arrhythmias. Within the first two hours after ingestion, the most common findings are an antimuscarinic syndrome (tachycardia, dilated pupils, delirium), drowsiness, and a wide QRS tachycardia that resembles ventricular tachycardia. Hypotension may occur because of vascular alpha-adrenergic blockade or direct cardiodepressant effects. Seizures, if multiple, may lead to metabolic acidosis and hyperthermia. The clinical laboratory can identify and quantify most of these drugs, but clinical decisions should not be based on serum concentrations. Prolongation of the QRS interval to greater than 0.12 sec is considered prognostic of severe toxicity (note that QRS prolongation may be absent with intoxication by amoxapine).

The differential diagnosis includes a variety of drugs and plants that produce atropine-like symptoms, especially the antihistamines and belladonna derivatives. Phenothiazines such as thioridazine (Mellaril) or chlorpromazine at extremely high concentrations may have cardiac effects resembling the antidepressants. Quinidine, procainamide, disopyramide, encainide, flecainide, propranolol, and antimalarials such as quinine, chloroquine, and quinacrine may also produce widening of the QRS complex and hypotension.

Treatment ■

SUPPORTIVE CARE

The treatment of cyclic antidepressant poisoning depends heavily on supportive care. *Protect the airway, assist ventilation, and control seizures.* Respiratory or metabolic acidemia resulting from coma and seizures can increase the free drug concentration and aggravate cardiac toxicity. Also, seizure activity may cause severe hyperthermia and rhabdomyolysis from excessive muscle activity.

Treat seizures first with diazepam, lorazepam, or midazolam. Phenytoin and phenobarbital are useful anticonvulsants but must be given very cautiously (over 15–20 minutes) because rapid injection may add to antidepressant-induced myocardial depression. General anesthesia may be necessary if the basic approach to anticonvulsant therapy is ineffective. Neuromuscular paralysis may be necessary to control muscular hyperactivity and hyperthermia.

Lidocaine and phenytoin may be effective for ventricular arrhythmias. Antiarrhythmics to be avoided include Type Ia (quinidine, procainamide, and di-

TABLE 77-1. *Symptoms and Signs of Cyclic Antidepressant Poisoning*

Mild/Moderate Intoxication
Sinus tachycardia
Mild hypertension
Dry mucous membranes
Delirium
Hyperreflexia
Myoclonic contractions
Mild QRS prolongation
Mydriasis
Urinary retention

Serious/Lethal Intoxication
Wide QRS bradycardia
Hypotension
Coma
Status epilepticus
Hyperthermia

sopyramide), Type Ic (flecainide, encainide), bretylium, and amiodarone. While physostigmine has been reported effective for delirium and tachycardia, it has also been associated with asystole and seizures and is no longer recommended.

Treat hypotension with IV fluids (hetastarch, saline, or lactated Ringer's, 10–20 ml/kg boluses) and sodium bicarbonate 1–2 mEq/kg (see next section). Because cyclic antidepressant poisoning produces alpha-adrenergic receptor blockade and prevents dopamine-induced norepinephrine release, the effects of conventional pressor therapy (dopamine) may be limited; norepinephrine infusion has been recommended in this setting.

Decontamination

Because of the potential for rapid onset of seizures and coma, ipecac syrup is contraindicated in cyclic antidepressant ingestion. Perform immediate gastric lavage and administer activated charcoal and cathartic (see Chapter 64). If the child is obtunded, protect the airway with an endotracheal tube before decontamination procedures.

SPECIFIC TREATMENT

Sodium bicarbonate (8.4%) effectively reverses cardiotoxicity by reversing acidosis and by supplying a hypertonic saline load that reverses sodium channel inhibition. Give 1–2 mEq/kg in boluses as needed to reverse hypotension and QRS interval prolongation. Maintain serum pH at least 7.45.

Dialysis and hemoperfusion have no recognized role because of the large volume of distribution of these drugs. In selected circumstances where conventional therapy has failed, partial cardiopulmonary bypass may theoretically be useful in supporting a patient until cardiac manifestations could become more manageable.

DISPOSITION

Admit symptomatic children to a monitored environment. The length of hospitalization may vary but should allow for 12–24 hours without symptoms. Observe asymptomatic patients until 8–12 hours postingestion.

Bibliography ∎

Crome P: Poisoning due to tricyclic antidepressant overdosage clinical presentation and treatment. *Med Toxicol Adverse Drug Exp* 1986; 1:261–285.

Kulig K: Management of poisoning associated with "newer" antidepressant agents. *Ann Emerg Med* 1986; 15:1039–1045.

Pentel PR, Benowitz NL: Tricyclic antidepressant poisoning management of arrhythmias. *Med Toxicol Adverse Drug Exp* 1986; 1:101–121.

78 Hallucinogens

S. Alan Tani

Hallucinogenic agents include a variety of naturally occurring and synthetic compounds (see Table 78-1). The mechanism of action depends on the compound and may include anticholinergic toxicity, sympathomimetic effects, and enhanced activity of brain neurotransmitters such as serotonin. In many cases, "toxic" effects are actually unpleasant psychic side effects after use of recreational doses. Among the most potent of these agents is lysergic acid diethylamide (LSD), which can produce intense hallucinations after ingestion of as little as 50–100 micrograms.

Clinical Findings ■

The clinical presentation depends on the specific agent (see Table 78-1). Hallucinations, altered sensory awareness, and altered time perception are common. With any of these compounds, recreational users may experience panic reactions characterized by anxiety, tachycardia, depersonalization, and acute paranoid psychosis. With overdose, excessive anticholinergic or sympathomimetic effects may be seen; seizures and hyperthermia may occur.

The differential diagnosis includes hypoglycemia, hypoxia, electrolyte imbalance, exertional heatstroke, and serious infections such as meningitis or encephalitis. Also consider functional psychosis or situational anxiety reaction.

Treatment ■

SUPPORTIVE CARE

Reassurance and psychological support are generally sufficient following a panic reaction or "bad trip." Put the patient in a quiet, darkened room, and display a calm, reassuring bedside manner. Diazepam (0.1–

TABLE 78–1. *Some Common Hallucinogens*

Agent	Comments
Lysergic acid diethylamide (LSD)	Intense visual hallucinations and time-space disorientation. Pupils usually widely dilated. Mild tachycardia and hypertension; hyperthermia rarely
Marijuana	Euphoria, altered time perception, heightened sensory awareness, sedation, tachycardia, conjunctival injection
Anticholinergics (jimson weed, Amanita muscaria, etc.)	Dilated pupils; dry, flushed skin, dry mouth; urinary retention; confusion; tachycardia; delirium. Hyperthermia may occur.
Amphetamines (MDA, MDMA ["Ecstasy"], cocaine, etc.)	Euphoria, tachycardia, hypertension, tremor, dilated pupils, diaphoresis, panic reactions, paranoia, Hyperthermia and seizures may occur.
Psilocybin	Found in psilocybin and paneolus mushrooms; effects similar to LSD. Ingestion of mushrooms typically causes vomiting.
Mescaline	Effects similar to LSD
Phencyclidine (PCP)	Vertical and horizontal nystagmus, alternating lethargy and agitation, tachycardia, hypertension. Seizures and hyperthermia may occur.

0.3 mg/kg orally) or another benzodiazepine may be used for severe anxiety or agitation. In general, avoid the use of antipsychotic phenothiazines and butyrophenones, because they may cause unwanted side effects such as dystonia or hypotension.

Treat medical complications such as tachycardia and hypertension with mild sedation or with combined alpha and beta blockers such as labetalol (0.1–0.2 mg/kg IV). Treat seizures with standard anticonvulsants. Treat hyperthermia aggressively (see Chapter 96) with tepid sponging, fanning, and neuromuscular paralysis if necessary.

DECONTAMINATION

Standard decontamination is indicated for skin, eye, or inhalation exposures. For ingested drugs, oral activated charcoal may be given without gut emptying if the ingested dose was relatively small. Avoid the use of ipecac except after large ingestions of marijuana or other hallucinogenic plants.

SPECIFIC TREATMENT

For anticholinergic delirium or agitation, consider physostigmine, 0.01–0.02 mg/kg IV. Caution: excessive use can cause bradycardia and seizures.

DISPOSITION

Patients having a pleasurable experience with no psychological or medical complications may be observed for 2–4 hours and discharged home with adequate supervision. Others may require psychiatric consultation or medical admission. In general, admit young children and rule out child abuse or neglect.

Bibliography ■

Kulberg A: Substance abuse: Clinical identification and management. *Pediatr Clin North Am* 1986; 11:325–361.

Welch MJ, Correa GA: PCP intoxication in young children and infants. *Clin Pediatr* 1980; 19:510–514.

79 Hydrocarbons

Suman Wason

Commonly encountered hydrocarbons can be categorized into the following groups:

1. Aliphatic petroleum distillates, such as diesel and fuel oils, gasoline, kerosene, mineral seal oil, petroleum naphtha, and petroleum ether
2. Natural oils, such as pine oil and turpentine
3. Aromatic hydrocarbons, such as benzene, toluene, and xylene
4. Halogenated hydrocarbons, such as carbon tetrachloride, trichloroethane, and trichlorethylene

The pulmonary toxicity of hydrocarbons is related to their viscosity, surface tension, and volatility. Products with the lowest viscosity and surface tension are associated with the greatest risk for pulmonary aspiration. Table 79-1 shows the toxic effects of the four groups of hydrocarbons.

Clinical Findings ■

INGESTION

Simple aliphatic hydrocarbons are not well absorbed from the GI tract. Rare findings have included bloody diarrhea, elevated hepatic transaminases, renal tubular toxicity, and mild hemolysis. These conditions are usually self-limited and do not require intervention.

Hydrocarbons from the other groups, such as natural oils, aromatic compounds, or chlorinated derivatives, are often well absorbed orally and may produce CNS depression, seizures, cardiac arrhythmias, and renal and hepatic damage.

ASPIRATION

The most common clinical findings after hydrocarbon aspiration are sudden coughing, gagging, and often spontaneous emesis. In cases of substantial aspiration, dyspnea, chest wall retractions, grunting, cyanosis, and hypoxia with lethargy may be present. Respiratory symptoms may progress during the first 24 hours and subside over 2–5 days. Fever and tachycardia may also be present early in the course of an aspiration pneumonia.

Laboratory findings include leukocytosis. Chest X-rays obtained early may be normal or may show minimal changes and have not been useful in the early detection of hydrocarbon pneumonitis. More useful in predicting hydrocarbon aspiration pneumonia have been clinical findings such as coughing, choking, lethargy, rhonchi, rales, retractions, cyanosis, tachypnea, fever, and leukocytosis.

INHALATION

Inhalation of hydrocarbons may produce hypoxia by displacement of oxygen from the alveoli or direct toxic effects of the hydrocarbon itself. Patients who have inhaled hydrocarbons may present with seizures, encephalopathy, and cardiac dysrhythmia. "Sudden sniffing death" may occur from dysrhythmias secondary to myocardial sensitization to endogenous catecholamines after acute inhalation of typewriter correction fluid.

The differential diagnosis is limited because almost invariably a history of hydrocarbon ingestion is available in patients who present with hydrocarbon pneumonia. In the absence of a history of hydrocarbon ingestion, consider pneumonia, foreign body aspiration, reactive airways disease, croup, and epiglottitis. Many drugs and toxins can produce coma, seizures, and cardiac dysrhythmias. Consider tricyclic antidepressants, cocaine, and amphetamines.

Treatment ■

SUPPORTIVE CARE

Ingestion

No specific treatment is required. Avoid maneuvers likely to result in vomiting.

TABLE 79–1. *Toxicity Risk Related to Type of Hydrocarbon*

	Pulmonary	Cardiac	CNS
Petroleum Distillates	+++	+	+
Natural Oils	+++	+	++
Aromatic	+	++	+++
Halogenated	+	+++	+++

Aspiration

Give supplemental oxygen. Endotracheal intubation and assisted ventilation may be required. Bronchodilators (beta$_2$-selective aerosols are preferred; see Chapter 15) may be indicated for patients with bronchospasm secondary to pneumonitis. Avoid epinephrine and other nonselective beta agonists because of the risk of ventricular dysrhythmias secondary to myocardial sensitization.

Inhalation

Treat seizures and coma as described in Chapter 63. Hyperactive patients may require sedation to avoid injury and precipitation of ventricular dysrhythmia by endogenous catecholamine secretion.

DECONTAMINATION

Ingestion and Aspiration

The vast majority of patients who have ingested hydrocarbons require no decontamination since systemic toxicity is very unlikely. When toxic compounds have been ingested, induce emesis or perform gastric lavage, and administer activated charcoal. GI decontamination, even with the placement of a cuffed endotracheal tube, may result in aspiration of the hydrocarbon into the lung. Clearly the risks and benefits must be weighed if it is felt that decontamination is necessary. (See also Chapter 64.)

Inhalation

Remove the patient from the exposure. Because of the inherent risk of dysrhythmia, patients should avoid intense activity.

SPECIFIC TREATMENT

Ingestion

No specific treatment is indicated unless a toxic hydrocarbon has been ingested (*e.g.,* organophosphate insecticide).

Aspiration

Neither antibiotics nor steroids are indicated for the initial treatment of chemical pneumonitis following hydrocarbon aspiration. Antibiotics have not been shown to be helpful unless a specific organism is identified, and steroids may be harmful by altering respiratory flora in favor of gram-negative organisms. Pneumatoceles may occur as a rare complication of hydrocarbon pneumonia; these usually resolve over days to weeks.

Inhalation

Hydrocarbon-induced seizures do not usually require anticonvulsant medication because of their short and benign nature. Cardiac dysrhythmias secondary to hydrocarbons are usually ventricular in origin and may be treated with lidocaine or esmolol.

DISPOSITION

Ingestion and Aspiration

Of children who are symptomatic (coughing, dyspnea) at the time of evaluation, few become asymptomatic during a four- to six-hour period of observation. Conversely, almost all patients who are asymptomatic at presentation remain asymptomatic. Therefore, admit all patients who have symptoms. Asymptomatic patients should be observed for four to six hours before being discharged. Routine chest X-rays are indicated only for symptomatic (and, therefore, admitted) patients.

Inhalation

Most patients will be asymptomatic by the time they are seen. Observe all patients and monitor for cardiac dysrhythmias for 2–4 hours. Discharge if they remain asymptomatic. No medical intervention is required, except for appropriate counseling.

Bibliography ■

Anas N, Namasonthia V, Ginsburg CM: Criteria for hospitalizing children who have ingested products containing hydrocarbons. *JAMA* 1981; 246:840–843.

Machado B, Cross K, Snodgrass WR: Accidental hydrocarbon ingestion cases telephoned to a regional poison center. *Ann Emerg Med* 1988; 17;804–807.

80 Iron Intoxication

William Banner, Jr., and Donald D. Vernon

Iron intoxication remains a significant problem in children because, unfortunately, iron and iron-containing vitamins are still perceived to have a low potential for toxicity. The keys to management of iron intoxication are to recognize the potential severity of these ingestions and to appreciate the role of good supportive care and aggressive decontamination.

Iron's early toxicity is related to GI corrosion, but as iron is absorbed it may directly produce a variety of effects, including coagulopathy and shock. Generally, the potential for severe toxicity exists after an ingestion of 60 mg/kg or more of elemental iron; death may follow untreated intoxication above 150 mg/kg of elemental iron. A single ferrous sulfate tablet (300 mg) contains 60 mg of elemental iron, so a 10-kg child may suffer serious intoxication after ingesting as few as 10 prenatal ferrous sulfate tablets.

Clinical Findings ■

Classically, iron intoxication progresses through four stages (Table 80-1). In the first stage, vomiting, gastric pain, diarrhea, and frank hemorrhage may occur because of severe GI irritation. Extensive loss of intravascular volume may occur as a result of "third spacing" of fluid into the gut lumen. Frequently, abdominal X-rays will show large distended loops of bowel with fluid-filled lumens; intact iron tablets are often visible. In experimental models, an increase in hematocrit is often seen in this stage.

The second stage is a period of relative stability, lasting from 4–36 hours. This probably represents a period of developing but unrecognized severe intoxication. Tachycardia and tachypnea associated with the developing acidosis, and mild obtundation from the circulatory effects of iron may all be present.

In the third stage, circulatory shock is most likely to lead to death. Shock is produced by hypovolemia from a generalized loss of capillary integrity (particularly, volume loss into the GI tract), a loss of venous tone, a decrease in myocardial contractility, and effects on cardiac conduction. Metabolic acidosis is probably caused by a combination of vascular compromise and liberation of hydrogen ion as iron is converted from ferric to ferrous iron. Iron may also inhibit oxidative metabolism. Coagulopathy may result from shock, tissue damage, and direct effects of iron on the coagulation cascade.

In the fourth phase, late manifestations affect the liver and the GI tract. Hepatitis may occur, although frank hepatic necrosis is extremely rare. Corrosive injury to the GI tract may lead to perforations or stricture formation; pyloric stenosis may occur up to 6 weeks after an ingestion.

Laboratory values taken shortly after ingestion may be misleading. Between 2–4 hours after the ingestion, obtain a complete blood count, blood glucose, bicarbonate, serum iron, and abdominal radiograph to assess the need for treatment (Table 80-2). Total iron-binding capacities may be spuriously elevated by severe iron intoxication and are not useful prognostically.

The differential diagnosis includes other causes of gastroenteritis with bloody diarrhea and hemodynamic compromise, such as mushroom poisoning, alkali or acid ingestion, some toxic plants, and arsenic, mercury, and other heavy metal salts.

Treatment ■

SUPPORTIVE CARE

Assess the adequacy of respiration and circulation. Endotracheal intubation may be needed for airway protection. Although chelation therapy is important in the management of iron ingestion, *aggressive treatment of shock, particularly adequate fluid administration, is the key to therapy.* In experimental models of iron intoxication, fluid infusions of up to 100 ml/kg have been needed to maintain intravascular volume. Central venous monitoring may be helpful. Since blood loss in the GI tract may be significant, obtain a crossmatch for blood products to

TABLE 80–1. *Stages in Iron Intoxication*

1. Gastrointestinal
2. Relative stability
3. Shock
4. Hepatic and gastric sequelae

correct coagulopathy. Sodium bicarbonate may reverse the severe metabolic acidosis.

Decontamination

Empty the stomach with ipecac-induced emesis or gastric lavage (see Chapter 64). Activated charcoal, while not contraindicated, does not bind iron and should be used only if other toxins might have been ingested.

Much controversy has been focused on what lavage fluids to use in gastric decontamination. Bicarbonate-containing fluids have been advocated to keep iron in an insoluble state to delay absorption, but excessive use of bicarbonate may cause hypernatremia and alkalosis. Deferoxamine has been advocated to bind iron in the stomach, although some studies suggest this may enhance absorption of the iron-deferoxamine complex, which may itself be toxic. Probably, lavage with a simple, standard fluid such as saline is the safest and most effective.

Occasionally, surgical removal of large concretions of iron pills is necessary. Continuous whole-bowel irrigation with balanced solutions (e.g., Colyte, GoLYTELY) may also be useful in selected patients with large numbers of tablets visible on X-ray.

SPECIFIC TREATMENT

The indications for chelation therapy with deferoxamine are controversial; Table 80-2 provides guide-

TABLE 80–2. *Indications for Chelation Therapy*

Serum iron > 500 μg/dl
Ingestion of >100 mg/kg of iron
Circulatory compromise
Severe gastroenteritis
Laboratory abnormalities
Bicarbonate < 15 mEq/l
WBC > 15,000/mm^3
Blood glucose > 150 mg/dl

lines. Patients with serum iron concentrations above 500 μg/dl should receive chelation therapy. Patients with major signs and symptoms of toxicity should also receive deferoxamine, even if the serum iron is less than 500 μg/dl. The treatment is unclear for patients with serum iron concentrations between 300 and 500 μg/dl and with no major manifestations of toxicity.

Deferoxamine may be given intramuscularly, although it is preferable to use the IV route. Give 10–15 mg/kg/hr by constant infusion. Caution: If IV deferoxamine is given rapidly, it may produce hypotension; this can generally be avoided by infusing the drug no faster than 15 mg/kg/hr. In severe poisoning cases, the infusion rate may be increased to 30–45 mg/kg/hr under carefully monitored circumstances.

The duration of chelation therapy is another source of controversy. Many authors rely on serum iron concentrations, which are generally accurate if deferoxamine concentrations are not excessive. The iron-deferoxamine complex has a characteristic orange-pink color, and the formation of so-called "vin rose" urine shows the continued presence of free chelatable iron in the circulation.

In addition to supportive care and chelation therapy, desperate measures have occasionally been tried in severe iron intoxication, including exchange transfusion, hemodialysis, and continuous arteriovenous hemofiltration. None has proven efficacy.

DISPOSITION

Low-dose iron ingestions (less than 20 mg/kg elemental iron), with a reliable history and no symptoms or signs of toxicity, can be managed by simple observation at home. Ingestions of 20–40 mg/kg may be treated with ipecac-induced emesis and close observation at home. Ingestions of more than 40–60 mg/kg require emergency department gut decontamination and at least 6–8 hours of monitoring of clinical status and serum iron concentrations. After resuscitation and stabilization, children in shock should be managed in an intensive care unit or transferred to a pediatric critical care center.

Bibliography ■

Banner WM, Tong T: Iron poisoning. *Pediatr Clin North Am* 1986; 33:393.
Proudfoot AT, Simpson D, Dyson EH: Management of acute poisoning. *Med Toxicol Adverse Drug Exp* 1986; 1:83.

81 Isoniazid

Suman Wason

Isoniazid (INH), which is about 90% bioavailable, is rapidly absorbed from the GI tract, mainly in the small intestine. Peak plasma concentrations occur 1–2 hours after oral dosage. Acetylation is a primary pathway of INH metabolism. The acetylator status is genetically determined: only 10–20% of Orientals are slow acetylators, compared to 50–60% of blacks and whites. The plasma half-life of INH is 1.1 ± 0.2 hours in fast acetylators and 3 ± 0.8 hours in slow acetylators.

INH produces toxicity as a result of its effects on brain GABA (gamma-aminobutyric acid) metabolism. GABA is synthesized from glutamic acid by the action of the pyridoxine-dependent enzyme glutamic acid decarboxylase. INH inhibits the activity of pyridoxal-5-phosphate (the active form of pyridoxine) and also depletes body stores of pyridoxine (vitamin B_6). This decreases brain GABA levels, resulting in a lowered seizure threshold. The acidosis that occurs after INH overdose is due to the interference of INH with nicotinamide-adenine dinucleotide, which is necessary for the metabolism of lactate to pyruvate.

Clinical Findings ■

Clinical effects occur thirty minutes to two hours after acute ingestion. Mild toxicity results in nausea, vomiting, dizziness, slurred speech, and hyperreflexia. Severe toxicity produces seizures, coma, and severe metabolic acidosis. Overdoses of 15 mg/kg of INH result in lowered seizure threshold. Overdoses approaching 35–40 mg/kg produce spontaneous seizures. While coma from INH may compromise respiratory function, some patients are treated with large doses of anticonvulsants for refractory seizures, thereby contributing to CNS and respiratory depression.

Therapeutic concentrations of INH are in the 5–8 mcg/ml range. Toxicity has occurred at concentrations as low as 20 mcg/ml.

Other drugs and chemicals that produce seizures must be excluded (see Table 63-8), such as tricyclic antidepressants, camphor, carbon monoxide, chlorinated hydrocarbons, local anesthetics, narcotics (meperidine, propoxyphene), stimulants (amphetamines, cocaine, phenylpropanolamine), theophylline, and organophosphate insecticides.

Treatment ■

SUPPORTIVE CARE

Maintain the airway, breathing, and circulation. In cases where a patient is actively seizing and the history of overdose is not yet known, give diazepam (0.1–0.3 mg/kg IV) because of its synergy with pyridoxine and GABA-agonist effects. Treat acidosis with bicarbonate, 1–2 mEq/kg IV.

Decontamination

Asymptomatic patients who have ingested potentially toxic amounts of INH should have prompt gastric lavage. Ipecac syrup is contraindicated since sudden seizure activity may occur. Follow gastric lavage by activated charcoal and a cathartic (see Chapter 64).

SPECIFIC TREATMENT

For patients who have had a seizure or are actively seizing, give pyridoxine, mixed as a 5% or 10% solution with water, IV over 10–20 minutes, in a dose equivalent in grams to the amount of INH ingested (if this amount can be estimated by history). When the amount of INH ingested is unknown, infuse pyridoxine in 5-g aliquots every 5–20 minutes until seizures cease.

Although the low protein-binding and small apparent volume distribution suggest that INH may be removable by dialysis and hemoperfusion, its short half-life and the antidotal efficacy of pyridoxine make these unnecessary in most cases of acute INH overdose.

DISPOSITION

Because of the potential for seizures, admit all symptomatic patients, as well as those who have ingested more than 15 mg/kg of INH.

Bibliography ■

Wason S, Lacouture P, Lovejoy FH: Single high-dose pyridoxine treatment for isoniazid overdose. *JAMA* 1981; 246: 1102–1104.

82 Lead

Michael Shannon

Lead is a ubiquitous heavy metal with significant clinical toxicity. Over the last two centuries, the use of lead in industry and in paints has led to the release of several tons of lead into the environment and a high level of exposure to children. (Table 82-1).

Lead exposure has a number of adverse health effects, particularly in children. Renal effects of chronic lead exposure are renal insufficiency and hypertension. Hematopoietic effects result from lead's ability to block key enzymes in the synthesis of the heme ring. The heme precursor, erythrocyte protoporphyrin (EP), rises as a result of this effect. CNS consequences of even low-level lead exposure in young children include compromise in cognition and development. All of these effects can be demonstrated at lead levels as low as 15 mcg/dl. However, clinical symptoms of serious lead poisoning in children are uncommon until whole blood lead levels exceed 80 mcg/dl.

Poisoning by organic lead occurs almost exclusively after inhalation of leaded gasoline and affects primarily the CNS, with symptoms that have little if any correlation with blood lead level.

While a toxic dose of lead cannot be established, positive lead balance occurs in children when daily lead intake exceeds 5 mcg/kg.

Clinical Findings ■

Overt signs and symptoms of lead intoxication are often absent until blood lead levels exceed 50–80 mcg/dl. At this range, children may exhibit behavioral changes or may complain of headache and malaise. Once lead levels exceed 80 mcg/dl, other symptoms such as abdominal pain (lead colic) appear. Lead levels greater than 100 mcg/dl are associated with lead encephalopathy (coma, seizures, or death).

With blood lead levels greater than 50 mcg/dl, the blood EP is almost invariably elevated. Microcytic anemia is often also present. The blood smear may be remarkable for basophilic stippling.

Radiographs may be helpful in diagnosis. Abdominal X-rays may reveal radiopaque particles, suggesting recent ingestion of a lead-containing substance. Long-bone films (distal radius/ulna or proximal tibia/fibula) may reveal growth arrest lines ("lead lines"), which indicate an exposure of at least several weeks' duration.

The diagnosis of lead poisoning relies on the measurement of a whole blood lead level. A serum lead level is inadequate since lead is primarily found in the erythrocyte.

Lead poisoning should be suspected in any child with severe abdominal pain of unclear origin, particularly if a history of pica is obtained. Consider the possibility of lead intoxication in the child presenting with behavioral changes, altered mental status, or seizures.

Treatment ■

SUPPORTIVE CARE

Patients with encephalopathy must be managed in an intensive care unit with airway protection and assisted ventilation if needed, avoidance of overhydration, and management of intracranial hypertension.

Decontamination

GI decontamination is necessary only if radiopaque material is evident on an abdominal radiograph. In this case, a mild cathartic (e.g., magnesium citrate, 4 mL/kg) should be given to promote expulsion of the material. Serial radiographs may be necessary to ensure removal of the material. Activated charcoal does not bind lead and is not recommended (see also Chapter 64).

Lead-containing foreign bodies retained in soft tissue have rarely been associated with lead absorption and systemic lead intoxication. In such cases, consider surgical removal of these foreign bodies.

377

TABLE 82-1. *Common Sources of Lead in Childhood*

Lead-based paint	Ingestion of paint chips
	Ingestion of dust released after renovation
	Inhalation of fumes after paint stripping
Soil, water	Ingestion
Air	Inhalation
Kitchenware	Ingestion of food cooked in glazed kitchenware or storage of acidic liquid in glazed containers
Old toys	Ingestion
Industry	Ingestion or inhalation of lead dust brought on the stained clothes of an adult caretaker

SPECIFIC TREATMENT

Immediate parenteral chelation therapy is warranted for lead levels ≥ 60 mcg/dl. Give CaNa$_2$EDTA in a dose of 1,000–1,500 mg/m^2/day (35–50 mg/kg daily). Because of its very short elimination half-life, EDTA is best given by continuous infusion, although frequent intramuscular injections are an alternative. BAL should be added to EDTA for lead levels ≥ 70 mcg/dl. BAL is given intramuscularly in a dose of 300–450 mg/m^2/day (about 12 mg/kg/day) in 4–6 divided doses. The first dose of BAL should always precede administration of EDTA by at least 4 hours.

Chelation therapy generally continues for 5 days; subsequent repeated chelation therapy is recommended if the post-chelation rebound lead level exceeds 50 mcg/dl. A 48-hour "honeymoon" without EDTA is necessary before further chelation therapy.

Because both lead and EDTA are nephrotoxic, monitor renal function closely. Obtain a pre-chelation urinalysis, BUN, and creatinine, and monitor these frequently during chelation. Watch urinalysis for the appearance of hematuria, glycosuria, or proteinuria. Keep urine specific gravity at less than 1.020 during chelation.

Many children, particularly those with lead levels less than 60 mcg/dl, have an unsatisfactory lead diuresis during the administration of EDTA. Therefore, an EDTA challenge test is often given first to test lead mobilizability. Typically, a single dose of 35–50 mg/kg of EDTA is given parenterally. Collect and measure 6–8 hours of urine for total lead. Calculate the excretion ratio as micrograms of lead excreted divided by the mg dose of EDTA given. A ratio of more than 0.50 identifies a child with mobilizable lead stores who will benefit from additional doses of EDTA.

In children whose lead levels are not elevated to a degree requiring hospitalization, eliminate or minimize further exposure to lead while the child is referred to a lead/toxicology clinic for outpatient therapy.

Bibliography ■

American Academy of Pediatrics: Statement on childhood lead poisoning. *Pediatrics* 1987; 79:457–465.

Centers for Disease Control: Childhood lead poisoning— United States: Report to the Congress by the Agency for Toxic Substances and Disease Registry. *MMWR* 1988; 37: 481–485.

Piomelli S, Rosen JF, Chisolm JJ, et al: Management of childhood lead poisoning. *J Pediatr* 1984; 105:523–532.

83 Methemoglobinemia

Michael Shannon

Methemoglobin is an abnormal hemoglobin that cannot carry oxygen; it differs from hemoglobin only in having the heme iron in the oxidized ferric (+3) state rather than the normal ferrous (+2) state.

Several naturally occurring and manmade agents can cause methemoglobinemia (Table 83-1). Everyone has a methemoglobin level of 1–3%; what prevents higher levels from occurring with daily exposure to oxidizing agents are endogenous and exogenous antioxidants (including glutathione, vitamin E, and vitamin C) and two enzymes that reduce methemoglobin back to hemoglobin.

Methemoglobinemia can be congenital or acquired. Congenital causes include the hemoglobinopathy M and congenital methemoglobin reductase deficiency. Acquired methemoglobinemia usually occurs after exposure to excessive amounts of an oxidizing agent. However, even a low oxidant exposure can produce methemoglobinemia in individuals with a mild deficiency of methemoglobin reductase and in infants (because fetal hemoglobin is more readily oxidized to methemoglobin).

Because methemoglobin cannot carry oxygen, the oxygen-carrying capacity falls, creating a functional anemia. A methemoglobin level of 30% will not be associated with symptoms in a person with a usual hemoglobin of 15 g/dL (15 gm%) because 10.5 gm% of functioning hemoglobin would still be present to maintain oxygenation. However, a 30% methemoglobin level in a child with a usual hemoglobin of 11 gm% would leave only about 8 gm% of functioning hemoglobin; such a low hemoglobin level may cause symptoms of hypoxia.

Clinical Findings ■

Methemoglobin levels correlate with clinical effects (Table 83-2). *Cyanosis is the cardinal feature of methemoglobinemia,* appearing with methemoglobin levels of as low as 10% (1.5 gm%). The cyanosis is due to the dark chocolate-brown color of methemoglobin and not to desaturated hemoglobin. A quick bedside test is to check the color of sampled blood on a piece of filter paper.

As methemoglobin levels rise above 30%, evidence of hypoxia appears as tachypnea, tachycardia, metabolic acidosis, and confusion. With levels above 50%, coma, seizures, and death may occur.

Methemoglobinemia does not cause a change in measured pO_2 or *calculated* oxygen saturation. Decreases in *measured* oxygen saturation are found only if the oximeter being used can detect methemoglobin. Pulse oximeters that measure oxygen saturation as the ratio between oxy- and deoxyhemoglobin cannot detect methemoglobin. Direct measurement of methemoglobin level is the specific diagnostic test.

The differential diagnosis includes conditions that may produce cyanosis due to increased deoxyhemoglobin concentration, such as pulmonary disorders (e.g., pneumonia, pulmonary embolus) and cardiovascular disorders (e.g., intracardiac shunting or shock). Other abnormal forms of hemoglobin that cannot carry oxygen (e.g., sulfhemoglobin) may also cause cyanosis. Appropriate diagnostic tests are an ECG, chest X-ray, arterial blood gas, complete blood count, and electrolytes.

Treatment ■

SUPPORTIVE CARE

In any cyanotic patient, ensure a patent airway and provide supplemental oxygen, with endotracheal intubation and assisted ventilation if needed.

Decontamination

GI decontamination is necessary only if the oxidant compound was ingested within the previous 4–6 hours. Induce emesis with syrup of ipecac or perform gastric lavage, then give activated charcoal. Multiple doses of activated charcoal appear to be beneficial with dapsone ingestion because it undergoes enterohepatic recirculation.

379

TABLE 83–1. *Common Agents Causing Methemoglobinemia*

Agent	Source
Acetanilid	Dyes, shoe polishes
Benzocaine	Topical anesthetics
Chlorates	Matches
Dapsone	Medications
Nitrates/nitrites	Well water, plant food, food, preservatives, "ice packs," medications
Phenacetin	Analgesics
Phenols	Cleansers
Pyridium	Bladder anesthetic
Sulfonamides	Medications

TABLE 83–2. *Correlation Between Methemoglobin Levels and Clinical Effect*

Levels (%)	Manifestations
10–15	Cyanosis appears; patient otherwise asymptomatic.
15–30	Worsening cyanosis without respiratory difficulty
30–40	Headache, dizziness, malaise, tachycardia, tachypnea
40–60	Dyspnea, acidosis, arrhythmias, coma, seizure
>70	Death

SPECIFIC TREATMENT

Methylene blue is the treatment of choice for significant methemoglobinemia. Give methylene blue for methemoglobin levels greater than 30% or in any patient with symptomatic evidence of significant hypoxia. It is given IV in a dose of 1–2 mg/kg (0.1 ml/kg of a 1% solution). This dose may be repeated once; however, because methylene blue is an oxidant at high doses and may itself induce methemoglobinemia, subsequent therapy must be cautious.

Because NADPH is generated primarily through the hexose monophosphate shunt, which requires the enzyme glucose-6-phosphate dehydrogenase (G-6-PD) for normal activity, patients with a G-6-PD deficiency will not respond to methylene blue therapy. In fact, they may develop acute hemolysis following methylene blue. Other causes for failure of methylene blue therapy are congenital deficiency of NADPH methemoglobin reductase and the presence of another abnormal hemoglobin (e.g., sulfhemoglobin).

For severe cases of methemoglobinemia that do not respond to methylene blue, exchange transfusion is effective at restoring hemoglobin levels to an adequate range.

DISPOSITION

Admit all patients with methemoglobin levels greater than 15% and all patients with clinical symptoms for oxygen, observation, and possible methylene blue therapy.

Bibliography ■

Curry S: Methemoglobinemia. *Ann Emerg Med* 1982; 11: 214–221.

Hall AH, Kulig KW, Rumack BH: Drug- and chemical-induced methaemoglobinaemia: Clinical features and management. *Med Toxicol Adverse Drug Exp* 1986; 1: 253–260.

Johnson CJ, Bonrud PA, Dosch TL, et al: Fatal outcome of methemoglobinemia in an infant. *JAMA* 1987; 257:2796–2797.

84 Nonsteroidal Anti-Inflammatory Drugs

Michael McGuigan

Nonsteroidal anti-inflammatory drugs (NSAIDs) are widely used prescription and over-the-counter analgesics. These drugs are a heterogenous group that can be classified by chemical structure (Table 84-1). The therapeutic actions are primarily mediated through inhibition of prostaglandin synthesis, as are some of the manifestations of acute toxicity, such as GI irritation and renal toxicity. The mechanisms of other toxic effects are poorly understood.

The diversity of NSAIDs precludes establishing a single toxic dose. For ibuprofen, doses exceeding 200 mg/kg may produce toxicity. For other drugs, approximate toxic doses are:

Piroxicam: 10 mg/kg
Indomethacin: 15 mg/kg
Mefenamic acid: 60 mg/kg
Phenylbutazone: a dose of 175 mg/kg resulted in death.

The NSAIDs can be roughly ranked by chemical class in ascending order of toxicity: arylalkanoic acids, arylcarboxylic acids, pyrazolones, and oxicams (Table 84-1).

Clinical Findings ■

Ingestions of carboxylic acid NSAIDs generally cause mild poisoning with GI signs (nausea, vomiting, abdominal pain) and CNS signs (drowsiness, headache). Massive ingestion may cause coma, hypotension, and renal failure. Mefenamic acid ingestion is often associated with convulsions.

The enolic acid NSAIDs generally cause more severe poisoning, characterized by coma, metabolic acidosis, convulsions, renal failure, and hepatitis. The clinical course may be prolonged because of the long serum elimination half-lives of these agents.

The choice of clinical laboratory tests depends on the expected severity of intoxication. For severely symptomatic cases, obtain a complete blood count, prothrombin time, blood glucose, BUN and creatinine, electrolytes, blood gases, hepatic transaminases, and urinalysis. Serum drug concentrations are not readily available and are not generally useful. A prognostic nomogram for ibuprofen is available, but its clinical usefulness has not been established.

The toxicologic differential diagnosis includes acetaminophen, salicylates, and iron.

Treatment ■

SUPPORTIVE CARE

GI irritation (bleeding and ulceration) may be treated with nonabsorbable antacids and H_2-receptor antagonists. Hypotension will generally respond to bolus

---

TABLE 84–1. *Nonsteroidal Anti-inflammatory Drugs*

Carboxylic Acids

Arylalkanoic Acids
Alclofenac, dicofenas, fenbufen, fenoprofen, fentiazac, flurbiprofen, ibuprofen, indomethacin, ketoprofen, naproxen, pirprofen, sulidac, suprofen, tiaprofenic acid, tolmetin

Arylcarboxylic Acids
Flufenamic acid, meclofenamic acid, mefenamic acid, tolfenamic acid

Enolic Acids

Pyrazolones
Azapropazone, feprazone, oxyphenbutazone, phenylbutazone

Oxicams
Piroxicam

Approximate relative toxicity: Oxicams > Pyralozones > Arylcarboxylic acids > Arylalkanoic acids

of IV crystalloids (saline or lactated Ringer's). Treat convulsions with standard drugs (see Chapter 26). Hypoprothrombinemia may respond to vitamin K.

Decontamination

Empty the stomach with ipecac syrup or gastric lavage; lavage is preferred if readily available (see Chapter 64). Induced emesis may mask the development of early GI signs of toxicity. Give activated charcoal and a cathartic.

SPECIFIC TREATMENT

There are no specific antidotes or special treatments. Repeated doses of activated charcoal may enhance elimination. There is no evidence to support the use of hemodialysis or hemoperfusion to remove the drugs.

DISPOSITION

Admit all symptomatic patients. Observe asymptomatic patients who have ingested a very large dose of NSAIDs for at least 6 hours for developing toxicity. After mefenamic acid ingestion, the observation period should be at least 12 hours because of the possibility of delayed-onset convulsions.

Bibliography ■

Hall AH, Smolinske SC, Conrad FL, et al: Ibuprofen overdose: 126 cases. *Ann Emerg Med* 1986; 15:1308–1313.

Vale JA, Meredith TJ: Acute poisoning due to non-steroidal anti-inflammatory drugs. Clinical features and management. *Med Toxicol Adverse Drug Exp* 1986; 1:12–31.

85 Opiates

Michael Shannon

Opiates are widely used as oral and parenteral analgesic agents. Their wide availability increases the potential for accidental ingestion by children. In adolescents and young adults, opiate use is almost always intentional, in the form of heroin abuse or ingestion of illegally obtained prescription opiates.

Heroin is the most common illegal opiate. Typically, heroin bought on the street has a purity averaging less than 5–10%. The most common heroin adulterants are quinine and cornstarch. While heroin is usually injected, nasal use (snorting) and smoking are also popular routes.

The primary therapeutic action of opiates is analgesia and euphoria due to stimulation of central opiate receptors. Chronic use of opiates results in tolerance, which may lead to increased use of the opiate. Another consequence of chronic opiate use is physical dependence and a withdrawal syndrome with abstinence.

Clinical Findings ■

Three somewhat distinct clinical syndromes can be caused by opiate exposure in children:

1. In *the young child* with accidental acute ingestion, characteristic signs and symptoms of opiate intoxication are altered mental status, respiratory depression, and miosis.
2. In contrast, *adolescents* are more likely to present with severe signs of intoxication, including coma, respiratory arrest, hypotension, and pulmonary edema (neurogenic pulmonary edema). A higher incidence of associated illnesses (hepatitis, phlebitis, bacteremia, endocarditis, acquired immunodeficiency syndrome) is also found in this group.
3. Withdrawal in *chronic opiate abusers* is characterized by agitation, abdominal pain, piloerection, tachycardia, and tachypnea. On physical exam, needle marks ("tracks") may or may not be present on patients suspected of opiate abuse.

Opiates can usually be detected in urine toxicologic analysis, although synthetic opiates such as fentanyl are often undetectable because they are chemically dissimilar to other opiates.

In patients with CNS depression and miosis, the differential diagnosis includes phenothiazines, clonidine, barbiturates, and other sedative-hypnotics, as well as cholinesterase inhibitors such as organophosphates and carbamates. Other potential diagnoses should include head injury, CNS infection, metabolic disturbances, and cerebrovascular events.

Treatment ■

SUPPORTIVE CARE

Focus immediate attention on airway protection and respiratory support. Endotracheal intubation may be necessary for severe respiratory depression or loss of a gag reflex. Cardiovascular support includes IV fluids for hypotensive patients.

Decontamination

Decontamination measures are unnecessary after injection or nasal application of opiates. However, in the case of opiate ingestion, induce emesis with syrup of ipecac or perform gastric lavage. Administer activated charcoal with a cathartic.

SPECIFIC TREATMENT

Naloxone is a specific opiate antagonist with no intrinsic opiate agonist effects. It will immediately reverse signs and symptoms of opiate intoxication. Give an initial dose of 0.1 mg/kg in children and 2 mg in adolescents. This dose may be repeated, generally to a maximal dose of 0.3 mg/kg in children and 8 mg in adults. Synthetic and semisynthetic opiates (e.g., codeine, propoxyphene, fentanyl) often require large doses of naloxone to reverse clinical signs of intoxication.

Because of its short duration of action (approximately 1–2 hr) naloxone must often be administered repeatedly. Naloxone may be given by continuous infusion, based on the dose of naloxone that must be administered over one hour to achieve a desired clinical effect.

Patients with mild opiate withdrawal may often be managed with calming and reassurance alone. Moderate to severe withdrawal symptoms may be treated with an oral benzodiazepine or an opiate. Methadone is effective and has a prolonged duration of action. The methadone dose is based on the extent of prior opiate abuse; typical starting doses are 10–20 mg orally.

DISPOSITION

Admit all patients with severe respiratory depression for overnight observation, regardless of how completely their symptoms resolve after naloxone. Refer patients with withdrawal for opiate detoxification, and ensure follow-up with a primary physician.

Bibliography ■

Cuddy P: Management of acute opioid intoxication. *Crit Care Quar* 1982:65–74.

King P, Coleman J Stimulants and narcotic drugs. *Pediatr Clin North Am* 1987; 34:349–352.

Mofenson HC, Caraccio TR: Continuous infusion of intravenous naloxone. *Ann Emerg Med* 1987;16:374–375.

86 Over-the-Counter Cold and Allergy Preparations

Olga F. Woo

The public spends millions of dollars each year for nonprescription cold and allergy products. Table 86-1 gives a system of classification, with usual dose recommendations. Multiple-drug combination products can also include other agents such as a cough suppressants (dextromethorphan) and analgesics (aspirin or acetaminophen).

SYMPATHOMIMETICS

Ephedrine and pseudoephedrine stimulate alpha- and beta-adrenergic receptors and also release norepinephrine from presynaptic neurons. Phenylpropanolamine is an alpha-receptor agonist with minimal beta-receptor activity. Phenylephrine is an alpha-receptor agonist. In general, serious toxicity is unlikely unless more than four times the maximum daily dosage has been taken. However, severe hypertension and intracerebral hemorrhage have occurred with relatively small overdoses of phenylpropanolamine in sensitive individuals. Phenylephrine is substantially hydrolyzed in the GI tract; small but unpredictable amounts are absorbed into the bloodstream.

The nasal decongestants are potent alpha-agonist vasoconstrictors that, like clonidine (see Chapter 74), can produce significant central alpha-2 effects. In young children, as few as several drops can cause CNS depression, hypotension, and bradycardia.

ANTIHISTAMINES

These agents vary in potency, but act similarly and antagonize histamine at H_1 receptors. Acute doses greater than 5–25 mg/kg may result in coma, seizures, and respiratory depression.

ANTICHOLINERGICS

Atropine and belladonna alkaloids block acetylcholine at muscarinic receptor sites. Doses greater than 175 ug/kg generally produce significant peripheral and central effects. Fatalities in children have oc-curred with doses as small as 1.6 mg, but other children have recovered after ingesting 600 mg.

Clinical Findings ◼

Overdosage may produce lethargy, drowsiness, ataxia, agitation, irritability, excitation, hallucinations, unusual behavior, tachycardia, hypertension, and cardiac dysrhythmias. Agents with predominantly alpha-agonist activity may produce hypertension with reflex bradycardia. Severe hypertension with phenylpropanolamine has resulted in intracranial hemorrhage and myocardial injury.

Anticholinergic agents commonly produce ileus, urinary retention and dilated pupils. Pupillary constriction may occur with alpha-agonist agents. Severe poisoning may produce seizures, coma, and respiratory arrest with all of these agents. Hyperthermia may also occur with all of these agents, especially if multiple seizures or prolonged muscular hyperactivity occur.

Routine drug screens and blood levels are not readily available. Specific requests are necessary to detect and measure these agents in the blood or urine.

Similar adrenergic cardiovascular stimulation is produced by drugs with sympathomimetic effects, such as amphetamines and related agents, anorexiants (phentermine, diethylpropion), beta-selective agonists (albuterol, metaproterenol, terbutaline), caffeine, theophylline, cocaine, LSD, phencyclidine, amantadine, and tricyclic antidepressants. Clonidine overdosage can mimic the clinical picture of topical vasoconstrictor decongestant overdose.

Treatment ◼

SUPPORTIVE CARE

Protect the airway and assist ventilation if necessary. Treat symptomatic hypertension with a short-acting

TABLE 86–1. *Over-the-counter Cold and Allergy Preparations Recommended Maximum Daily Dosage*

Agent Class	Recommended Maximum Daily Dosage
Sympathomimetic	
Oral	
Ephedrine	2 mg/kg
Pseudoephedrine	4–6 mg/kg
Phenylpropanolamine	1–3 mg/kg
Topical	
Naphazoline	
Oxymetazoline	0.025%: 1–3 drops twice a day
Phenylephrine	0.125–0.25%: 1–3 drops q 3–4 hr
Tetrahydrozoline	
Antihistamine	
Brompheniramine	0.5 mg/kg
Carbinoxamine	0.2–0.4 mg/kg
Chlorpheniramine	0.3–0.4 mg/kg to 24 mg
Cyclizine	3 mg/kg to 200 mg
Dimenhydrinate	5 mg/kg
Diphenydramine	5 mg/kg to 300 mg
Methdilazine	16 mg
Pheniramine	3–5 mg/kg
Pyrilamine	3–5 mg/kg
Tripolidine	1–4 mg/kg
Anticholinergic	
Atropine	0.5–1 mg

agent such as phentolamine (0.05–0.1 mg/kg IV), nifedipine (0.1–0.2 mg/kg PO), or nitroprusside (0.5–5 μg/kg/min IV). Manage tachyarrhythmias with lidocaine or a beta blocker (propranolol 0.05–0.1 mg IV or esmolol 25–50 μg/kg/min IV). Do not treat reflex bradycardia with atropine because it may worsen hypertension. Treat seizures with diazepam and/or phenobarbital.

Decontamination

Induce emesis with syrup of ipecac, or perform gastric lavage (see Chapter 64). If blood pressure is elevated, do not empty the stomach, but give oral activated charcoal and a cathartic (unless diarrhea exists). There is no evidence that repeat doses of activated charcoal or dialysis procedures enhance the elimination of these drugs.

SPECIFIC TREATMENT

There is no single specific antidote for sympathomimetic overdoses. Drug treatment is directed at antagonizing alpha-mediated vasoconstriction or blocking beta-stimulatory effects. Physostigmine may effectively antagonize many of the effects of the anticholinergics and antihistamines, but its duration of action is short and it may cause seizures and bradyarrhythmias.

DISPOSITION

Observe asymptomatic patients for at least 4–6 hours. Symptoms can be delayed for 3–4 hours with the sympathomimetic agents and as late as 6–12 hours with agents that have anticholinergic activity, and in patients with decreased bowel activity. Admit patients whose vital signs do not normalize within six hours.

Bibliography ■

Bale JF, Fountain MT, Shaddy R: Phenylpropanolamine-associated CNS complications in children and adolescents. *Am J Dis Child* 1984; 138:683–685.
Soderman P, Sahlberg D, Wiholm BE: CNS reactions to nose drops in small children. *Lancet* 1984; 1:573.

87 Pesticides (Organophosphates and Carbamates)

Olga F. Woo

Organophosphate and carbamate insecticides are among the most common pesticides involved in pediatric poisonings. Table 87-1 summarizes other important pesticide categories, their toxic effects, toxic doses, and treatment. Many liquid products are formulated with a petroleum distillate solvent such as toluene or xylene. These hydrocarbons may be listed as inert ingredients, but they can have inherent harmful effects of their own and can add to product toxicity.

Organophosphate and carbamate insecticides inhibit the enzyme acetylcholinesterase and cause acetylcholine to accumulate at the neuromuscular junction site of skeletal muscle, preganglionic synapses of the autonomic ganglia, parasympathetic postganglionic sites, and CNS receptors. Carbamates do not cross the blood-brain barrier well, and central effects are generally absent or minimal.

The toxicity range is wide, and data on human toxic doses for these compounds are sparse, especially in

TABLE 87–1. *Other Pesticides and Their Toxicity*

Class	Toxic Symptoms
Insecticides	
Chlorinated hydrocarbons (Endrin, lindane, chlordane, methoxychlor)	Nausea, vomiting, disorientation, weakness, paresthesias (1 g can cause seizures)
Pyrethrum and related	Hypersensitivity reactions, nausea, vomiting, seizures (rare). Lethal dose is >1 g/kg.
Herbicides	
Paraquat and diquat	Vomiting, diarrhea, respiratory failure (paraquat), brainstem hemorrhage (diquat), renal and hepatic injury. 10–50 ml concentrate may be fatal. Hemoperfusion may be effective.
Chlorphenoxy (2,4-D, 2,4,5-T)	Gastritis, hypotension, hyperthermia, metabolic acidosis
Dinitrophenol	Sweating, hyperthermia, seizures
Fungicides	
Pentachlorophenol	Similar to dinitrophenol
Dithiocarbamates	Can cause disulfiram-alcohol reaction
Others	
Methyl bromide	Seizures, ventricular arrhythmias
Metaldehyde	Vomiting, salivation, seizures; toxic dose is 25–50 mg/kg.
Diethyltolumaide (DEET)	Ataxia, seizures
Roenone	Vomiting, lethargy, respiratory depression

children. Severe poisoning may occur in a small child after ingesting as little as 5 ml of a home veterinary product, Dermaton Dip (chlorpyrifos 24.5%). Highly lipophilic organophosphate compounds such as fenthion may produce prolonged symptoms. All of these agents are well absorbed across the skin.

Clinical Findings ■

Organophosphate and carbamate insecticides stimulate peripheral and central muscarinic and nicotinic receptors (Table 87-2). These compounds are well absorbed by all routes of exposure and can produce isolated muscarinic symptoms at the localized site: miosis and blurry vision; rhinorrhea; bronchoconstriction, wheezing, and increased pulmonary secretions; sweating and muscle twitching on the skin. Oral ingestions produce a constellation of symptoms of intoxication, depending on the balance of muscarinic and nicotinic receptor stimulation. At low doses, muscarinic receptor activity generally dominates, producing cholinergic symptoms that can be remembered by the acronym DUMBELS (Table 87-2). Higher doses stimulate nicotinic and central receptor activity, which may result in tachycardia, hypertension, muscular weakness, ataxia, apnea, seizures, and coma. Death is due to respiratory and cardiovascular depression. Carbamate insecticide poisoning is seldom severe, and the duration of intoxication is generally short.

Serum and red blood cell (RBC) cholinesterase activity can be measured to confirm cholinesterase inhibition. RBC cholinesterase more accurately reflects true cholinesterase activity but serum cholinesterase activity may be depressed sooner. A depression of 25% activity or greater indicates organophosphate toxicity. In carbamate insecticide poisoning, the measurements are less useful because reversal of enzyme inhibition occurs rapidly.

The differential diagnosis of lethargy, bradycardia, and miosis includes narcotics, clonidine, and parasympathomimetics (physostigmine, pilocarpine). Consider intoxication by phenothiazines, phencyclidine, or Lomotil if tachycardia is present instead of bradycardia. Severe sedative-hypnotic poisoning may also produce miosis, hypotonia, coma, and respiratory depression, but heart rate is generally normal.

TABLE 87–2. *Signs and Symptoms of Organophosphate and Carbamate Toxicity*

Muscarinic Receptor Stimulation "DUMBELS"
  Diarrhea, Urination, Miosis, Bradycardia/bronchospasm, Emesis, Lacrimation, Salivation

Nicotinic Receptor Stimulation
  Pallor, tachycardia, hypertension, hyperglycemia, muscle weakness, fasiculations, twitching, paralysis (especially respiratory muscles)

CNS Receptor Stimulation
  Agitation, ataxia, seizures, coma

Examples of Common Organophosphates and Carbamates

  *Organophosphates**
  Highly toxic: TEPP, demeton,† disulfoton,† mevinphos, methyl parathion, chlorfenvinphos, methamidophos, bomyl

  Moderately toxic: dichlorvos, demeton-methyl, propetamphos, chlorpyrifos, cythioate, fenthion, diazinon, malathion

  Carbamates
  Highly toxic: aldicarb,† methomyl

  Moderately toxic: methiocarb, propoxur, carbaryl

---

* Insecticides listed in descending toxicity.
† Agent is systemically taken up by the plant and can be toxic if eaten.

Treatment ■

SUPPORTIVE CARE

Protect the airway and assist ventilation if necessary. Treat seizures with diazepam and/or phenobarbital. Correct hypotension with fluid therapy; vasopressors are seldom necessary.

Decontamination

Induce emesis with syrup of ipecac or perform gastric lavage, and administer activated charcoal (see Chapter 64). Repeat doses of activated charcoal may hasten the elimination of chlorinated hydrocarbon compounds (e.g., lindane).

Remove all affected clothing, and thoroughly wash the skin with soap and water.

SPECIFIC TREATMENT

Administer antidotal therapy with atropine to reverse cholinergic excess as soon as possible. Atropine will not reverse nicotinic symptoms such as muscle weakness and respiratory paralysis; therefore, pralidoxime must also be given in organophosphate poisoning.

In children less than 12 years old, give 0.05 mg/kg of atropine initially, and 0.02 to 0.05 mg/kg repeated every 10–30 minutes until signs of atropinization develop (dry mouth, dry and flushed skin, dilated pupils, tachycardia). The total dose of atropine required may be exceedingly large in severe poisonings; as much as 100 mg has been reported.

The pralidoxime dose is 25 to 50 mg/kg infused IV over 15–30 minutes and repeated after 1–2 hours if needed, then at 8–12-hour intervals until nicotinic symptoms are reversed (normal sinus rate, if tachycardia was a dominant sign; increased muscle strength; normal respirations). More frequent doses of pralidoxime may be necessary in severe poisonings.

Carbamate poisoning is quickly reversed with atropine, and mild poisoning may not require treatment because symptoms usually resolve spontaneously after 6–8 hours. In more severe poisonings with highly toxic compounds such as aldicarb, large and frequent doses of atropine may be required. It is controversial whether pralidoxime administration may increase carbamate insecticide toxicity, although in most cases pralidoxime is unnecessary.

Disposition ■

Observe asymptomatic patients for at least 4–6 hours before discharge from the emergency department. Observe symptomatic patients for an additional 24–48 hours after treatment and recovery to ensure that no rebound occurs when the effects of atropine and pralidoxime have subsided.

Bibliography ■

Gehlbach SH, Williams WA: Pediatric pesticide poisonings in North Carolina: Epidemiologic observations. *South Med J* 1977; 70:12–14.

Mortensen ML: Management of acute childhood poisonings caused by selected insecticides and herbicides. *Pediatr Clin North Am* 1986; 33:421–445.

88 Phencyclidine

S. Alan Tani

Phencyclidine (PCP) is a dissociative anesthetic and hallucinogenic agent. Doses of 1–5 mg result in euphoria; doses as low as 20 mg have caused death.

Clinical Findings ■

PCP in low doses results in hallucinations and nystagmus. Serious overdoses cause severe agitation, combativeness, and unusual displays of strength. Coma, respiratory depression, and a wide-eyed stare are seen in massive overdose. Other significant findings include hypertension, tachycardia, and hyperthermia. Large patients seriously intoxicated with PCP often require six-point restraints and may pose a significant risk to emergency department personnel.

Consider the presence of other drugs of abuse, such as amphetamines or cocaine, and other causes of psychosis or coma. Carefully examine for evidence of trauma.

Treatment ■

SUPPORTIVE CARE

Maintain an airway and support ventilation, if necessary. Major cardiac arrhythmias, severe hypertension, or shock may occur and require further supportive care in the most serious overdoses. Manage seizures with standard anticonvulsants. Refractory seizures may require general anesthesia. Treat hyperthermia aggressively with external cooling or neuromuscular paralysis. Rhabdomyolysis and secondary renal failure, common complications of seizures and hyperthermia, require urinary alkalinization and occasionally hemodialysis.

Decontamination

Standard decontamination is indicated for skin, eye, or inhalation exposure. If PCP is ingested, perform gastric lavage and follow with activated charcoal and sorbitol (see Chapter 64). Do not administer ipecac because of the risk of increased agitation and seizures.

SPECIFIC TREATMENT

Hard or soft restraints are often required. Minimize external stimuli by gently covering the eyes with gauze and paper tape. Do not place the patient in a dark room because of the need for close observation. Severe agitation may be managed with diazepam, haloperidol, or lorazepam. Hemodialysis or charcoal hemoperfusion do not remove significant amounts of PCP.

Disposition ■

Observe mildly symptomatic patients in the emergency department for 4–8 hours and discharge to psychiatry or home with adequate supervision. Admit patients with continued symptoms or evidence of hyperthermia or rhabdomyolysis to the intensive care unit, or transfer to a pediatric critical care center.

Bibliography ■

McCarron MM, Schulze BW, Thompson GA, et al: Acute phencyclidine intoxication: Incidence of clinical findings in 1,000 cases. *Ann Emerg Med* 1981; 10:237–242.

Welch MJ, Correa GA: PCP intoxication in young children and infants. *Clin Pediatr* 1980; 19:510–514.

89 Phenothiazines and Related Antipsychotic Agents

Mary Ellen Mortensen

Phenothiazines, thioxanthenes, and butyrophenones inhibit dopamine receptors and decrease catecholamine synthesis in the CNS. These agents lower the seizure threshold and depress vasomotor reflexes. Extrapyramidal syndromes (EPS) are occasionally seen soon after therapy is started. These movement disorders consist of acute dystonic reactions (more common in children), akinesia, and akathisia. Peripheral signs consist of anticholinergic effects and initial adrenergic effects due to blocked catecholamine uptake, progressing to alpha-adrenergic blockade. Anticholinergic signs and sedation may be more prominent with phenothiazines; EPS may be more prominent with butyrophenones.

Neuroleptic malignant syndrome (NMS), a rare but potentially life-threatening complication of antipsychotic therapy, is characterized by muscle rigidity, severe hyperthermia, and altered mentation (confusion progressing to coma).

Clinical Findings ■

Patients usually present within 6–24 hours after overdose. In addition to the clinical signs listed in Table 89-1, patients may have pupillary constriction (alpha-adrenergic blockade). Significant respiratory depression is uncommon even in massive overdose. Acute dystonic reactions may be accompanied by hyperpyrexia. Affected patients are at risk for rhabdomyolysis, myoglobinuria, and subsequent renal failure. In massive overdose, quinidine-like cardiotoxicity may occur, producing QRS and QT interval prolongation, hypotension, and AV block.

Drug levels are not clinically useful except to confirm the diagnosis.

In the differential diagnosis, consider other drugs that produce anticholinergic signs (antihistamines) and cardiac dysrhythmias (tricyclic antidepressants). Other drugs causing coma include narcotics, barbiturates and other sedative-hypnotic agents, and al-cohol. Rule out CNS trauma or infections, and metabolic disturbances. During acute dystonic reactions, patients remain awake and responsive, differentiating this condition from a seizure.

Treatment ■

SUPPORTIVE CARE

Maintain a patent airway and assist ventilation, if needed. Monitor blood pressure and cardiac rhythm. If hypotension is unresponsive to IV fluids, a vasopressor may be needed. Treat hyperthermia aggressively (see Chapter 96).

Monitor urine output for myoglobin if rigidity or hyperthermia are present.

TABLE 89–1. *Presenting Signs of Antipsychotic Drug Overdose*

Anticholinergic
 Dry mucous membranes and skin, diminished GI
  motility, urinary retention, tachycardia

Cardiovascular
 Hypotension, vasodilation, direct myocardial
  depression (quinidinelike), prolonged QRS, PR, and
  QT intervals

CNS
 Miosis (small pupils)
 Sedation/stupor/coma
 Decreased seizure threshold
 Extrapyramidal syndromes (movement disorders)
  Acute dystonic reactions (oculogyric crisis,
   opisthotonos, torticollis, facial grimacing or
   trismus, abdominal wall muscle rigidity)
 Akinesia (parkinsonian)
 Akathisia (restlessness, discomfort)
 Neuroleptic malignant syndrome
 Dysarthria, dysphagia
 Hypothermia or hyperthermia

Decontamination

Induce emesis or, preferably, perform gastric lavage. Administer activated charcoal with a cathartic (see Chapter 64).

SPECIFIC TREATMENT

If quinidine-like cardiotoxicity is present, administer IV sodium bicarbonate 1–2 mEq/kg boluses.

EPS: Acute dystonic reactions usually respond promptly to diphenhydramine (Benadryl) 1–2 mg/kg IV or benztropine (Cogentin) 0.01–0.03 mg/kg IM. Oral treatment for an additional 48–72 hours is needed to prevent recurrence.

NMS: Treat hyperthermia aggressively, using neuromuscular paralysis if necessary. Dantrolene 0.5 mg/kg IV may be useful if rigidity is resistant to neuromuscular paralyzing agents.

Hemodialysis and hemoperfusion are ineffective for drug removal.

Disposition ■

Admit all symptomatic patients. Observe asymptomatic patients for at least 4–6 hours.

Bibliography ■

Knight ME, Roberts RJ: Phenothiazine and butyrophenone intoxication in children. *Pediatr Clin North Am* 1986; 33:299–310.

90 Salicylates

Michael McGuigan

Salicylates are available in many nonprescription and prescription products, including cold medications, analgesics, rubs, stomach medications, and antipyretic agents. The two most common forms of salicylate are acetylsalicylic acid (aspirin) and methylsalicylate (oil of wintergreen). One ml of oil of wintergreen has the same salicylate content as 1.4 g of aspirin.

Salicylate is directly irritating to the GI mucosa and may cause bleeding. Once absorbed, salicylates exert a concentration-dependent inhibition of intracellular enzymes. Oxidative phosphorylation is uncoupled, resulting in increased cellular oxygen consumption and excessive production of heat and carbon dioxide. Inhibition of other enzymes interferes with oxygen utilization and leads to anaerobic metabolism with production of excess lactic acid. Salicylates also interfere with lipid metabolism, causing increased production of ketone bodies and contributing to metabolic acidosis. Altered glucose metabolism may cause hyperglycemia or hypoglycemia. Direct stimulation of the respiratory center, combined with compensatory hyperventilation in response to metabolic acidosis, results in respiratory alkalosis.

Acute clinical toxicity may be predicted from the ingested dose of salicylate (if known): less than 150 mg/kg is associated with no systemic toxicity; 150–300 mg/kg produces mild to moderate poisoning; 300–500 mg/kg causes serious toxicity; and doses greater than 500 mg/kg are often lethal. Chronic salicylate poisoning may result from ingestion of more than 100 mg/kg/day for two or more days.

Clinical Findings ■

Early after acute ingestion, the presenting clinical findings may not accurately predict the severity of the overdose. Common findings include nausea, vomiting, and hyperpnea. Lethargy, disorientation, seizures, and coma may occur, but are often delayed several hours. Dehydration and hyperpyrexia are relatively uncommon after acute ingestion. In chronic intoxication, clinical findings are similar, except that dehydration, electrolyte imbalance, coma, and convulsions are more common. Pulmonary edema may occur, but is more common in adult salicylism.

Laboratory determination of electrolytes and arterial blood gases will reveal respiratory alkalosis and metabolic acidosis with an elevated anion gap (Chapter 63). Severe acidemia is more common with chronic intoxication. Blood glucose levels may be elevated initially and then may fall below normal. The prothrombin time is often prolonged.

The serum salicylate concentration should be measured in all cases of suspected salicylate poisoning. For acute ingestions, the estimated severity of poisoning can be obtained by plotting a six-hour postingestion level on the salicylate nomogram (see Figure 90-1); however, *the nomogram is invalid if the salicylate product is enteric-coated or if the intoxication is chronic.* In these cases, severe toxicity may be expected with serum salicylate levels as low as 50–60 mg/dl (500–600 mg/liter).

Salicylate intoxication should be considered, regardless of the history, in any patient with non-focal neurologic abnormalities, dyspnea/tachypnea, or acid-base abnormalities. Disease entities that may be confused with salicylism include diabetic ketoacidosis, acute bronchospasm, meningitis, and encephalitis. Other toxicologic causes of acidosis include methanol, ethylene glycol, iron, isoniazid, and cyanide.

Treatment ■

SUPPORTIVE CARE

Maintain a patent airway. Assisted ventilation and supplemental oxygen may be required if pulmonary edema or aspiration is present. Provide sufficient fluids to replace losses, normalize electrolytes, and ensure adequate urine output (forced diuresis is not required).

393

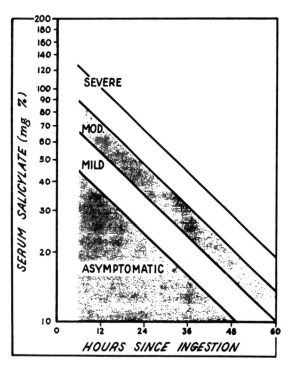

SERUM SALICYLATE (mg %)

SEVERE

MOD.

MILD

ASYMPTOMATIC

HOURS SINCE INGESTION

FIGURE 90–1. Nomogram for acute salicyate poisoning.

Decontamination

Empty the stomach with ipecac syrup or gastric lavage (see Chapter 64). Lavage is preferred if readily available. Give activated charcoal and a cathartic. If the ingested dose of salicylate exceeds 300 mg/kg, one or two additional doses of charcoal are recommended. Additional repeated smaller doses of activated charcoal have been shown to enhance salicylate elimination from the body, but the utility and safety of this procedure has not been established in children. Massive ingestion of sustained-release or enteric-coated aspirin may be treated with whole-bowel irrigation (see Chapter 65).

SPECIFIC TREATMENT

Give sodium bicarbonate if the salicylate level is elevated or if there is metabolic acidosis. The initial

TABLE 90–1. *Indications for Hemodialysis in Salicylate Intoxication*

Clinical Findings
Severe delirium; coma, convulsions; pulmonary edema; aspiration pneumonia

Salicylate Level
Acute overdose with level > 100 mg/dl (1,000 mg/liter, 7.2 mmol/liter).
Chronic intoxication with level > 60 mg/dl (600 mg/liter, 4.3 mmol/liter)

Therapeutic Failure
Persistent acidemia

dose is 1–2 mEq/kg over 1 hour; repeat as needed to maintain serum pH above 7.4, plasma bicarbonate above 18 mmol/liter, and urine pH above 7–8. Caution: Fluid overload and hypernatremia may occur; give bicarbonate in hypotonic fluids to achieve a total sodium content of no more than 140 mEq/liter of solution.

Hemodialysis is recommended for severe intoxication (Table 90-1). Although hemoperfusion is also effective, it does not provide rapid correction of acid-base and fluid abnormalities.

Disposition ■

Admit all symptomatic patients with any degree of acidosis or elevated salicylate levels. Admit asymptomatic patients who have ingested enteric-coated products.

Bibliography ■

Gaudreault P, Temple AR, Lovejoy FH: The relative severity of acute versus chronic salicylate poisoning in children: A clinical comparison. *Pediatrics* 1982; 70:566–569.
Temple AR: Pathophysiology of aspirin overdose toxicity with implications for management. *Pediatrics* 1978; 62(suppl):873–876.

91 Sedative-Hypnotic Drugs

Michael D. Reed

The barbiturate and nonbarbiturate sedative-hypnotics (Table 91-1) represent a diverse group of pharmacologic agents that possess similar toxicologic properties. This class of compounds includes the barbiturates (e.g., phenobarbital), benzodiazepines (e.g., diazepam), chloral hydrate, ethchlorvynol, glutethimide, methaqualone, meprobamate, and others.

All sedative-hypnotic drugs depress the CNS; many also possess muscle-relaxant and anticonvulsant properties. The continuum of clinical effects (i.e., muscle relaxation to sedation to hypnosis to coma) are dose related. Although very unusual in young children, chronic use/abuse of these agents for variable time periods is associated with a psychological and/or physical addiction that can be associated with an abstinence syndrome.

Clinical Findings ■

Sedation, lethargy, somnolence, ataxia, mental confusion (i.e., variable changes in level of consciousness), poor muscle tone, and depressed reflexes are common. Children usually present as very lethargic or asleep after an accidental ingestion of these agents; in more serious intoxications, patients may present comatose or in respiratory arrest. Hypotension and hypothermia are common in severe overdose. With the possible exception of phenobarbital, serum concentrations of these agents are of limited utility for directing therapy or for prognostication.

The differential diagnosis includes alcohol, phenothiazines, antidepressants, antihistamines, opiates, and other depressants. Rule out hypoglycemia, hypothermia, head trauma, and serious CNS infection.

TABLE 91–1. *Clinical Features Often Associated With Sedative-Hypnotic Intoxication*

Drug	Clinical Features
Barbiturates Phenobarbital, pentobarbital, secobarbital, others	Prolonged coma, especially with phenobarbital; continuous charcoal dosing important; severe overdose may benefit from hemoperfusion.
Benzodiazepines Diazepam, chlodrazepoxide, clonazepam, temazepam, triazolam, others	Generally mild intoxication with large margin of safety; newer short-acting agents (e.g., triazolam) can cause respiratory arrest after even small overdose.
Other Agents Glutathimide	Cyclic coma, anticholinergic features
Ethchlorvynol	Pearlike breath odor, pulmonary edema after IV use
Chloral hydrate	Alcoholic breath odor, arrhythmias may be seen

Treatment ■

SUPPORTIVE CARE

Maintain the airway, and intubate and assist ventilation if necessary. Monitor ECG, blood pressure, and temperature, and perform rewarming (see Chapter 95) if necessary. Treat hypotension initially with IV fluid (10–20 ml/kg). If a patient remains hypotensive after rewarming and two bolus doses of normal saline (20 ml/kg total), institute vasopressor infusion (i.e., dopamine). Insertion of a Swan-Ganz catheter and/or arterial pressure lines may be necessary to monitor therapy. Depending on the agent ingested, prolonged coma (longer than two weeks) has been described, requiring prolonged supportive care and extensive monitoring for fluid/electrolyte balance, aspiration pneumonia, and pulmonary edema.

Decontamination

Empty the stomach with emesis or gastric lavage (see Chapter 64). Use caution, depending on the patient's current or impending level of consciousness. Give activated charcoal; if the child refuses it, insert an oro- or nasogastric tube for charcoal dosing. Repeated dose of charcoal (see Chapter 65) may enhance elimination.

SPECIFIC TREATMENT

At present, there is no specific antidote for these drugs, although the benzodiazepine antagonist flumazenil is undergoing experimental trials. Attempts to augment body removal of these agents by extracorporeal measures (e.g., hemodialysis, hemoperfusion) have produced poor results, due to the high lipophilic nature and extensive tissue distribution of most of these drugs. Phenobarbital has a small volume of distribution and may be effectively removed with hemoperfusion (see Chapter 65). Forced alkaline diuresis (pH above 7.5) may also augment body removal of phenobarbital and mephobarbital.

Disposition ■

Admit all symptomatic children to the intensive care unit and place them on continuous cardiopulmonary monitoring, or transfer them to a pediatric critical care center. Asymptomatic or mildly symptomatic children who have ingested a long-acting benzodiazepine may be admitted to the ward; discharge them if they are stable or improving after 4–6 hours of observation and after evaluating the family environment.

Bibliography ■

Bertino JS Jr, Reed MD: Barbiturate and nonbarbiturate sedative hypnotic intoxication in children. *Pediatr Clin North Am* 1986; 33:703–722.

92 Theophylline Intoxication

Pierre Gaudreault

In children, theophylline and its derivatives are mainly prescribed for the treatment of asthma and neonatal apnea. However, theophylline (or caffeine, a related drug with similar toxicity) can also be found in certain over-the-counter medications such as cold medicine or wake-up pills. Although theophylline poisoning is not one of the most common causes of childhood intoxication, it is a serious one: up to 35% of the patients reported in the literature who developed seizures died or suffered significant sequelae.

Theophylline affects primarily the GI system, the cardiovascular system, and the CNS. Nausea and vomiting result from stimulation of the vomiting center in the medulla oblongata and irritation of the gastric mucosa.

Several factors are implicated in the generation of cardiac arrhythmias:

1. Theophylline decreases the ventricular fibrillation threshold, the result of an increase in cyclic AMP or a decrease in adenosine synthesis.
2. Theophylline increases the cardiac conduction velocity nonuniformly, which favors the reentry phenomenon.
3. Theophylline increases catecholamine liberation.
4. Reduced oxygen supply to the myocardium, secondary to a fall in the coronary blood flow and an increase in oxygen demand by the cardiac muscle, induces a relative ischemia that favors arrhythmias.
5. The hypokalemia often seen with theophylline intoxications can enhance dysrhythmias.

The mechanism responsible for the stimulation of the CNS is thought to be related to the blockade of adenosine synthesis.

There is no lethal dose established for theophylline in humans. Factors such as the patient's age and health at the time of the incident and the ingestion of other products influence the severity of the intoxication. However, acute ingestion of more than 10 mg/kg of theophylline is likely to induce signs of toxicity; acute ingestion of more than 50 mg/kg is likely to cause seizures.

Clinical Findings ■

Toxic signs and symptoms appear usually within 1–2 hours after the ingestion, although the onset of seizures may be delayed for several hours. Most patients present with GI symptoms such as nausea and vomiting, but some patients present with seizures as their first sign of toxicity.

Theophylline can induce both supraventricular and ventricular dysrhythmias. Sinus tachycardia, multifocal atrial tachycardia, atrial flutter and fibrillation are among the supraventricular arrhythmias encountered. Ventricular arrhythmias range from premature ventricular contractions to ventricular tachycardia and fibrillation. In children and adolescents, life-threatening arrhythmias have been reported only when serum concentrations exceeded 50 μg/ml. Hypoxemia, hypercapnia, and acidemia significantly increase the likelihood of arrhythmias.

Hemodynamic changes are dose dependent. At low doses, theophylline induces a transitory hypertension secondary to an increase in cardiac output and total peripheral resistance. At high doses, stimulation of beta$_2$ receptors reduces total peripheral resistance, provoking a fall in the blood pressure.

CNS manifestations range from agitation, tremors, and hypertonicity to seizures. Convulsions are usually generalized but can be focal. Following an acute overdose (i.e., one large single ingestion), most patients with seizures have peak serum concentrations above 80–100 μg/ml. However, one study reported two patients who seized with serum concentrations around 50 μg/ml. *Patients who receive theophylline chronically (i.e., more than one dose) or have a previous history of seizures may seize with serum concentrations below 50 μg/ml.*

Severe theophylline intoxication can induce hypokalemia, hyperglycemia, hypophosphatemia, metabolic acidosis, and respiratory alkalosis. Hyperglycemia is secondary to an increase in gluconeogenesis and glycogenolysis mediated by catecholamines. Hypokalemia seems to be secondary to an intracellular shift of potassium ions due to the hyperglycemia and also to direct beta$_2$ receptor stimulation.

Nausea and vomiting usually occur with serum concentrations above 20 μg/ml. Life-threatening arrhythmias and seizures may occur with serum concentrations above 50 μg/ml and are highly likely when concentrations exceed 100 μg/ml. This correlation between theophylline serum concentrations and serious side effects is less clear in chronically intoxicated patients.

In addition, pre-existing cardiac disease or epilepsy may increase the susceptibility to theophylline toxicity. After acute ingestion, especially with sustained-release preparations such as Theo-Dur®, serum levels may continue to rise for 12–24 hours.

Treatment ■

SUPPORTIVE CARE

Maintain a patent airway and adequate ventilation. Supraventricular tachycardia usually does not necessitate treatment, unless it is associated with significant hemodynamic changes.

Drugs such as lidocaine, procainamide, digoxin, and verapamil have been tried in the treatment of theophylline-induced arrhythmias, but have been ineffective or even harmful. Adequate correction of hypoxemia, acidosis, and hypokalemia is essential and should further reduce the risk of arrhythmias.

Treat seizures promptly and aggressively. Diazepam is the drug of choice, at IV doses of 0.3 mg/kg (maximum: 10 mg/dose). If seizures do not stop rapidly or if they recur, give phenobarbital 15–20 mg/kg IV over 20–30 minutes. A second dose of phenobarbital may be given if seizures are not controlled within 30 minutes. Phenytoin should not be used, because it is ineffective for theophylline-induced seizures and has caused harmful effects in animal studies.

Propranolol is the drug of choice for both supraventricular and ventricular arrhythmias. Give IV doses of 0.02 mg/kg (maximum: 1 mg/dose) slowly and repeat every 5 to 10 minutes until arrhythmias are stopped or a maximum of 10 mg is reached. Caution: Propranolol can cause bronchospasm in asthmatic patients.

Hypotension, which is probably due to beta$_2$-mediated vasodilation, has responded poorly to fluid administration, metaraminol bitartrate, dopamine, and norepinephrine. Propranolol with its beta$_2$-blocking effect has successfully controlled hypotension.

Decontamination

Empty the stomach with emesis or lavage (see Chapter 64). Activated charcoal is an essential part of the treatment of theophylline intoxications. *Give every patient with a theophylline overdose activated charcoal, regardless of the alleged time of ingestion.* The acute ingestion of a large amount of drug or the ingestion of a sustained-release preparation may prolong absorption and delay the time to achieve peak serum concentrations.

Recent data have demonstrated that the repeated administration of activated charcoal every 4–6 hours significantly enhances the elimination of theophylline. Give a dose of 1 g/kg of body weight every 4–6 hours until the patient has evacuated a stool containing charcoal and theophylline serum concentrations are less than 30 μg/ml. Patients with repeated vomiting may be given fractionated doses orally or via gastric tube. If the patient still cannot tolerate the activated charcoal, 50 mg of ranitidine (1–2 mg/kg) may be given IV before giving subsequent doses of charcoal.

Forced diuresis will not significantly increase theophylline elimination. Exchange transfusion and peritoneal dialysis are inefficient and contraindicated. Hemoperfusion is the technique of choice for the rapid removal of theophylline. Hemodialysis is less efficient than hemoperfusion and should be used only if hemoperfusion is unavailable. Consider hemoperfusion if shock and arrhythmias persist despite beta-blocker therapy, if seizures persist despite adequate anticonvulsive therapy, or if theophylline serum concentrations are above 100 μg/ml.

Disposition ■

Patients presenting with cardiac arrhythmias, seizures, or hypotension or with theophylline serum concentrations above 40 μg/ml should be admitted to an intensive care unit or transferred to a pediatric critical care center. Patients presenting with only mild GI symptoms and serum concentrations of 20–40 μg/ml may be observed in the emergency department and discharged when the side effects have abated, a stool containing charcoal has been evacuated, and serum concentrations are declining. Remember that serum concentrations may continue to rise over 12–24 hours, especially after ingestion of sustained-release products.

Bibliography ■

Gaudreault P, Guay J: Theophylline poisoning. Pharmacological considerations and clinical management. *Med Toxicol Adverse Drug Exp* 1986; 1:169–91.

Olson KR, Benowitz NL, Woo OF, et al: Theophylline overdose: Acute single ingestion versus chronic repeated overmedication. *Am J Emerg Med* 1985; 3:386–94.

IX
Environmental Emergencies

93 Animal Bites

Michael L. Callaham

Animal bites are a common problem, accounting for about 1% of all emergency department visits in the United States. The annual incidence of dog bites is 300–700 per 100,000 population; most of the victims are children, who are particularly prone to bites about the head, face, and hands. About 90% of bites are inflicted by dogs, about 5% by cats, and the rest by humans and other animals. About 10% of bite victims seen in EDs require suturing, and 1% require hospitalization. Although in the United States few people are killed by animal bites each year, this is a major problem in developing and tropical countries. Even in the United States, about 10 people a year are killed by dogs, 10 times more than those who die of rabies.

Etiology and Pathophysiology ■

Animals harbor more than 100 microorganisms in their mouths, and these plus the resident skin flora of the victim usually contaminate the wound. In addition, because few animal teeth are very sharp, bite wounds are often crushing or tearing injuries as well. An attack by a large animal can inflict injury to deep structures and can cause major trauma. Whether or not the wound becomes infected depends primarily on wound toilet, but the host's immune defenses, the contaminating organism, and the bite location are also important.

Clinical Findings ■

The diagnosis of bite is generally easy and is provided by the history and the physical evidence of a wound. Bite wounds should be carefully inspected for the degree of contamination, foreign bodies, dirt, invasion of deep structures such as bone, vessels, nerve, and tendon, and depth. The diagnosis of infection is more difficult and is usually a clinical diagnosis based on redness, tenderness, swelling, and production of pus, *especially if these are increasing over time* (the first three are common in the first day or two after wound repair).

Ancillary Tests ■

See Table 93-1. Laboratory tests are seldom useful in animal bites. In the fresh uninfected wound, none are indicated; cultures and gram stains taken at this time are very inaccurate and predict neither the occurrence of infection nor the infecting organism. In infected wounds, cultures and gram stains are similarly inaccurate and rarely influence the choice of antibiotic therapy, which must be started before culture results are available. Therefore, cultures should be obtained only in cases of resistance to initial antibiotic treatment or in patients with other risk factors (i.e., diabetes, immune suppression, sepsis, bone or joint involvement, etc.). When cultures are obtained, both aerobic and anaerobic cultures are needed.

The white blood count and sedimentation rate are also unhelpful, even when infection is present, because management is never based on their results. Instead, *management is determined by the clinical appearance and severity of the wound and the toxicity of the patient (including vital signs)*. The WBC is not predictive of the nature or severity of infection.

X-rays are indicated in two situations. The first is the infant who has been bitten about the head or face by a carnivore; these animals have sharp canine teeth that can penetrate bone and cause osteomyelitis, meningitis, cranial abscess, etc. The second is in the case of bites of the hand, where X-rays can indicate bone involvement, air in the joint space, deep space infection (by the presence of gas in tissues), or osteomyelitis. Such X-rays are indicated only when the bite wound is deep; superficial bites and contusions do not need X-rays.

TABLE 93-1. *Indications for Laboratory Tests in Bite Wounds*

X-ray

Deep bite wounds of the hand (fractures, osteomyelitis, air in joint)

Cranial and facial bites in infants (bony penetration)

Cultures

Never indicated in fresh uninfected wounds.

Infected wounds only if resistant to initial antibiotic treatment or with multiple risk factors.

WBC and/or sed rate (ESR)

Not indicated; management should be based on clinical factors.

TABLE 93-2. *Summary of Animal-Bite Wound Treatment*

Mandatory (All Wounds)

1. Ensure appropriate tetanus immunization (check status of primary series).
2. Irrigate wound with several hundred ml of normal saline or 1% povidone-iodine solution, using a 12 ml syringe and 19 g needle or commercial 10–20 psi irrigation set.
3. Debride crushed and devitalized tissue.
4. Assess and treat for rabies if needed.
5. Assess risk factors to decide on further treatment.
6. Do not culture fresh wounds.
7. Do not give prophylactic antibiotics for routine bite wounds.

Selected Wounds Only

1. Suture all skin wounds unless high risk (e.g., hand wounds, high-risk species, immunosuppressed patient).
2. Culture infected wounds only if
   They fail to respond to initial antibiotic therapy, they are very high risk, there is evidence of systemic sepsis.
3. Consider
   Delayed primary closure of high-risk wounds (close in 72 hours if still uninfected),
   Prophylactic antibiotics in high-risk wounds (unproven value; must be given as early as possible, which means first dose must be parenteral).

(Adapted with permission from Callaham M: *Animal Bites*. In Callaham M, ed: *Current therapy in emergency medicine*. Toronto, B. C. Decker Inc. 1987.)

Treatment ■

PREHOSPITAL

If the victim is more than an hour from treatment, clean the wounds at the scene. Early cleansing reduces the chance of bacterial wound infection and can kill rabies and other viruses. It is adequate to use potable water, but ordinary hand soap will add some bactericidal, virucidal, and cleansing properties. *Avoid alcohol, hydrogen peroxide, and other disinfectants, which in their commonly available concentrations are harmful to normal tissue.* After the wound has been cleansed thoroughly, cover it with sterile dressings or a clean, dry cloth. Wounds of the hands or feet require immobilization after cleansing.

EMERGENCY DEPARTMENT

Wound toilet is more important to a good outcome than any other treatment (Table 93-2). Further treatment is based on a judgment of the risk factors present (Table 93-3). Most bite wounds are low risk and should be sutured, since healing is much faster with primary repair and scars are much smaller. If the wound has several risk factors, do not suture it, or suture with delayed primary repair (after 72 hours).

Cat bites are high risk, with an infection rate of up to 50%, perhaps because most are deep, small punctures that cannot be irrigated and many of them occur on the hand. *All cat bites of the hand deserve prophylactic antibiotics.*

Human bites are alleged to be very high risk, but the literature is biased by its concentration on deep human bites of the extensor surfaces of the hand (the so-called "closed-fist injury," incurred by the high-speed collision of a clenched, closed fist with a hu-man mouth). Human bites in other anatomic areas have an infection rate of about 10%, the same as dog bites; on the face, lips, or ears, the infection rate of human bites inflicted by others is under 3%. In children, human bites are particularly benign. Interestingly, through-and-through oral bites that are self-inflicted (due to seizures or injury) seem to have a high infection rate and may warrant prophylactic antibiotics. Even a patient with a closed-fist injury (which should always be suspected in the case of a laceration over a knuckle, especially in a young male, regardless of stated history) can be treated as an outpatient if the wound is less than 12 hours old and uninfected. Treatment consists of good wound toilet, antibiotic coverage, a bulky immobilizing "mitten" dressing, elevation, and careful follow-up within 24 hours.

Prophylactic antibiotics are not indicated in typical dog bite wounds, which are low risk. Appropriate use of antibiotics on the basis of risk factors will result

TABLE 93–3. *Animal-Bite Risk Factors for Infection*

High Risk		
Location	Hand, wrist, or foot	
	Scalp or face in infants (high risk of cranial perforation)	
	Over a major joint (possibility of perforation)	
Wound Type	Punctures (impossible to irrigate)	
	Tissue crushing that cannot be debrided (typical of herbivores such as cows, horses)	
Patient	Asplenic	
	Altered immune status (chemotherapy, AIDS, immune defect)	
	Diabetic	
	Chronic corticosteroid therapy	
	Prosthetic or diseased cardiac valve (consider systemic prophylaxis)	
	Prosthetic or seriously diseased joint (consider systemic prophylaxis)	
Species	Domestic cat	
	Large cat (deep punctures can penetrate joints, cranium)	
	Human (hand wounds only)	
	Primates (anecdotal evidence only)	
	Bat, skunk	
Low Risk		
Location	Face, scalp, ear, and lip (all should be sutured and will do very well)	
Wound Type	Large clean lacerations that can be thoroughly cleansed; the larger the laceration and the better the cleansing, the lower the infection rate	
Species	Rodents	

(Adapted with permission from Callaham M: *Animal Bites.* In Callaham M, ed: *Current therapy in emergency medicine.* Toronto, B.C. Decker Inc. 1987.)

in giving them to a small subset of bite victims, with a good cost-benefit ratio. To be effective, prophylactic antibiotics must reach the tissues as early as possible; therefore they must be given soon after the patient arrives at the facility. Handing the patient or parent a prescription to be filled later that day is worthless. If the wound is more than an hour old and the patient is to receive antibiotics, the wound should be thoroughly scrubbed with a moist gauze to break up the coagulum that protects bacteria from the antibiotic.

In addition to prophylactic use in carefully selected high-risk situations, antibiotics are of course useful whenever there is sign of established infection.

The choice of antibiotic is the same whether given for prophylactic or therapeutic reasons. For dog bites, dicloxacillin is the most effective and least costly choice (Table 93-4). It covers the broad range of possible pathogens (which are always unknown to the physician at the start of treatment), including *Streptococcus, Staphylococcus,* and a variety of aerobic and anaerobic species. Dicloxacillin is a good choice for cat bites, too, which often include *Pasteurella.*

In human bites, *Eikenella corrodens* is a consideration; this requires the addition of penicillin to the above regimen. In diabetics, hand infections seem to have an unusually high incidence of gram-negative infections, so that the addition of parenteral aminoglycosides or use of a second-generation cephalosporin (such as cefuroxime) is probably wise.

Complications and Caveats ■

Rabies is always a concern in animal bites; manage according to Figure 93-1. It is very helpful to know the incidence of rabies in common local species; in many parts of the United States, there has been no rabies in dogs or cats for decades. On the other hand, rabies is common in bats, skunks, and foxes.

If immunoprophylaxis is indicated, give 20 IU/kg of human rabies immune globulin immediately to produce passive protection. Infiltrate half the dose around the wound, then give the other half IM. If the risk is very high and the wound is about the face or neck, a dose of 40 IU/kg may be more effective, but

TABLE 93–4. *Oral Antibiotics for Bite Wounds*

Treatment duration: maximum 5 days for prophylaxis, until clinically free of infection for infected wounds

	Antibiotic	Dosage	Maximum Dosage
Organism Known	Treat according to specific antibiotic sensitivities of cultured organism.		
*Organism Unknown**	Dicloxacillin (cheapest), cephalexin, or cephradine	50 mg/kg/day in 4 divided doses	500 mg PO 4 times/day
If Penicillin-Allergic	Erythromycin	30–50 mg/kg/day in 4 divided doses	500 mg PO 4 times/day
Cat Bites (high likelihood of *Pasteurella multocida*†)	Penicillin V or dicloxacillin	50–100 mg/kg/day in 4 divided doses	500 mg 4 times/day
If Penicillin-Allergic	Erythromycin	30–50 mg/kg/day in 4 divided doses	500 mg PO 4 times/day
If Resistant to Initial Treatment, Culture and Consider	Cefaclor	25–40 mg/kg/day in 3 divided doses	1 g PO in 3 doses
Human Bites of Hand Organisms Include Gram-Positives, *Staphyloccocus aureus,* and *Eikenella corrodens*	Dicloxacillin plus penicillin	50–100 mg/kg/day in 4 divided doses	500 mg 4 times/day
If Penicillin-Allergic	Cefaclor	25–40 mg/kg/day in 3 divided doses	1 g PO in 3 doses
Deep Infection or Compromised Host	*Consider:* Parenteral antibiotics such as second- or third-generation cephalosporins.		
More Expensive Alternatives for Special Situations Can Be Used in all Types of Wounds but Are Unnecessary in Most	Augmentin (amoxicillin plus clavulanate)	20–40 mg of amoxicillin in 3 doses	500 mg PO t.i.d.
	Ceftriaxone	25 mg/kg IM b.i.d.	1 g IM once a day

* This regimen will be effective for most potential pathogens. No one antibiotic will cover all.
† Penicillin is excellent for *Pasteurella* but is not optimal for many other significant pathogens; dicloxacillin and cephalexin have a much broader spectrum but less efficacy against *Pasteurella*. Amoxicillin/clavulanic acid has a good spectrum and is effective for *Pasteurella* but is much more expensive and has far more side effects.
(Adapted with permission from Callaham M: *Animal Bites.* In Callaham M, ed: *Current therapy in emergency medicine.* Toronto, B.C. Decker Inc. 1987.)

this is controversial; consult an infectious-disease expert.

At the same time, begin active immunization with human diploid cell vaccine (HDCV), 1 ml IM on days 1, 3, 7, 14, and 28. This is a very effective vaccine; 25% of recipients have local redness and tenderness, but allergic and other serious reactions are very rare.

Disposition ■

Most animal bite wounds can be managed on an out-patient basis, if uninfected and seen within the first 12 hours after injury. The first follow-up visit can be at least three days later and, with a very reliable patient, at the time of suture removal (if any). Carefully instruct all patients and parents to seek medical care immediately if there are any signs of infection. See Chapter 143 for home-care wound instructions.

Evaluate patients with one or more risk factors more frequently, even if the wound is uninfected. In this situation, schedule the first follow-up visit within three days.

Infected wounds need close follow-up. Usually a return visit in several days is appropriate. In some cases, the clinician may be unsure whether the patient needs to be admitted or not, or the patient or family may be very unreliable. In this case, 24-hour follow-up by the same clinician is appropriate to ensure that the infection is responding to treatment.

Whether infected or not, bite wounds of the hand that penetrate bones, joints, or tendons mandate hos-

Rabies prophylaxis

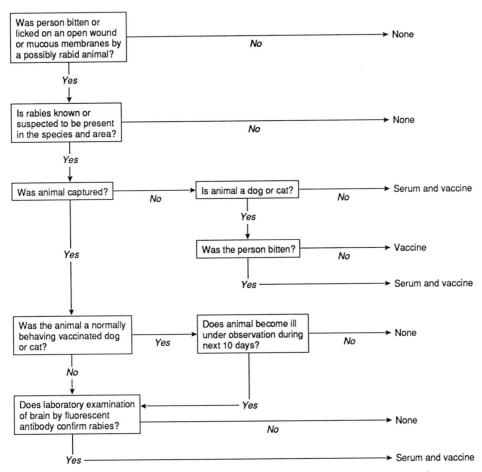

FIGURE 93–1. Postexposure rabies prophylaxis algorithm. (Reproduced with permission from Corey L, Hattwick M: Treatment of persons exposed to rabies. *JAMA* 1975;232:273)

pital admission (Table 93-5). Most infected bite wounds of the hand also mandate admission, especially when tenosynovitis or deep-space infection is present. Occasionally, very superficial cellulitis that does not involve any deep structures in the hand can be safely managed in very reliable outpatients.

Although sepsis from an animal bite is rare, any such patient obviously requires admission and immediate infectious disease consultation, because organisms may be unusual and resistant to common antibiotics.

TABLE 93–5. *Indications for Hospital Admission*

Hand bite:
    Involvement of bone, joint, tendon
    Deep-space infection or tenosynovitis
Sepsis from animal bites
Cranial injuries in infants
Severe wound infection causing systemic toxicity
Major trauma inflicted by large animals

Bibliography ■

Boenning DA, Fleisher GR, Campos JM: Dog bites in children: Epidemiology, microbiology, and penicillin prophylactic therapy. *Am J Emerg Med* 1983; 1(1):17–21.

Brook I: Microbiology of human and animal bite wounds in children. *Pediatr Infect Dis J* 1987; 6:29–32.

Callaham M: Controversies in antibiotic choices in bite wounds. *Ann Emerg Med* 1988; 17(12):1321–1330.

Callaham M: Wild and domestic animal bites. In: Auerbach PS, Geehr EC, eds: *Management of wilderness and environmental emergencies,* 2nd ed. New York: Macmillan, 1989.

Doan-Wiggins L: Animal bites and rabies. In: Rosen P, Baker FJ, Braen GR, et al, eds.: *Emergency medicine: Concepts and clinical practice,* 2nd ed. St. Louis: CV Mosby, 1988, pp. 965–974.

Goldstein EJC, Barones MF, Miller TA: *Eikenella corrodens* in hand infections. *J Hand Surg* 1983; 8:563–567.

Guy RJ, Zook ES: Successful treatment of acute head and neck dog bite wounds without antibiotics. *Ann Plast Surg* 1986; 17:45–48.

Lindsey D, Christopher M, Hollenbach J, et al: Natural course of the human bite wound: Incidence of infection and complications in 434 bites and 803 lacerations in the same group of patients. *J Trauma* 1987; 27:45–48.

Ordog GJ; The bacteriology of dog bite wounds. *Ann Emerg Med* 1986; 15:1324–1329.

Rosen RA: The use of antibiotics in the initial management of recent dog bite wounds. *Am J Emerg Med* 1985; 3:19–23.

Schweich P, Fleisher G: Human bites in children. *Pediatr Emerg Care* 1985; 1:51–53.

Worlock P, Boland P, Darrell J, et al: The role of prophylactic antibiotics following hand injuries. *Br J Clin Pract* 1980; 34:290–292.

94 Aquatic Hazards

Terrance J. Zuerlein and Paul S. Auerbach

The oceans and bodies of fresh water that cover the earth are unquestionably a great wilderness. Within this realm dwell four-fifths of all living organisms, many of them hazardous to humans. The largest concentration of noxious marine organisms is in warm temperate and tropical seas. To avoid needless unpleasant contact, be intelligently aware and respect the territorial rights of sea life.

Aquatic hazards can be grouped as follows, in order of increasing frequency:

1. *Shocks:* Electrical injuries from rays and electric eels
2. *Trauma:* Crushing and lacerating trauma from such sea life as sharks, barracuda, and moray eels
3. *Poisoning:* Induced by toxins generated within the fish or planktonic toxins ingested by the fish
4. *Stings:* By spicules or spines, with or without accompanying toxin envenomation, by a variety of invertebrates and vertebrates. Stings make up the majority of aquatic hazards.

Children are particularly prone to aquatic emergencies for several reasons:

1. Children often have not learned respect for the hazards of aquatic settings and sometimes are left unattended too long near water.
2. Bites, intoxications, envenomations, or stings that are trivial in adults may be catastrophic in children. Systemic reactions to toxins that can prove unpredictable in adults are even more so in children, who have limited hemodynamic and metabolic reserves. Multisystem trauma in children may occur with serious bites (e.g., sharks), requiring a high degree of urgency in transport and treatment.
3. Removing spines and spicules is far more difficult in children. It often requires sedation and, occasionally, general anesthesia.

Treatment ■

Table 94-1 presents general treatment principles. Tables 94-2, 94-3, and 94-4 provide specific management based on the injury category.

TABLE 94–1. *Aquatic Hazards: Treatment Principles*

1. Parents and caregivers should stay calm.
2. Approach the child gently, with the child either on the parent's lap or restrained.
3. If time and clinical condition allow, explain to the child and parents the nature of the problem and the planned course of treatment.
4. Use sedation (chloral hydrate 25–75 mg/kg/dose q 8 h PO/PR) or parenteral analgesia (meperidine 1–1.5 mg/kg/dose, max: 100 mg, plus hydroxyzine 0.5–1 mg/kg/dose q 4 h) for painful procedures such as extraction and debridement.
5. Consider general anesthesia if involved areas are extensive.
6. Check immunization history. Tetanus toxoid 0.5 ml IM may be warranted. Consider tetanus immunoglobulin, 250–500 units IM.
7. Have a high index of urgency when tissue loss occurs (e.g., shark).
8. Consult or transport to appropriate pediatric resources (e.g., poison control, children's hospital).
9. Admit for close observation and monitoring when systemic reactions are unpredictable or dangerous.
10. Gastric evacuation and activated charcoal/catharsis are warranted for many ingestion intoxications.
11. Prophylactic antibiotics may be indicated for penetrating trauma.
12. Epinephrine 1:100,000, 0.01 mg/kg = 1 ml/kg IV should be administered for systemic hypotension associated with anaphylaxis.

TABLE 94–2. *Aquatic Hazards: Shocking and Traumatogenic*

Type	Species	Source of Injury	Clinical Signs/ Symptoms	Treatment
Shocking	Marine stargazers, electric rays, Amazonian electric, eel	Electrical discharge is reflexively produced on contact, of 8–220 volts and low amperage.	Stunned appearance and cutaneous burns or abrasions	Symptomatic/supportive
Traumato-genic	Sharks, barracuda, moray eels	Lacerations by sharp teeth and crushing injury by powerful jaw musculature	Massive tissue loss and even amputation are possible. Considerable hemorrhage with resultant hypovolemic shock	Use compression for external hemorrhage. Avoid arterial-occlusive tourniquets.
				Attain IV access, administer crystalloid, blood or colloid.
				MAST garment may be needed in older children.
				Evaluate for evidence of cervical, intrathoracic, or intra-abdominal trauma.
				Transport to trauma center for surgical intervention if necessary.
				Do *not* close wounds without thorough exploration, debridement, and irrigation.
				Administer tetanus toxoid and immunoglobulin.
				Antibiotics are warranted for shark bites: Cefoperazone (25–100 mg/kg/day ÷ q 12 h) Gentamicin (5–6 mg/kg/day ÷ q 8 h) *or* Trimethoprim-sulfamethoxazole (10 mg/kg/day ÷ q 12 h, based on the trimethoprim component)
				Culture wounds only when clinical evidence for infection exists.

SHOCKS AND TRAUMA

These injuries are less common but more sensationalized than are poisonings and stings. They do, however, account for significant morbidity and mortality. Even a low-dose electric shock may be incapacitating or lethal in a young child, and secondary drowning may occur. Multiple-system internal injury is not uncommon in children attacked by biting sea life.

The key to successful intervention is rapid assessment, stabilization, and transport to appropriate tertiary care if necessary. See Table 94-2.

POISONINGS

Poisonings by eating a fish or planktonic toxins within the fish are fairly common. Symptoms are primarily GI and neurologic and vary from mild to profound and lethal. Toxin-mediated illness is largely dose dependent, so children of low body mass are particularly at risk for more serious reactions. See Table 94-3.

STINGS

Stings make up the largest single group of aquatic hazards. The predominant difficulties with aquatic stings are cutaneous manifestations and pain. Anaphylaxis may occur and, rarely, death may follow cardiovascular collapse and multisystem organ failure. See Table 94-4.

Prevention ■

Infants, toddlers, and young children should be supervised near water. The entire family should avoid

(text continues on page 413)

TABLE 94–3. *Aquatic Hazards: Poisonous*

Category	Toxin Origin	Species	Clinical Signs/Symptoms	Treatment	Comment
Ichthyocrino-toxication	Glandular secretions of foam or slime	Pufferfish, lamprey, moray eel	Nausea, vomiting, diarrhea, abdominal pain, weakness	Empty stomach. Symptomatic/supportive	
Tetrodotoxica-tion	Varies with reproductive cycle and feeding habits	Pufferfish, porcupine fish, sunfish, mola	Tingling of mouth and eventually entire body. Salivation, weakness, nausea, vomiting, diarrhea, muscle twitching, paralysis, convulsions, respiratory insufficiency, death	Empty stomach using alkaline lavage. Activated charcoal. Symptomatic/supportive. Admission warranted.	This neurotoxin is one of the most potent known, with the fatality rate exceeding 50% in the full syndrome.
Ichthyootoxica-tion	Fish gonads	Sturgeon, salmon, pike, carp, catfish, perch, sculpin	Nausea, vomiting, diarrhea, abdominal pain, thirst, dry mouth, fever, headache, hypotension, paralysis	Empty stomach. Symptomatic/supportive. Admission advisable.	
Ichthyohepato-toxication	Fish liver	Skate, ray, mackerel, porgy, sandfish, tropical shark	Nausea, vomiting, diarrhea, abdominal pain, tingling mouth, visual disturbances, delirium, respiratory distress, coma, death	Empty stomach. Symptomatic/supportive. Admission warranted.	Resembles hypervitaminosis A
Ciguatera fish poisoning	Marine dinoflagellate that ascends the food chain	Barracuda, snapper, jack, parrotfish, grouper	GI distress followed by numbness/tingling. Cold feels hot and vice versa. Headaches, vertigo, ataxia are common. Rash, pruritus. Bradycardia, hypotension, and respiratory failure rarely occur.	Empty stomach. Charcoal/catharsis. Symptomatic/supportive. Mannitol may be efficacious. Admission warranted.	The most common foodborne disease associated with fish ingestion. Cooking does not destroy this toxin.

Ichthyoallyein-otoxication	Concentrated in fish heads	Sturgeon, chub, mullet, goatfish, rabbitfish	Dizziness, lack of coordination, itching, burning throat, hallucinations	Symptomatic	
Clupeotoxic fish poisoning	Plankton that ascends the food chain	Herring, sardine, tarpon	GI complaints followed by headache, vertigo, hypotension, paralysis, respiratory distress, convulsions, coma, and not uncommonly death.	Empty stomach. Charcoal/catharsis. Symptomatic/supportive. Admission warranted.	These plankton proliferate in summer months and cause colored "tides."
Paralytic shellfish poisoning	Plankton that ascends the food chain	Sand crab, mussel, clam, oyster, scallop	Lip, gum, and tongue burning, spreading to rest of body. Numbness, headache, incoherence, and weakness follow. Respiratory paralysis with death possible.	Empty stomach. Charcoal/catharsis. Symptomatic/supportive. Admission warranted.	Occurs with improper fish preservation or refrigeration
Scombroid poisoning	Bacteria-enhanced decomposition of fish, to histamine and histidine	Tuna, mackerel, bluefish, ocean salmon, dolphin, mahi-mahi	Pseudo-allergic reaction with flushing, headache, nausea, vomiting, diarrhea, urticaria, bronchospasm, and possibly hypotension	Empty stomach. For the allergic component: diphenhydramine (1–2 mg/kg IV) cimetidine (20–40 mg/kg/d ÷ q 6 h) epinephrine 1: 100,000, 0.01 mg/kg IV, or 1: 1,000, 0.01 mg/kg sub Q	

TABLE 94–4. *Aquatic Hazards: Stinging*

Category	Sting Origin	Species	Clinical Signs/Symptoms	Treatment	Comment
Sponges	Spicules	Fire sponge	Pruritic dermatitis, erythema multiforme, or anaphylactoid reactions. Stiff joints possible. Vesiculation and desquamation may occur.	Remove spicules with adhesive tape. Apply 5% acetic acid soaks. Steroids: prednisone 1 mg/kg PO, methylprednisolone 1 mg/kg IV.	Steroids may worsen primary reaction but should alleviate secondary inflammation.
Coelenterate	Nematocyst stinging cells discharge on contact with victim's body surface.	Fire coral, Portuguese man-o'-war, true jellyfish, coral, anemone	Pruritus, paresthesias, burning sensation. Linear whiplike nematocyst contact site. Blistering, edema, and ulceration may occur. Severe envenomation may lead to GI or anaphylactic symptoms, coma, or death.	Pain control with naloxone-reversible narcotics (IV/IM) meperidine 1–2 mg/kg, morphine 0.1–0.2 mg/kg.	Fresh water will stimulate untriggered nematocysts.
				Rinse the wound with *sea water*.	
				Apply 5% acetic acid (vinegar) soaks. Isopropyl alcohol 40–70% may be used.	
				Papain (meat tenderizer) yields variable results.	
				Antihistamines may be given.	
				Remove remaining nematocysts by shaving the area.	
				Lidocaine HCl 2.5% or benzocaine 14% may be soothing.	
				Tetanus prophylaxis is in order.	
		Box jellyfish, sea wasp	May lead to rapid decompensation	In addition to above, apply a proximal venous-lymphatic occlusive constriction bandage if an extremity is involved.	Loosen every 10 minutes for 90 seconds.
				For known box jellyfish (*Chironex fleckeri*) sting, specific antivenin is available: 1 ampule over 5 minutes IV or 3 amps IM. Anticipate anaphylaxis and pretreat with antihistamine.	

Corals	Exoskeleton	All	Raised red welts and local pruritus. May progress to cellulitis with ulceration.	Scrub vigorously with soap and water. Apply diluted hydrogen peroxide. Tetanus prophylaxis Manage with sterile wet to dry or dilute antiseptics.	
Mollusks	Bites or stings	Oyster, clam, cone shell, mussel, snail, squid, octopus	Local ischemia, pruritus, numbness, paresthesias. Blurred vision, dysphagia, ataxia, and weakness may occur. Muscular paralysis may lead to respiratory failure. Cerebral edema, coma, disseminated intravascular coagulation, and cardiac failure are possible with severe envenomations.	Attain veno-lymphatic occlusion with elastic bandages. Tetanus prophylaxis Symptomatic/supportive Admission warranted.	
Echinoderms	Spines	Starfish, sea urchin	Burning, redness, swelling, and aching. May get muscular paralysis and respiratory distress; occasionally death	Immerse in hot water to tolerance (45°C) for 30–90 minutes. Remove embedded spines. Symptomatic/supportive Admission advisable with neuromuscular involvement.	
Vertebrates Stingrays	Spines at base of tail	Stingray	Pain, edema, and bleeding at the laceration site. May have nausea, vomiting, diarrhea, tachycardia, syncope, muscle cramps, hypotension, arrhythmias, and rarely, death	Irrigate with sterile saline or sea water. Immerse in hot water to tolerance. Remove embedded spines. Narcotic analgesia. May use lidocaine without epinephrine for local infiltration or nerve block. Tetanus prophylaxis and antibiotics as for shark bite	One of most common stinging venomous injuries Do not exceed 5 mg/kg.

TABLE 94–4. Aquatic Hazards: Stinging *(continued)*

Category	Sting Origin	Species	Clinical Signs/ Symptoms	Treatment	Comment
Catfish	Dorsal and pectoral fin spines inject venom	Both marine and fresh water	Stinging, throbbing, or scalding with radiation up the affected limb. Initial ischemia and pallor progress to swelling and redness. Muscle spasm and fasciculation may occur.	Same as for stingray punctures	
Scorpion fish	Dorsal, pelvic, and anal spines	Lionfish, scorpion fish, stonefish	Immediate intense pain severe enough to cause delirium. Systemic effects may evolve and are similar to stingray envenomation.	Same as for stingray punctures. A stonefish antivenin against Indo-Pacific species is available.	Healing may require up to 6 months.
Sea snakes	Maxillary fangs	Pelagic sea snakes	Notable lack of local reaction. Initial complaints include euphoria, malaise, or anxiety. Muscle aching and an ascending flaccid or spastic paralysis follow. Speech and swallowing are impaired. Muscle twitching, spasm, and trismus develop. Vision may fail and the patient may lapse into a coma. Myoglobinuria occurs 3–6 hours post-bite.	Principles the same as with terrestrial bite Apply pressure with elastic wrap to sequester venom. Keep the extremity dependent and seek a source of antivenin from local poison control agency. Polyvalent sea snake antivenin is most effective if given within 8 hours. Admission is warranted.	No sea snakes live in the Atlantic Ocean or Caribbean Sea.

endemic and high-risk areas. Children should be kept away from "dead" beach animals or suspicious objects from the sea. Seafood must be cleaned, refrigerated, and prepared properly to avoid poisonous ingestions.

Educating both children and adults in coastal areas will lead to a healthy respect for the sea and its abundant life.

Bibliography ■

Anderson BS, Sims JK, Wiebenga NH, et al: The epidemiology of ciguatera fish poisoning in Hawaii, 1975–1981. *Hawaii Med J* 1983; 42:326.

Anker RL, Straffon WG, Loiselle DS, et al: Retarding the uptake of "mock venom" in humans. Comparison of three first-aid treatments. *Med J Aust* 1982; 1:212.

Auerbach PS, Yajko DM, Nassos PS, et al: Bacteriology of the marine environment: Implications for clinical therapy. *Ann Emerg Med* 1987; 16:643.

Auerbach PS, Halstead BW: Hazardous aquatic life. In: Auerbach PS, Geehr EC, eds: *Management of wilderness and environmental emergencies,* 2nd ed. St. Louis: CV Mosby, 1989, pp. 933–1028.

Behling AR, Taylor SH: Bacterial histamine production as a function of temperature and time of incubation. *J Food Sci* 1982; 47:1311.

Blakesly ML: Scombroid poisoning: Prompt resolution of symptoms with cimetidine. *Ann Emerg Med* 1983; 12: 104.

Boyd W: Sea-wasp antivenom in a toddler. *Med J Aust* 1984; 104:504.

Burnett JW, Rubinstein H, Calton GJ: First aid for jellyfish envenomation. *South Med J* 1983; 76:870.

Fusetani N, Sato S, Hashimoto K: Occurrence of a water-soluble toxin in a parrotfish (*Ypsicarus ovifrons*) which is probably responsible for parrotfish liver poisoning. *Toxicon* 1985; 23:105.

Moss SS: Shark feeding mechanisms. *Oceanus* 1981/1982; 24:23.

Prescott BD: "Scombroid poisoning" and bluefish: The Connecticut connection. *Conn Med* 1984; 48:105.

95 Cold Temperature Emergencies

Alan M. Gelb

Hypothermia is defined as a core body temperature of ≤ 35°C (95°F). The actual freezing of tissue is *frostbite*. Other specific local complications of exposure to cold that do not involve the freezing of tissue are *immersion ("trench") foot* and *chilblains* (pernio).

In all age groups, hypothermia is more common in males than females. In children ages 10 to 14, boys predominate 8 to 1. Neonatal hypothermia has been correlated with poverty, home deliveries, and lack of medical assistance. Mortality rates vary greatly in different series, ranging from 12–71%.

Etiology ■

Both environmental and host factors can be responsible for the development of hypothermia and cold injuries. Hypothermia results from decreased heat production, and/or increased heat loss, and/or impaired thermoregulation. Table 95-1 presents common causes of hypothermia and associated mechanisms for cold injury.

Neonates are specifically at risk because of the following:

Exposure during childbirth and resuscitation
Rapid evaporative heat loss, in ambient temperatures, especially if not dried
Underdeveloped thermoregulatory mechanisms
Increased surface area to body mass
Decreased subcutaneous tissue.

In older children, inadequate clothing due to child neglect or prolonged activity in cold-weather sports may pose major environmental risks.

Infants and children may also develop iatrogenic hypothermia during resuscitation and emergency department procedures because of exposure and/or the infusion of large quantities of unwarmed blood or crystalloid. Provide warm blankets or heating lamp whenever possible and administer fluids warmed to 37°C when rapid infusion is anticipated.

Normal children can often withstand severe cold, but neonates and children with certain underlying conditions (see Table 95-1) may be at high risk for hypothermia even with ambient temperatures above 80°F.

Pathophysiology ■

HYPOTHERMIA

As body temperature decreases, three phases of physiologic change occur:

1. During the initial phase, from 37°–32°C (98.6°–90°F), homeostatic mechanisms attempt to maintain body temperature. Peripheral vasoconstriction decreases heat loss through capillaries in the extremities. The metabolic rate is increased, and shivering increases heat production.
2. Below 32°C (90°F), protective mechanisms begin to fail, with alterations in all organ systems. Vasoconstriction is conserved, but shivering stops. Diminished mental status impairs the individual's ability to seek warmth.
3. Below 24°C (75°F), the patient becomes essentially cold-blooded. All thermoregulatory mechanisms cease, and the patient becomes the same temperature as the environment. Cardiorespiratory function stops.

LOCAL COMPLICATIONS

The major causes of *frostbite* are intense vasoconstriction and ice crystallization of intra- and extracellular water. A vicious cycle of cellular injury, increased tissue pressure, decreased perfusion, and tissue freezing then follows. Areas most commonly affected are the distal extremities, ears, nose, cheeks, and chin. The severity of injury is proportional to not only the ambient temperature, but also wind chill, increased humidity, duration of exposure, and clothing.

Frostnip is a superficial, localized, reversible freezing of tissue that resolves without permanent injury.

414

TABLE 95–1. *Causes of Hypothermia and Cold Injury*

Exposure
  Low temperature IHL
  High wind IHL
  Low humidity IHL
  Inadequate clothing IHL
  Submersion IHL
  Resuscitation IHL

Physical Acclimatization and Condition
  Diaphoresis IHL
  Decreased subcutaneous tissue IHL, DHP
  Starvation DHP
  Age extremes IHL, DHP, ITR

Drugs (Therapeutic and Toxic Doses)
  Alcohol IHL, DHP, ITR
  Barbiturates DHP, ITR
  Narcotics DHP, ITR
  Sedatives DHP, ITR
  General anesthetics DHP, ITR
  Tricyclics IHL, DHP, ITR
  Phenothiazines IHL, DHP, ITR
  Lithium ITR

Infection
  Sepsis IHL, ITR
  Meningitis, encephalitis ITR
  Pneumonia (including tuberculosis) ITR
  Peritonitis ITR
  Endocarditis ITR

CNS Disorders
  Seizure IHL, ITR
  Paralysis, paralysis, paresis DHP, ITR
  CNS infarct, hemorrhage, or tumor ITR
  Anorexia nervosa IHL, ITR

Metabolic and Endocrine Disease
  Hypothyroidism DHP, ITR
  Hypoglycemia DHP, ITR
  Diabetic ketoacidosis DHP, IHL, ITR
  Arenal insufficiency DHP
  Uremia ITR
  Hypopituitarism DHP, ITR
  Hepatic failure ITR

Other
  Erythrodermas (eczema, psoriasis) IHL
  Trauma (hypotension, hypovolemia) IHL, ITR
  Malignancy (Hodgkin's carcinomatosis) ITR
  Iatrogenic (treatment of burns, cold parenteral fluids, ice applied to injuries) IHL

DHP = decreased heat production
IHL = increased heat loss
ITR = impaired thermoregulation

If not caught in this early phase, frostnip may progress to frostbite.

Both *immersion (trench) foot* and *chilblains* (pernios) probably result from sympathetic deregulation and cold-induced vasculitis rather than actual ice crystallization in tissue.

Clinical Findings ■

HYPOTHERMIA

The clinical presentation of hypothermia may be obvious or subtle. In the child found unconscious in the snow, the diagnosis is not difficult. The diagnosis may be delayed or missed because the temperature is not taken in the emergency department, the coolness of the child's body goes unrecognized, or the temperature is read at 35°C (95°F), the lowest recording on most hand-held thermometers. *Whenever hypothermia is suspected, low-reading thermometers (e.g., rectal probes) must be used.*

In general, the clinical findings in hypothermia develop predictably as core body temperature falls (Table 95-2). Signs and symptoms may reflect a predisposing or underlying condition or illness.

Poor feeding and lethargy may be presenting signs in hypothermic neonates and infants. The physical exam may disclose a somewhat rigid child, with hardened, erythematous skin and peripheral edema. Infants presumed to have sudden infant death syndrome should always have a core temperature determination. *If the core temperature is less than 30° C (86° F), the patient is hypothermic, not dead, until warmed* (see treatment below).

Other presenting signs and symptoms in children and adolescents include slurred speech, ataxia, poor judgment, and shivering in mild hypothermia. As the core temperature falls, blood pressure, pulse, and respirations decrease. Mentation becomes increasingly impaired between 32°C and 28°C, followed by coma and sluggish or absent reflexes in severe hypothermia (less than 20°C).

LOCAL COMPLICATIONS

Frostbite is classified, similar to a burn, according to the depth of tissue destruction (Table 95-3). The initial appearance and sensation of the affected area may not correlate well with the extent of injury. Involved tissue initially appears white, yellow, or blue; paresthesias, decreased sensation, or locally anesthetic areas may be present. The skin may feel frozen with softer underlying tissue, or woody hard. An accurate prognosis may require 24–48 hours, and actual demarcation of devitalized tissue may require 3–6 weeks.

Immersion (trench) foot may occur in any individual with prolonged exposure to wetness and temperatures above freezing. Clinically, the involved

TABLE 95–2. *Clinical Findings in Hypothermia*

Stage	Core Temperature	Cardiovascular Pulse–BP–Other	Neurologic	Respirations	Musculoskeletal	Other
Mild	35°C (95°F)	↑, ↑ or →, NSR	Dysaarthria	Increased	Shivering maximum	Senses cold, diuresis begins
Moderate	32°C (89.6°F)	↓, ↓ or →, NSR	Apathy and confusion	Unchanged or decreased	Rigidity and edema	Oxygen consumption decreased 25%
	30°C (86°F)	↓, ↓, Possible atrial fib	Stupor or irritability	Decreased	Shivering stops, urine output declines	Lose thermoregulation
Severe	28°C (82.4°F)	↓, ↓, Possible vent tach or fib	Unconscious, dilated pupils	Decreased	Rigidity may resolve	Oxygen consumption decreased 25%
	26°C (78.8°F)	↓↓, ↓↓, Cardiac output 50% of normal	No response to pain, areflexic	Possible pulmonary edema	Stiffness, edema, cyanosis	Renal blood flow decreased by 50%
	18°C (64.4°F)	Asystole	Flat EEG	Apnea	Similar to rigor mortis	Survival has been reported

NSR, normal sinus rhythm.

areas are indistinguishable from frostbite, but these lesions usually have a more favorable prognosis.

Chilblains (pernios) are usually seen in young women or adolescent girls. These lesions are erythematous or bluish plaques or nodules on the dorsal surfaces of the distal extremities. Often, chilblains are associated with localized burning or pruritis and occur after new or repeated exposure to cold, damp, windy weather.

Ancillary Data ■

Hypothermic patients require extensive laboratory investigation. Table 95-4 presents laboratory data commonly found in hypothermia, frequent associated problems, and recommended treatment. Laboratory abnormalities may be due to a predisposing condition, hypothermia itself, or one of the complications of hypothermia.

Controversy exists about the correction of arterial blood gases. Uncorrected values are read by machines at 37°C, but the actual pO_2 and pCO_2 are lower and the pH higher at hypothermic body temperatures.

Serum glucose is often elevated in acute hypothermia but decreased in chronic hypothermia. Cold-induced glycosuria may be present at normal or even low serum glucose levels. *A rapid bedside dipstick blood glucose determination is imperative to ensure immediate dextrose administration in appropriate patients,* since hypothermia may mask the signs of hypoglycemia. Even if hyperglycemia initially exists, serial glucose determinations are necessary because serum glucose usually falls during rewarming.

TABLE 95–3. *Classification of Frostbite*

Based on appearance more than 24 hours after rewarming (see text)

Degree	Symptoms	Signs	Duration
First	Paresthesia, burning	Mottled, hyperemic, edematous	1–2 weeks
Second	Paresthesia, burning	Clear bullae progressing to eschar	3–4 weeks
Third	Anesthesia	Blue bullae; hard, gray skin; loss of subcutaneous tissue	2–3 months
Fourth	Anesthesia	Vesicles, bullae, ulceration, eschar, gangrene, autoamputation	2–3 months

TABLE 95–4. *Laboratory Results in Hypothermia*

Test	Result	Associated Problem	Treatment Notes
pO_2	Decrease	Cold-induced bronchorrhea, decreased cough and gag, aspiration pneumonia	Supplemental oxygen, careful suctioning, and antibiotics
pCO_2	Decrease	Decreased metabolic rate	Consider supplemental CO_2 if pCO_2 less than 20.
	Increase	Decreased respiratory drive	Consider increasing tidal volume or respiratory rate.
pH	Decrease	Lactic acidosis, hypoventilation	Do not give bicarbonate
	Increase	Possible iatrogenic hyperventilation	Decrease tidal volume or respiratory rate.
WBC	Decrease	Sepsis, sequestration	Cover all patients for sepsis, regardless of WBC.
	Increase	Infection, dehydration	
Hct	Decrease	GI bleed, previous anemia	Transfuse as needed.
	Increase	Dehydration	Hydration with crystalloid as needed
Platelets	Decrease	Sequestration, DIC	Common in neonates, corrects with rewarming. Verify with fibrin split product levels.
K^+	Increase	Rhabdomyolysis, renal failure	Draw confirmatory CPK, treat conservatively. Consider dialysis.
	Decrease	Alcoholism, diuretics, acidosis	May self correct. Treat conservatively, repeat test frequently.
Glucose	Increase	Catecholamine-induced glycogenolysis	Self corrects on rewarming
	Decrease	Glycogen depletion	Glucose administration
Amylase	Increase	Pancreatitis	Hypothermia may mimic clinical findings (ileus).
PT	Increase	DIC	Verify with fibrin split product levels.
BUN, creatinine	Increase	Dehydration, decreased clearance	Poor indicators of volume status
Toxicology screen	Positive	Overdose	Decreased hepatic and renal clearance

The ECG may reveal prolongation of the PR, QRS, and QT intervals due to slowed conduction. Additionally, an Osborn (J) wave may be seen as a widened hump at the end of the QRS complex (Figure 95-1). These findings are neither prognostic nor diagnostic in the hypothermic patient, and may occur in cardiac or central nervous system ischemia as well as a variety of other conditions. Monitoring the cardiac rhythm closely is far more important in this situation than interpreting ECG morphology. Dysrhythmias are common below 30°C (86°F).

Infection is a common predisposing factor in children with hypothermia. Culture blood, urine, CSF, and sputum. Obtain a chest X-ray.

Studies to assess associated underlying conditions may be individualized. Thyroid and adrenal function tests, cardiac enzymes, toxicology screens, cervical spine series, and computerized tomography of the head may be indicated.

Treatment ∎

BASIC PRINCIPLES

The first task is resuscitation and stabilization; then, definitive evaluation can be made and diagnosis-specific therapy can be instituted (Figure 95-2).

TREATMENT CAVEATS

Use the patient's rectal probe temperature to guide further therapy. Below 28°C (82°F), resuscitation in hypothermic patients differs from conventional protocols:

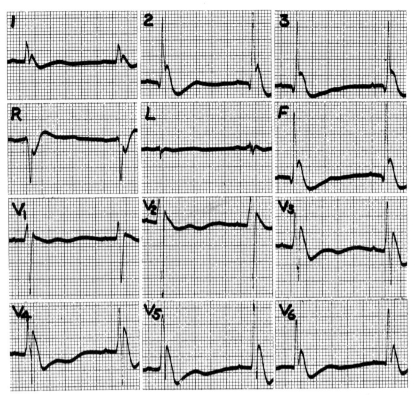

FIGURE 95–1. Electrocardiographic changes in hypothermia. Note "J" deflection maximal in midprecordial leads. (Reproduced with permission from Marriot JL: *Practical Electrocardiography.* Baltimore: Williams & Wilkins; 1981:305)

1. Avoid adrenergic medications, since their efficacy at this temperature range is low and precipitation of ventricular fibrillation is likely.
2. Give bretylium tosylate 5 mg/kg prophylactically.
3. Avoid inserting intracardiac catheters and nasogastric tubes until the core temperature is above 28°C (82°F), since mechanical stimulation of the heart may induce dysrhythmias.
4. Extracorporeal blood rewarming by cardiopulmonary bypass or femoral-femoral dialysis should replace chest compressions as quickly as possible. This is the most effective way of raising core temperature and may be less likely to induce ventricular fibrillation.

2. Give naloxone (0.4–2 mg IV) for altered mental status.
3. Give $D_{25}W$ 2 ml/kg for hypoglycemia or bedside dipstick <100 mg%.
4. Provide infection-specific or broad-spectrum antibiotic coverage after cultures are obtained.

Undertake rewarming carefully because of the risk of acidosis, decreased blood pressure, and dysrhythmias. With standard treatment, core body temperature should increase 1–2°C per hour. Determine which rewarming method to use by the degree of hypothermia and the patient's clinical presentation (Table 95-5).

INITIAL FLUIDS AND DRUGS

In all patients, begin D_5NS *warmed to 40° C (104° F)*.

1. Use maintenance rates for normotensive individuals; bolus D_5NS 20 ml/kg for hypotension.

TREATMENT OF LOCAL COMPLICATIONS

Rapidly warm areas of possible frostbite using a water bath heated to 40–42°C (104–108°F). Keep the bath at this temperature for no longer than 30 minutes. *If appropriate frostbite treatment is impossible, such as*

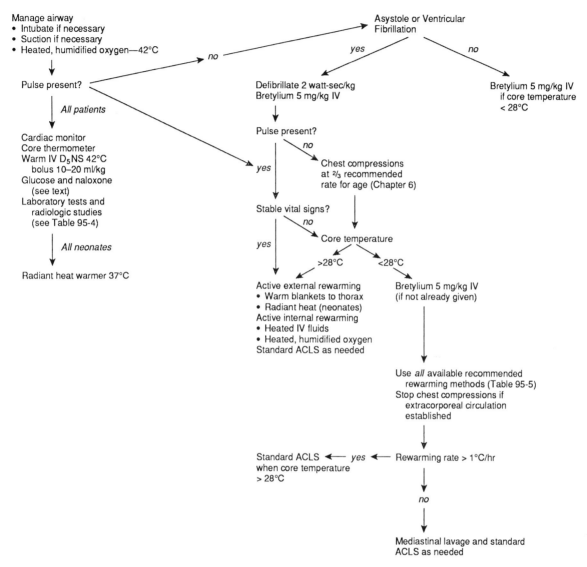

FIGURE 95–2. Hypothermia algorithm.

in the woods, leave areas frozen, since refreezing after initial rewarming significantly worsens the prognosis.

Wrap affected areas loosely with sterile dressings. Do not rupture bullae. Ensure tetanus immunization and give prophylactic penicillin for all but first-degree frostbite.

Treat immersion foot by removing all layers of clothing and drying affected areas. Do not rub the skin or soak in water. Elevate affected areas and protect them from trauma. Antibiotics are indicated only for documented infection.

Treat chilblains simply by warming affected areas at room temperature and elevating them. Soaking these lesions may lead to increased pruritis or pain.

Disposition ■

Patients with core temperature less than 35°C (95°F) require hospitalization. Those with core temperature below 33°C (91.4°F) are best managed in a pediatric-equipped intensive care unit, or should be transferred to a pediatric critical care center expeditiously.

Admit all patients with frostbite and immersion foot for aggressive local care. Patients with chilblains do not require admission.

TABLE 95–5. *Rewarming Techniques*

Category	Method	Advantages	Disadvantages	Comments
Passive external (T = 33–35°C)	Wrap in dry blanket	Noninvasive, simple, maintains peripheral vasoconstriction	Slow, useless if patient <30°C (poikilothermic)	Useful in mild, chronic hypothermia
Active external (T = 30–32°C)	Wrap in dry warmed or electric blanket	Noninvasive, simple	Thermal burns possible with electric blanket	Wrap thorax only.
	Radiant heat warmer (37°C)	Maintains accessibility for monitoring and resuscitation	May cause peripheral vasodilatation, decreases BP	Useful in neonates and infants
	Warm water immersion (40°)	None	Lack access to patient, peripheral vasodilatation, decreases BP	Not recommended
Active internal (T < 30°C)	Heated humidified oxygen (42°C)	Noninvasive, simple, safe, and very effective	Requires specialized equipment	Mandatory, may use with mask or tracheal intubation
	Heated intravenous fluids (42°C)	Simple, safe	Requires blood warmer or microwave	Useful adjunct, do not use in central line.
	Heated gastric lavage (42°C)	Availability	Aspiration, induced electrolyte abnormalities	Not recommended
	Heated peritoneal lavage (42°C)	May remove drugs in overdose patients	Invasive, may induce hypokalemia	Do not use in stable patients; limited usefulness.
	Hemodialysis (40°C)	Very effective, improves blood flow, may remove drugs	Invasive, requires specialized equipment, requires anticoagulation	Use only in arrested patients and those not responding to other methods.
	Cardiopulmonary bypass (40°C)	Very effective, improves blood flow, improves oxygenation		
	Mediastinal lavage (40°C)	Very effective, permits open chest cardiac massage	Invasive, requires left tube thoracostomy or thoracotomy	Use only in arrested patients where hemodialysis or bypass is unavailable or ineffective.

Parental training in all cases of exposure-induced hypothermia is essential. If child neglect or child abuse is suggested by the clinical presentation, notify appropriate authorities.

Bibliography ■

Danzyl DF. Accidental Hypothermia. In: Rosen P, Baker II JF, Barkin RM, Braen GR, Dailey RH, Levy RC, eds. Emergency Medicine: concepts and clinical practice. 2nd ed. St. Louis: C.V. Mosby, 1988:663.

Kaplan M, Eidelman AI. Improved Prognosis in Severely Hypothermic Newborn Infants Treated by Rapid Rewarming. J Pediatr 1984; 105:470.

Robinson M, Seward PN. Environmental Hypothermia in Children. Pediatr Emerg Care 1986; 2:254.

Shaw JF, Frostbite. In: Rosen P, Baker II JF, Barkin RM Braen GR, Dailey RH, Levy RC eds. Emergency Medicine: concepts and clinical practice. 2nd ed. St. Louis: C.V. Mosby, 1988;609.

Sofer S, Yagupsky P, Hershkowits J, Bearman JE. Improved Outcome of Hypothermic Infants. Pediatr Emerg Care 1986; 2:211.

96 Heat Illness

Alan M. Gelb

Heat illness accounts for more than 4,000 deaths each year in the United States. Both the very young and the very old are at increased risk for complications caused by elevated environmental temperatures.

Heat illness is an adverse response to environmental heat. Fever may be present or absent in patients with heat illness. Heat cramps, heat exhaustion, and heatstroke are syndromes of increasing severity that result from the body's physiologic response to heat stress.

Etiology ■

Both host and environmental factors play important roles in causing heat illness (Table 96-1). Because of several inherent physiologic differences, children have a higher risk than adults of developing heat illness:

1. Increased surface area to mass, resulting in greater heat transfer from the environment to the child
2. Greater metabolic heat production per kg during exercise
3. Diminished sweating capacity
4. Diminished ability to increase cutaneous blood flow during exercise
5. Slower acclimatization to warm weather

Infants are often placed at risk when they are left in cars without adequate ventilation. Neonates and infants wrapped in multiple layers of clothing on warm summer nights may also develop heat illness.

Older children participating in athletics during hot, humid weather without adequate water intake are at risk, as are adolescents who use stimulants such as amphetamines, cocaine, and PCP.

Pathophysiology ■

As body temperature increases, two homeostatic adjustments occur: *vasodilatation* (with heat loss due to conduction, convection, and radiation) and *sweat-*ing. At environmental temperatures above body temperature, evaporation of sweat is essential for heat loss to continue. When humidity reaches 75–90%, sweat evaporation declines and ceases, and body temperature increases.

Failure of these adaptive mechanisms results in the clinical syndromes of heat cramps, heat exhaustion, and heatstroke. *Heat cramps* are a relatively mild disorder caused by exertion and sweating in patients with adequate water replacement but salt depletion. *Heat exhaustion* involves depletion of both water and salt. *Heatstroke* is similar to heat exhaustion, but is much more severe because of loss of CNS thermoregulation. Body temperatures often surpass 40°C (104°F). Thermal cellular damage then causes widespread organ system dysfunction (Table 96-2).

Clinical Findings (TABLE 96-3) ■

HEAT CRAMPS

Heat cramps are caused by exercising vigorously in hot and often dry weather. The water lost in sweat has been replaced by the consumption of large quantities of salt-free water. Severe cramps occur, primarily in the legs and abdomen. Muscle fasciculations may be present. Other systemic signs and symptoms of heat illness are absent.

HEAT EXHAUSTION

Heat exhaustion is more severe and may progress to heatstroke, a potentially fatal disorder. It occurs after the patient has been sweating without replacing water or salt. Symptoms may be due to dehydration, salt depletion, or both. Weakness, anorexia, headache, muscle cramps, nausea, and vomiting are common. Small infants may appear irritable; older children may appear giddy or agitated. The physical signs of dehydration (Chapter 22) are usually present. Coma and seizures do not occur; when present, they suggest either heatstroke or a separate underlying etiology.

TABLE 96–1. *Risk Factors in Heat Illness*

Host Factors
  Increased Heat Production
Athletics
Seizures
Infection
Stimulants
Delirium
Salicylate poisoning
Neuroleptic malignant syndrome
Malignant hyperthermia
  Decreased Heat Loss
Decreased Sweating
  Anticholinergic drugs (antihistamines)
  Abnormal skin (burns, cystic fibrosis)
  Dehydration
Decreased cutaneous blood flow
  Congestive heart failure
  Hypotension
  Obesity
Overdressing
  Neonates and infants
  Athletic uniforms

Environmental Factors
  Weather Conditions
High temperature
High humidity
Low wind velocity
  Specific Locations
Automobiles
Hot tubs
Tents

HEATSTROKE

Patients with heatstroke have a history of exposure to an environmental heat source or internal heat production due to pre-existing illness. High temperature (usually above 40°C) and severe CNS impairment (seizure, coma, delirium, or posturing) are universal. A history of environmental heat exposure must be sought from the parents of neonates and infants. Tachycardia and tachypnea are present; hypotension is common. The skin is usually hot, red, and dry. Diaphoresis is rare. Bizarre neurologic abnormalities occur, including anisocoria, fixed pupils, focal findings, tremor, oculogyric crisis, and nuchal rigidity.

Often, heatstroke cannot be distinguished from CNS infection in a child with fever and altered mental status. Distinguishing between the two is especially difficult in the infant, who even with meningitis may not present with clinical findings of meningeal irritation.

Ancillary Data ■

HEAT CRAMPS

If mild and straightforward, no laboratory tests are necessary. For severe heat cramps, obtain serum sodium, potassium, and glucose determinations.

If the diagnosis is unclear, in children with severe muscle cramps or fasciculations an arterial blood gas and serum calcium will rule out hyperventilation, metabolic alkalosis, and hypocalcemia as causes of tetany.

HEAT EXHAUSTION

Laboratory studies include complete blood count, electrolytes, BUN, creatinine, glucose, urinalysis, serum glutamic-oxaloacetic transaminase (SGOT), and lactic dehydrogenase (LDH). SGOT and LDH levels greater than several thousand units with myoglobinuria should prompt more aggressive therapy for heatstroke.

HEATSTROKE

Table 96-4 reviews common laboratory abnormalities, significance, and treatment. Chest X-ray and lumbar puncture are usually necessary. When neurologic findings are unilateral, computerized axial tomography may be indicated to exclude a mass lesion, prior to lumbar puncture. Serial electrolyte determinations are essential in management.

Treatment ■

HEAT CRAMPS

Once the diagnosis is established, place the child at rest in a cool environment. Give an oral 0.1% salt solution (¼ tsp salt in 1 quart water) at 20 ml/kg. For clinical dehydration or inability to tolerate oral salt solutions, give 0.9% NS 20 ml/kg IV.

HEAT EXHAUSTION

Treat as for heat cramps with rest, cool environment, and 0.9% NS IV, 10–20 ml/kg, over the first hour. Monitor temperature, electrolytes, BUN, creatinine, and urinalysis. For a temperature above 40°C, lack of cooling with hydration, major CNS abnormalities, or persistent hypotension, treat for heatstroke.

TABLE 96–2. *Organ System Dysfunction in Heatstroke*

Organ System	Pathologic Finding	Clinical Finding
CNS	Cerebral edema Neuronal degeneration Ventricular petechiae	Seizures, coma, focal findings, posturing, etc. (see text)
Skeletal muscle	Rhabdomyolysis	Weakness, pain, tenderness
Cardiac muscle	Subendocardial hemorrhage	Dysrhythmias, infarction
Kidneys	Acute tubular necrosis Interstitial nephritis Renal hemorrhage	Renal failure
Hepatobiliary	Cholestasis Centrolobular necrosis Hypofibrinogenemia	Jaundice, bleeding, encephalopathy
Hematologic/vascular	Fibrinolysis Intravascular thrombi Thrombocytopenia	Disseminated intravascular hemorrhage
Skin	Obstructed sweat glands	Anhydrosis, vesicular rash
GI	Mucosal ulceration	GI hemorrhage

HEATSTROKE

Initial Resuscitation

1. *Manage airway,* intubate for seizures or coma, and give supplemental 100% oxygen. Attach cardiac monitor.

2. *Start a large-bore venous line* with 0.9% NS and rapidly give 20 ml/kg. Additional fluid administration at 10–20 ml/kg is guided by serial assessment of volume status. Urinary output through a Foley catheter is a sensitive measure of volume and perfusion; establish output of 1 ml/kg/hr.

TABLE 96–3. *Clinical Findings in Heat Illness*

	Heat Cramps	Heat Exhaustion	Heatstroke
History of Exercise	Yes	Variable	Variable
Water Intake	Adequate	Variable	Inadequate
Salt Intake	Inadequate	Inadequate	Inadequate
Muscle Cramps	Severe	Variable	Variable
Diaphoresis	Present	Variable	Usually absent
Core Temperature	Normal or slightly elevated	Variable, <40°C	Elevated, usually >40°C
Hemodynamics	Normal	Orthostatic hypotension common	Hypotension and tachycardia common
Respirations	Normal	Normal	Increased
CNS Alterations	None	Minor	Severe
Differential	Tetany	CNS infection, malaria, malignant neuroleptic syndrome, malignant hyperthermia, thyroid storm, status epilepticus, DKA	

TABLE 96–4. *Laboratory Abnormalities in Heatstroke*

Test	Result	Significance	Management
Sodium	Increased	Water depletion > salt depletion	Start all patients on 0.9% NS, adjust as serial electrolytes dictate.
	Decreased	Salt depletion > water depletion	
Potassium	Increased	Renal failure and/or rhabdomyolysis is present.	May require dialysis if renal failure is present
	Decreased	Respiratory alkalosis may be present.	Replace only in the setting of acidosis.
Hemoglobin	Increased	Caused by volume depletion and hemoconcentration	Responds to volume replacement
	Decreased	Suspect DIC with possible GI bleeding.	Transfuse as necessary.
WBC	Increased	Caused by stress, hemoconcentration, or infection	Evaluate for sepsis.
BUN, creatinine	Increased	If BUN/creatinine is >20, dehydration present 10–20, suspect renal failure <10, suspect rhabdomyolysis	Monitor volume replacement, consider mannitol and furosemide to maintain urine output.
SGOT, SGPT	Increased	Elevation to several thousand consistent with heat exhaustion; continued rise to tens of thousands indicates heatstroke (due to hepatocellular damage).	
CPK	Increased	Rhabdomyolysis present, myocardial damage if CPK-MB elevated	Anticipate myoglobinuric-induced renal failure; consider mannitol and bicarbonate.
Calcium	Decreased	Caused by rhabdomyolysis	Replace only for cardiac complications.
Phosphorus	Decreased	Caused by respiratory alkalosis	Replace only for level <1.0 mg/dl.
Glucose	Increased	Caused by stress, DKA	Treat only for DKA
	Decreased	Serious, indicates possible preterminal state	Administer $D_{25}W$ ml/kg IV if Dextrostix low.
PT, PTT	Prolonged	Common in heat illness; decreased fibrinogen and platelets indicate DIC	Treat only for DIC (see Chapter 90).
Urinalysis	Casts	Caused by dehydration and tubular damage	See management for increased BUN and creatinine, above.
	Myoglobin	Indicates rhabdomyolysis	
ECG	Abnormal rhythms and morphology	Rarely indicates true myocardial infarction	Most changes reverse with cooling, but treat as per ACLS protocol.
ABG	Metabolic acidosis	Lactic acid accumulation due to cellular damage	Controversial; sodium bicarbonate may worsen heat illness.

3. *Begin cooling* by exposing the patient, covering (not immersing) him or her with cool water, and fanning to accelerate heat loss by evaporation. Place core temperature probe in rectum.

Treat Complications

1. *Consider cold potassium-free peritoneal dialysis* if initial cooling is ineffective.
2. *Control shivering* with diazepam 0.1–0.3 mg/kg IV q 20 min × 3 initially.
3. *Seizures unresponsive to cooling.* Treat as described in Chapter 26 with diazepam 0.1–0.3 mg/kg IV, then diphenylhydantoin at 20 mg/kg over 20 minutes IV.
4. *Consider antibiotics,* pending culture results.
5. See Table 96-4 for management of other complications.

Evaluate Precipitating Events

1. Consider infectious or metabolic etiologies.
2. Consider child abuse or neglect.

Disposition ■

Children with heat cramps may be sent home to rest for 2–3 days. Observe those with heat exhaustion at least 12 hours in the hospital and admit if any clinical or laboratory abnormalities persist. Admit all patients with heatstroke to a critical care unit with pediatric capability, or consider transfer to a pediatric critical care facility.

Patients experiencing heat illness are predisposed to recurrent problems. Educating parents and coaches can help prevent these recurrences.

Bibliography ■

American Academy of Pediatrics, Committee on Sports Medicine: Climatic heat stress and the exercising child. *Pediatrics* 1982; 69:808.
Beyer CB: Heat stress and the young athlete. *Postgrad Med* 1984; 76:109.
Callaham M: Heat illness. In: Rosen P, Baker II JF, Barkin RM, et al, eds: *Emergency medicine: Concepts and clinical practice,* 2nd ed. St. Louis: CV Mosby, 1988:693.
King K, Negus K, Vance JC: Heat stress in motor vehicles: A problem in infancy. *Pediatrics* 1981; 68:579.
Robinson MD, Seward PN: Heat injury in children. *Pediatr Emerg Care* 1987; 3:114.

97 Lightning Injuries

Mary Ann Cooper

Lightning injuries cause more deaths each year in the United States than tornadoes, earthquakes, and floods put together. Each year, 150–200 deaths occur, with nearly five times that many total injuries. Most injuries occur during the thunderstorm months (May through October) and during the afternoon, when people are outside working or playing. It is not uncommon for a single lightning strike to cause multiple injuries and fatalities: almost 30% of fatalities occur in groups of two or more.

In the past, more males have been injured than females, perhaps because they have been more involved in outdoor work and recreational activities. Few epidemiologic statistics exist for children, although several cases of injuries to both children and fetuses have been reported. Injuries range from psychological and learning disabilities to superficial burns to cardiac arrest and brain damage with permanent disability.

Etiology and Pathophysiology ■

Injuries may occur from five mechanisms:

1. Direct strike
2. Sideflash or splash, in which the current splashes from a tree or another person onto the victim
3. Contact voltage, in which the victim is touching the object hit by the lightning stroke
4. Ground current, in which the stroke hits the ground and spreads through the first few inches of the surface radially outward to include persons at some distance from the strike
5. Rarely, by setting the victim's clothing afire.

A direct strike may cause more damage and is probably more often fatal, although there is no hard evidence to support this.

While lightning follows the same laws of physics that other electrical phenomena do, it causes very different injuries than high-voltage electrical currents. Fatalities from lightning are a result of cardiac arrest.

Unlike high-voltage electrical injuries, in which deep, extensive burns are the rule, burns from lightning injuries are usually quite superficial. The duration of exposure to the current of a lightning strike is so incredibly short (about $\frac{1}{10,000}$–$\frac{1}{1,000}$ of a second) that tissue breakdown, such as an entry or exit burn, seldom occurs. Instead, the current tends to flow around the surface of the victim in a so-called "flashover effect."

Clinical Findings ■

The most important clinical findings in the victim of lightning strike include cardiac, neurologic, and cutaneous manifestations. *Unlike high-voltage electrical injuries, where severe deep burns may occur, burns tend to be a minor part of the lightning victim's problems.* Far more common is the patient in cardiac arrest or with permanent neurologic damage.

About 1,000 people each year are injured by lightning, with a mortality of about 20–30%. The primary cause of death is cardiac arrest secondary to the lightning strike.

Rhythms seen after lightning injuries include asystole, ventricular fibrillation, and occasionally various blocks and premature contractions. The ECG will often show nonspecific ST wave changes, which may persist for months. Sometimes these patterns mimic a myocardial infarction pattern with inferior, anterior, or lateral changes, but more often the changes are diffuse and nonspecific. If arrhythmias occur, antiarrhythmic drugs are indicated. The patient may be bradycardic or tachycardic, or may have a normal rhythm and ECG pattern.

A surprisingly common presenting picture is the patient who is unconscious or combative and has cool, mottled, usually pulseless lower (65%) and sometimes upper (30%) extremities. This is probably due to a vascular and sympathetic nervous system instability that usually resolves spontaneously over a period of hours and does not require specific therapy, other than routine neurovascular checks.

Seizures may occur because of direct injury to the brain or as a result of cardiopulmonary arrest and hypoxia. Computerized scanning of the brain may be indicated to rule out subdural, epidural, or intracerebral hemorrhage or to follow cerebral edema. *Routine use of anticonvulsants for all lightning victims is not indicated unless there are indications of seizure activity.* Fluid restriction, however, is indicated in almost all cases to decrease the effect of cerebral edema, if present.

Occasionally, the patient will complain of blindness, tinnitus or deafness, or inability to move an extremity. These often resolve but may be permanent in some cases. Almost all victims have amnesia for some part of the event and anterograde amnesia for several days, similar to a patient who has been treated with electroconvulsive therapy. Late sequelae include sleep disturbances, storm phobias, and trouble with mentation and attitude. Children especially tend to exhibit psychiatric sequelae, although they may often improve with time and sometimes psychotherapy.

Nearly half of all victims have ruptured eardrums on presentation. Cataracts, common with high-voltage electrical injuries near the eyes, are also common with lightning strikes to the shoulders or above, but may take as long as two years to develop. Dilated pupils cannot be used as an indication of brain death, since numerous eye injuries (such as retinal detachment and optic nerve damage and atrophy) have been reported. Numerous other eye problems, including iritis, iridocyclitis, corneal ulcer, and uveitis, may also occur.

Cutaneous manifestations of a lightning strike are usually superficial burns. Rarely do deep burns, similar to high-voltage electrical burns, occur. Burns may appear linear, punctate, or featherlike (the feathery markings are not true burns and usually pass within a few hours to days). The linear and punctate burns may require minimal burn therapy but should have tetanus prophylaxis. Occasionally, the hair may be singed off a strip of the victim's head while the underlying skin is uninjured.

As the lightning flashes over the victim, it often blows his or her clothes and shoes apart, leaving the victim nearly nude. Sometimes the lightning's force may cause the victim to be thrown or to suffer injuries similar to those seen in explosions, with blunt injuries to the head, thorax, abdomen, or extremities, including fractures and dislocations.

Several cases of pregnant victims have been reported. About half the fetuses were born living and well, about one quarter were stillborn, and about one quarter were aborted. There are not enough cases to make any conclusions or predictions of survival by trimester of injury.

Ancillary Data ■

Ordering ancillary tests should be guided by the severity of the patient's injuries. Generally, all patients should have an ECG. Cardiac monitoring may be indicated for several hours to days. Cardiac enzymes may be useful but may not show a change for several hours after the injury, consistent with cell breakdown and release of creatinine phosphokinase and other substances.

A complete blood count may be indicated as a baseline. While myoglobinuria and hemoglobinuria are rare with lightning injuries, it is still worth observing new urine for pigments and testing it for myoglobin a few hours after the patient presents. If the urine is found to be pigmented, then baseline BUN and creatinine determinations are essential. Fluid loading in these cases will necessitate continued monitoring of urine output, pigmentation, and specific gravity. Other lab tests may be indicated by the patient's condition.

X-ray examinations also should be guided by the patient's condition. Any patient with a deteriorating level of neurologic function requires computerized scanning of the brain to rule out an intracranial lesion.

Treatment ■

1. Address the patient's airway and circulatory status.
2. Institute resuscitation protocols (Chapter 6) if the patient is in cardiac arrest. Begin immediate CPR on any victim in cardiac arrest. Cardiac monitoring is essential to rule out arrhythmia.
3. Establish an IV line. Fluid restriction is usually the rule for lightning victims, especially those who have a cardiac arrest, because of the incidence of cerebral edema and the low incidence of deep burns requiring fluid loading.
4. If shock is present and there is a reason to suspect that it may be because of hypovolemia or blunt injury, initiate fluid resuscitation.
5. Some patients present with initial hypertension, which usually resolves in a few hours without therapy. If no peripheral pulses are palpable, use a Doppler to evaluate the blood pressure, since extreme spasm of the peripheral vessels often makes the pulses difficult to find despite normal underlying blood pressure.
6. Institute spinal precautions if the patient fell, was thrown, or suffered a blunt injury.
7. Treatment of seizures should focus on the cause and its correction, whether it is intracranial hemorrhage, hypoxia, electrolyte abnormality, hy-

poglycemia, or blunt injury. Use routine therapy (Chapter 26) to control seizures after correctable causes have been ruled out or controlled.

8. Treat ruptured tympanic membranes conservatively, with removal of debris and referral to an otolaryngologist.

9. Ensure that a thorough eye evaluation is done to establish a baseline, should cataracts become a problem in the future.

10. Superficial burns require little therapy other than tetanus prophylaxis. In the rare case of deep burns, fluid loading, fasciotomies, and mannitol or furosemide diuresis may be necessary to maximize tissue salvage and avoid renal damage (see Chapter 61).

11. Treat blunt injuries routinely.

Disposition ■

The patient who has had a cardiac arrest will need admission to the intensive care unit. Probably all children with injuries other than simple skin manifestations require hospital observation. Patients who have continuing confusion, cardiac arrhythmias or other cardiac damage, pigmented urine, or paresis always need admission, observation, monitoring, and treatment, usually in the intensive care unit or transfer to a pediatric critical care center. Alert victims who can carry on a conversation (despite the fact that they are amnesic for the event and may have anterograde memory defects for the next few days) can probably be observed overnight on a pediatric ward.

Follow-up referral may be necessary for dysesthesias, psychological problems, or tympanic membrane rupture.

Bibliography ■

Cooper MA: Lightning injuries. In: Auerbach P, Geehr E, eds: *Management of wilderness and environmental injuries.* St. Louis: CV Mosby, 1989.

Dollinger SJ, O'Donnell JP, Staley AA: Lightning-strike disaster: Effects on children's fears and worries. *J Consult Clin Psychol* 1984; 52:1028–1038.

Harwood SJ, Catrou PG, Cole GW: Creatinine phosphokinase isoenzyme fractions in the serum of a patient struck by lightning. *Arch Intern Med* 1978; 138:645–646.

Kotagal S, Rawlings CA, Chen S, et al: Neurologic, psychiatric, and cardiovascular complications in children struck by lightning. *Pediatrics* 1982; 70:190–192.

Myers GJ, Colgan MT, VanDyke DH: Lightning-strike disaster among children. *JAMA* 1977; 238:1845–1846.

Noel LP, Clarke WN, Addison D: Ocular complications of lightning. *J Pediatr Ophthalmol Strabismus* 1980; 17:245–246.

Ravitch MM, Lane R, Safar P, et al: Lightning stroke. *N Engl J Med* 1961; 264:36–38.

Stanley LD, Suss RA: Intracerebral hematoma secondary to lightning stroke: Case report and review of the literature. *Neurosurgery* 1985; 16:686–688.

Yost JW, Holmes F: Myoglobinuria following lightning stroke. *JAMA* 1974; 228:1147–1148.

98 Radiation Injury

David W. Griffin

The recent disasters at Three Mile Island and Chernobyl have heightened our awareness of potential radiation emergencies, whether as a consequence of accident or inappropriate exposure. The Joint Commission on Accreditation of Hospitals now requires hospitals to have specific procedures to deal with such emergencies; physicians must be similarly prepared to recognize, treat, triage, and ensure appropriate patient disposition.

Etiology and Pathophysiology ■

Ionizing radiation comes in four forms:

1. *Alpha* particles are positively charged, heavy, and easily shielded by the outer layer of skin or even a sheet of paper. Plutonium, uranium, and radium emit alpha particles.
2. *Beta* particles, which are electrons, are more penetrating and thus can produce more injury. Carbon-14 emits beta particles.
3. *Gamma and X-rays* are purely electromagnetic radiation, with no mass. They can deeply penetrate body tissues and can cause significant injury.
4. *Neutrons* are neutral particles that also can penetrate tissues deeply to cause significant injury. Neutrons are released in nuclear explosions, reactor accidents, and particle accelerators.

Ionizing radiation is measured in *rads* (radiation absorbed dose), while its effective dosage to humans is measured in *rems* (roentgen equivalent in man). A rem equals a rad for gamma rays, X-rays, and beta particles, but because of its increased relative biologic effectiveness (RBE), neutron irradiation results in a rem dosage of twice the rad exposure.

Radiation of all forms excites molecules and produces free radicals, which then disrupt enzymes, nucleic acids, and protein functions. Transient cellular dysfunction and/or cell death ensue. In general, tissues with the greatest turnover rate are the most radiosensitive. Thus, the rapidly dividing cells of the reproductive, hematopoietic, and GI systems are at highest risk. Lymphocytes, although they do not have a particularly high mitotic rate, are quite radiosensitive and serve as a convenient biologic marker to follow after exposure.

Children are at particular risk from radiation exposure because of their growth and potential longevity. Their more rapidly dividing cells are more susceptible to radiation effects. Also, some radiation effects are cumulative and delayed; these effects may manifest years after exposure.

Clinical Findings ■

CONTAMINATION

External contamination (the presence of radioactive particulates on the skin) and internal contamination (the presence of radioactive particulates within the body) result from exposure to or ingestion or inhalation of alpha or beta particles. Contamination could occur because of accidental or excessive radioisotope administration in a medical setting, exposure to natural environmental sources, or exposure to fallout from a nuclear plant mishap.

With external contamination, radioactivity levels are present and measurable on the skin surface. Internal contamination should be suspected from the history or the presence of measurable radioactivity in mouth or nasal secretions.

External contamination is not an emergency in itself, but often is accompanied by more serious problems such as thermal injuries or trauma. Internal contamination, although less common, is of more emergent concern; effective treatment requires prompt institution of the measures described in the Treatment section below.

LOCALIZED IRRADIATION

With the more common use of radioactive sources for industrial and medical purposes, the chances of accidental or excessive exposure to electromagnetic

TABLE 98–1. *Dose–Effect Relationships of Radiation Exposure*

<100 rads	Asymptomatic, but potential chromosomal aberrations in cultured lymphocytes and potential depression of lymphocytes
100 rads	Prodromal stage with nausea and vomiting in 10%
100–400 rads	Hematopoietic syndrome within 2–3 weeks after exposure
400 rads	50% fatalities within 60 days without intensive support
600 rads	GI syndrome within 7–10 days after exposure
3500 rads	Acute encephalopathy and cardiovascular collapse

irradiation have increased. Gamma or X-ray exposure, if localized to a small area of the body, will cause mainly local manifestations. Localized radiation burns may be the only physical finding. Radiation burns, which resemble thermal burns, typically present 7 to 60 days after exposure and rarely before several hours.

The key to the proper ED response to localized irradiation is *recognition,* as no radioactivity is present from the irradiation. Depending upon the extent and quantity of exposure, there may or may not be any systemic findings. Unexplained thermal burns, bruising, or bleeding may follow days after exposure, with the child and parent unaware of its occurrence. Thus, the differential diagnosis of these signs must include unappreciated radiation exposure and child abuse.

WHOLE BODY IRRADIATION

A large, single exposure of penetrating radiation to the whole body results in *acute radiation syndrome (ARS).* The dose determines the effects in a fairly standard fashion (Table 98-1). ARS is typically divided into four phases:

1. Prodromal
2. Latent
3. Manifest illness
4. Recovery.

The prodromal phase is an acute, toxic period that begins within minutes to hours after exposure and lasts for days. It quiesces into the latent phase, a period of relative well-being lasting days to weeks. Manifest illness then surfaces as a result of the initial radiation injury, with eventual progression to recovery or death.

Most victims will present to the ED in the prodromal phase. Signs and symptoms include anorexia, nausea, vomiting, diarrhea, intestinal cramps, salivation, and dehydration. These directly result from GI and CNS dysfunction secondary to acute radionecrosis and release of vasoactive substances.

The prodromal phase usually occurs with acute dosages greater than 100 rads and almost always with doses greater than 400 rads. Generally, the quicker the onset and the longer the presence of prodromal symptoms, the higher the radiation exposure. For exposures of less than 400 rads, the usual onset is 2–6 hours and lasts 48 hours. For doses of 400–1,000 rads, the onset begins within 2 hours and may persist through the latency period into manifest illness. Exposures of 3,500 rads or more may result in an immediate and profound prodromal phase with hypotension, convulsions, and prompt death (the cardiovascular/CNS syndrome).

With the regression of the prodromal phase into the latency phase, the patient has a period of relative but deceptive well-being that typically lasts days to weeks.

Manifest illness then appears either as a predominantly hematopoietic or GI syndrome again, in a dose-dependent fashion. Hematopoietic changes occur with dosages above 100 rads; the GI tract becomes involved at dosages above 600 rads. With damage to the hematopoietic system, lymphocytes decrease or disappear within hours, granulocytes within days, and platelets within 10 days. If there is sufficient exposure for the GI syndrome, vomiting, diarrhea, malabsorption, and electrolyte disturbances recur a week after the prodromal phase regresses. This time, however, the mechanism involves disrupted epithelial cell junctions and decreased cell production in the small intestine. With appropriate medical support, the patient will then pass into the recovery phase.

Treatment ■

After diagnosis, there are four components of ED care of radiation injury (Table 98-2).

Treatment advice is available around the clock from the Radiation Emergency Assistance Center/Training Site (REAC/TS) in Oak Ridge, Tennessee. REAC/TS can be contacted by calling Oak Ridge Hospital, (615) 482-2441.

Disposition ■

The key to proper disposition of radiation accidents is *prevention.* Political and economic issues cloud

TABLE 98–2. *ED Protocol for Radiation Exposure Victims*

1. **Emergency medical management** with stabilization of victim(s). Fluid resuscitation may include blood components if necessary.
2. **Decontamination**
   (a) Monitor for radiation, with a designated holding area available if present.
   (b) External decontamination proceeds with attention to wounds first.
   (c) Internal decontamination requires prompt radionuclide identification and may require specific blocking, chelating, dilutional, or purging techniques.
3. **Collection** of biologic materials
   (a) Samples of nails, hair, body fluids, wound secretions
   (b) Swabs of orifices
   (c) Type and crossmatch, chromosomal analysis of peripheral lymphocytes, HLA typing, and sequential blood counts
4. **Triage,** with isolation indicated for those likely to progress to the hematopoietic or GI syndrome.

TABLE 98–3. *Prognosis Based on Lowest Lymphocyte Count Within 48 Hours*

1500–3000	No injury
1000–1500	Significant injury but good prognosis
<1000	Severe injury, isolation indicated
<100	Grave prognosis in absence of bone-marrow transplantation

our ability to prevent radiation exposure from nuclear explosions or reactor mishaps. But proper institution of shielding and safety precautions in industrial and medical settings can prevent the great majority of radiation accidents of lesser magnitude.

For children who sustain significant radiation exposure, proper disposition must be determined. Patients judged to be at risk for the hematopoietic syndrome (on the basis of the clinical history, the speed of onset of the prodromal phase, and the rate of white blood cell decline) should be hospitalized in reverse isolation for their own protection and observation. Inpatient treatment, usually at a regional center, may include skin engraftment, antibiotics, and potentially bone-marrow transplants. Those with lesser exposures may be followed as outpatients.

Key prognostic features in the Chernobyl experience were:

1. Clinical history of proximity and duration and type of exposure
2. Presence and speed of onset of the prodromal phase
3. Presence and extent of skin burns
4. Rate of white blood cell decline (Table 98-3)

All children who have experienced significant radiation exposure must be closely followed for the development of malignancy for the rest of their lives.

Bibliography ■

Conklin JJ, Walker RI, Hirsch EF: Current concepts in the management of radiation injuries and associated trauma. *Surg Gynecol Obstet* 1983; 156:809–829.

Fleischer G, Ludwig S, eds: *Textbook of pediatric emergency medicine.* Baltimore: Williams & Wilkins, 1988.

Gale PG: Immediate medical consequences of nuclear accidents. *JAMA* 1987; 258:625–628.

Geiger HJ: The accident at Chernobyl and the medical response. *JAMA* 1986; 256:609–612.

Hendee WR: Management of individuals accidentally exposed to radiation or radioactive materials. *Semin Nucl Med* 1986; 16:203–210.

Hubmer KF, Fry SA, eds: *Medical basis for radiation accident preparedness.* New York: Elsevier-North Holland, 1980.

Leonard RB, Ricks RC: Emergency department radiation accident protocol. *Ann Emerg Med* 1980; 9:462–470.

Milroy WC: Management of irradiated and contaminated casualty victims. *Emerg Med Clin North Am* 1984; 2:667–686.

National Council on Radiation Protection and Measurements: *Management of persons accidentally contaminated with radionuclides.* Washington DC, Report 65, 1980.

99 Submersion Injuries

James S. Seidel

Submersion injuries are common in the United States and are the second leading cause of death from unintentional injuries in childhood. Submersion injuries cause about 7,000 deaths each year in the United States; most occur in fresh water (80%), in lakes, ponds, quarries, and swimming pools. Two-thirds of those who drown in swimming pools are under age three.

For every death from submersion, there are 10 nonfatal injuries. An estimated 700 spinal-cord injuries occur annually associated with submersions; most of these are from diving, surfing, and water-skiing. In adolescents and young adults, fatal submersion injuries are commonly associated with water sports and alcohol abuse.

Submersion injuries are more common in males than females, and deaths are significantly more common in blacks and Native Americans.

The past 10 years have seen an increase in the use of residential hot-tub spas. About 1,100 people with spa or hot-tub injuries require emergency treatment each year; most are teens and adults, and many such injuries are associated with alcohol use. The spa's high temperature, combined with moderate levels of alcohol in the bloodstream, leads to drowsiness and eventually somnolence and submersion of the victim. Some victims are young infants and children who become trapped under a hot-tub cover or are held under the water by the filtering system.

Drowning may be defined as death after submersion in a liquid. *Near-fatal submersion* is recovery of vital signs following a submersion injury. *Secondary drowning* is death occurring 24 hours to days after a near-fatal submersion injury, usually secondary to pulmonary edema. *Post-immersion syndrome* refers to complications of a submersion injury that may involve multiple systems (pulmonary edema, hyperthermia, cardiac rhythm disturbances, cerebral edema, renal failure, GI bleeding, etc.).

Etiology ■

The etiology of submersion injuries includes one or more of the following risk factors:

1. Lack of an effective safety barrier around a pool or body of water. This barrier should have a self-closing gate and no lateral slats in the fence. In all drownings where there was a fence around the pool, the gate was either unlatched or opened
2. Lack of appropriate supervision of infants and children. The children are left with an older sibling, or there is a misunderstanding about which adult is supervising the children
3. Inability to swim. Young children who take swimming classes are not "drown-proofed"
4. Disobedience. The child goes into the water without letting an adult know
5. Medical illness, such as a seizure
6. Participation in water sports while under the influence of alcohol
7. Diving, surfing, or water-skiing injuries
8. Hyperventilation while swimming, which leads to a vasoconstriction of the cerebral blood vessels, a decrease in cerebral blood flow, and loss of consciousness while in the water
9. Child abuse. Submersion injuries that occur in unusual places (bathtubs, buckets, toilets, etc.) should be investigated to rule out intentional trauma.

Pathophysiology ■

Submersion injuries are the result of an initial hypoxic insult that may affect multiple organ systems. Victims of submersion injuries generally have a period of breath-holding after their head is submersed in the liquid. There is generally a period of struggling, followed by closure of the airway and resultant hypoxia that leads to unconsciousness. The airway may be initially protected by laryngospasm and by the diving reflex, which causes closure of the airway and protects perfusion of the heart, lungs, and brain.

Research in animal models has demonstrated that a large amount of water (more than 22 ml/kg) must be aspirated before profound disturbances of fluid and electrolytes occur. This rarely occurs in humans; about 15–20% of submersion victims are so-called "dry drownings" and aspirate very little fluid.

Although there are theoretical differences between submersion in fresh and salt water, the clinical picture is the same because of the relatively small amounts of fluid in the lungs. Hypoxia results from airway occlusion and the resultant atelectasis; loss of surfactant-producing cells leads to poor lung compliance. Shunting of blood from the affected portions of the lung contributes to the hypoxia.

The two major alterations in body homeostasis seen in submersion injuries are *hypoxia* and *acidosis.* If these are not corrected in a timely manner, multiple end-organ failure may ensue. The CNS is the weakest link in the hypoxic chain.

Hypothermia may occur very rapidly in a child submerged in cold water. Although hypothermia may cause organ dysfunction, it may also provide some protection against hypoxic injury. Children lose heat rapidly by radiation and conduction to the cold environment, and struggling and shivering may add to heat loss. When the core body temperature is reduced, the metabolic requirements of the heart and CNS are reduced. The preservation of the reserves of adenosine triphosphate in the brain may further protect membrane permeability. The heart rate may be dramatically reduced and disturbances of cardiac rhythm may be evident.

Clinical Findings and Treatment ■

PREHOSPITAL CARE

If the patient is still in the water when the rescue team arrives, pay careful attention to a controlled removal of the victim from the water. Maintain a neutral position of the spine and ensure airway patency by using the jaw thrust. If the victim is on a flotation device and the rescuer must await a boat or additional personnel to remove the patient, initiate ventilation using mouth-to-mouth or mouth-to-nose-and-mouth ventilations. If the child is pulseless, chest compressions may be difficult to perform and may not be useful while the victim is still in the water. Do not initiate CPR if the victim can be removed from the water quickly.

After the patient is removed from the water, continue spinal immobilization with the use of a backboard and stiff neck collar. Sandbags may also be used to stabilize the neck. Pay immediate attention to restoring ventilation and perfusion. *Effective CPR in the field is the key to a good outcome.* Early endotracheal intubation is preferred for management of the apneic and pulseless child with a submersion injury.

IV access is often difficult in young children. If starting an IV will significantly delay transport of the patient or if the time to start an IV is longer than the transport time, transport the patient immediately to the nearest appropriate emergency department. The endotracheal tube may be used to deliver resuscitation drugs en route to the hospital.

Also, remember to warm the hypothermic patient. Wet clothing may be removed en route to the hospital and replaced with sheets and blankets.

Initiate CPR on all patients in the field unless it is obvious that the patient is dead. This may be difficult to determine in the field if the core temperature is low. Children with low core temperatures may have no palpable pulses or may have cardiac rhythm disturbances that are resistant to therapy. Hypothermic submersion patients should receive effective CPR and passive rewarming until their arrival in the ED.

Any infant or child that has had a true submersion in a liquid should be transported to the nearest ED. Even patients who appear well may have late pulmonary complications.

EMERGENCY DEPARTMENT MANAGEMENT

If CPR is in progress, follow guidelines for resuscitation presented in Chapter 6. Place the patient on a mechanical ventilator with the lowest possible positive inspiratory pressure and an appropriate amount of positive end expiratory pressure (PEEP) to maintain the airway. The use of PEEP is important in these patients, who generally have poor airway compliance. Assess the effectiveness of chest compressions by feeling for a femoral pulse.

Rewarm hypothermic patients, but proceed slowly to avoid further acidosis and "rewarming shock" or "afterdrop" with overly aggressive active external rewarming, as outlined in Chapter 95 and Table 95-5.

Reassess the patient frequently, and continuously monitor the cardiac and respiratory status until the patient is transferred to the inpatient service.

PROGNOSIS

Although there are no absolute predictors of outcome of any resuscitation, presenting CNS status may be the best. Most studies have shown that children who arrive in the ED in full arrest have poor outcomes.

Several tools may be used to assess the patient's neurologic status, such as the Glasgow Coma Scale (Figure 16-1) and the AVPU method of assessment (A = Alert, V = responds to verbal stimuli, P = responds to painful stimuli, U = unresponsive). The Modell-Conn Classification correlates different neurologic stages with prognosis (Table 99-1).

TABLE 99–1. *Conn-Modell Neurologic Classification of Submersion Victims*

Neurologic Category	Description	Prognosis
A (alert)	Alert and fully conscious	Good
B (blunted)	Obtunded, stuporous but arousable, responds to pain	Fair to good
C (coma)		
C1 (decorticate)	Flexion response to pain	Poor to fair
C2 (decerebrate)	Extensor response to pain	Poor to fair
C3 (flaccid)	Flaccid, no response to pain	Poor

Ancillary Data ■

Assessment of the submersion injuries includes analysis of arterial blood gases (ABG), serum electrolytes, BUN, and creatinine (serum sodium and potassium abnormalities are rarely of clinical significance). A complete blood count and urine analysis may also provide useful data. Coagulation studies may be indicated if bleeding from the GI tract is noted. After initial ABG, pulse oximetry is usually adequate.

A chest radiograph may be initially normal or may show a pattern of pulmonary edema; it should be repeated if the patient remains in the ED for an hour or more or if the patient's pulmonary status changes. X-rays of other areas are indicated if abnormalities of bones are palpated. An ECG is indicated in patients who have evidence of a rhythm disturbance.

Complications ■

Many complications may occur after resuscitation from a submersion injury. A few of the more common ones are listed in Table 99-2.

Disposition ■

All patients with significant submersion injuries require hospital admission. Some may be best managed in centers with pediatric intensive care units, pediatric nurses, and pediatric subspecialists; this is particularly

TABLE 99–2. *Multisystem Complications of Submersion Injuries*

Pulmonary
Hypoxia and direct effect of any aspirated water may produce pulmonary edema in about 15% of near-drowning cases. This may take up to 24 hours to evolve. Poor lung compliance and mechanical ventilation may lead to pneumothorax or interstitial emphysema.

Cardiac
Rhythm disturbances may develop and are more common in patients who have aspirated fluid. Most rhythm disturbances are the result of hypoxia and/or hypothermia and will resolve with treatment of the underlying disorder.

Neurologic
Severe neurologic damage occurs in 12–27% of near-drowning patients. Patients who arrive in the ED in asystole are at risk for a poor outcome or death.

Renal
Renal failure is uncommon but can occur. It is usually secondary to hypoxia but may be precipitated by hemoglobinuria or myoglobinuria.

GI
GI bleeding may be secondary to hypoxia of the bowel, stress, or CNS damage.

important for the patient who may need respiratory therapy or is at risk for multisystem disease. Arrange for critical care transport as soon as possible, since rapid transport to definitive care after the initial resuscitation may improve outcome.

Bibliography ■

Conn AW, Barker GA: Freshwater drowning and near-drowning: An update. *Can J Anaesth* 1984; 31:S38–44.

Frates R: Analysis of predictive factors in the assessment of warm-water near-drowning in children. *Am J Dis Child* 1981; 135:1006–1008.

Giammona ST: Drowning: Pathophysiology and management. *Curr Probl Pediatr* 1971; 1:1.

Modell JH: *The pathophysiology of drowning and near-drowning.* Springfield, Ill.: Charles Thomas, 1971.

Peterson B: Morbidity of childhood near-drowning. *Pediatrics* 1977; 59:364–370.

Robinson M, Seward P: Submersion injury in children. *Pediatr Emerg Care* 1987; 3:44–49.

Seidel JS, Henderson DP: *Prehospital care of pediatric emergencies.* Los Angeles: Los Angeles Pediatric Society, 1987.

100 Plant and Mushroom Poisoning

*Edward C. Geehr and Delmer J. Pascoe**

Of the 30,000 identified plants in the world, about 700 are suspected to be poisonous. Plants and mushrooms rank third, behind cleaning substances and analgesics, as the most commonly reported items of toxic ingestion or exposure. As many as 170,000 plant ingestions may occur annually (about 95,000 are reported). Brightly colored berries and flowers of common house and garden plants attract children; over 85% of all plant ingestions involve children less than 6 years old. Although major morbidity secondary to plant or mushroom ingestion does occur, fatalities are rare.

Basic Principles ■

1. An astounding amount of misunderstanding accompanies poisonous-plant identification and nomenclature. Common names are widely used incorrectly. For example, "yew" is a common name normally referring to a species of Taxus. *Taxus canadensis* is commonly called "ground hemlock" and is lethal. "Hemlock" is applied to four genera of plants, one of which is not lethal.
2. Toxicity cannot be determined by genus alone. Similar toxins can be isolated from plants with vast botanical differences. Poisonous plants can vary greatly, owing to environmental factors, seasonal variations, horticultural manipulation, and regional variations. Plants east of the Mississippi are similar to those in Europe.
3. Gardeners are using more cultivated exotics. Many prized cultivated ornamentals are extremely dangerous.
4. With the popularity of hiking, back-to-nature movements, and the harvesting of natural foods, plant poisonings are more common. Inexperienced gatherers often mistake poisonous plants for edibles, harvest plants out of their edible season, or improperly prepare plants that require specific preparation.
5. Teas, extracts, herbals, and home remedies may contain toxic elements. The literature cites nutmeg, jimsonweed, foxglove, hellebore, ginseng, pennyroyal, pokeweed, and tansy as plants used in potentially toxic herbal preparations and extracts. Clinical syndromes for herbal toxicity include psychoactive, anticholinergic, cardiotoxic, and hepatotoxic forms.
6. Most plant poisonings occur in or near the home or yard. Some common nontoxic houseplants are listed in Table 100-1.

Clinical Findings ■

HISTORY

The history should include the following elements:

1. Time of ingestion
2. Amount consumed
3. Initial symptoms
4. Time between ingestion and onset of symptoms
5. Method of preparation (e.g., raw, cooked, boiled, stewed)
6. Others who ate the plant and their symptoms

PHYSICAL EXAM

Few clear-cut toxidromes relate to plant poisonings; syndromes are often mixed or variable. Thus, rushing to therapy using an "antidote" based on a presumptive diagnosis can cause clinical deterioration rather than improvement. Moreover, changes in behavior or mental status should not always be attributed to plant toxins. Always rule out traumatic or infectious etiologies whenever appropriate. Table 100-2 presents a differential diagnosis of plant intoxications by early symptoms.

* Deceased

TABLE 100–1. *Nontoxic Houseplants*

The following have *not* been reported to cause illness. An asterisk (*) indicates that other species may be toxic.

African violet (*Saint pauliaionatha*)
Air plant (*Kanlanchoe pinnata*)
Aluminum plant (*Pilea cadierei*)
Aralia, false (*Dizygotheca elegantissima*)
Aralia, Japanese (*Fatsia japonica*)
Asparagus fern (*Asparagus plumosus*)
Baby's breath (*Gypsophilia paniculata*)
Baby's tears (*Helxine* or *Soleirolia soleirolii*)
Begonia (*Rex begonia*)
Bird of paradise* (*Strelitzia reginae*)
Bird's Nest fern (*Asplenium nidus*)
Boston fern (*Nephrolepsis exalta, N. bostoniensis*)
Bromeliad family
California poppy (*Eschscboizia californica*)
Camelia (*Camellia japonica*)
Cast iron plant (*Aspidistra elatior*)
Chinese evergreen (*Aglaonema modestum*)
Coffee tree (*Coffee arabica*)
Coleus
Cornstalk plant (Dracaena fragrans)
Coral berry* (*Aechamea fulgens, Ardisia crispa*)
Crape myrtle (*Lagerstromea indica*)
Creeping charlie* (*Pilea nummularifolia*) or Swedish ivy (*Plectranthus australis*)
Crocus* (spring-blooming only)
Croton
Dahlia
Dogwood (*Cornus*)
Donkey's tail (*Sedum morganianum*)
Dragon tree (*Dracaena draco, D. marginata*)
Easter cactus (*Schlumbergeria bridgesii*)
Easter lily (*Lilium longiflorum*)
Echeveria: Mexican snowball, painted lady, plush plant
Emerald ripple (*Peperomia caperata*)
Fern sword (*Nephrolepsis cordifolia, exaltata*)
Fiddleleaf fig (*Ficus lyrata*)
Fig tree (*Ficus benjamina*)
Forget-me-not (*Myosotis alpestris, M. sylvatica*)
Forsythia
Fuchsia
Gardenia
Geranium* (*Pelargonium*)
Gloxina (*Sinningia speciosa*)
Grape ivy (*Ciccus rhombifolia*)
Hawaiian ti plant (*Cordyline terminalis*)
Hawthorne berry (*Crataegus*)
Hibiscus
Honeysuckle berry (*Lonicera*)
Ice plant
Impatiens walleriana
Jasmine (*Jasminum rex*), Madagascar jasmine (*Mephanotis floribunda*)
Kalanchoe: maternity plant, monkey plant, panda bear plant
Lace plant, Madagascar (*Aponogeton sentralis*)
Lady's slipper (*Cypripedium, Paphiopedidum*)

Lipstick plant (*Aeschynanthus radicans*)
Maidenhair fern (*Adiantum*)
Mangold, African/American/tall (*Tagetes*)
Moon cactus (*Gymnocalycium*)
Mother-in-law's tongue, snake plant (*Sansevieria trifasciata*)
Mother of pearls (*Grapetopetalum paraguayens*)
Mountain ash berry (*Sorbus*)
Natal palm (*Carissa grandiflora*)
Norfolk Island pine (*Araucaria heterophylla*)
Old man cactus (*Cephalocereus senilis*)
Olive tree (*Olea europaea*)
Orchid (*Cattleya, Cymbidium, Oncidium*)
Oregon grape (*Malionia aquifollium*)
Palm bamboo (*Chamaedorea erumpeus*), paradise (*Howea* or *Kentia forsterana*), parlor (*Chamaedora elegans* or *Kentia*), sentry (*Howea belmoreana*)
Pansy flower (*Viola*)
Passion vine (*Passiflora*)
Peanut cactus (*Chamaecereus sylvestri*)
Pellionia
Peony flower (*Paeonia*)
Pepetomia
Petunia
Phlox
Piggyback plant (*Tolmiea menziesii*)
Pigmy date palm (*Phoenix roebelenii*)
Pocketbook (*Calceolaria herbeohybrida*)
Polka dot or Freckle-face plant (*Hypoestes sanguinolenta*)
Prayer plant (*Maranta leuconeura*)
Pussy willow (*Salix discolor*)
Pyracantha berry
Queen's tears (*Billbergia nutans*)
Rabbit's foot fern (*Davallia fejeensis*)
Raphiolepsis
Rainbow plant (*Billbergia sandersii*)
Rosary pearls (*Senecio rowleyanus*)
Rosary vine (*Ceropegia woodii*)
Roses (*Rosa*)
Rubber plant (*Ficus elastica*)
Schefflera plant (*Brassaia* or *Schefflera actinophylla*)
Sedum
Sensitive plant (*Mimosa pudica*)
Silver Heart (*Peperomia marmorata*)
Snake Plant, mother-in-law's tongue (*Sansevieria trifasciata*)
Snapdragon (*Antirrhinum majus*)
Spider plant (*Antbericum, Chlorophytum comosum*)
Staghorn fern (*Platycerium bifurcatum*)
Starfish flower (*Stapelia*)
String of beads* (*Senecio rowleyanus, S. herreianus*)
String of hearts (*Ceropegia woodii*)
Swedish ivy (*Plectranthus australis*) or creeping Charlie
Tahitian bridal veil (*Gibasis geniculata, Tripogandra multiflora*)

TABLE 100–1. Nontoxic Houseplants (*continued*)

Umbrella tree (*Schefflera actinophylla*)
Vagabond plant (*Vriesea*)
Velvet plant, purple (*Gynura aurantiaca*)
Venus's flytrap (*Dionaea muscipula*)
Violet (*Viola*)
Wandering Jew (*Tradescantia albiflora*)

Wandering Jew—red and white (*Zebrina pendulla*)
Wax plant (*Hoya exotica*)
Yucca
Zebra plant (*Aphelandre squarrosa*)
Zinnia

Ancillary Data ■

Baseline laboratory data in symptomatic children includes a urinalysis (for specific gravity, red cell casts, protein, and crystals), BUN/creatinine (to establish baseline renal function), and glucose (to rule out hypoglycemia). Other tests will depend on the anticipated toxicities of individual plant or mushroom toxins. Samples of emesis or gastric lavage fluid should be saved for toxicologic analysis or, in the case of mushroom ingestions, for microscopic examination to look for characteristic spores.

TABLE 100–2. *Differential Diagnosis of Plant Intoxications by Early Symptoms*

	Dieffenbachia	Wisteria	Saponin	Resin	Taxine	Protoanemonin	Misc. Gastrointestinal	Toxalbumin	Solanine	Oxalate	Colchicine	Digitalis	Aconite	Veratrum	Veratrine	Nicotine	Atropine	Cicuta	Cyanide	Akee	Lantana
Burning sensation in mouth	X		(X)	X	X						X										
Salivation	X		X											X		X		X			
Immediate nausea and emesis		X	X	X	X	X	X				X		X	X	X	X		X	X		
Delayed emesis								X	X	X	X									X	X
Abdominal pain			X	X	X	X		X	X	X	X	X									
Diarrhea			X	X	X	X	X	(X)	X	X	X										
Mydriasis				X													X				X
Visual disturbances												(X)		X			X				
Depression or coma								X		X				X						X	X
Headache									X	X		X	X								
Paresthesias			X										X		X						
Tremors or convulsions													X					X	X	X	
Psychoses																	X				
Rash					X	X											X				
Hyperthermia																	X				
Tachycardia																X	X				
Bradycardia										X			X	X	X						
Hypotension							X							X	X						
Arrhythmias					X			X				X	X								
Dry mouth								(X)									X				
Dyspnea													X				X		X		

(Reproduced with permission from Lampe KF, Fagerstrom R: Plant toxicity and dermatitis. Baltimore: Williams & Wilkins, 1968)

TABLE 100–3. Common Poisonous Plants

Common Name	Scientific Name	Plant Characteristics	Toxic Signs and Symptoms	Treatment
Acorns (see Oak)				
Akee	*Blighia sapida*	The white aril of the mature fruit is edible, but the fruit wall, the black seeds, and the unripe or rancid spoiled fruit are highly toxic.	Vomiting, convulsions, and coma appear 6–24 hours after ingestion. The toxic state may begin with convulsions and coma.	Glucose is important because peptides produce hypoglycemia. Acidosis is a consistent finding.
Almond (see Seeds of Fruit)				
Angel's Trumpet (Moon Flower)	*Datura sp.*	All parts of these plants are poisonous, especially the seeds and leaves.	Anticholinergic intoxication—hallucinations, sensory flooding, delirium, visual disturbances, alternating levels of consciousness, and toxic delirium	Avoid phenothiazines, which may potentiate anticholinergic affects.
Apple seeds, crab apple (see Seeds of Fruit)				
Apricot seeds (see Seeds of Fruit)				
Autumn crocus	*Colchicum autumale*	The entire plant of the autumn crocus is toxic and contains colchicine.	Burning in the mouth, abdominal cramps, nausea, diarrhea, kidney failure, CNS depression, and circulatory collapse	
Azalea, kaimia, mountain laurel, mountain ivy, rhododendron (see Rhododendron)				
Baneberry (Snakeberry, Doll's Eyes)	*Actaea sp.*	All parts of the baneberry are toxic, particularly the roots and berries.	Poisonous glycosides cause severe stomach cramps, headaches, rapid pulse, vomiting, delirium, dizziness, and circulatory failure.	
Belladonna (see Nightshade)				
Be-still-tree (Yellow Oleander)	*Thevetia peruviana*	Yellow oleander is considered the most common cause of poisoning in Hawaii. This entire plant is toxic and contains cardiac glycosides.	Vomiting, dizziness, convulsions, and cardiac depression	

Common name (Scientific name)	Toxic portion	Symptoms	Treatment
Bittersweet (Blue Nightshade) *Solanum dulcamara*	The leaves and unripe fruit of this plant are toxic. Bittersweet contains solanine, a steroid alkaloid.	Burning sensation in the throat, nausea, vomiting, diarrhea, dizziness, weakness, chills, dilated pupils, coma, and convulsions	Obtain baseline liver function tests and watch for liver failure.
Black cherry, wild cherry (see Seeds of Fruit)			
Black locust *Robinia pseudoacacia*	The inner bark, young leaves, twigs, and seeds of the black locust contain phytotoxins.	Burning of the mouth and throat accompanied by abdominal pain. Headache, nausea, vomiting, diarrhea, and hemorrhagic gastritis occur hours later. Allergic reactions may be severe. Delayed systemic effects include hypotension, seizures, and coma.	
Bleeding heart *Dicentra sp.*	All portions of this plant are toxic and contain protopine and other alkaloids.	Mucous membrane irritation, abdominal pain, and vomiting. Cardiac toxicity has been described.	
Bloodroot *Sanguinaria canadensis*			
Buttercup (Ranunculus family; see Delphinium)			
Caladium, colocasia *Caladium sp.*	The leaves and roots contain calcium oxalate crystals.	Burning and edema of the mucous membrane. Poisoning may also cause airway obstruction.	Topical measures for severe burning include cold compresses and a mixture of 2% viscous lidocaine and diphenhydramine elixir.
Cannabis, hemp (see Chapter 78)			
Castor bean *Ricinis communis*	Castor bean seeds contain ricin and are highly toxic.	Burning of the mouth and throat accompanied by abdominal pain. Headache, nausea, vomiting, diarrhea, and hemorrhagic gastritis occur hours later. Allergic reactions may be severe. Delayed systemic effects include hypotension, seizures, and coma.	Obtain baseline liver function tests and watch for liver failure.

(continued)

TABLE 100–3. Common Poisonous Plants (*continued*)

Common Name	Scientific Name	Plant Characteristics	Toxic Signs and Symptoms	Treatment
Cherry (see Seeds of Fruit)				
Chinaberry tree	*Meliz azederach*	Although the berries are the most toxic part of this tree, tea made from the leaves contains a saponin and a toxic alkaloid.	Nausea, vomiting, and bloody diarrhea. Depression or excitement, mental confusion, stupor, convulsions, ataxia, paralysis, dilated pupils, and respiratory difficulties are also seen.	
Chrisimas rose	*Helleborus niger*	The toxic portions of this plant are the leaves and roots, which contain cardiac glycosides.	GI upset, weakness, cramps, ataxia, excitability, circulatory collapse, convulsions, and death	
Crab's eye (see Rosary Pea)				
Crocus (see Autumn Crocus)				
Coyotillo		The fruits and seeds are toxic.	Paralysis a few days after ingestion	
Cyanogenic plants		Amygdalin-producing plants include plum, apricot, cherry, laurel, peach, wild black cherry, jetberry bush, bitter almond, apple seeds, crab apple seeds, elderberry, loquat, cassava root, and hydrangea.	Cyanogenic glycosides (amygdalin) are hydrolyzed in the GI tract and liberate hydrocyanic acid (cyanide ion).	(See cyanide poisoning, chapter 76.)
Daffodil (Jonquil; see Narcissus)				
Daphne (Spurge Laurel)		All parts of this plant are toxic, especially the berries.	Ulceration of the throat and GI tract, hematemesis, internal bleeding with bloody diarrhea, weakness, coma, and death. Kidney damage can occur.	
Death camas (Black Snakeroot)	*Zygadenus intermedius*	The entire Zygadenus plant is toxic, particularly the bulb, which contains zygadenine.	Salivation, muscular weakness, GI upset with pain, vomiting, diarrhea, hypotension, difficulty in breathing, coma, and death	Atropine may reverse symptomatic bradycardia.

Delphinium (Larkspur)	*D. consolida*	The entire *D. consolida* plant, especially the seeds, contains the toxic compound of delphinine (similar to aconitine).	Death may occur within six hours. Symptoms include tingling and burning of the mouth, tongue, and lips and numbness. Generalized paresthesia occurs. Nausea, vomiting, salivation followed by a dry mouth, sweating (with cold, clammy skin), tinnitus, myocardial depression and arrhythmias (supraventricular tachycardia and conduction disturbances) may appear.	Cardiac monitoring is essential.
Dieffenbachia (Dumbcane)			Swelling of the mucous membranes and tongue due to ingestion of dieffenbachia may cause airway obstruction. The swelling may leave the victim speechless (hence the name dumbcane). Symptoms of nausea, vomiting, and diarrhea may indicate the presence of additional toxins.	Treat as for caladium exposure.
Duranta (see Pokeweed)				
Elderberry (Elder, Black Elder)	*Sambucus sp.*	The roots, stems, and leaves of the elderberry plant contain toxic alkaloids and cyanogenic glycosides. Children have been poisoned by using the stems for blowguns, popguns, and whistles.		
Elephant's ear	*Colocasia antiquorum*	The leaves and stems of this plant are dangerous if eaten in quantity.	Severe burning of the throat is to some extent due to the needle-like calcium oxalate crystals, as in caladium. In severe cases, swelling of the mouth and tongue may cause choking.	Treat as for caladium exposure.
English ivy	*Hedera helix*	The leaves and berries of English ivy are toxic, containing saponin glycosides.	Excitement, difficulty in breathing, CNS and cardiovascular toxicity, and coma	

(continued)

TABLE 100–3. Common Poisonous Plants (*continued*)

Common Name	Scientific Name	Plant Characteristics	Toxic Signs and Symptoms	Treatment
False helebore	*Veratrum*	The roots, leaves, and seeds of Veratrum plants are toxic; they all contain veratrum.	Salivation, gastroenteritis, weakness, difficulty in breathing, rapid pulse, and convulsions	
Foxglove	*Digitalis purpurea*	The leaves and seeds of the foxglove plant are toxic.	Poisoning symptoms are identical to those of digitalis poisoning: cardiac irregularities, gastric upset, confusion, nausea, diarrhea, severe headaches, tremors, convulsions, and death.	Treat as for digitalis overdose. Successful immunotherapy with digoxin FAB fragments has been reported (see Chapter 72).
Golden chain	*Laburnum anagyroides*			
Kentucky coffee tree	*Gymnocladus dioica*	The Kentucky coffee tree bean has been used as a coffee substitute, but the flowers and seeds of this plant contain the alkaloid cytisine.	Excitement, stomach and intestinal irritation, nausea, severe vomiting, diarrhea, irregular pulse, convulsions, coma, and death	
Green hellebore (see False Hellebore)				
Heavenly blue glory (see Morning Glory)				
Henbane	*Hyoscyamus niger*	Atropine, hyoscyamine, and hyoscine are the toxic alkaloids found throughout this plant.	Dry mouth, headache, nausea, rapid pulse, convulsions, and delirium	Treat as for any atropine-like poisoning (see Chapter 63).
Holly berries	*Ilex sp.*	When eaten in quantity, the berries (red or black) of native and cultivated holly shrubs and trees are toxic.	Vomiting, diarrhea, and stupor. Ingestion of 20–30 berries by a child may produce severe and even fatal CNS depression.	
Horse chestnut, buckeye	*Aesculus sp.*	Leaves, flowers, young sprouts, and seeds of the horse chestnut are toxic.	Nervous twitching of muscles, weakness, lack of coordination, dilated pupils, vomiting, diarrhea, depression, paralysis, and stupor	

Common name	Scientific name	Toxic parts	Symptoms	Treatment
Hyacinth	*Hyacinthus orientalis*	The hyacinth bulb is toxic.	Intense gastroenteritis, vomiting, and diarrhea	
Hydrangea		The leaves and buds of the hydrangea contain cyanogenic glycosides.	Nausea, vomiting, diarrhea, dyspnea, weakness, ataxia, fibrillary twitching, stupor, coma, convulsions, and death	Treat as for other forms of cyanide poisoning (see Chapter 76).
Iris (Blue Flag)		Toxic portions of the iris include the leaves and roots, both of which contain resin.	GI upset and blistering of the lips	
Jack-in-the-pulpit (Arums; see Dieffenbachia)				
Jequirity bean (see Rosary Pea)				
Jerusalem cherry	*Solanum pseudocapsicum*	The leaves and unripe fruit of this tree are toxic, with solanine as the toxic alkaloid.	Leaf ingestion causes cardiac depression with bradycardia. Berry ingestion produces a scratchy feeling in the mouth, nausea and vomiting, abdominal pain, and diarrhea (melena). Dizziness, weakness, salivation, sweating, headache, and convulsions occur.	Atropine may reverse bradycardia.
Jessamine, night blooming and day blooming	*Gestrum sp.*	The berries and sap of these plants are toxic. The maturity of the berry determines the nature of the toxic substance. Unripe berries contain solanine; mature berries contain tropane alkaloids (atropinelike).	Gastroenteritis	Anticholinergic symptoms may require therapy.
Jimsonweed	*Datura stramonium*	All parts of the jimsonweed, especially the leaves and seeds, contain atropine and hyoscine (scopolamine).	Thirst, pupil dilation, dry mouth, redness of skin, headache, hallucinations, nausea, rapid pulse, fever, hypertension, delirium, convulsions, coma, and death	Treat for anticholinergic poisoning (see Chapter 63).

(continued)

TABLE 100–3. Common Poisonous Plants (*continued*)

Common Name	Scientific Name	Plant Characteristics	Toxic Signs and Symptoms	Treatment
Lantana		The unripened fruit of the lantana shrub is most toxic, and all species are suspected of being poisonous.	GI irritation, muscular weakness, circulatory collapse, and death	
Larkspur (see Delphinium)				
Laurel, mountain laurel	*Kalmia latifolia*	The entire laurel plant is toxic. Mountain laurel, azaleas, and rhododendrons contain grayanotoxins that exhibit toxicity similar to the steroid alkaloids in false hellebore and death camas.	Salivation, emesis, and paresthesias. Hypotension, bradycardia, muscular weakness, and incoordination may occur.	Reversal of symptoms expected in 24 hours.
Lily-of-the-valley		The toxic portions of lily-of-the-valley include the leaves, flowers, and roots.	Toxic ingredients are cardiac glycosides that produce a digitalis effect.	
Lobelia, indian tobacco, cardinal flower		All parts of this plant contain toxic alkaloids.	Nausea, vomiting, weakness, stupor, tremors, convulsions, coma, and death.	
Lucky bean (see Rosary Pea)				
Mayapple, mandrake		The foliage, roots, and green fruit of the mayapple are toxic; they all contain resin.	Severe gastroenteritis and vomiting.	
Milk bush (Euphorbia)		The milky sap of the spurge family may cause a primary irritant dermatis.	Gastroenteritis is the most common symptom upon ingestion.	

Mistletoe	*Phoradendron serotinum*	While all parts of this plant are toxic, the berries are usually involved, causing GI irritation.	Ingesting a few berries is not a cause for alarm, but death has been reported following consumption of a large number of berries.	
Monkshood	*Aconitum sp.*	All parts of this plant contain aconitine.	Numbness of the lips and tongue, visual disturbances, bradycardia, hypotension, vomiting, respiratory irregularities, paralysis, convulsions, and death in a few hours	Temporary cardiac pacing may be required.
Moon flower (see Angel's Trumpet)				
Morning glory	*Ipomoea violacea*	The toxic part of this plant is the seeds, which contain LSD and are ingested for psychedelic experiences. From 50 to 200 seeds produce euphoria and hallucinations.	GI symptoms, nausea, and acute and chronic psychotic reactions	
Mushrooms (see Mushroom Poisoning in this chapter)				
Narcissus		The narcissus bulb is toxic.	Gastroenteritis, diarrhea, vomiting, tremors, and convulsions	
Nicotiana (Tobacco)		Severe poisoning and death have occurred from eating Nicotiana leaves, both cooked and uncooked. Children have become ill from sucking the flowers.	Severe vomiting, diarrhea, slow pulse, dizziness, collapse, and respiratory failure	

(continued)

TABLE 100-3. Common Poisonous Plants (*continued*)

Common Name	Scientific Name	Plant Characteristics	Toxic Signs and Symptoms	Treatment
Nightshade (Wild Tomato, Potato, Climbing Nightshade)	*Solanum sp.*	All parts of this plant are toxic; poison can be absorbed from the leaves and by ingesting the berries. Solanine and other compounds are the toxic elements.		See also Jerusalem Cherry.
Oak	*Querius sp.*	Acorns, young shoots, and leaves of the oak tree are mildly toxic.		
Oleander		The entire oleander plant is toxic.	GI upset, bloody diarrhea, depressed respirations, bradycardia, and death	See Foxglove.
Peach (See Seeds of Fruit)				
Pearly gates (see Morning Glory)				
Philodendron, monstera, arum family (see Dieffenbachia)				
Pigeonberry (see Pokeweed)				
Plum (see Seeds of Fruit)				
Poinciana, bird of paradise		The green seed pods of this cultivated shrub are toxic.	Mild to severe GI symptoms	The well-known bird of paradise of the banana family is considered nonpoisonous.
Poinsettia		The juice of the leaves, the flowers, and the stem of the poinsettia are toxic.	GI irritation. The sap can produce skin irritation.	
Poison hemlock	*Conium maculatum*	The toxic leaves, stems, and fruit of this hemlock are often mistaken for parsley or anise.	Nausea, emesis, salivation, drowsiness, paresthesia, ataxia, dilated pupils, slow pulse, muscle weakness, paralysis, respiratory depression, coma, convulsions, and death	Respiratory support and cardiac pacing may be required.

Poison ivy, poison oak, poison sumac			Contact with the plant causes dermatitis in susceptible people.	
Pokeweed	*Phytolacca americana*	This is one of the most dangerous plants. Poisonings are caused by ingestion or by preparation without proper or complete boiling. This plant is used commonly as a home remedy. The roots and leaves are toxic, the fruit and seeds less so.	Burning sensation in the mouth, nausea, vomiting, diarrhea, abdominal cramps, visual disturbances, and respiratory and circulatory depression	
Potato	*Solanum tuberosum*	Only the ripe tuber of the plant is edible. The toxic alkaloid solanine, found in both unripe and spoiled potatoes and in potato sprouts, has caused severe poisonings.	Headache, mental confusion, stomach pain, paralysis, vomiting, shock, circulatory and respiratory depression, cardiac depression, and death	See Jerusalem Cherry.
Precatory bean (see Rosary Pea)				
Privet, ligustrum		The entire privet plant is toxic.	Nausea, vomiting, and diarrhea	
Purge nut, physic nut	*Jatropha curcas*	Fruit, seeds, and sap from all parts of this plant are toxic.	Nausea, violent vomiting, bloody diarrhea, and coma from a few minutes to several hours after ingestion. Three seeds are sufficient to cause severe symptoms.	
Pyracantha		Although the orange-red berries are not very toxic, ingesting a large number may produce toxicity.	Gastroenteritis	
Rhododendron		The entire rhododendron plant is toxic.	See Laurel.	

(*continued*)

TABLE 100-3. Common Poisonous Plants (continued)

Common Name	Scientific Name	Plant Characteristics	Toxic Signs and Symptoms	Treatment
Rhubarb	Rheum rhabarbarum	The blade of the rhubarb leaf contains a highly poisonous soluble oxalate.	Stomach pains and cramping, burning of the mouth and throat, nausea, vomiting, difficulty in breathing, tetany, convulsions, hypotension, coma, and death	Hypocalcemia may be refractory to treatment. Treatment is directed at correcting hypocalcemia while maintaining a brisk diuresis. Consider gastric lavage with 0.15% calcium hydroxide solution.
Rosary pea	Abrus precatorius	The seeds of this plant are shiny red and black and extremely toxic. One seed, if chewed, can be fatal.		See Castor Bean.
Seeds of fruit		The seeds of almonds, apples, apricots, cherries, chokeberries, loquats, peaches, and plums contain amygdalin, a cyanogenic compound. The lethal dose of hydrocyanic acid in adults is approximately 50 mg, in children 20 mg.	Seed kernels are high in cyanide (apricot, 0.1–2.8 mg/g; peach, 0.6–1.6 mg/g), as are the leaves (1.4–3.7 mg/g).	Treat as for other forms of cyanide exposure (see Chapter 76).
Skunk cabbage		The leaves and root stocks of skunk cabbage are toxic because they contain calcium oxalate crystals.	Irritation of the mucosa and edema of the tongue, throat, and mouth	Monitor for respiratory obstruction.
Snow-on-the-mountain (Spurge)	Euphorbia margenta	The milky sap is toxic.	Gastroenteritis if ingested or skin irritation on contact. Severe intoxication may lead to cardiovascular collapse.	See Milk Bush.
Sweet pea	Lathyrus	The seeds and peas of this plant are toxic.	Slow and weak pulse, shallow breathing, convulsions, paralysis, and skeletal deformities (lathyrism)	
Thorn apple (see Jimsonweed)				

Common name	Scientific name	Description	Symptoms	Notes
Tung nut	*Aleurites fordii*	The nut of this plant is the part usually involved in poisonings, although the entire plant is toxic. One seed can cause severe poisoning.	Nausea, vomiting, cramps, diarrhea, and tenesmus. More severe symptoms include pyrexia, tachypnea, irregular respiration, dilated pupils, severe headache, paresthesias, and cyanosis.	
Water hemlock, cowbane	*Cicuta maculata*	The entire plant is toxic; it contains cicutoxin, especially in the fleshy, hollow rootstock. It is among the most poisonous of plants. Ingestions are common due to its similarity to anise, wild parsnips, and wild artichokes.	Vomiting, diarrhea, abdominal cramps, frothing at the mouth, salivation, dilated pupils, delirium, seizures, respiratory depression, and death	One mouthful of the root is sufficient to kill an adult.
Wisteria		The elongated wisteria pods and their seeds are toxic.	Severe gastroenteritis, stomach pain, diarrhea, and collapse	Two seeds can cause serious illness in a child.
Yellow jessamine (South Carolina state flower)	*Gelsemium sempervirens*	The entire plant is toxic, especially the nectar and roots. Children have been severely poisoned by chewing the leaves or sucking the nectar. Sometimes honeybees make poisonous honey and are poisoned themselves. The rootstock is used as a source for some medicinal preparations.	Sweating, depression, muscular weakness, convulsions, and paralysis of motor-nerve endings are symptoms of poisoning.	Respiratory support
Yew	*Taxus sp.*	Most parts of the yew plant contain the toxic alkaloid taxine. Seeds are edible in small quantities.	Diarrhea, vomiting, trembling, pupil dilation, difficulty in breathing, muscular weakness, convulsions, and coma	

TABLE 100-4. Clinical Spectrum of Common Types of Mushroom Poisoning

Group	Toxins	Principal Mushrooms	Onset of Symptoms	Symptoms	Treatment and Duration of Illness
Type A—Toxins Causing Cellular Destruction—Delayed Onset					
I	Cyclopeptides (amanitins)	*Amanita bisporigera* *A. ocreata* *A. phalloides* *A. verna* *A. virosa* *Galerina autumnalis* *G. marginata* *G. venenata* *Lepiota sp.*	6–24 hr (typically 10–14 hr)	Abdominal pains, nausea, vomiting, and diarrhea lasting 1+ days; short remission of symptoms, then recurrence of pains with jaundice, renal shutdown, convulsions, coma, and death.	Maintain fluid and electrolyte balance. Follow liver and renal parameters and blood sugar. Death may occur between 4–7 days, or recovery may take 2 weeks.
II	Gyromitrin, monomethylhydrazine (MMH)	*Gyromitra esculenta* and others	6–12 hr	Bloated feeling, nausea, vomiting, watery (or bloody) diarrhea, abdominal pains, muscle cramps, faintness, loss of coordination, and, in severe cases, convulsions, coma, and death.	Pyridoxine HCl 25 mg/kg IV titrated with patient's symptoms. Follow methemoglobin and free hemoglobin levels and hepatic parameters.
Type B—Toxins Affecting the Autonomic Nervous System—Rapid Onset					
III	Muscarine and other muscarinic compounds	*Clitocybe dealbata* *C. cerussata* and perhaps *C. illudens* (*Omphalotus olearius*) and others; *Inocybe, most sp.*	0.5–2 hr	PSL syndrome (perspiration, salivation, and lacrimation), blurred vision, abdominal cramps, watery diarrhea, constriction of pupils, fall in blood pressure, slow pulse.	Atropine 0.02 mg/kg IV repeated prn for symptomatic bradycardia and secretions compromising the airway. Symptoms subside within 6–24 hours. Death reported only in people with concurrent disease.

IV	Coprine (Antabuselike)	*Coprinus atramentarius, Clitocybe clavipes*	About 30 minutes after drinking alcohol; as many as 5 days after eating mushrooms.	Flushing of face and neck, distention of neck veins, swelling and tingling of hands, metallic taste, tachycardia and hypotension; later nausea, vomiting, and sweating.	Avoid elixirs and tinctures. Propranolol may be necessary to control arrhythmias. Recovery usually spontaneous within 2–4 hours.

Type C—Toxins Affecting the CNS—Rapid Onset

V	Ibotenic acid, Muscimol (isoxazoles)	*Amanita muscaria A. pantherina* and others	0.5–2 hr	Dizziness, incoordination, staggering (intoxication); muscular jerking and spasms; hyperkinetic activity; comalike deep sleep and "visions."	Do *not* give atropine unless definite cholinergic symptoms are present. Do *not* intubate unless there is actual respiratory distress. Recovery in 4–24 hours.
VI	Psilocybin and Psilocin (indoles)	*Psilocybe cubensis P. balocystis* and others	30–60 (180) min	Pleasant or apprehensive mood; unmotivated laughter; hilarity; compulsive movements; muscle weakness; drowsiness; "visions" while awake; then sleep.	Diazepam rarely necessary. Reassurance for apprehension. Recovery within 6 hours.

Type D—Toxins Affecting the GI Tract—Rapid Onset

VII	Diverse, mostly unknown	Many species from diverse genera	0.5–2 (4) hr	Principally nausea, vomiting, diarrhea, and abdominal pain	Careful attention to fluid and electrolyte replacement. Death is rare. Recovery time varies according to species from 1 hour to several days or a week.

(Reproduced with permission from Mitchell DH: Amanita mushroom poisoning. Ann Rev Med 1980; Volume 31)

Treatment ■

After ensuring that the patient's airway, breathing, and circulation (ABCs) are stabilized, toxin removal is essential. If the patient has not vomited, administer 15 ml of syrup of ipecac with copious amounts of water. For unresponsive patients, perform gastric lavage with adequate airway protection. Following gastric emptying, give activated charcoal (0.5–1 g/kg in 6–8 oz water). If diarrhea is not a feature of the poisoning, cathartics are indicated.

The most common serious sequela in children who ingested toxic plants or mushrooms is dehydration due to vomiting, diarrhea, and third-space losses. Thus, pay meticulous attention to the state of hydration (tearing, mucous membranes, skin turgor and color) and to objective measures such as pulse, blood pressure, and urinary output. Children may require vigorous volume replacement based on the above assessment (see Chapter 22).

Common Poisonous Plants ■

Table 100-3 presents common poisonous plants in America, with their characteristics, toxic signs and symptoms, and their special treatment considerations.

Prevention ■

1. Know the dangerous plants in your area, yard, and home.
2. Keep plants, seeds, fruit, and bulbs away from infants. Store bulbs in a safe place.
3. Teach children to keep plants and plant parts out of their mouths.
4. Know the plants and the plant parts used by children as playthings.
5. Keep children from sucking nectar from flowers or from making tea from leaves.
6. Know the plant before eating the fruit. If children are included in harvesting, allow them to collect only the very well known berries. Do not allow them to eat any that are not served to them. Remember, it takes far fewer berries to poison a child than an adult.
7. No safe rules exist for visually differentiating edible plants from poisonous ones. Do not rely on pets, birds, and squirrels, or on expert mushroom identifiers ("There are old mushroom hunters. There are bold mushroom hunters. There are no old, bold mushroom hunters").

TABLE 100–5. *Treatment of Mushroom Poisoning*

Gastric Decontamination
A. Emesis, if not already adequate from poisoning itself. Ipecac syrup 15–30 ml followed by 250–500 ml oral liquids
B. Gastric lavage if patient is unconscious or convulsing. Large-bore gastric tube (34 French or larger) until clear
C. Activated charcoal, 0.5–1 g/kg in water every 6 hours
D. Catharsis, if not already adequate; magnesium sulfate 250 mg/kg PO

Enhancement of Elimination
Forced diuresis to obtain urine output of 3–6 ml/kg/hr with oral or IV fluids. Add furosemide 1 mg/kg/hr IV p.r.n.

Supportive Measures
A. Maintain respiration with adequate airway, oxygen, and rarely, *in extremis,* ventilatory support.
B. Maintain blood pressure with IV fluids and, if necessary, vasopressors.
C. Maintain blood sugar and electrolytes.
D. Follow hepatic and renal parameters for at least 48 hours.
E. Sedatives (e.g., diazepam) for anxiety, hysteria, hallucinations, or convulsions, which may occasionally occur in children.

Drug Intervention
Specific therapy with drug intervention is rarely required, and then *only* when the type of poisoning is diagnosed.

Mushroom Poisoning ■

Mushroom poisonings have caused many deaths in the United States and Europe. The *Amanita phalloides* group (commonly called "death cap" and "destroying angel") cause 95% of the fatalities. About 100 of the 2,000 mushroom species known in the United States are poisonous. Even trained mycologists may confuse toxic varieties with edible ones because of the variations among species. Thus, the hazards of gathering and eating wild mushrooms are considerable, and the outcome may be fatal.

CLINICAL FINDINGS

Table 100-4 summarizes common types of mushroom poisoning. *Amanita phalloides* is listed under Type A, Group 1, and because of its clinical importance it is described in more detail below.

Consider the possibility of mushroom poisoning if the patient presents in the late summer or early autumn with GI symptoms. Inquire about mushroom intake.

The clinical course has two phases:

1. *The GI phase* follows the latent period of 10–14 hours after ingestion. Note: The classic latent period may be absent if a rapid onset of symptoms is actually the manifestation of another mushroom eaten with *Amanita phalloides.* Characteristics of the GI phase are violent abdominal pain, vomiting, diarrhea (choleralike), hematuria, fever, tachycardia, hypotension, and rapid volume depletion with electrolyte imbalance.
2. *The hepatic and renal phase* manifests itself after an apparent remission that lasts 1–3 days. Laboratory studies become abnormal and the patient's symptoms include jaundice with elevation of liver enzymes, renal shutdown with elevation of BUN and creatinine, coagulopathy, and coma. Death from liver or renal failure occurs in 4–7 days.

Radioimmunoassay for amatotoxin can be done on samples of gastric juice, blood, or urine. The toxin can be detected in duodenal aspirates 36 hours after ingestion.

TREATMENT

For general principles of treatment of mushroom poisoning see Table 100-5. For specific treatment of different groups of mushrooms see Table 100-4.

Bibliography ■

Geehr EC: Toxic plant ingestions; Poisonous mushrooms. In: Auerbach PS, Geehr EC, eds: *Management of wilderness and environmental emergencies,* 2nd ed. St. Louis: CV Mosby, 1989.

Goldfrank L: Herbal medicine. *Hospital Physician* 1982; 18: 64–86.

Hardin JW, Arean JM: *Human poisoning from native and cultivated plants,* 2nd ed. Durham, NC: Duke University Press, 1974.

Kingsbury JM: Phytotoxicology. In: Doull J, Klassen CD, Amdur MO, eds: *Toxicology.* New York: Macmillan, 1980.

Lampe K: *Common poisonous and injurious plants.* US Department of Human Services, Public Health Services, Food and Drug Administration, Bureau of Drugs, Division of Poison Control. HHS Publication No. (FDA) 81-7006, 1981.

Lincoff G, Mitchel DH: *Mushroom poisoning: A handbook for physicians and mushroom hunters.* New York: Van Nostrand Reinhold, 1977.

Litovitz TL, Schmitz BF, Matyunas N, et al: 1987 annual report of the American Association of Poison Control Centers National Data Collection System. *Am J Emerg Med* 1988; 6:479–515.

Mitchel DH: Amanita mushroom poisoning. *Annu Rev Med* 1980; 31:51–57.

101 Wilderness Emergencies

Michael Young and Kenneth W. Kizer

Wilderness emergencies are injuries and illnesses occurring during recreational activities in sparsely settled areas, with rescue times of two or more hours. Wilderness medicine includes environmental physiology, mountain medicine, aerospace and marine medicine, plant toxicology, and traditional medicine in outback situations; some of these subjects are covered in Chapters 93–100.

Epidemiology ■

Unintentional injury is the leading cause of death in children. In 1978, over 6,000 sports deaths were reported; about 25% were wilderness deaths. In 1982, about 1.8 million recreational injuries required emergency department treatment; 600,000 of them in children. Injury rates from recreational activities are higher than those at most other locations, including school. Table 101-1 indicates injury rates and location by age category. Among the over-5 age group, recreational areas are more frequent locations for injuries than school and home locations combined.

Injury rates increase steadily from infancy to a peak during adolescence. While overall injury rates are higher in non-white and poorer children, the opposite is true for wilderness injury, perhaps because children of higher socioeconomic status have greater exposure to wilderness activities.

In about half the cases of wilderness injury among adolescents, a major predisposition is mind-altering drugs, especially alcohol. In younger children, the major predispositions involve inadequate supervision, poor training, and substandard equipment. Death rates increase with the degree of energy devoted to the activity and with high-technology equipment.

Injury by Sport ■

SKIING AND WINTER SPORTS

Downhill skiing is the best-studied recreational activity causing pediatric injury. Ski injury rates at downhill areas are about 25% higher in children than adults, and result in 50,000 pediatric ED visits a year in the United States. Children suffer more neck and back injuries than adults. Spiral fractures of the distal tibia are the most common pediatric injuries. With better equipment, significant knee and femur injuries appear to be increasing, while tibia-fibular injuries are decreasing. Head injury is associated with nearly all skiing fatalities. Competitive skiing creates an increase in both the frequency and severity of injury.

In children, the most common causes of injury are inadequate or poorly fitted equipment, followed by poor judgment and fatigue. Improperly adjusted or inadequate bindings are the most frequent equipment problems for children and may be a preventable factor in up to 75% of pediatric ski injuries.

Nordic (cross-country) skiing injury is less well reported. Sprains of the ankle and upper extremity are common. Rescues may be complicated by the more remote setting, combined with high injury severity. A long rescue time can predispose to hypothermia, and significant injuries may be occult. Thus, a high level of urgency is imperative in field and ED management of backwoods ski trauma.

About 47,000 wilderness injuries were associated with *toboggans, sleds, disks, and tubes* in 1982 in the United States. Falling off and colliding with trees were the usual mechanisms. CNS and spine injury cause the most significant morbidity and mortality, although lacerations and fractures are the most common injuries. Simple preventive measures include adequate supervision and use of designated areas.

Several hundred fatalities a year occur in *snowmobiles;* one-fourth of injuries are suffered by drivers under 18 years of age. Speeding and not wearing helmets increase riders' vulnerability. Contusions and lacerations account for 40% of injuries, followed by fractures (30%), sprains (20%), and concussions (3%). As in Nordic skiing, a life-threatening injury may occur hours from a hospital, and cold injury and transport delay worsen the outcome. Alcohol use is associated with nearly half of snowmobile injuries. Snowmobile victims require the most expectant approach in the field and in the hospital; assume major trauma until proven otherwise. Preventive measures

454

TABLE 101–1. *Types of Injury by Age Group*

Location of Injury	Percentage			
	Under 1 year	1–4 years	5–9 years	10–14 years
Home	82	60	13	9
Road	6	12	17	15
School	0	0	16	11
Recreational	0	13	45	45
Other	12	15	9	20

(Reproduced with permission from Troop PA: Accidents to children: An analysis of inpatient admission. Public Health 1986; 100: 281)

include mandatory helmet use, minimum skills requirements for driving, and abstention from drugs and alcohol.

MOUNTAINEERING AND HIKING

There are about 100,000 active mountain climbers in the United States; if casual mountain hiking is included, the number may be several million. In the European Alps, there are over 500 mountain fatalities a year, many involving adolescents. Snow avalanche is the biggest single killer.

Hiking also has many potential hazards. Orthopedic injuries secondary to hiking at summer camp are a major cause of visits to camp physicians. In the mountains, falls or slips are the leading cause of morbidity and mortality. Hypothermia, lightning injury, drownings during stream crossings, sun and fire exposure, and altitude illness are also significant risks for hikers.

ALL-TERRAIN VEHICLES

In 1985, more than 85,000 all-terrain vehicle injuries required ED visits. Nearly half occurred in children under 16 years, and 19% were in children under 12. More than 600 deaths have been reported, and the injury rate has increased in recent years. Risk factors for injury include alcohol use, lack of helmets, driver inexperience, lack of concentration, and excess speed. Head injury, severe facial and dental wounds, long-bone fractures, and dislocations occur, as well as significant numbers of abdominal catastrophes and spinal cord injuries. Preventive strategies include total vehicle recall, community education, formal licensing requiring drivers to be older than 16, mandatory helmet use, and vehicle modifications.

TRAIL-BIKE INJURIES

There are about 600 trail-bike deaths a year in children in the United States. Recently bikes with fat tires and more rugged construction have become popular for dirt and trail riding. Like those in street bikes, trail-bike injuries are often caused by poor judgment, inadequate bike maintenance, and lack of helmets. Education of families and communities should emphasize skills teaching, supervised riding, helmet use, compulsory bike maintenance, and protective clothing.

Injury by Mechanism ■

STINGS AND ENVENOMATIONS

Arthropod bites are common backwoods nuisances that occasionally become major emergencies. About 25,000 people suffer severe acute reactions each year. Illness is caused either by direct transmission of disease, such as malaria, or by envenomation with powerful toxins. The important venomous classes of arthropods include Insecta (insects), Arachnida (spiders, scorpions, ticks, and mites), Chilopoda (centipedes), and Diplopoda (millipedes).

Almost everyone has suffered insect envenomation from bees, wasps, and ants of the order Hymenoptera. Local pain, erythema, and swelling, followed by itching, are the most common reactions to Hymenoptera stings. But about 0.4% of the population has an allergy to Hymenoptera venom that may result in severe local reactions or in anaphylaxis. Urticaria, respiratory distress, and hypotension may develop suddenly. Time of onset of anaphylaxis is usually 15 minutes to 6 hours from envenomation (see Chapter 17). Uncommon delayed reactions include serum sickness, acute glomerulonephritis, thrombocytopenia, and nonspecific toxic reactions such as fever, nausea, vomiting, and diarrhea.

The manifestations of arachnid envenomation are variable. Black widow spiders are ubiquitous in the continental United States, and their venom is more toxic than many snake venoms. The black widow bite is often painless, but in less than an hour severe local and systemic signs develop. Local pain is followed by severe cramping of the thorax, back, and abdomen. Hypertension, respiratory compromise, diaphoresis, nausea and vomiting, headache, and paresthesias may occur. Death ensues in 5% of untreated cases. Children with systemic manifestations require hospital admission for observation and treatment.

Like the black widow, the brown recluse spider is found in nearly all parts of the United States. Bites generally occur indoors in the warmer months; they are more common in children. The clinical picture is typically mild, but lesions may become necrotic with bullae and a hemorrhagic edge, ultimately leaving an eschar. Death may result from vomiting, dehydration, and hemolysis. Major systemic reactions include seizures, headache, fever, hematuria, chills, and a petechial rash. Hospital admission is imperative when systemic findings are present.

Tarantula bites generally cause only local pain. Stings by most scorpion species are similar in severity to those of the Hymenoptera, although envenomation by the *Centruroides sculpturatus* may be life threatening, especially in young children.

Tick bites may lead to Lyme disease, Rocky Mountain spotted fever, and rarely tick paralysis. In the latter condition, ascending paralysis similar to Guillain-Barré develops 4–7 days after tick attachment, with death in 10% of patients. Removing the tick resolves symptoms.

Centipedes have fangs, but envenomation rarely leads to serious systemic reactions. Millipedes secrete irritating and toxic substances that may create local tissue damage.

Treatment

ED treatment of arthropod bites requires meticulous local cleaning, reassurance, and routine tetanus prophylaxis. Patients with anaphylaxis need aggressive management (see Chapter 17). Spider-bite therapy remains controversial. Antivenom is useful for severe black widow bites. Severe muscle spasms may respond transiently to intravenous calcium gluconate or benzodiazepines.

Steroids are indicated when patients have systemic reactions to brown recluse bites. Dapsone (2 mg/kg PO once daily) in children may be as effective as recluse antivenom in reducing local necrosis.

SNAKE BITES

Two species of poisonous snakes (pit vipers and coral snakes) in the United States are responsible for 8,000 bites and 20 deaths each year. Most of the victims are 10–19 years old, and most bites happen near home, often while snakes are being handled. Bites most commonly involve the lower extremities.

The clinical response to envenomation can be graded objectively and used to guide antivenom administration (see Table 101-2). Table 101-3 presents fundamentals of field and ED treatment of snake bite. Management of envenomations from coral snakes and pit vipers is identical, although different antivenoms are used.

HIGH-ALTITUDE ILLNESS

High-altitude illness is a common wilderness problem that includes a spectrum of ailments, from acute mountain sickness (AMS) to the more serious high-altitude pulmonary edema (HAPE) and high-altitude cerebral edema (HACE). Acute mountain sickness occurs in 30% of those who are rapidly exposed (less than 2–3 days) to 3,000 meters altitude and in 75% of those exposed to 4,500 meters. At high altitudes, the reduced partial pressure of oxygen impairs cellular metabolism and causes hyperperfusion and hyperventilation. Either or both mechanisms may be responsible for mountain sickness. Table 101-4 outlines clinical findings, treatment, and prevention for the three major forms of high-altitude illness.

SOLAR INJURIES

Excess sun exposure can cause sunburn, photokeratoconjunctivitis, and retinal damage. Wind may be an important exacerbating factor. Chronically, sun exposure may increase the risk of non-melanotic skin

---

TABLE 101–2. *Clinical Grading of Snakebite Envenomations*

Grade	Clinical Findings	Treatment
0	Fang marks but no local or systemic reactions	No antivenom Observe for 6 hours.
1 (minimal)	Local swelling, no systemic reaction	2–5 vials of antivenom (slowly over 5 minutes, then quickly if no reaction)
2 (moderate)	Swelling beyond the bite site, systemic reactions, laboratory changes	5–10 vials of antivenom
3 (severe)	Marked local reaction, severe symptoms, and laboratory changes	10–20 vials of antivenom

TABLE 101–3. *Management of Snakebites*

Field
1. Immobilize involved extremity. Identify snake if possible. If snake is dead, bring to ED.
2. If greater than 30 minutes from medical care, apply constricting band 3 inches above bite if bite is fresh. Incise through bite, carefully avoiding underlying vascular, musculotendinous, and neural structures; apply suction for 60 seconds.
3. Keep extremity at heart level.
4. Do not apply heat or cold.

Hospital
1. Apply cardiac monitor.
2. Obtain blood for disseminated intravascular coagulation studies (prothrombin time, bleeding time, fibrinogen, fibrin split products, platelets), electrolytes, blood gases. Perform ECG.
3. Assess need for antivenom (see Table 101–2).
4. Ensure epinephrine and diphenhydramine are immediately available for severe serum reaction.
5. Emphasize meticulous local care, including cleaning and debridement.
6. Immobilize extremity at heart level. Fasciotomies are rarely indicated.
7. Admit for observation.
8. Consider ampicillin 150 mg/kg/d.
9. Contact Oklahoma City Poison Information Center (303) 629-1123 for information on obtaining antivenom, antivenom doses for small children, and for expert consultation.

cancer by 78% and may cause cataracts. Risk factors include light skin, prolonged exposure, high altitude, and reflection from water and snow.

The diagnosis of *sunburn* is apparent often several hours after exposure. Children are more susceptible than adults. Sensitivity to sunlight is increased by sulfonamides and their derivatives, such as trimethoprim-sulfamethoxazole, most tetracyclines, and barbiturates. Prevention requires reflective clothing and meticulous use of sunscreens. Table 101-5 describes the European system of sun protective factor (SPF) now used in the United States as a rough guide for skin protection requirements.

Field treatment consists of cool compresses to reduce pain. The effectiveness of systemic steroids for treatment of sunburn is unproven. Nonsteroidals that inhibit prostaglandin synthesis are useful if used early in superficial sunburn. Avoid topical agents that may sensitize the skin, leading to allergic eczematous reactions.

Eye injury from sun exposure is usually superficial and reversible. Snow blindness from a superficial inflammation (photophthalmia) may have no warning symptoms. Irritation develops after a delay of hours, leading to extreme pain and photophobia. Severe cases may be disabling for several days and can result in corneal ulceration.

Sunglasses, ideally with sideshields, can prevent all forms of acute sun-related eye injuries. Sunglasses are especially important at elevations above 2,500 meters or when sun exposure is intensified by reflection from water or snow, or with prolonged exposure at sea level. Lenses must block at least 90% of ultraviolet radiation.

Mainstays of treatment are cold compresses, systemic analgesia, hourly use of topical steroid ointment or eye drops, and patching for the first 12–24 hours. Ophthalmologist follow-up is recommended.

DEHYDRATION

Acute volume depletion is an important and common wilderness emergency. Exercise, cold or heat, and high altitude may combine to create fluid replacement needs of five times normal maintenance levels. Cold and altitude exposure suppress thirst, and the wilderness setting often makes fluid consumption difficult. Even mild dehydration predisposes children to hypothermia, hyperthermia, excessive fatigue, and exacerbation of acute mountain sickness. To avoid dehydration, fluid intake and urine output must be monitored closely in children. If food is also eaten frequently, most hypotonic solutions, including water, are probably adequate. Ensure fluid intake every 1–2 hours during the day at high altitude, during substantial exertion, and in any extreme weather.

Treatment ■

Treatment of backwoods emergencies is often complex, and preparation is key (see section on Wilderness Planning and Rescue). Successful first aid may depend more on wilderness skills than sophisticated medical treatment. Improvisation, ingenuity, and resourcefulness are essential. *Above all, keep treatment simple, act conservatively, and never take unnecessary risks.*

Most mountain and hiking injuries occur in the afternoon or early evening, a time when fatigue may stress the entire party. In addition, heat equilibrium on mountain trips is often in delicate balance. Stopping a group in the wind or dampness can precipitate hypothermia. Hypoxia from altitude, stress, and cold may impair judgment.

With evacuation times of six or more hours in remote settings, survival is less likely. Among pediatric deaths in backwoods locations, free falls are the usual mechanism, with associated head injury (90% of

TABLE 101–4. *Clinical Spectrum of High-Altitude Illness*

Condition	Clinical Findings	Prevention/Treatment
Acute mountain sickness	Headache, worse in morning and with exercise; anorexia, nausea, insomnia, periorbital edema, retinal hemorrhage, oliguria, Cheyne-Stokes sleep breathing	Ascend 300 m/day above 2500 m Acetazolamide, 5–10 mg/kg/day divided b.i.d. Dexamethasone, 0.15 mg/kg/day divided q.i.d. Descend 300 m Rest, small meals, fluids
High-altitude pulmonary edema	Lassitude, fatigue, cough, worsening dyspnea Pink, frothy sputum Tachypnea, tachycardia, rales, low-grade fever	Acetazolamide, dexamethasone (as above) Descend immediately. Rest, oxygen NO NARCOTICS Diuresis may be dangerous In ED: intubation, PEEP, and ICU admission
High-altitude cerebral edema	Headache, lassitude in 24–48 hours; ataxia, altered mental status, papilledema; confusion, hallucinations, coma, death.	Descend immediately Oxygen Dexamethasone, 0.15 mg/kg/day In ED: head CT scan, tox screen

cases), lung injury (30%), and abdominal injury (40%, usually lacerations of the liver and spleen).

In the ED, evaluation and treatment are based on principles of care appropriate for major blunt trauma (see Trauma section). In most wilderness injuries, a lower threshold for admission to the hospital is indicated, especially when frostbite, inadequate nutrition, and wound management are presenting problems.

Wilderness Planning and Rescue ■

Preparing for backwoods activities is the key to preventing and treating wilderness emergencies. Anticipating likely problems permits a purposeful approach to untoward events. Appropriate anticipatory

TABLE 101–5. *Skin Types and Necessary Sunscreen Protection*

Skin Type	Sensitivity to UV	Sunburn History	SPF (Sun Protective Factor)
I	Very sensitive	Burns easily, never tans	15 or more
II	Very sensitive	Burns easily, tans minimally	15 or more
III	Sensitive	Burns moderately, tans gradually and uniformly	10 to 15
IV	Moderately sensitive	Burns minimally, tans well	6 to 10
V	Minimally sensitive	Rarely burns, tans profusely	4 to 6
VI	Insensitive	Never burns, black	none indicated

TABLE 101–6. *A Generic Wilderness Medical Kit*

The items listed here are not meant to be all-inclusive or necessary for every wilderness outing. Instead, this list is meant to serve as a starting point that will be modified according to the likely needs of the specific outing.

Medical guidebook or reference book
Pencil or pen with notepad
First-aid report forms
Flashlight (preferably waterproof)
Band-aids, assorted sizes
Butterfly bandages or Steri-Strips, assorted sizes
2" × 2" and 4" × 4" sterile gauze pads
Sterile eye patches
2" and 4" rolled gauze
2" and 4" elastic wraps
Otoscope
Ophthalmoscope
Moleskin or molefoam
Cravat cloth (triangular bandages)
2" rolls of adhesive tape
Large safety pins
#11 scalpel blades and handle
Paper clips and matches
Surgical forceps (tweezers)
Scissors
Thermometer (low-reading)
Finger splint
Tongue blades
Oral airway
Cotton swabs (Q-tips)
Sterile eyewash
Tincture of benzoin
Sunscreen (preferably with SPF of 10 or greater)
Insect repellent
Water disinfectant (e.g., Potable Aqua or 2% tincture of iodine)
Snakebite kit (elastic wrap, razor blade, suction cup)
#8 or #10 angiocaths (×2)
10 ml and 30 ml syringes
Disinfectant solution (e.g., povidine-iodine or benzalkonium chloride solution)
70% Isopropyl alcohol
5% Acetic acid solution (e.g., vinegar)
Adolph's Meat Tenderizer (unseasoned)
Powdered electrolyte mix (e.g., Gatorade)
Aspirin, 325-mg tablets
Acetaminophen, 325-mg tablets
Codeine, 15-mg or 30-mg tablets (with or without acetaminophen)
Antacid (e.g., Mylanta or Gaviscon)
Steroid cream (e.g., hydrocortisone 1% or triamcinolone 0.1%)
Polysporin or bacitracin ointment

Proparacaine eye drops
Antibiotic eye drops (e.g., sulfacetamide 10% or chloramphenicol 0.5%)
Cortisporin or VoSol otic solution
Decongestant-antihistamine combination tablets (e.g., Actifed or Drixoril)
Oxymetazoline (0.05%) decongestant spray
Sulfamethoxazole with trimethoprim, double-strength tablets
Dicloxacillin, 250-mg or 500-mg capsules
Tetracycline, 250-mg or 500-mg capsules
Cephalexin or other cephalosporin, 250-mg capsules
Ampicillin or amoxicillin, 250-mg capsules
Metronidazole, 250-mg tablets
Diphenhydramine, 25-mg tablets
Epinephrine with needle/syringe (e.g., Ana-kit or EpiPen)
Diazepam, 5-mg tablets
Antidiarrheal agent (e.g., diphenoxylate/atropine or loperamide tablets)
Prednisone, 10-mg tablets
Ibuprofen, 200-mg or 600-mg tablets
Antinauseant (e.g., prochlorperazine 5 mg or 10 mg, or promethazine, 25-mg tablets)
Acetazolamide, 250-mg tablets
Anti–motion sickness medication (e.g., Transderm Scop patches or meclizine, 25-mg tablets)
Antifungal cream (e.g., clotrimazole or zinc undecenoate cream)
Chloroquin

For Extended or Very Isolated Trips
Suture kit and sutures
Foley catheter
Nasogastric tube
Incision and drainage kit
Injectable morphine or meperidine
Chloramphenicol tablets
Injectable antibiotic (e.g., cefoxitin, gentamicin, or clindamycin)
Injectable xylocaine
Cimetidine or other H2 blocker
Oil of cloves
Stethoscope
Sphygmomanometer
Sterile lubricant jelly
Sterile gloves
Sterile needles and syringes

guidelines for the novice and the veteran back-woodsperson include:

1. Vaccinations and pharmacologic prophylaxis where indicated. Examples are tetanus boosters, chloroquine for malaria, gamma globulin for

hepatitis, and trimethoprim-sulfamethoxazole for diarrhea.

2. Dental fitness
3. Insect repellent
4. Water disinfectant

5. Appropriate footwear and protective clothing. Rain and cold often occur unexpectedly and pose major hazards.
6. Sunglasses
7. Physical conditioning. Cardiovascular and muscular fitness for wilderness activities helps prevent common overuse syndromes and fatigue-related accidents.
8. Experienced leadership. The leader must ensure that the outing does not exceed anyone's abilities.
9. Trip plan, including evacuation
10. Knowledge of endemic hazards
11. Notification of local authorities or a responsible party, when appropriate, about the complexity or duration of a trip. Information must include trip plan, number in party, duration of outing, and potential medical or environmental problems.
12. Wilderness medical kit. This vital piece of equipment should be tailored to the environment encountered, the background and medical training of group members, the size of the party, the duration of the outing, time and distance from sophisticated medical care, and any pre-existing medical problems. The suggested contents are listed in Table 101-6.

In addition to capable prospective organization, well-orchestrated field care and timely transport are keys to optimal treatment of serious wilderness emergencies. For all but minor medical maladies, it is prudent to promptly evacuate any ill or injured person. Delaying transport may allow the victim to deteriorate dangerously or may permit weather or other environmental conditions to change and hinder safe later evacuation. *A reliable evacuation plan must be determined before the trip begins.*

Helicopter rescue has become increasingly popular in the European Alps and parts of the United States, but the role of helicopter search and rescue in the wilderness is sometimes marginal and dangerous. Ground retrieval is often the most dependable and least risky method of evacuation, especially with small victims who are more easily carried.

Bibliography ■

Barbarh G: Management control of aeromedical evacuation systems. *Aviat Space Environ Med* 1988; 59:172–175.

Eitzen M: Arthropod envenomations in children. *Pediatr Emerg Care* 1988; 4:266–271.

Johnson T: Acute mountain sickness. *N Engl J Med* 1988; 319:841–845.

Kraus J: Morbidity and mortality from injuries in sports and recreation. *Annu Rev Public Health* 1984; 5:163–192.

Mallory S: Sunburn, sun reactions and sun protection. *Pediatr Ann* 1987; 16:77–84.

Noakes T: The danger of an inadequate water ingestion during prolonged exercise. *Eur J Appl Physiol* 1988; 57:210–219.

Paulson J: Epidemiology of injuries in adolescents. *Pediatr Ann* 1988; 17:84–96.

Sewell CM: Children's skiing injuries in Australia. *Med J Aust* 1987; 146:193–195.

Waller J: *Injury Control.* Boston: Lexington Books, 1985.

Wilkerson J, ed: *Medicine for Mountaineering.* Seattle: The Mountaineers, 1987.

Williamson J, ed: *Accidents in North American mountaineering.* New York: American Alpine Club, 1988.

X
Organ
System
Disorders

102 Metabolic and Electrolyte Disorders

Ronald A. Dieckmann

Acid-Base Disorders ■

Acid-base status is defined by serum pH, and is maintained within a very narrow range of normal (between 7.35 and 7.45). The relationship of pH and carbon dioxide tension (pCO_2), and serum bicarbonate (HCO_3^-) is established by the equations:

$$pH = pK + \frac{\sim HCO_3^- \text{ (Base)}}{H_2CO_3 \text{ (Acid)}}$$

$$H+ + HCO_3^- \leftrightarrow H_2CO_3 \leftrightarrow H_2O + CO_2$$

Acid-base disorders are of four types:

1. Respiratory acidosis
2. Respiratory alkalosis
3. Metabolic acidosis
4. Metabolic alkalosis

The pH, pCO_2, and HCO_3^- characteristics of these entities are shown in Table 102-1. Often, mixed acid-base disturbances occur. Serum pH can be rapidly altered through changes in *ventilation* and corresponding pCO_2. Serum pH is altered more slowly through *metabolic processes,* primarily renal HCO_3^- losses and H^+ production.

RESPIRATORY ACIDOSIS

Many diverse conditions can depress ventilation and increase pCO_2, by decreasing either the rate of respiration or the tidal volume. Respiratory acidosis is sometimes a sign of rapidly impending respiratory failure. Emergent therapy is required in the pre-arrest state to avert major complications or death. Chapter 14 presents the diagnosis and treatment of respiratory acidosis and respiratory failure.

RESPIRATORY ALKALOSIS

Respiratory alkalosis occurs when ventilation is increased and pCO_2 depressed. Serum pH can rise above 7.60, with pCO_2 <10 mm Hg. Clinical findings include paresthesias of the fingers, toes, and perioral region, muscle cramps, chest pain, dyspnea, and syncope. Occasionally, carpopedal spasms develop; rarely, seizures and cardiac dysrhythmias occur. The most common childhood conditions causing respiratory alkalosis are psychogenic hyperventilation syndrome, poisoning, and CNS disorders with central neurogenic hyperventilation. Common poisons are salicylates and sympathomimetic drugs.

Treatment is usually directed at the underlying disorder. In the patient with hyperventilation syndrome, specific measures to calm the child and to slow respirations are needed. Usually, gentle reassurance will suffice; rarely, pharmacologic sedation is necessary. Rebreathing into a paper bag has unproven value and may be dangerous. First, exclude other conditions causing tachypnea (e.g., DKA, hypoxia).

METABOLIC ACIDOSIS

Metabolic acidosis is the most common acid-base disorder. Underlying causes are legion (see Table 102-2); classification is usually based on the presence or absence of a calculated anion gap, as determined by the formula:

$$Na + K - (Cl + HCO_3) = \text{Anion Gap}$$

In children, a high anion gap (16 ± 4) indicates the presence of nonmeasured anions, especially sulfates, phosphates, lactates, or other organic anions. The most common conditions producing metabolic acidosis with a high anion gap are represented by the mnemonic SALAD (Salicylates, Alcohols, Lactic acidosis, Azotemia, and DKA).

Clinical findings in metabolic acidosis are usually those of the precipitating condition, but acidosis itself may be responsible for anorexia, vomiting, lethargy, and abdominal pain. Examination usually reveals

TABLE 102–1. *Laboratory Values in Acid-Base Disturbances*

	pH	pCO$_2$	HCO$_3^-$
Respiratory acidosis	↓	↑↑	↑
Respiratory alkalosis	↑	↓↓	↓
Metabolic acidosis	↓	↓	↓↓
Metabolic alkalosis	↑	↑	↑↑

Double arrows signify primary disturbance. Compensatory mechanisms may correct pH to near-normal. Mixed acid-base disturbances are common.

compensatory tachypnea and tachycardia, and sometimes fever.

Laboratory data are useful. Arterial blood gas measurements may show metabolic acidosis or a mixed acid-base picture (e.g., salicylism causes respiratory alkalosis and metabolic acidosis). Other laboratory tests include serum Na, K, Cl, CO$_2$, BUN, creatinine, glucose, and toxicology screen. Urine pH may be useful in suspected renal tubular acidosis. A frequent laboratory finding is mild hyperkalemia, due to intracellular and renal exchange of H$^+$ for K$^+$ ions.

Treatment of metabolic acidosis is controversial. Reversing the underlying pathophysiology is key. *Therapy with bicarbonate for metabolic acidosis has no proven benefit to outcome and may be hazardous* (see Chapter 6). Metabolic acidosis mediates a host of metabolic adjustments in disease that may ultimately preserve homeostasis. Bicarbonate may interfere with intrinsic homeostatic mechanisms and

TABLE 102–2. *Common Causes of Metabolic Acidosis*

High Anion Gap Acidosis
  Salicylates
  Alcohols (ethanol, methanol, isopropyl, ethylene, glycol)
  Lactate
    Hypovolemia
      Dehydration
      Hemorrhage
    Hypoxia
  Azotemia
  Diabetic ketoacidosis

Normal Anion Gap Acidosis
  Renal tubular acidosis
  Enteric losses through fistulas, enterostomies
  Drugs (amphotericin, acetazolamide, ammonium chloride)

create other metabolic derangements, including increased respiratory acidosis.

Therefore, give bicarbonate only with great caution, at low doses, and only in the child who is well ventilated and can blow off the increased carbon dioxide tension generated by bicarbonate.

Calcium Disorders ■

Chapter 103 presents diagnosis and treatment of hypocalcemia and hypercalcemia.

Glucose Disorders ■

Chapter 103 presents the diagnosis and treatment of hypoglycemia. Chapter 23 addressed hyperglycemia.

Sodium Disorders ■

Disorders of serum sodium are the most common childhood electrolyte disturbances. Usually, acute gastroenteritis and dehydration are responsible (see Chapter 22). Other etiologies for hyponatremia and hypernatremia are listed in Table 102-3.

HYPONATREMIA

Low serum sodium (Na <135 mEq/L) may reflect low, normal, or (rarely) increased body sodium, de-

TABLE 102–3. *Common Causes of Abnormalities in Serum Sodium*

Hyponatremia
  Hyperosmolality
  Dehydration
    Gastroenteritis
    Burns
  Water intoxication
  Medications
    Diuretics
    Antineoplastics
  Congestive heart failure
  Hepatic failure
  Acute renal failure
  Cystic fibrosis
  Syndrome of inappropriate antidiuretic hormone
  Mineralocorticoid deficiency

Hypernatremia
  Dehydration
    Gastroenteritis
    Increased insensible water losses
  Sodium poisoning
  Diabetes insipidus

pending on the water content of the extracellular space (ECS). Sodium loss usually occurs with water loss and contraction of the ECS, such as in gastroenteritis. However, absolute water gain and expansion of the ECS, without change in sodium (e.g., water intoxication), may cause hyponatremia. These are the most common causes of hyponatremia. Rarely, intrinsic regulatory systems controlling mineralocorticoids and antidiuretic hormone (ADH) go awry, and hyponatremia results (see Chapter 103).

Clinical findings in hyponatremia are determined by the rate and degree of decrease in serum sodium, but they are not well correlated with specific serum levels. Seizures and coma may occur with rapid sodium decreases, and shock may develop from accompanying losses of volume. When the fall in sodium concentration is slow (over days), signs and symptoms are less specific. Anorexia, nausea, cramps, and lethargy may be present, along with clinical signs of confusion, changes in respiratory pattern, myoclonus, and hyporeflexia.

Laboratory data guide the specific treatment, in concert with clinical assessment of overall volume status. Serum Na, K, Cl, CO_2, BUN, creatinine, glucose, osmolality, and urinalysis with urine Na and osmolality are helpful for differential diagnosis. Table 102-4 summarizes serum and urine sodium measurements in common hyponatremic conditions. *When hyperglycemia is present, serum sodium concentration is predictably decreased 1.6 mEq/L for every 100 mg% increase in glucose.*

TABLE 102–4. *Serum and Urinary Sodium Levels in Common Abnormalities of Serum Sodium*

Condition	Na Serum	Na Urine	Osm Serum	Osm Urine
Hyponatremia				
Hyperosmolality	↓	↓	↑	↑
Dehydration	↓	↓	↓	↑↑
Water intoxication	↓	↑	↓	↓↓
CHF	↓	↓	↓	↑
Acute renal failure	↓	↑	↓	↓↑
SIADH	↓	↓	↓	>Osm serum
Hypernatremia				
Dehydration	↑	↓	↑	↑↑
Na poisoning	↑	↑	↑	↑
Diabetes insipidus	↑	↓	↓	↓↓

Treatment

When ECS is contracted, immediate rehydration with parenteral isotonic saline and/or oral rehydration therapy is indicated. When ECS is normal or increased in hyponatremia, water restriction is the preferred treatment and is based on hydration status and calculated daily fluid and electrolyte requirements (see Chapter 22).

HYPERNATREMIA

High serum sodium (Na >145 mEq/L) may be present with low, normal, or increased body sodium, depending on ECS water volume. While numerous conditions can produce hypernatremia (Table 102-3), gastroenteritis and acute dehydration is the usual cause.

Clinical findings in hypernatremia are usually those of dehydration. Acute hypernatremia typically manifests early CNS changes (weakness and listlessness to seizures and coma). Circulatory insufficiency in hypernatremia occurs later than with similar degrees of volume loss in hyponatremia.

Laboratory evaluation may help distinguish less common etiologies and guide specific therapy.

Treatment

As with hyponatremia, initial treatment is determined by clinical assessment of volume status. When ECS is contracted, begin isotonic saline rehydration at 10–20 ml/kg bolus, then change to oral rehydration and hypotonic rehydration (usually $D_5\frac{1}{2}NS$) to reduce serum sodium 10–15 mEq/L/day, over 48 hours. Too-vigorous sodium reduction can result in brain edema and CNS hemorrhage (Chapter 22). When ECS is normal or increased, measure both serum and urine sodium and osmolality to assist differential diagnosis (Table 102-5). In most cases, parenteral administration of D_5W, without added sodium, is the mainstay of treatment.

Potassium Disorders ■

HYPOKALEMIA

Low serum potassium (K <3.5 mEq/L) is an uncommon pediatric emergency. Usually, hypokalemia is secondary to metabolic alkalosis, and intracellular buffering of K^+ ions in the ECS with H^+ from the intracellular space (ICS). Interpretation of serum potassium must include evaluation of acid-base status. *A 0.1 change in pH causes a 0.6 mEq/L alteration in serum potassium.* Most body potassium is in the

TABLE 102–5. *Common Causes of Abnormalities in Serum Potassium*

Hypokalemia
Alkalosis
Sustained vomiting
Diarrhea and dehydration
Cystic fibrosis
Diuretics
Renal tubular acidosis
Diabetic ketoacidosis
Mineralocorticoid excess

Hyperkalemia
Laboratory error
Acidosis
Renal failure
Potassium poisoning
Rhabdomyolysis
Mineralocorticoid deficiency

ICS, where concentrations are 150 mEq/L, compared to ECS concentrations of only 3.5–5 mEq/L. While serum levels do not reflect body potassium, rapid changes in serum potassium may have major effects on membrane potentials and cardiac conductivity. Also, normal serum potassium levels may be present in conditions with severe ICS potassium depletion (e.g., DKA and profound dehydration).

Clinical findings in hypokalemia occur at levels <3.0 mEq/L. Muscle weakness, abdominal distention, and ileus may occur. More severe levels of hypokalemia produce paralysis, hyporeflexia, rhabdomyolysis, and cardiac dysrhythmias. A particularly dangerous hypokalemic state develops when a digitalized child has low serum potassium; the hypokalemia places the child at increased risk for drug toxicity.

Laboratory evaluation of hypokalemia includes serum Na, KCl, CO_2, glucose, BUN, and creatinine. Sometimes arterial blood gases and urine Cl and K are needed to establish a specific diagnosis. Urine findings can often distinguish hypochloremia (Cl urine <10 mEq/L), mineralocorticoid excess (Cl urine >20 mEq/L), and renal potassium wasting (K urine >20 mEq/L). ECG findings in hypokalemia include depressed ST segments, decreased T waves, and increased U waves, but are not closely tied to serum levels.

Treatment is directed at the underlying etiology. Often, this involves only the correction of alkalosis. Parenteral potassium replacement must be done slowly and cautiously, at rates no greater than 0.25 mEq/kg/hour, to avert the harmful effects on myocardial conduction. An ECG monitor is imperative. Higher rates may require a central venous catheter,

and administration is best accomplished in the intensive care unit. Estimated deficits in potassium are most safely replaced over a 48-hour period, emphasizing the oral route when possible. Extravasation of potassium solutions subcutaneously is extremely painful. Occasionally, peripheral IV administration is painful, requiring reduction in flow rates, a second IV, or central administration.

HYPERKALEMIA

Hyperkalemia (serum K >5.0 mEq/L) usually develops as a secondary effect of metabolic acidosis, or because of acute renal failure or potassium poisoning. Other etiologies may occur (Table 102-5). Sometimes, reported hyperkalemia is factitious, caused by hemolysis of the blood specimen.

Clinical findings are neuromuscular, with paresthesias, weakness, and paralysis. The most dreaded complication of hyperkalemia is cardiac toxicity. ECG manifestations parallel rising potassium levels: peaked T waves, widening QRS complex, and increasing PR interval develop first, progressing to heart block, ventricular tachycardia, and ventricular fibrillation (see Figure 102-1).

Treatment for hyperkalemia is based on the clinical condition and ECG features:

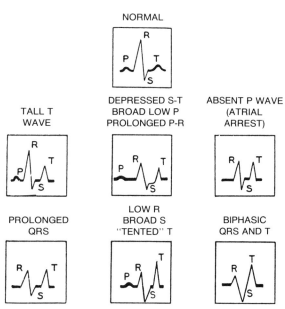

FIGURE 102–1. Effect of high serum potassium on the ECG. (Reprinted with permission. Lipman BS, Dunn M, Massie E: *Clinical Electrocardiography.* Chicago: Year Book Medical Publishers, Inc., 1984:271)

TABLE 102–6. *Treatment of Hyperkalemia*

Intervention	Dose	Route	Onset of Action	Duration of Effect	Comment
Calcium chloride, 10%	50 mg/kg	Slow IV	Immediate	1 hour	Reverses membrane toxicity
Sodium bicarbonate, 8.4%	2–3 mEq/kg	IV	Minutes	15–30 minutes	Buffers K intracellularly
Dextrose $D_{50}W$ (>2 yr) $D_{25}W$ (<2 yr)	1 ml/kg 2 ml/kg	IV	Minutes	1 hour	Facilitates intracellular K transport
Insulin	1 unit of regular insulin per 5 g dextrose	IV	Minutes	1 hour	Use after dextrose to augment intracellular K transport.
Sodium polystyrene sodium (Kayexalate)	1 g/kg 1.5–2 g/kg	PO PR	1–2 hours	2–4 hours	Cation exchange resin. Use laxative with PO form. PR form needs 30–45 min retention time.
Dialysis		Peritoneal dialysis Hemodialysis	Variable Immediate	Variable Variable	Indicated with renal failure and severe hyperkalemia

1. If serum K is <6.5 mEq/L, the patient is asymptomatic, and the ECG shows only peaked T waves, remove all potassium and correct the underlying cause.
2. If serum K is >7.0 mEq/L and the ECG shows prolonged conduction intervals, treat with dextrose, insulin, and sodium bicarbonate, plus Kayexalate.
3. If serum K is >8.0 mEq/L, or cardiac dysrhythmias are present, initiate treatment with calcium, dextrose, insulin, and sodium bicarbonate while arranging for ICU admission or immediate dialysis. Add Kayexalate after parenteral treatments.

Table 102-6 presents specific drugs, doses, onset of action, and duration of essential treatment modalities in severe hyperkalemia.

Bibliography ■

Finberg L: Treatment of dehydration in infancy. *Pediatr Rev* 1981;3:113–116.

Guskin AB, Baluarte HJ, Prebis JW, et al: Serum sodium abnormalities in children. *Pediatr Clin North Am* 1982; 29:907–932.

Levine MM, Pizarro D: Advances in therapy of diarrheal dehydration. *Adv Pediatr* 1984; 31:207.

103 Endocrine Disorders

Felix A. Conte and Melvin M. Grumbach

Adrenal Insufficiency ■

Acute adrenocortical insufficiency can be a life-threatening endocrine emergency. It usually results from a combined deficiency of both aldosterone and cortisol; an isolated deficiency of glucocorticoid or mineralocorticoid is rare.

PATHOPHYSIOLOGY

The physiologic secretion of cortisol is modulated by adrenocorticotropic hormone (ACTH) secreted by the pituitary gland. The pituitary gland is stimulated by corticotropin-releasing factor (CRF) secreted by the hypothalamus. The secretion of both CRF and ACTH is regulated by the concentration of plasma cortisol; in addition, a variety of neural stimuli, neuropeptides, and biogenic amines influence CRF release.

Recent data in prepubertal children indicate that the adrenal gland secretes about 9 mg (± 2.3 mg) of cortisol/m² of body surface area per day. Cortisol is secreted episodically and exhibits diurnal variation (highest in the morning and lowest in the evening). In response to stress, fever, anesthesia, and trauma, cortisol secretion increases to 3–15 times (30–140 mg/m² of body surface area per day). Among its many other actions, cortisol stimulates gluconeogenesis, thus helping to maintain glucose homeostasis. It is also critical to the maintenance of vascular tone.

Aldosterone is the other major hormone secreted by the adrenal gland. Its secretion is modulated by the renin-angiotensin system in response to hyponatremia, hyperkalemia, and volume depletion. Aldosterone stimulates the reabsorption of sodium from the proximal convoluted tubule while promoting the excretion of potassium.

Doses of cortisol or its equivalent exceeding 15 mg/m²/day parenterally, or 25 mg/m²/day orally when given in divided doses around the clock for more than 10–14 days, invariably result in inhibition of ACTH secretion and, as a consequence, adrenal suppression. The degree of suppression of cortisol secretion is a function of the dose of glucocorticoid given, its biologic activity, and its half-life, as well as the timing, route, and the duration of therapy (Table 103-1). Abnormalities at the level of the hypothalamus, pituitary gland, or adrenal gland can result in adrenal insufficiency.

CLINICAL FINDINGS

Acute adrenal insufficiency should be suspected in the child presenting with a history of vomiting leading to progressive dehydration, hypoglycemia, and vascular collapse. Increased pigmentation involving the buccal mucosa, gums, flexor surfaces, or areas exposed to sunlight in older children, or the genital region in infants, may be a clinical clue to increased ACTH and, consequently, melanin production. In infancy, ambiguous male genitalia or an apparent male with nonpalpable gonads with the above clinical picture would suggest acute adrenal insufficiency secondary to a salt-losing form of congenital adrenal hyperplasia.

The biochemical hallmarks of acute adrenal insufficiency are hypoglycemia, hyponatremia, hyperkalemia, and metabolic acidosis. In contrast, patients with "pure" cortisol deficiency manifest weakness, fatigue, hypotension, and hypoglycemia; plasma electrolytes are usually normal, although hyponatremia with normal potassium levels can occur secondary to the absence of the permissive effect of cortisol on free water clearance.

In the older child, adrenal insufficiency is characterized by a progressive, insidious increase in the pigmentation of the skin at the flexor surfaces or in areas exposed to sun, as well as at the line between the gums and the teeth. Patients complain of fatigue and weakness, postural hypotension, salt craving, nausea, vomiting, diarrhea, and progressive weight loss. Alopecia and monilial lesions affecting the skin and nails may be found in autoimmune Addison's disease. Progressive depletion of adrenal reserve or stress may finally result in acute adrenal insufficiency in these patients. The differential diagnosis is presented in Tables 103-2 and 103-3.

TABLE 103–1. *Steroids Used in Treatment of Endocrine Emergencies*

Glucocorticoid Equivalents (Anti-inflammatory)

Cortisone	25
Hydrocortisone	20
Prednisone	5
Methyl-predniolone	4
Dexamethasone	0.7

Mineralocorticoids
0.1 mg of 9-α-fluorohydrocortisone = 2.5 mg of DOCA*

Time Taken to Achieve Maximal Plasma Cortisol Levels

Cortisone acetate	Oral: 2 hr
	IM: 18–24 hr
Hydrocortisone sodium succinate (Solu-Cortef)	IM: 30 min–2 hr
	IV: Immediate

Plasma Half-life of Various Steroids

Cortisone†	30
Cortisol	90
Prednisone†	60
Prednisolone	200
Dexamethasone	200

Relative Mineralocorticoid Activity of Adrenal Steroids as DOCA Equivalents

DOCA‡	1
Hydrocortisone	20
Cortisone	20
Prednisone	50
Prednisolone	50
Dexamethasone	

* DOCA onset of action—2 hr (currently not available)
† Cortisone and prednisone are both metabolically inactive and are converted to cortisol and prednisolone by the liver
‡ DOCA duration of action up to 24 hr; average, 16 hr

DIAGNOSIS

Rely on the signs and symptoms, as noted above. Serum electrolytes will reveal hypoglycemia, hyponatremia, hyperkalemia, metabolic acidosis, and azotemia, except in patients with isolated cortisol deficiency (where only hypoglycemia may be present) or isolated mineralocorticoid deficiency (where only the electrolyte abnormalities may be present). The concentration of plasma cortisol is low, and ACTH and renin levels are elevated. The plasma 17-hydroxyprogesterone level is >1,000–2,000 ng/dl in patients with congenital adrenal hyperplasia due to 21-hydroxylase deficiency. In patients with hyper-

TABLE 103–2. *Differential Diagnosis of Acute Adrenal Insufficiency in Infancy*

Congenital adrenal hyperplasia
Hemorrhage into the adrenals
Congenital adrenal hypoplasia
Isolated cortisol deficiency/hypopituitarism
Congenital unresponsiveness to ACTH
Isolated salt loss/pseudohypoaldosteronism (end organ resistance to aldosterone)
Biosynthetic errors in aldosterone metabolism

kalemia, an ECG may reveal high peaked T waves and/or an arrhythmia. A chest X-ray may reveal a small heart, an enlarged thymic shadow, and/or calcified adrenal glands.

TREATMENT

1. Give oxygen if necessary.
2. Give hydrocortisone sodium succinate 50–100 mg/m² by rapid IV push. If there is no response (improved perfusion, blood pressure, etc.), the dose may be repeated. Thereafter, add 50–100 mg/m²/day of hydrocortisone sodium succinate to the infusion (may also be given in divided 6-hour bolus doses).

TABLE 103–3. *Differential Diagnosis of Acute Adrenal Insufficiency in Childhood and Adolescence*

Autoimmune adrenalitis (may be associated with diabetes mellitus, oophoritis, hypoparathyroidism, hypothyroidism, pernicious anemia, malabsorption, chronic active hepatitis, vitiligo, alopecia, or mucocutaneous candidiasis)
Congenital adrenal hyperplasia
Adrenoleukodystrophy (bronze Schilder's disease)
Congenital adrenal hypoplasia
Infection—tuberculosis
Hemorrhage into the adrenals (Waterhouse-Friderichsen syndrome)
Neoplasia
Isolated cortisol deficiency/hypopituitarism
    Idiopathic
    Secondary to a suprasellar mass lesion and its therapy
    Secondary to an inherited disease or anomaly (i.e., septo-optic dysplasia, midline defect, etc.)
Congenital unresponsiveness to ACTH
Secondary to iatrogenic suppression of adrenal function by pharmacologic glucocorticoid therapy

3. Treat hypoglycemia, if present. Give 1–2 ml (0.25–0.5 g)/kg of 25% glucose IV (maximum dose, 25 g) and continue glucose infusion to maintain normoglycemia (4–8 mg/kg/min).
4. Infuse normal saline IV to expand volume and correct hypotension (20 ml/kg in first hour). Thereafter, adjust the rate for correction of sodium, water deficit, and maintenance. If the child is not severely volume-depleted and does not require acute volume expansion, use 5% glucose in normal saline in physiologic amounts.
5. If symptomatic (arrhythmia) hyperkalemia is present, follow the acute treatment guidelines presented in Chapter 102.
6. If the blood pressure does not respond to fluids and cortisol, pressor agents may be necessary.
7. Admit the child for inpatient evaluation and further treatment.

Hypocalcemia ■

Hypocalcemia is a concentration of serum calcium of less than 8 mg/dl (7 mg/dl for preterm infants) during the first few days of life. Thereafter, levels of less than 8.5 mg/dl are uncommon in normal children.

PATHOPHYSIOLOGY

Normal serum calcium ranges from 8.5–10.5 mg/dl (4.5–5.5 mEq/L). About 47% of serum calcium is protein bound, primarily to albumin. Protein-bound calcium is physiologically inactive. Ionized calcium has an action on membrane permeability, neuromuscular function, and bone metabolism. The serum calcium is regulated by the vitamin D endocrine system. A decline in ionized calcium stimulates parathyroid hormone secretion. Parathyroid hormone along with vitamin D increases calcium absorption in the intestine and works with parathyroid hormone to increase calcium release from bone into blood. Parathyroid hormone also acts to increase phosphate excretion and reduce calcium loss by the tubules.

Magnesium has a permissive effect on parathyroid secretion; hence, hypomagnesemia results in decreased parathyroid hormone secretion. Calcitonin, a hormone secreted by cells in the thyroid gland, acts to diminish bone reabsorption and calcium release and hence to lower serum calcium. The neonate is particularly predisposed to hypocalcemia, due to the limited secretory capacity of the parathyroid gland during this period, as well as diminished renal responsiveness and elevated calcitonin levels. *In childhood, a deficiency of vitamin D, either because of decreased intake, hepatocellular disorders and fat malabsorption, or an inherited abnormality in vitamin D metabolism or action, can result in hypocalcemia and rickets.* Defects in parathyroid hormone secretion, metabolism, and action also cause hypocalcemia in infancy and childhood.

CLINICAL FINDINGS

The clinical symptoms of hypocalcemia are due to neuromuscular instability. In infancy, tetany as manifested by twitching, tremors, and frank convulsions. Also seen are lethargy, weakness, laryngospasm, and rarely carpopedal spasm. Chvostek's sign (facial contraction on tapping the facial nerve near the angle of the jaw) may be elicited in normal newborns, and hence is nondiagnostic. Prematurity, asphyxia, maternal diabetes, or maternal hyperparathyroidism increase the risk of neonatal hypocalcemia.

All infants with congenital heart disease involving the aortic arch (DiGeorge syndrome) and those with renal disease should be screened and followed closely for hypocalcemia. In the older child, hypocalcemia may manifest with muscle cramps, weakness, lethargy, listlessness, apathy, paresthesias (tingling) of the fingers and toes, personality changes, carpopedal spasm, laryngospasm, and convulsions. If hypocalcemia is chronic, diarrhea, malabsorption, keratitis, and lenticular opacities, as well as poor enamel formation of the teeth, may be observed.

Patients with chronic mucocutaneous candidiasis should be screened for hypocalcemia secondary to autoimmune hypoparathyroidism. Patients with pseudohypoparathyroidism manifest with bradymetacarpal dwarfism, mental retardation, and cutaneous calcifications. Patients with rickets have widening of the ends of long bones or prominence of the costochondral junctions of the ribs (rachitic rosary) on physical examination.

The signs of hypocalcemia are the Chvostek sign, the Trousseau sign (inflating a cuff to 15 mm Hg or more above the systolic blood pressure for 1–2 minutes results in carpal spasm), and the peroneal sign (tapping the peroneal nerve leads to plantar flexion of that foot). The differential diagnosis of hypocalcemia is presented in Tables 103-4 and 103-5.

ANCILLARY DATA

In infancy, a calcium level <8 mg/dl in full-term infants and 7 mg/dl in premature infants is diagnostic of hypocalcemia. Obtain electrolytes, BUN, phosphate, alkaline phosphatase, pH, 25(OH)D, 1,25(OH)$_2$D, and parathyroid hormone levels to determine the etiology of the hypocalcemia, as well as a CBC including a total lymphocyte count, and immunologic function studies to rule out DiGeorge

---

TABLE 103–4. *Differential Diagnosis of Hypocalcemia in Infancy*

Prematurity or asphyxia
Maternal diabetes
Congenital heart disease, absent parathyroid glands, and thymic hypoplasia (DiGeorge's syndrome)
Maternal hyperparathyroidism
Idiopathic hypoparathyroidism (transient or permanent)
Vitamin D deficiency or dependency (rickets)
Renal disease
Furosemide therapy
Citrate administration during exchange transfusion
Hypomagnesemia
Hypoproteinemia (total serum calcium decreased but not ionized fraction)

---

syndrome. An ECG may show prolongation of the QT interval and, in rare instances, partial heart block. In the patient with congenital heart disease, a chest X-ray will determine if the thymus is present.

In the child with hypoparathyroidism, the calcium level is usually <8 mg/dl and the phosphorus >7 mg/dl. Alkaline phosphatase levels are normal, as are BUN, creatinine, magnesium, urinalysis, electrolytes, pH, and serum proteins. The parathyroid hormone levels are low in relation to the serum calcium level.

In patients with rickets and hypocalcemia, the phosphorus level, while usually low, may be normal; however, alkaline phosphatase levels are markedly elevated, 25-hydroxy-vitamin D levels are low (except in inherited forms of rickets), and roentgenograms of long bones demonstrate the classic metaphyseal changes of rickets.

TABLE 103–5. *Differential Diagnosis of Hypocalcemia in Childhood*

Idiopathic hypoparathyroidism (may be associated with Addison's disease and candidiasis)
Post-thyroidectomy (usually transient unless the parathyroid glands have been removed or damaged)
Pseudohypoparathyroidism
Rickets (early phase)
Chronic renal failure
Malabsorption (celiac disease, sprue, pancreatic insufficiency, biliary atresia, regional enteritis)
Fleet enema retention (phosphate levels markedly elevated)
Renal tubular acidosis
Hypomagnesemia
Respiratory or metabolic alkalosis (total serum calcium normal but ionized fraction decreased)
Hypoproteinemia

Patients with pseudohypoparathyroidism have hypocalcemic tetany, basal ganglia calcification, hyperphosphatemia, and high parathyroid hormone levels. They also may have a typical phenotype (short stature, obesity, round facies, short 4th and 5th metacarpals and metatarsals, and subcutaneous calcifications).

TREATMENT OF NEONATAL TETANY OR HYPOCALCEMIC SEIZURES

1. The usual dose of 10% calcium gluconate is 1 ml/kg. Dilute the 10% calcium gluconate and administer IV very slowly (less than 1 ml/min).
2. Monitor the effects of the infusion constantly by ECG or stethoscope. Discontinue the infusion if bradycardia ensues.
3. Discontinue the calcium infusion when seizures are terminated (usually after 1–3 ml).
4. Toxic reactions may be avoided if the maximum dose does not exceed 2 ml/kg of 10% calcium gluconate at one time.
5. If necessary, IV calcium may be repeated 3 or 4 times in 24 hours to control seizures.
6. After seizures are controlled, add calcium to the infant's formula so that the calcium-to-phosphorus ratio in the formula is 4:1. Each gram of calcium gluconate contains 90 mg of elemental calcium; thus, 4 g of 10% calcium gluconate *or* 1 g of calcium carbonate (40% calcium by weight) should be added to one liter of Similac 60/40 PM (Ca/P content 400 mg/200 mg), a low-phosphate formula. Monitor serum calcium and phosphate closely. Adjust the calcium supplement to maintain the serum calcium and phosphorus in the normal range.
7. Infants who cannot be treated by oral calcium administration may be treated with repetitive bolus injections of calcium as needed, or by continuous IV infusion. In neonates, doses of 2–5 ml/kg (18–45 mg/kg) of 10% calcium gluconate per 24 hours have been given in the 24-hour infusion. Use a continuous cardiac monitor and evaluate calcium twice daily to avoid inadequate or too-vigorous calcium therapy. Label the IV tubing with calcium to prevent admixture with incompatible solutions (bicarbonate and phosphate) or inadvertent escalation of the infusion rate. Calcium infusion can cause necrosis of the liver if given via an umbilical vein into the portal system. Whenever possible, treatment of hypocalcemia in neonates should consist of orally administered calcium gluconate in addition to a low-phosphate formula.
8. Use extreme caution when giving calcium to patients on digitalis or those who are hypokalemic.
9. Suspect hypomagnesemic tetany in patients with

tetany in the absence of hypocalcemia, or if symptoms are not relieved by appropriate amounts of calcium. The normal magnesium level varies from a mean of 1.5 mEq/L in premature infants to a mean of 2 mEq/L in adults. Suspect acute hypomagnesemic tetany in patients whose magnesium levels are below 1.3 mEq/L in the neonatal period or 1.6 mEq/L thereafter. This can be treated initially with an IM injection of magnesium sulfate (0.1 ml/kg of a 50% solution of $MgSO_4$). Determine serum magnesium levels every 12 hours to monitor the need for further therapy. For chronic therapy, use oral magnesium in divided doses as magnesium chloride, or citrate or lactate (2–4 mEq/mg/kg/day) in divided doses to a maximum of 1 g mg/day.

TREATMENT OF HYPOCALCEMIA DUE TO HYPOPARATHYROIDISM IN CHILDHOOD

1. Tetany or seizures are an indication for IV calcium administration. Dilute a 10% solution of calcium gluconate and give *slowly* with ECG monitoring. Discontinue the IV injection when the tetany or seizures stop. The usual dose is 1 ml/kg of 10% calcium gluconate, to a maximum of 20 ml.

2. In children and adolescents, vitamin D therapy will usually prevent the recurrence of tetanic symptoms or convulsions, even though the concentration of serum calcium may still be below normal. If the patient has recurrent tetanic or convulsive episodes during the initial phase of therapy, give repetitive bolus doses of 10% calcium gluconate slowly.

3. Hypoparathyroidism and pseudohypoparathyroidism require treatment with vitamin D. Use a loading dose of 5,000–10,000 U/kg/day for 3–7 days to initiate a rise in calcium. Monitor the serum calcium daily, and when the calcium level rises to 8 mg/dl, cut the dose of vitamin D back to a maintenance dose of 1,000–2,000 U/kg/day and titrate to maintain the calcium level between 8–9 mg/dl.

4. Crystalline dihydrotachysterol may be used in place of vitamin D. It has a more rapid onset of action and a shorter half-life (50 hours). One milligram of dihydrotachysterol has at least the equivalent effect of 3 mg of vitamin D (1 mg of vitamin D = 40,000 U).

5. Oral calcium supplements may be useful early in the therapy for hypocalcemia, especially since the effects of vitamin D may be delayed for several days. Doses of elemental calcium of 20–50 mg/kg (maximum, 1 g/day) can be given in three to four divided doses per day.

6. Use aluminum hydroxide gel or preferably calcium carbonate to lower the phosphate levels in the initial stages of therapy.

7. Refer the child to his primary care provider or a pediatric endocrinologist for continued therapy.

Hypoglycemia ■

Hypoglycemia is a plasma glucose level <45 mg/dl in an infant or child, regardless of whether symptoms are present. A plasma glucose level <25 mg/dl in premature and small-for-date infants for the first 72 hours, and 35 mg/dl in term infants defines hypoglycemia. Whole blood glucose levels are 15% lower than plasma or serum levels, and venous blood has a glucose concentration 10% lower than capillary blood. Specimens collected in tubes without fluoride will undergo glycolysis, which will lower the glucose significantly on a time-dependent basis.

PATHOPHYSIOLOGY

The level of glucose in the blood is a function of intake, gluconeogenesis, glycogenolysis, and utilization. Glucose production and utilization is higher in infants (5–7 mg/kg/min) than in adults. Furthermore, the brain, whose primary metabolic fuel is glucose, represents one-third to one-sixth of the total body weight in infants. *Hence, an abnormality in production or utilization of glucose manifests more readily in infancy or childhood than in adults.*

CLINICAL FINDINGS

The prompt diagnosis and treatment of hypoglycemia is critical, since hypoglycemia, especially in infants, can cause irreparable brain damage. The symptoms of hypoglycemia are related to either epinephrine secretion (i.e., sweating, pallor, tachycardia) or manifestations of neuroglycopenia such as seizures and coma. In the neonate, symptoms may be less specific and may include tremors, cyanosis, apnea or irregular respirations, lethargy, apathy, limpness, refusal to eat, eye rolling or crossing, a high-pitched cry, congestive heart failure, and seizures of any type.

Transient hypoglycemia in the first few days of life is commonly seen in low-birth-weight infants, the smaller of twins, and infants born to toxemic mothers. Infants born to mothers with gestational or frank diabetes mellitus may develop beta cell hyperplasia in utero secondary to elevated blood glucose levels during gestation. Post-delivery, hyperinsulinism may result in transient or prolonged hypoglycemia. Infants with CNS disorders such as hemorrhage or infection, those with severe erythroblastosis, and those with sepsis or severe asphyxia are also at risk for transient hypoglycemia.

TABLE 103–6. *Differential Diagnosis of Hypoglycemia in Infancy*

Hormone Deficiencies
  Isolated growth hormone deficiency
  Hypopituitarism (may be associated with microphallus, midline defects, hepatomegaly with an elevation in conjugated bilirubin and transaminases, and optic nerve hypoplasia)
  Cortisol deficiency due to congenital adrenal hypoplasia, hyperplasia, or ACTH unresponsiveness

Hyperinsulinism
  Beta cell hyperplasia
  Nesidioblastosis
  Islet cell adenoma
  Beckwith syndrome
  Autoimmune hypoglycemia

Hereditary Defects in Carbohydrate, Amino Acid, and Fatty Acid Metabolism
  Glycogen storage disease, Types I and III
  Glycogen synthetase deficiency
  Fructose-1, 6-diphosphate deficiency
  Pyruvate carboxylase deficiency
  Phosphoenolpyruvate carboxykinase (PEPCK) deficiency
  Galactosemia
  Maple syrup urine disease
  Methylmalonic acidemia
  Carnitine deficiency

Persistent or recurrent hypoglycemia in the neonatal period suggests an abnormality in the secretion of a glucoregulatory hormone or a hereditary defect in carbohydrate, amino acid, or fat metabolism (Table 103-6). After infancy, consider other causes of hypoglycemia (Table 103-7).

The history should include details of the pregnancy and neonatal status, the age of onset of symptoms, and the relationship to meals and periods of starvation or illness. Morning hypoglycemia in a growth-retarded child or one with a midline defect (i.e., cleft lip or palate, optic hypoplasia, or microphallus) suggests hypopituitarism (including growth hormone

TABLE 103–7. *Other Causes of Hypoglycemia in Toddlers and Children*

Ketotic hypoglycemia (accelerated starvation)
Drug-induced hypoglycemia (ethyl alcohol, salicylates, oral hypoglycemic agents, propranolol)
Reye's syndrome
Hepatitis
Leucine sensitivity (a form of hyperinsulinism)
Insulin overdose

and/or ACTH deficiency) as an etiology for the hypoglycemia. Marked hepatomegaly suggests an abnormality in glycogen metabolism, although hepatomegaly can be found in patients with hyperinsulinism as well as patients with hypopituitarism. The presence of ketones in the urine militates against the diagnosis of hyperinsulinism and suggests the possibility of either a hormone deficiency, an enzymatic defect in gluconeogenesis or glycogenolysis, or the diagnosis of accelerated starvation.

Obtain a 24-hour glucose profile on a patient with suspected hypoglycemia. With a documented spontaneous hypoglycemic episode, obtain plasma insulin, cortisol, growth hormone, blood gas (metabolic acidosis), lactate, and pyruvate, as well as urinary ketones and organic acids. These laboratory determinations will help to ascertain the etiology of the hypoglycemia quickly. In particular, a plasma insulin level >12 μU/ml in the face of a glucose concentration <40 mg% or a ratio of glucose:insulin <3:1 is diagnostic of hyperinsulinism. Growth hormone levels rise in response to hypoglycemia and are normally high in the neonatal period, so that growth hormone levels <7–10 ng/ml associated with hypoglycemia are strongly suggestive of deficiency. Likewise, cortisol levels increase with hypoglycemia, so that a low cortisol level is highly suggestive of ACTH or adrenal insufficiency. Elevated lactate and pyruvate levels may be found in patients with hereditary defects in gluconeogenesis.

TREATMENT

Neonates

In high-risk neonates, monitor blood glucose every 2 hours for the first 12 hours of life, then every 6 hours for up to 48 hours. In the clinically asymptomatic neonate, treat a low plasma glucose immediately with a feeding of 10% glucose followed by repeat glucose determinations. If the plasma glucose does not stabilize above 45 mg% or if the infant becomes symptomatic, IV glucose therapy is indicated.

Give 1–2 ml (0.25–0.5 g/kg) per kg of 25% glucose over 2–4 minutes, preferably in a peripheral vein. Follow the initial bolus of glucose with an infusion of 6–10 mg/kg/min of glucose. Adjust the rate and concentration of glucose in the infusion to maintain the glucose >45 mg/dl and <120 mg/dl. Add sodium (3 mEq/100 Kcal) and potassium (1–2 mEq per 100/Kcal) to the daily infusion to prevent electrolyte imbalances. When the glucose level stabilizes above 45 mg% for 24–48 hours, the rate of infusion may be gradually reduced over the next 24–48 hours, while plasma glucose levels are maintained. Oral feedings are given as tolerated.

Suspect hyperinsulinism in patients who require >12 mg/kg/min of glucose to raise and sustain the glucose level >45 mg%. If the glucose levels cannot be sustained or stabilized >45 ng% despite vigorous IV glucose therapy because of hyperinsulinism, diazoxide 5–15 mg/kg/day by mouth in 3 divided doses may need to be instituted.

Toddlers and Older Children

As in the neonate, first draw a plasma sample for glucose, insulin, growth hormone, cortisol, lactate, and ketone bodies. Always obtain the first urine for ketone bodies. Then give 1–2 ml (0.25 g/kg to 0.5 g/kg) of 25% glucose IV (maximum total dose, 25 g). Thereafter, maintain the patient on an infusion of 10% glucose in 0.25% normal saline at a rate sufficient to maintain the blood glucose level between 45–120 mg/dl, and compatible with the child's fluid requirements. If there is no immediate therapeutic response to parenteral glucose (i.e., cessation of seizure activity and/or arousal from coma), consider giving cortisol 50–100 mg/m^2 by IV push. If no response ensues thereafter, it would suggest that the hypoglycemia is a secondary phenomenon or that severe hypoglycemia has resulted in cerebral edema.

After the patient is stabilized, the etiology of the hypoglycemic episode must be sought to effectively treat and prevent recurrence.

When an IV line cannot be established rapidly in a hypoglycemic patient with altered mental status (e.g., seizures, coma), use glucagon 0.03–0.1 mg kg (not to exceed 1 mg) IM for *temporary* elevation in serum glucose. Start IV glucose as soon as feasible.

Bibliography ■

Aynsley-Green A: Hypoglycemia in infants and children. *Baillieres Clin Endocrinol Metab* 1982; 2:1.

Aynsley-Green A, Soltesz G: Hypoglycemia in infancy and childhood. In: *Current reviews in paediatrics,* vol. 1. Edinburgh: Churchill-Livingstone, 1985.

Burke CW. Adrenocortical insufficiency. *Baillieres Clin Endocrinol Metab* 1985; 14:4.

Chamberlin P, Meyer WJ III: Management of pituitary-adrenal suppression secondary to corticosteroid therapy. *Pediatrics* 1981; 67:245.

Heymond MW: Hypoglycemia in infants and children. *Endocrinol Metab Clin North Am* 1989; 18:211–253.

LaFranchi S: Hypoglycemia of infancy and childhood. *Pediatr Clin North Am* 1987; 34:961.

Sönksen PH, Lowy C. Endocrine and metabolic emergencies. *Baillieres Clin Endocrinol Metab* 1980; 9:435–639.

Stanley CA, Baker L: Hyperinsulinism in infants and children: Diagnosis and therapy. *Adv Pediatr* 1976; 32:315.

Styne DM: *Pediatric endocrinology for the house officer.* Baltimore: Williams & Wilkins, 1988.

Tsang RC, Venkataroman P: Pediatric parathyroid and vitamin D-related disorders. In: Kaplan SL, ed: *Clinical pediatric and adolescent endocrinology.* Philadelphia: WB Saunders, 1982.

104 Dermatologic Disorders

Mary L. Williams and Ilona J. Frieden

The febrile child with a rash and the child with a pruritic rash are the dermatologic presentations most likely to seek urgent pediatric care. The most common causes of these rashes are hypersensitivity reactions and infectious diseases. This chapter describes important and common entities, their diagnostic hallmarks, and a plan for their acute management (see Table 104-1 to 104-5).

Hypersensitivity Reactions ■

URTICARIA (HIVES)

Clinical Findings

Urticaria is an IgE-mediated immunologic reaction. Skin lesions are characteristic: *wheals* (pale, flat-topped plaques) due to edema in the upper dermis, surrounded by a *flare* of erythema due to vasodilatation. Lesions are intensely pruritic, multiple, and symmetrically distributed. They vary in size from small and round to giant geographic plaques. By definition, these lesions are evanescent, disappearing or shifting contours over 2–12 hours. Urticarial reactions may be accompanied by more massive, deeper cutaneous edema (angioedema) and involvement of the airway, producing laryngospasm and/or bronchospasm.

Diagnosis

Diagnosis rests upon clinical recognition. The presence of scaling, vesiculation or blisters, petechiae or hemorrhage, is not compatible with urticaria. In uncertain cases, outline the margins of the lesions to document changing shape over a few hours.

Differential Diagnosis

1. Erythema multiforme: Lesions are fixed and show a predilection for acral sites and palms/soles.

Presence of "target" lesions or blisters is characteristic.
2. Vasculitis (including Henoch-Schönlein purpura): Lesions are fixed and show a predilection for lower extremities or dependent sites; purpura ("palpable purpura") is characteristic.
3. Infectious exanthems and nonurticarial drug eruptions: Lesions are fixed and tend to be smaller and more numerous.
4. Papular urticaria due to insect bites: Lesions are fixed and asymmetrically distributed and may exhibit a central puncta.

Acute Treatment

1. *Airway:* Management of airway involvement takes precedence over treatment of skin lesions.
2. *α-adrenergics:* Aqueous epinephrine is of no benefit in uncomplicated urticaria because of its brief duration of action (<3 hrs); hives invariably recur. Sus-Phrine (1:200) produces a somewhat longer duration of action (6 hours); in severe cases it may be given as a single injection (0.005 ml/kg SC, to a maximum single dose of 0.15 ml). Institute antihistamine therapy concurrently to prevent rebound flares.
3. *Antihistamines:* Antihistamines are the mainstay in the management of urticaria. Their main purpose is to *prevent* the development of new lesions. Titrate the dose of antihistamine to suppress the appearance of new hives. Continue therapy until the patient has been hive-free for 3–5 days, then reduce the dose gradually in quantity and frequency to maintain the hive-free state. Monitor toxicity (CNS depression) in patients receiving high-dose and/or combination therapy. Hives may persist for several weeks, requiring continued antihistamine therapy.
4. *Corticosteroids:* Topical steroids are of no benefit in acute urticaria. Systemic steroids may suppress the appearance of new hives but are indicated only in severe cases inadequately controlled by or re-

TABLE 104-1. Antibiotics for Superficial Skin Infections

	Indications	Dose
Penicillin V	B-Streptococcus	25,00 u/kg/da
		PO divided q6h
		Adult dose 1 g/da
Dicloxacillin	Staphylococcus aureus	25 mg/kg/day
		PO divided q6h
		Adult dose 1–2 g/da
Erythromycin	Staphylococcus aureus (most strains)	30 mg/kg/da
		PO divided q6h
	B-streptococcus	Adult dose 1 g/da
Cephradine or cephalexin	Staphylococcus aureus	25 mg/kg/da
		PO divided q6h
		Adult dose 1–2 g/da

quiring high doses of antihistamines, and where an infectious cause has been excluded. Prednisone, 1–2 mg/kg PO given as a single A.M. dose, may be initiated in these patients, with a slow taper over 2–3 weeks.

5. *Search for antigenic cause:* Inquire into the probable antigen causing the allergic reaction. Obtain a careful history of drugs (prescription and OTC) ingested in the preceding week; discontinue all nonessential drugs. Inform patients/parents that they may be allergic to these drugs and advise that they may be at risk for an anaphylactic reaction with future usage. Seek evidence for a systemic infection as cause, especially streptococcal disease. Obtain a dietary history; foods commonly asso-

ciated with urticarial reactions are shellfish, nuts, and strawberries.

CONTACT DERMATITIS

Clinical Findings

Contact dermatitis is a local skin reaction due to a foreign substance's direct contact with the skin. The nature of these reactions may be *irritant* (i.e., due to the agent's noxious qualities, such as chemical burns from lyes or acids) or *allergic,* usually delayed-type or cellular hypersensitivity reaction. These reactions are eczematous (i.e., characterized histopathologically by varying degrees of edema within the epidermis).

Clinically acute eczemas (such as poison ivy [*Rhus*] dermatitis) are characterized by pruritic, red, edematous plaques that may vesicate or blister within 48–72 hours. The distribution of lesions is determined by sites of antigenic contact (e.g., linear streaks due to brushing against *Rhus*). Lesions begin to appear 24–72 hours after exposure and persist for 2–3 weeks. Subacute and chronic eczemas are characterized by ill-defined, erythematous, scaly patches with lichenification (accentuation of skin markings). Determining the precise antigenic cause may entail considerable detective work, including allergy (patch) testing, which usually requires referral to a dermatologist.

Treatment

1. *Corticosteroids:* In localized eruptions, topical corticosteroids may provide symptomatic relief but probably do not shorten the duration of lesions. For extensive eruptions or severe exposure in sensitized patients, systemic corticosteroids are required. The initiating dose should be sufficient to suppress new lesions (e.g., prednisone 2 mg/kg

TABLE 104-2. Antihistamines for Dermatologic Conditions

	Dose	Comment
Diphenhydramine	5–7 mg/kg/da	Indicated for urticaria or pruritis; at higher doses observe for CNS toxicity (depression or stimulation)
	PO divided q6h	
	Adult dose: 50–75 mg/q.d.	
Hydroxyzine hydrochloride	2–4 mg/kg/da	Indicated for urticaria or pruritis; at higher doses observe for CNS toxicity (depression or stimulation)
	PO divided q6h	
	Adult dose: 25–75 mg/q.d.	
Cyproheptidine	0.25 mg/kg/da	Indicated for urticaria
	PO divided q8h	

TABLE 104–3. *Topical Corticosteroids for Dermatologic Conditions*

Body Site	Potency		
	Low	Moderate	High
Face/groin	Hydrocortisone 1%	Hydrocortisone 2½%	Desonide 0.05%
Body	Hydrocortisone 1% or 2½%	Desonide 0.05%	Triamicinolone 0.1%
		Triamcinolone 0.025%	Fluocinonide 0.05%
			Amcinonide 0.1%*

Therapeutic Principles

Ointments usually more potent than creams

Creams: Use on red, acutely inflamed, or weeping skin.

Ointments: Use on dry, scaly, lichenified skin.

Lotions or gels: Use on scalp.

Avoid use of high-potency steroids for prolonged periods and on sensitive areas (e.g., face, flexures, groin).

* Prescribe small amount (15 g) for use on small areas.

PO in a single A.M. dose) and continued long enough to prevent rebound flares (e.g., 2–3 weeks). A simple regimen is prednisone 2 mg/kg for 5–7 days; then 1 mg/kg for 5–7 days, then ½ mg/kg/day for 5–7 days (adult dose, 60, 40, and 20 mg, respectively).

2. *Antihistamines:* Antihistamines are useful for pruritis.
3. *Wet dressings:* Soft cloths soaked in Burrow's solution 1:40 with cool water and applied to lesions for 20–30 minutes, or cool oatmeal baths will relieve itching, will help dry vesiculating lesions, and will help prevent secondary infection.
4. *Search for antigenic cause:* A history of topical exposure during the 4–5 days preceding the onset

of the rash is usual. When *Rhus* dermatitis is suspected, launder clothing worn during the exposure.

ERYTHEMA MULTIFORME

Clinical Findings

Erythema multiforme (EM) is believed to be an immune-complex mediated immunologic reaction. Skin lesions are multiple, symmetrically distributed, annular, erythematous plaques, often predominantly over acral surfaces. Characteristic lesions with central duskiness (target lesions) or central bullae (iris lesions) tend to be few in number and are found es-

TABLE 104–4. *Antifungals for Dermatologic Conditions*

	Dose	Comments
Systemic		
Griseofulvin	15–20 mg/kg/day	Single PO dose given with meals
Topical		
Ketoconazole Cream	Once daily only	
Miconazole Cream	b.i.d. (OTC)	Effective against both yeasts and dermatophytes
Clotrimazole Cream or Lotion	b.i.d.	
Nystatin Cream	b.i.d. (OTC)	Ineffective against dermatophytes. Less effective than imidazoles against yeasts
Tolnaftate Cream	b.i.d. (OTC)	Ineffective against yeasts. Less effective than imidazoles against dermatophytes

pecially on elbows and knees and palms and soles. Mucous membrane lesions include erythema and erosions.

EM has minor and major forms. In the minor form, disease is limited to the skin or one mucosal surface without systemic symptoms; the process is self-limited and therapy is generally not required or helpful. In the major form (Stevens-Johnson syndrome), systemic symptoms are present and more than one mucosal surface is involved. Toxic epidermal necrolysis (TEN), the most severe end of the spectrum, is characterized pathologically by full-thickness epidermal necrosis and clinically by widespread blistering and denuded skin. Lesions are extremely painful and are accompanied by systemic toxicity and high mortality. TEN is almost always drug-induced.

Diagnosis

Diagnosis usually rests upon clinical grounds. Skin biopsy may be useful for confirmation of diagnosis. Where TEN is suspected, perform an immediate biopsy using frozen section.

Differential Diagnosis

1. Urticaria: Borders of lesions shift within 12 hours. Lesions are not bullous. Mucous membranes are spared.
2. Vasculitis: Lesions show hemorrhage or petechiae (palpable purpura) and blisters occur only on a hemorrhagic base. Lesions are most numerous on legs and dependent areas.
3. Other drug eruptions/viral exanthems: Lesions are smaller and more monomorphous.
4. Staphylococcal scalded skin syndrome (SSSS): Skin tenderness is characteristic. Blisters are more superficial than in TEN (i.e., intraepidermal rather than subepidermal). Diagnosis is established by a Tzanck preparation (acantholytic cells in SSSS) or by skin biopsy using frozen sections.

Treatment

1. Patients with severe disease, particularly those with erosions or mucosal involvement, require hospitalization. Monitor fluid and electrolyte balance closely. Observe patients for signs of infection and consider cultures (e.g., skin, blood).
2. *Skin care:* For bullous skin lesions, use tepid wet compresses with dilute Burrow's solution (1:20) in tepid tap water, 20 min b.i.d., followed by applications of silver sulfadiazine (Silvadene) cream. Sulfamylon should be avoided since it can exacerbate or precipitate sulfonamide-induced EM.

TABLE 104–5. *Antiviral Agents for Dermatologic Conditions*

	Dose	Comments
Acyclovir	Oral: 200 mg 5×/day	Pediatric oral dose 30 to 50 mg/kg/day (not fully established)
	IV: 15 to 30 mg/kg/day divided t.i.d.	Use parenterally if patient is neonate, immunocompromised, or toxic.

3. *Mucous membrane care:* Oral lesions may be gently debrided using chlorhexidene oral solution or 30% hydrogen peroxide, diluted 1:9.
4. *Eye care:* Ocular lesions are a potentially devastating complication of Stevens-Johnson syndrome. Consult an ophthalmologist if eye lesions are present. There currently is no evidence that either systemic or intraocular steroids can prevent progression of ocular disease. Avoid sulfa-containing eye drops.
5. *Corticosteroids:* Topical steroids are ineffective. Systemic corticosteroids have not been shown to be beneficial and may increase the risk of infection.
6. *Search for antigenic cause:* EM is triggered by either infection or drugs. The most common infectious agents are Type I or II *Herpes simplex* and *Mycoplasma pneumoniae.* Patients on antiepileptics, sulfonamides, or other antibiotics should be suspected of having drug-induced disease. Discontinue the offending agent, and observe the patient closely during the first 72 hours for progression to TEN.

ATOPIC DERMATITIS

Clinical Findings

Atopic dermatitis is a subacute to chronic, recurrent, eczematous dermatitis occurring in genetically predisposed ("atopic") individuals. Many patients have elevated serum IgE levels, or positive scratch and radioallergosorbent test (RAST) tests to common allergens, and other IgE-mediated diseases (e.g., allergic rhinitis, asthma). Dry skin, abrupt changes in environmental temperature, stress, and bacterial skin infection are important causes of flares in many patients.

Lesions are characterized by ill-defined erythematous patches or plaques with scaling and increased skin markings (lichenification). They are intensely pruritic. Distribution patterns differ depending upon age (face, scalp, and extensor extremities in infants; flexures and dorsum of hands and feet in children; hands and flexures in adults), but at any age, any sites may be involved. Vesicles, pustules, or serous crusts are usually indicative of secondary infection.

Diagnosis

Diagnosis is established by history and physical examination. Skin biopsy is not helpful, nor is total serum IgE, which is elevated in a variety of skin diseases. Obtain a skin culture from pustules or moist, weeping areas.

Treatment

1. *Corticosteroids:* Topical steroids are the mainstay of therapy. Therapy may be initiated with a moderate- to high-potency steroid (e.g., triamcinolone 0.1%) cream or ointment. Once the acute flare has subsided (5–7 days), substitute a lower-potency steroid (e.g., triamcinolone 0.025% or hydrocortisone 2½% or 1%, in order of decreasing potency), usually in an ointment. Use a nonfluorinated moderate- or low-potency steroid on the face. Superpotent topical steroids (e.g., Diprolene, Temovate) are rarely, if ever, indicated in the management of pediatric atopic dermatitis.

   Systemic corticosteroids (e.g., prednisone 1–2 mg/kg/day, in a single A.M. dose) may give prompt relief to acute flares, but severe rebound flares are common. In children with widespread, severe, recalcitrant atopic dermatitis, consider brief hospitalization for intensive topical therapy and a family rest.
2. *Antihistamines:* Antihistamines are commonly used to relieve itching. Administration one hour before bedtime may result in lessened nighttime scratching.
3. *Wet dressings:* Acutely eczematous eruptions may be quieted using soft cloths soaked in cool tap water or a dilute (1:40) Burrow's solution for 20–30 minutes q.i.d., followed by liberal application of topical steroids. Maximal benefit is achieved within 48–72 hours in most cases; continued therapy after this time may be overly drying. In some patients, a cool bath using oilated Aveeno (oatmeal) may serve as a substitute.
4. *Antibiotics:* Acute flares of atopic dermatitis are commonly precipitated or accompanied by skin infection. *Staphylococcus aureus* and less often streptococcus are the most common organisms. Begin therapy with oral erythromycin, cephradine, or dicloxacillin while awaiting culture results; antibiotics are indicated during severe flares or if serous crusting or pustules are present.
5. If punctate erosions or vesicles are present, consider the diagnosis of eczema herpeticum caused by infection with *Herpes simplex* virus. This can be confirmed by demonstration of multinucleated giant cells on Tzanck preparation, by direct immunofluorescent antibody smear of lesional skin, and by viral culture. Treatment is with either oral or IV acyclovir, depending on the severity of infection.

Infectious Diseases ■

SYSTEMIC INFECTIONS

Etiology

Exanthems are skin eruptions, usually generalized, caused by an acute bacterial or viral infection (see Table 104-6).

Clinical Findings

The age of the child, time of year, exposure history, knowledge of current illnesses in the community, history of previous exanthems, and medication history are essential historical information. Inquire about a history of prodromal symptoms, fever, and the anatomic progression of the rash.

The most important part of the physical examination is a global evaluation of how ill (toxic) the child appears to be. Then assess the morphology and distribution of the rash. Examine mucous membranes carefully for the presence of enanthem as well as for cheilitis, glossitis, and conjunctivitis. Pay special attention during the exam to the lymph nodes, liver, and spleen, and for signs of meningeal irritation. The extent of laboratory evaluation will depend on the specific etiology suspected, as well as the toxicity of the child. In children with mild exanthemic illnesses, it may be appropriate not to do any laboratory tests.

Differential Diagnosis

1. Drug eruptions: Exanthem-like reactions to drugs are common. Drugs that often cause such reactions include antibiotics and anticonvulsants; antihistamines, decongestants, and antipyretics are rarely responsible.
2. Still's disease (juvenile rheumatoid arthritis): A generalized rash consisting of multiple erythematous macules in a generalized distribution is often present in the afternoon or evening in association with fever; it disappears by morning. Arthritis is usually present, and lymphadenopathy and splenomegaly are common.
3. Henoch-Schönlein purpura: A generalized papular or urticarial eruption is usually accompanied by

palpable purpuric lesions on the legs and/or buttocks.
4. Urticaria and erythema multiforme: See sections
above.

SUPERFICIAL BACTERIAL INFECTIONS: IMPETIGO AND ECTHYMA

See Chapter 118.

Clinical Findings

Impetigo represents a bacterial infection of the outer
epidermis. Virulent strains of *S. aureus* and beta-hemolytic streptococcus may infect normal skin (primary impetigo). Less virulent strains of staphylococci
may superinfect dermatitic skin (secondary impetigo). Lesions are characterized by superficial erosions with a honey-colored crust, and are most common on the face and exposed sites on extremities.
Some strains of *S. aureus* produce a toxin that causes
fragile blisters filled with polymorphonuclear leukocytes and organisms (bullous impetigo). Ecthyma
represents a full-thickness epidermal infection.
Round, heavily crusted lesions are surrounded by an
erythematous rim and mild tenderness.

Confirm bacterial infection by culturing pustules
or wet, weeping lesions, and determine antibiotic
sensitivities.

Treatment

1. *Antibiotics:* Begin oral erythromycin, dicloxacillin,
   or cephradine (Table 104-1), pending culture results. Topical muperocin is an alternative for children with limited disease. Other topical antibiotics
   (e.g., Bacitracin, Polysporin, Neosporin) are ineffective.
2. *Local skin care:* Aggressive efforts to remove impetigo crusts are traumatic to the child and do not
   hasten healing. Crusts will separate easily once the
   infection is brought under control and no new
   transudation occurs. Gentle loosening of crusts
   using warm compresses may then be initiated.

SUPERFICIAL FUNGAL INFECTIONS

Clinical Findings

Superficial fungal infections may be divided into
dermatophyte and yeast infections. The presentation
of dermatophyte infections (tineas) depends on the
body site affected, the virulence of the organism, and
the immune reactivity of the host. The most common
presentation of tinea capitis is dandruff-like scaling
with minimal alopecia. Less common presentations
include large areas of alopecia filled with broken-off
hairs ("black-dot" tinea capitis) and circumscribed
areas of boggy edema, pustulation, and alopecia
(kerion). The hallmark of tinea infections elsewhere
on the body is annular lesions, usually few in number,
with a tendency toward central clearing and an active,
scaly or papulopustular border. Intertriginous tineas
show maceration with scaling. Yeast infections, commonly due to *Candida,* present with a "beefy red"
dermatitis and peripheral (satellite) pustules.

Diagnosis

In black-dot tinea capitis, establish a positive diagnosis either by KOH preparation of affected hairs or
through fungal culture (which requires 2–4 weeks)
before treatment is initiated. Because organisms are
few in kerions and isolation is difficult, make the diagnosis on clinical grounds and initiate therapy. Diagnosis of tineas elsewhere on the body or candida
infections can be readily confirmed by KOH examination. Most tinea capitis infections are due to *Tri-
chophyton tonsurans,* an endothrix infection that
does *not* fluoresce under ultraviolet (Wood's) light.

Differential Diagnosis

1. Dandruff (seborrheic dermatitis): Diffuse scaling
   without hair loss. Rare after infancy in preadolescent children.
2. Alopecia areata: Smooth oval or round patches of
   hair loss without broken hairs or scaling.
3. Pityriasis alba: Round, hypopigmented, and often
   mildly scaly lesions. Indistinct, not accentuated
   margins; no central clearing.
4. Nummular (atopic) eczema: Red, round, scaly, and
   often numerous lesions; no central clearing or active border.

Treatment

1. Tinea capitis: Systemic griseofulvin is the drug of
   choice (Table 104-6). Black-dot infections must
   be treated until cultures are negative (usually 12–
   20 weeks). While kerions represent self-limited
   infections, if extensive, suppress the inflammatory
   reaction with systemic steroids (e.g., prednisone
   1–2 mg/kg/day) to prevent scarring alopecia. Se-
   lenium sulfide (2%) shampoo may decrease con-
   tagion. Topical antifungals are of no benefit in tinea
   capitis. Infected children should not share combs,
   hats, or other headgear. Examine and culture all
   family members.

TABLE 104–6. *Exanthems*

Disease (etiology)	Usual Age	Season	Prodrome	Morphology
Measles (rubeola virus)	Infants to young adults	Winter/spring	High fever, URI Sx, conjunctivitis	Erythematous macules and papules, become confluent
Rubella (rubella virus)	Adolescents/ young adults	Spring	Absent or low-grade fever, malaise	Rose pink papules, not confluent
Erythema infectiosum (parvovirus B19)	5–15 yr	Winter/spring	Usually none	Slapped cheeks; reticulate erythyma or maculopapular
Enteroviral exanthems (coxsackie, echo, other enteroviruses)	Young children	Summer/fall	Fever (occ.)	Extremely variable; maculopapular, petechial, purpuria, vesicular
Hand-foot-mouth syndrome (several Coxsackie viruses)	Children	Summer/fall	Fever (occ.), sore mouth	Grey white vesicles 3–7 mm on normal or erythematous base
Adenovirus exanthems (adenoviruses)	5 mo–5 yr	Winter/spring	Fever, URI Sx	Rubelliform, morbilliform, Roseola-like
Chickenpox (varicella-zoster virus)	1–14 yr	Late fall/ winter/spring	Usually none	Macules, papules rapidly become vesicles on erythematous base, then crusts
Roseola (?herpesvirus 6)	6 mo to 3 yr	Spring/fall	High fever for 3–5 days	Maculopapular rash appears *after* fever declines
Lyme disease (borrelia carried by ticks)	School age	Summer, geographical distribution	None	Erythema chronicum migrans
Rocky Mountain spotted fever (Rickettsia rickettsii carried by ticks)	Any age	Summer	Fever, malaise	Maculopapular and petechial rash
Kawasaki disease	6 mo–6 yr	Winter/spring	High fever, irritability	Polymorphous—papular, morbiliform, erythema with desquamation
Gianotti-Crosti syndrome (hepatitis B, CMV, cosackie E-B, etc.)	1–6 yr	Any season	Usually absent	Papules or papulovesicles; may become confluent
Scarlet fever (B-streptococcus)	School-age children	Fall to spring	Acute onset with fever, sore throat	Diffuse erythema with sandpaper texture
Staph scalded skin syndrome (*Staphylococcus aureus*/epidermolytic toxin)	Infants	Any season	None	Abrupt onset, tender erythroderma
Toxic shock syndrome/staph toxin	Adolescents/ young adults	Any season	None	Macular erythroderma
Meningococcemia/ meningococcus	<2 yr	Winter/spring	Malaise, fever, URI symptoms	Papules, petechiae, purpura

Distribution	Associated Findings	Diagnosis	Special Management
Begins on face and moves downward over whole body	Koplik's spots, toxic appearance, photophobia, cough, adenopathy, high fever	Usually clinical; acute/conv. hemeagglutin (HAI) serology	Report to public health
Begins on face and moves downward	Postauricular and occipital adenopathy; headache, malaise	Rubella IgM or acute/conv. HAI serology	Report to public health; check for exposure to pregnant women.
Usually arms/legs; may be generalized	Rash waxes and wanes for several weeks; occasional arthritis, headache, malaise	Usually clinical; acute/conv. serology	
Usually generalized, may be acral	Low-grade fever; occ. myocarditis, aseptic meningitis, pleurodynia	Usually clinical; viral culture from throat, rectal swabs in selected cases	If petechiae or purpura, *must consider* meningococcemia
Hands/feet most common; diaper area; occ. generalized	Oral ulcers, (occ.) fever, adenopathy	Same as enteroviral exanthems	
Generalized	Fever, URI symptoms, occasionally pneumonia	Viral isolation or acute/ conv. seroconversion	
Often begins on scalp or face; more profuse on trunk than extremities	Pruritus, fever, oral lesions, occ. malaise	Usually clinical; Tzanck preparation or direct immunofluorescence	Antihistamines for itching; aspirin contraindicated (Reye's syndrome)
Trunk, neck; may be generalized, last hours to days	Cervical and postauricular adenopathy	Clinical	
Trunk, extremities	Fever; late complication— arthritis cardiac, neurologic	Serology	Penicillin for children younger than nine; tetracycline for older children
Wrists, ankles, palms, soles; trunk later	CNS, pulmonary, cardiac lesions	Serology	Treat on presumptive clinical grounds
Generalized, often with perineal accentuation	Conjunctivitis, cheilitis, glossitis, peripheral edema, adenopathy	Clinical	Admit to hospital for IV gamma globulin, salicylates
Face, arms, legs, buttocks, spares the torso	Occasional lymphadenopathy, hepatomegaly, splenomegaly	Clinical; hepatitis B and E-B serologies	
Facial flushing with circumoral pallor, linear erythema in skin folds	Exudative pharyngitis, palatal petechiae, abdominal pain	Throat cultures	Penicillin IM or oral erythromycin
Diffuse with perioral, perinasal scaling	Fever, conjunctivitis, rhinitis	Clinical; culture of *S. aureus* from systemic site (not skin)	Neonate; if blistering present, hospitalize for IV nafcillin and fluid/ electrolyte Rx.
Generalized	Hypotension; fever, myalgias, diarrhea/ vomiting	Clinical case definition criteria isolation *S. aureus,* cervix, etc.	Treatment of hypotension, admit to hospital; antibiotics to eradicate staph
Trunk, extremities, palms, soles	Temp >40°C, meningismus, circulatory collapse	Clinical, blood culture, spinal tap	Immediate IV penicillin in ED, treatment for shock, if present

TABLE 104-7. *Treatment of Scabies With Lindane*

Contraindications

Lindane should *not* be used in malnourished or premature infants, in situations where there are large areas of denuded skin, in pregnant or nursing women, or in patients unable to understand the following instructions:

Instructions to Patients

Do not bathe before application.

Apply a thin coat of medicine (1 ounce/adult/ treatment) from the neck down over the entire body. Leave it on for 8 hours, then take a bath or shower.

Wash all bedding, towels, and any clothes worn within 72 hours of treatment in the hot-water cycle of the washing machine.

Itching may continue for up to two weeks despite adequate treatment. Do not retreat itchy areas.

2. Tinea Corporis/Facei/Cruris/Pedis and Candida infections: Topical antifungals are effective (Table 104-4). A mild topical steroid (e.g., 1% hydrocortisone cream) in conjunction with an antifungal may be desirable in inflammatory Candida infections. The combination steroid/antifungal preparations Mycolog and Lotrisone are not indicated for Candida diaper dermatitis because their corticosteroids are too potent for use in this area.

Scabies ■

CLINICAL FINDINGS

Scabies is a hypersensitivity reaction to skin infestation with the *Sarcoptes scabiei* mite. Affected individuals usually present with an intensely pruritic rash, often more symptomatic at night. Other family members are often symptomatic. Lesions are polymorphous and include papules, wheals, vesicles, pustules, nodules, crusts, and excoriations. The most characteristic lesion of scabies, the burrow, is a tiny threadlike hyperkeratotic lesion, which may be subtle. The distribution of lesions in an important clue to diagnosis: in infants, the medial insteps of the feet and the axilla; in older children and adults, the wrists, palms and interdigital web spaces, the periumbilical area, and the penis. Burrows are usually found only on palms/soles (infants) or finger webs, wrists, nipples, and penis (older children and adults). The back and head are usually spared, except in infants.

DIAGNOSIS

Search carefully for burrows, which are pathognomonic for scabies, and scrape the lesion for the microscopic presence of mites, eggs, and/or feces. If a scraping is negative, but lesions are typical in morphology and distribution, treatment may be initiated on clinical grounds.

DIFFERENTIAL DIAGNOSIS

The differential diagnosis of scabies commonly includes papular urticaria due to other insect bites, pruritic exanthems, drug eruptions, atopic dermatitis, and dry skin eczema.

TREATMENT

1. *Scabicides:* Lindane is the treatment of choice in most situations, but give careful instructions for use because of potential neurotoxicity if used incorrectly (Table 104-7). Treat the entire family simultaneously to avoid reinfestations. For infants under one year of age and for pregnant or nursing mothers, 5–10% precipitated sulfur in petrolatum is the treatment of choice. It should be applied daily for three successive days. In infants only, treatment should include the head. Examine patients treated with sulfur in two weeks to ensure clinical response.
2. *Fomites:* Treatment for fomites (Table 104-3) is recommended but is of secondary importance to ascertaining and treating affected human contacts.
3. *Pruritis:* Antihistamines and oatmeal baths may be used to treat pruritis.
4. *Antibiotics:* Treat secondary infection if present with an oral antibiotic (see above).
5. *Corticosteroids:* Patients still uncomfortable after the above measures may benefit from a brief burst of oral corticosteroids (e.g., prednisone 1–2 mg/ kg single A.M. dose for 3–5 days).

Head Lice ■

Head lice are an infestation of the scalp caused by the louse *Pediculus capitis*. The gray insect is 2–3 mm long and lives within 1 cm of the scalp. Affected individuals usually present with severe itching of the scalp, and they may also have noticed live lice or eggs (nits) in the hair. Findings on physical examination may include excoriations, pyoderma, and occipital adenopathy.

DIAGNOSIS

Nits or actual lice can be identified with a magnifying glass or on low-power lens on a microscope. Nits are oval-shaped with a caplike cover (operculum) and are firmly attached to the hair shaft with a cementlike substance. The presence of nits within 5 mm of the scalp is presumptive evidence of active infection with head lice, even in someone who has previously been treated.

DIFFERENTIAL DIAGNOSIS

The differential diagnosis includes scalp pyoderma without lice and seborrheic dermatitis. It also includes hair casts, concretions along the hair, and accretions of keratin, which resemble nits but do not have the characteristic operculum and do not cause itching.

TREATMENT

1. *Pediculocides:* Permethrin 1% cream rinse (NIX) is the only effective single-application pediculocide. It is applied to hair that has been washed and towel-dried, and is left on for 10 minutes. It is about twice as expensive as other available treatments. Synergized pyrethrins (A-200, RID, R&C) are also effective for treatment, and are available over the counter. They are applied in the same way as permethrin rinse, but should be reapplied in one week. Lindane shampoo is no longer an effective treatment for head lice. Lindane lotion can be applied overnight to the scalp, with treatment repeated in one week, but this has no significant advantage over other treatments. *Treat all family members, even if they are asymptomatic, to prevent reinfestation.*

2. *Fomites:* Lice can survive for 3–10 days away from humans on inanimate objects. Combs and brushes should be washed in hot, soapy water. Hats, coats, sheets, towels, and pillowcases should be washed, dry cleaned, or pressed with a hot iron.

3. *Nit Picking:* The nits that remain after treatment are not infectious, but may prohibit the child's return to school. Nits can be removed with a fine-toothed comb. If this is ineffective, the hair can be soaked in equal parts of vinegar and water for 15 minutes, to loosen their attachments.

Bibliography ■

Adzick NS, Kim SH, Bondoc CC, et al: Management of toxic epidermal necrolysis in a pediatric burn center. *Am J Dis Child* 1985; 139:499–502.

Barton LL, Friedman AD: Impetigo: A reassessment of etiology and therapy. *Ped Dermatol* 1987; 4:185–188.

Bierman FZ, Gersory WM: Kawasaki disease: Clinical perspective. *J Pediatr* 1987; 111:789–793.

Carson DS, Tribble PW, Weart CW: Pyrethrins combined with piperonyl butoxide (RID) vs 1% permethrin (NIX) in the treatment of head lice. *Am J Dis Child* 142:768–769.

Crosson FJ, Black SB, Trumpp CE, et al: Infections in day-care centers. *Curr Probl Pediatr* 1986; 16:125–184.

Cherry JD: Cutaneous manifestations of systemic infections. In: Feigin RD, Cherry JD, eds: *Textbook of pediatric infectious diseases,* 2nd ed. Philadelphia: WB Saunders, 1987, pp 786–817.

Cherry JD: Viral exanthems. *Curr Probl Pediatr* 1983; 13:1–44.

Hanifin JM: Basic and clinical aspects of atopic dermatitis. *Ann Allergy* 1984; 52:386–393.

Krowchuck DP, Lucky AW, Primner SI, et al.: Current status of the identification and management of tinea capitis. *Pediatrics* 1983; 72:625–631.

Rasmussen JE: Recent developments in the management of patients with atopic dermatitis. *J Allergy Clin Immunol* 1984; 74:771–776.

Reeves JR: Head lice and scabies in children. *Pediatr Infect Dis J* 1987; 6:598–602.

Tinea capitis: Current concepts. *Pediatr Dermatol* 1985; 2:324–337.

105 Gastrointestinal Disorders

Colin D. Rudolph

This chapter addresses pancreatitis, hepatitis, Reye's syndrome, and acute cholecystitis. Other important GI disorders are discussed elsewhere: colic in Chapter 28; diarrhea in Chapter 29; constipation in Chapter 30; vomiting in Chapter 31; GI bleeding in Chapter 32; swallowed foreign body in Chapter 33; abdominal pain in Chapter 40; abdominal trauma in Chapter 56; and anorectal disorders in Chapter 106.

Pancreatitis ■

Pancreatitis is a process of autodigestion of the pancreas resulting from the premature activation of precursor proteolytic enzymes within the pancreas. Obstruction of the pancreatic duct, drugs or toxins, and infection are frequent etiologies. Pancreatitis usually occurs in children older than 5 years of age, but occasionally occurs in infants and children of all ages.

ETIOLOGIES

1. *Blunt abdominal trauma* accounts for 10–35% of all cases of acute pancreatitis in children. If pancreatic damage is suspected, obtain immediate surgical consultation and admit the patient to the hospital for observation and serial serum amylase values (see Chapter 56).
2. *Drugs,* including valproate, azathioprine, L-asparaginase, prednisone, tetracycline, thiazides, furosemide, oral contraceptives, and others.
3. *Infections,* including coxsackievirus, Echovirus, Epstein-Barr virus, mumps, Mycoplasma pneumoniae, and malaria.
4. *Obstruction of the pancreatic duct* can result from cholelithiasis. Ascariasis is one of the most common causes of acute pancreatitis in children from endemic regions. Congenital anomalies such as choledochal cysts and intraduodenal duplications can also cause pancreatic obstruction.
5. *Metabolic abnormalities* associated with an increased incidence of pancreatitis in childhood include hyperparathyroidism, cystic fibrosis, vitamin

A deficiency, and hyperlipidemia types I, IV, and V.
6. *Hereditary pancreatitis* presents at a mean age of 10–12 years. Suspect if multiple nonalcoholic family members have a history of pancreatitis. Other causes of pancreatitis must still be excluded.
7. *Alcoholism* is the major cause of pancreatitis in adults. Consider this etiology in adolescent patients.

CLINICAL FINDINGS

Pancreatitis typically presents with a history of mild to severe, constant, sharp to gnawing supraumbilical pain, sometimes radiating to the back. Nausea and vomiting and low-grade fevers are common. Occasionally there is jaundice.

Physical exam will reveal a tender abdomen with voluntary guarding. A rigid abdomen with rebound tenderness is present in more severe cases. Bluish discoloration around the umbilicus or flanks provides ominous evidence of intraabdominal hemorrhage.

Absolute criteria for diagnosis of acute pancreatitis include either an increase in two pancreatic enzymes (amylase, immunoreactive trypsin or lipase) to more than three times normal, or evidence of acute pancreatitis by ultrasound, CT, or surgical exploration. *In children, a clinical diagnosis of acute pancreatitis can usually be established from the history, physical examination, and serum amylase of more than three times normal.*

Other conditions associated with hyperamylasemia include chronic pancreatitis, mesenteric infarction (such as with volvulus), and perforation of the stomach or duodenum.

ANCILLARY DATA

Obtain a hematocrit, WBC, amylase, glucose, liver function tests, albumin, calcium, BUN, and type and crossmatch, as well as a chest and abdominal radiograph. Plain radiographs of the abdomen may reveal a distended small intestinal loop near the pancreas (sentinel loop) or a paralytic ileus. The psoas margins may be obscured. Free intraperitoneal air indicates perforation of the bowel. If there is any question regarding the diagnosis, obtain other diagnostic tests, including an abdominal ultrasound or CT scan.

TREATMENT AND DISPOSITION

There is no specific treatment for acute pancreatitis. Treatment is mainly supportive and focuses on recognizing and treating complications, including pain, pleural effusion, respiratory distress syndrome, hypovolemia, hemorrhagic pancreatitis, pancreatic pseudocyst, renal failure, hyperglycemia, and hypocalcemia.

1. Monitor oxygen saturation with pulse oximetry.
2. Begin rehydration and correction of electrolyte imbalances immediately in the ED (see Chapters 8 and 22). Send blood specimens for appropriate analysis, as indicated.
3. Give the patient nothing orally; consider a nasogastric tube to decompress the stomach and evacuate intestinal secretions.
4. Administer analgesia (meperidine HCl, 1–2 mg/kg IM) as required.
5. Consider bladder catheterization to monitor perfusion and response to hydration, if the patient is severely hypovolemic or septic.
6. In cases of blunt abdominal trauma or severe hypovolemia, obtain surgical and gastroenterologist consultations. If pancreatitis is documented, an emergency endoscopic retrograde cholangiopancreatography (ERCP) may be necessary. Emergency partial pancreatectomy is indicated if the pancreatic duct has been damaged. Do not perform ERCP during an acute episode of pancreatitis for any other indication.
7. Admit all patients with acute pancreatitis for observation.
8. Findings associated with a complicated or severe course (if present within the first 48 hours) include WBC >15,000 cells/mm^3; glucose >180 mg/dl; BUN >45 mg/dl; arterial pO$_2$ <60 Torr; calcium <8.0 mg/dl; serum albumin <3.2 gm/dl; aspartate aminotransferase (AST) or alanine aminotransferase (ALT) >200 units/L.

Hepatitis ■

Hepatitis refers to inflammation of the liver, a relatively common GI disorder of childhood. Causes are multiple and most are self-limited infectious conditions (usually hepatitis A).

ETIOLOGIES

1. *Hepatitis A virus* is spread by the fecal-oral route. Person-to-person transmission is the most common mode, but foodborne and waterborne epidemics occur. Transmission in day-care centers is common. Transmission by blood transfusion is rare. Anicteric infection is more common in children infected before 5 years of age; most adolescents and adults manifest jaundice.

   The incubation period is 15–50 days. The presence of anti-HAV IgM antibodies provides serologic confirmation of hepatitis A infection. Anti-HAV IgM antibodies are present at the onset of illness through the first 2–4 months.
2. *Hepatitis B virus* is transmitted from person to person by direct contact with blood or secretions. Infection can occur from blood transfusion, birth exposure, sexual intercourse, or open wound contact with blood or secretions containing hepatitis B virus. Hepatitis B infection is much more common in IV drug users, prostitutes, and hemophilia patients. The incubation period is 50–180 days. A positive hepatitis B surface antigen (HBsAg) provides serologic confirmation of hepatitis B contagiousness. HBsAg is present in cases of acute hepatitis or in hepatitis B carriers. Persons of Asian, Pacific Island, or Alaskan Eskimo descent and persons born in Haiti or sub-Saharan Africa are most likely to be carriers. In some cases of acute hepatitis, the HBsAg has disappeared and antibody to surface antigen (anti-HBs) has not yet appeared. In these cases, IgM anti-HBC antibody is present.
3. *Other viral infections* including Epstein-Barr virus (EBV), rubella virus, echovirus, herpesvirus, rheovirus, coxsackievirus, adenovirus, and cytomegalovirus (CMV) all can cause acute hepatitis. Most of these viral infections are classified as "non-A, non-B hepatitis." One distinct transfusion-related non-A, non-B hepatitis virus has recently been identified. Post-blood transfusion hepatitis usually occurs 2–12 weeks after transfusion.
4. *Other infections* associated with acute hepatitis include leptospirosis, yellow fever, malaria, Q fever, visceral larva migrans, and amebic liver abscess.
5. *Drugs* of many types can cause mild to severe hepatitis. Obtain a careful history of medications, including vitamins. Liver damage can be caused by therapeutic doses of some medications, including oral contraceptives, oxacillin, cimetidine, ranitidine, azathioprine, furosemide, phenytoin, valproate, and others. Overdoses of acetaminophen, iron, vitamin A, and aspirin can cause severe hepatitis. Acquired hypersensitivity reactions present with hepatitis associated with fever, rash, arthralgias, and eosinophilia.

6. *Toxins,* including phosphorus, arsenic, carbon tetrachloride, tetrachloroethylene, and trichloroethane, produce severe hepatitis. Obtain a careful history of possible toxin exposure to prevent recurrent exposures.

CLINICAL FINDINGS

Hepatitis is usually associated with anorexia, malaise, and fatigue. Jaundice and an enlarged, tender liver are the most common signs of disease. Obtain a careful history of possible toxin exposure or medication ingestion. Similarly, a history of recent shellfish ingestion, travel, or exposure to infectious agents may be significant. Any alteration in mental status such as irritability or lethargy may signal fulminant hepatitis or Reye's syndrome (see below). Findings of ascites or a small, hard, nontender liver are more suggestive of chronic hepatitis.

ANCILLARY DATA

Laboratory tests indicating ongoing hepatocellular injury include AST and ALT. Values >2,000 IU/l are uncommon in acute hepatitis and warrant further studies to ensure that the patient does not have submassive or fulminant hepatitis. Bilirubin may be normal or mildly elevated in acute hepatitis. Serum alkaline phosphatase is often only mildly elevated. Large elevations of bilirubin and alkaline phosphatase suggest the possibility of extrahepatic obstruction, requiring further evaluation. A normal prothrombin time, ammonia, and glucose ensure that the liver is adequately maintaining protein synthesis, detoxification, and glucose production. *Abnormal liver function tests in infants less than 1 year old are more likely to represent metabolic or structural liver disease and must be evaluated more carefully by a pediatrician.* This evaluation can usually be performed as an outpatient, assuming that the patient is otherwise well and without signs of severe hepatic necrosis.

Specific serologic tests include anti-HAV IgM and IgG antibodies; hepatitis B surface antigen (HBsAg) and antibody (anti-HBs), and IgM anti-hepatitis core antibody (IgM anti-HBC).

TREATMENT AND DISPOSITION

Differentiating acute, chronic, and fulminant hepatitis is essential to ED management.

Acute hepatitis usually results from infection and is rarely life-threatening. Inform patients of potential complications and address public health concerns (limiting exposure to other individuals and ensuring appropriate prophylaxis of contacts).

ED management of chronic hepatitis is generally limited to the recognition and early management of secondary complications of variceal bleeding, hepatic encephalopathy, and spontaneous peritonitis.

Fulminant hepatitis is a life-threatening illness that requires prompt recognition and referral to a pediatric critical care center.

Specific therapy is limited. There is no evidence that any interventions influence the rate of recovery from hepatitis. Discontinue suspected causative drugs.

Hospitalize the patient if IV fluid administration is required, if the patient cannot tolerate oral fluids, if synthetic liver function is significantly compromised, or if complications are present (see below).

Most patients can be discharged. Fatigue is common; encourage rest and allow school absence. Anorexia and nausea are also common. Ingesting fatty foods may worsen nausea; if so, they should be avoided. Ensure adequate hydration.

FOLLOW-UP AND PROPHYLAXIS

The most important concerns in the management of acute hepatitis are follow-up and prophylaxis of other exposed individuals.

Follow-up is required to ensure that the hepatitis resolves and does not progress to hepatic failure. Advise parents to return for evaluation if the patient has any suggestion of unusual behavior, lethargy, or dehydration. Weekly physical exams and determination of bilirubin and SGOT are indicated until the hepatitis resolves. Mental status changes suggest the development of a fulminant hepatitis (see below). If bilirubin or SGOT are elevated for more than 2 months, consider chronic hepatitis and refer to a pediatric gastroenterologist.

Prophylaxis for Hepatitis A

1. Observe enteric precautions. If hospitalization is required, patients with diarrhea or incontinence or those who are not toilet-trained should have private rooms and enteric precautions for 1 week after the onset of jaundice.
2. Give all household contacts 0.02 ml/kg of immune globulin (IG) IM as soon as possible after exposure. Serologic testing is not required. Treatment more than 2 weeks after the last exposure is not indicated.
3. In day-care centers with children who are not toilet-trained, if HAV infection is identified in a child or in the household contacts of two of the enrolled children, give 0.02 ml/kg IG to all employees and enrolled children.

Prophylaxis for Hepatitis B

1. Give hepatitis B IG (HBIG) 0.06 ml/kg IM within 1 week to infants less than 12 months of age who are in close contact with a household member with acute HBV infection, then vaccinate with the hepatitis B vaccine (0.5 ml IM) within 7 days and at 1 and 6 months. Breastfeeding does not increase the risk of HBV infection and need not be discontinued.
2. Vaccinate children older than 12 months only if the household member with HBV infection becomes a carrier.
3. Needlestick exposure with HBsAg-positive blood results in infection in 6–12% of cases. Exposure of susceptible persons to blood that tests positive or is from a high-risk group requires the administration of HBIG within 1 week of exposure (0.06 ml/kg IM, maximum 5 ml). Administer HB vaccine (1 ml) within 7 days and at 1 and 6 months. If the blood source is negative or the source is low-risk, HB vaccine administration alone is adequate.
4. After needlestick exposure from a needle contaminated with non-A, non-B hepatitis, give IG 0.06 ml/kg, although the efficacy is uncertain.

COMPLICATIONS

Fulminant Hepatitis

Fulminant hepatitis or submassive hepatic necrosis results from etiologies similar to acute hepatitis. Transaminase values over 5,000 IU/L are an ominous sign. Bilirubin may not be elevated in the early stages of hepatic failure.

Immediately hospitalize for evaluation any patient with an elevated ammonia or prothrombin time. Consider the possibility of hepatic failure or Reye's syndrome in all patients with altered mental status and treat as follows:

1. Assess mental status and the stage of coma (see Reye's syndrome below). Carefully document liver size. Determine serum ammonia, bilirubin, prothrombin time, fibrinogen, transaminases, and glucose.
2. Obtain emergent gastroenterologist consultation. Admit to the intensive care unit or arrange immediate transfer to a pediatric critical care center.
3. Perform an emergency head CT to determine if intracranial hemorrhage has occurred or if there is evidence of raised intracranial pressure (see Chapter 50 for management of increased ICP).
4. Correct coagulopathy with vitamin K (see Chapter 19).
5. All patients with hepatic failure are at risk for hypoglycemia. Give 10% dextrose IV to provide 5 mg/kg/min of glucose.
6. Treat hyperammonemia with oral neomycin (50 mg/kg/d divided q 6 h) and lactulose (15–30 ml PO q 4 h).
7. Perform liver biopsy as soon after admission as feasible.

Chronic Hepatitis

Refer patients with chronic hepatitis to a pediatric gastroenterologist. However, the following complications associated with chronic hepatitis may present in the ED and require urgent treatment:

1. *Hepatic encephalopathy.* Alterations in mental status in a patient with chronic hepatitis may result from the encephalopathy associated with end-stage liver failure. Exclude meningitis and sepsis. Patients require admission to the hospital for specific and symptomatic treatment.
2. *GI bleeding* due to varices. Management is described in Chapter 32.
3. *Spontaneous bacterial peritonitis* occurs in patients with ascites due to chronic liver disease. Any patient with a fever and increasing ascites, with or without abdominal tenderness, requires a *diagnostic* paracentesis for aerobic and anaerobic culture. WBC >300 cells/mm³ suggests peritonitis, requiring hospitalization for IV administration of ampicillin and cefotaxime.

Reye's Syndrome ■

Consider Reye's syndrome in any patient with vomiting and altered mental state. Reye's syndrome typically occurs during recovery from an antecedent viral illness (in particular, varicella and influenza B). Aspirin ingestion may increase the incidence. Hereditary metabolic defects, including urea-cycle enzyme deficiency states, systemic carnitine deficiency, and organic acidemias, may present with a Reye's-like illness. Erroneous assumptions of drug ingestions may delay diagnosis and treatment.

CLINICAL FINDINGS AND ANCILLARY DATA

Physical examination reveals hepatomegaly without jaundice. The stages of coma are as presented in Fig. 50-1.

Laboratory findings reveal mild to markedly elevated ALT and AST, prolonged prothrombin time, mild to markedly increased ammonia, bilirubin <3 mg/dl, and mild to severe hypoglycemia. If the bilirubin is >3 mg/dl, consider another diagnosis, such as early fulminant hepatic failure

TREATMENT

Treatment requires ED stabilization and immediate admission to an intensive care unit or transfer to a pediatric critical care center. A pediatric gastroenterologist, neurologist, and neurosurgeon must be available, since diagnosis and treatment may require liver biopsy, placement of an intracranial monitoring device, and serial EEGs. Initial measures include the following:

1. Perform endotracheal intubation for airway protection, respiratory irregularity or insufficiency, or transport. Maintain neuromuscular paralysis to minimize intracranial pressure elevations.
2. Give maintenance IV 10% glucose solution with appropriate electrolytes to provide 70% of daily fluid requirements (see Chapter 22).
3. Give vitamin K, 1 mg IV if <1 year or 5 mg IV if >1 year.
4. Initiate treatment for hyperammonemia with oral neomycin (50 mg/kg/d divided q 6 h) and lactulose (15–30 ml PO q 4 h).
5. Control intracranial pressure elevation as described in Chapter 50. Intracranial pressure monitoring is indicated in any patient achieving Stage 3 coma.

Cholecystitis ■

Acute cholangitis is rare in children. It occurs most commonly in patients that have undergone biliary tract surgery for congenital abnormalities of the bile ducts or in patients with hemolytic disease resulting in cholelithiasis. Acalculous cholecystitis occurs in otherwise well children.

CLINICAL FINDINGS AND ANCILLARY DATA

Fever with jaundice and right upper quadrant pain are the hallmarks of cholecystitis. Jaundice may be absent early in the presentation. Nausea and vomiting are common. The abdominal pain is increased with deep inspiration or coughing during light palpation over the right upper quadrant (Murphy's sign). The tender gallbladder may be palpable.

Laboratory findings include leukocytosis and mild elevations in bilirubin and alkaline phosphatase, SGOT, and SGPT. Amylase may be mildly elevated in cases of cholecystitis, without significant evidence of pancreatitis. Differential diagnosis includes pneumonia, hepatitis, acute appendicitis, perforated duodenal ulcer, and abdominal sickle-cell crisis. In sexually active adolescents, consider gonococcal perihepatitis (Fitz-Hugh-Curtis syndrome). Adnexal tenderness will be present on physical exam.

In the initial evaluation, include a plain abdominal and a chest radiograph. Obtain surgical and gastroenterology consultations. Obtain abdominal ultrasound; in patients with acute cholecystitis, gallstones can usually be demonstrated, and the gallbladder wall is thickened. Sensitivity and specificity of ultrasound are 90% and 95%, respectively. Biliary scintigraphy is more sensitive (97%) but less specific (90%) than ultrasound. Usually, a combination of these tests can provide a reliable diagnosis.

Treatment requires rapid correction of dehydration, nasogastric intubation (see Chapter 22), and hospital admission. Prophylactic antibiotic treatment (cefazolin and gentamicin) is not clearly beneficial but is often recommended. Early cholecystectomy is the treatment of choice in most otherwise well children.

Bibliography ■

Fitzgerald JF, Angelides A, Wyllie R: The hepatitis spectrum. *Curr Prob Pediatr* 1981; 11:1–51.

Plotkin SA et al: *Report of the Committee on Infectious Diseases.* Elk Grove Village, Ill.: American Academy of Pediatrics, 1988.

Weizman Z, Durie PR: Acute pancreatitis in childhood. *J Pediatr* 1988; 113:24–29.

106 Anorectal Disorders

Colin D. Rudolph

Common anorectal disorders discussed in this chapter include anal fissure, abscess, hemorrhoids, and prolapse of the rectum. Constipation is addressed in Chapter 30 and GI bleeding in Chapter 32.

Clinical Findings ■

When a child presents with a complaint related to the anorectum, elicit a basic *history* from the parent or child about the usual stooling pattern, the composition and appearance of stools, diet, pain with defecation, blood in or around stools, drugs, and past medical history. For a breastfeeding infant, ask about the mother's diet and drug and medical history.

Physical assessment is best performed with the child in a knee-chest position. First, gently separate the buttocks and inspect the anus for position, presence of fissures, hemorrhoids, fistula, skin tags, or perianal cellulitis. Next, perform digital examination by introducing a well-lubricated finger slowly with constant pressure against the anal sphincter. When properly performed, *rectal examination is not a painful procedure.* Palpation may reveal an abscess, polyp, or perirectal mass. Obtain stool to test for occult blood.

Specific Conditions ■

ANAL FISSURES

Anal fissures are tears or splits in the mucosa of the anal canal. They can be secondary to the passage of hard stools or to inflammation and erosion of perianal skin. Anal fissures often cause painful defecation and bleeding; this often results in stool withholding, leading to constipation and exacerbation of the damage to the anal canal mucosa, then the eventual passage of a large, firm fecal mass.

Focus treatment on softening the stools. This can be accomplished with dioctyl sodium sulfosuccinate (5–10 mg/kg/24 h) or mineral oil (see Chapter 30). Advise special attention to perineal hygiene and rec-

ommend sitz baths. Topical anesthetic creams are not very helpful in infants but may decrease the pain associated with stooling in older children with anal fissures. If fissures do not heal in 2 months, obtain surgical consultation. Recurrent anal fissures that are resistant to treatment should alert the physician to the possibility of an underlying causative factor, such as Crohn's disease or sexual abuse.

ABSCESS AND FISTULA

Anal abscess and fistula result from fissures or infection of the perianal ducts and glands. An abscess forms in subcutaneous tissues and extends to the perianal skin, resulting in fistula formation. Incision and drainage of abscess and fistula is indicated. To prevent damage to the anorectal sphincter, the ED physician or pediatrician usually should consult a surgical specialist with detailed knowledge of anorectal anatomy. Often this procedure requires general anesthesia and operating room care. Consider immunodeficiency and Crohn's disease in patients with an anal abscess or fistula that does not respond to initial treatment.

PERIANAL CELLULITIS

Both group A and B hemolytic streptococci are increasingly recognized as a cause of perianal cellulitis. Intense erythema and tenderness of the perianal skin is the major finding. Often there is a history of recent pharyngitis. Culture the skin for hemolytic streptococci prior to treatment with penicillin V (25,000 U/kg divided q.i.d. for 2 weeks).

PRURITUS ANI

Pruritus ani is itching of the perianal skin. Most cases are due to either poor hygiene or excessive hygiene. Frequent vigorous washing with irritant soaps causes contact dermatitis. Discourage topical applications of deodorants and ointments. Tight clothing, non-absorptive underclothes, and obesity promote perianal perspiration and warmth; this environment fosters infection with Candida, causing itching.

Treatment requires avoiding tight clothing, and careful cleansing after defecation. Cleansing with moist cotton followed by careful drying with a soft cloth or hair dryer is most effective. Applying nonmedicated talcum powder to maintain a dry environment is sometimes useful. In cases where alterations in hygiene do not lead to resolution of the problem, exclude other infections, such as pinworms, trichomonads, scabies, and pediculosis. Pruritus ani also occurs with psoriasis, atopic eczema, diabetes mellitus, and liver disease.

HEMORRHOIDS

Hemorrhoids are rare in children. When they do occur, they are almost all external. Treatment with sitz baths, stool softeners, and topical anesthetics such as 2% Xylocaine ointment provides increased comfort with stooling. Occasionally, hemorrhoids occur in children with portal hypertension; therefore, the physical examination must always include a careful evaluation for splenomegaly, which may suggest portal hypertension.

RECTAL PROLAPSE

Rectal prolapse occurs when the mucosa or the entire wall of the rectum protrudes through the anus. It usually occurs in children less than 2 years of age. The most common predisposing factor is constipation, but rectal prolapse may be the presenting problem in patients with cystic fibrosis or celiac disease. Rectal prolapse is also relatively common in children with severe malnutrition and in patients with spina bifida.

Prolapse usually occurs during straining with stooling. The prolapsed rectum is usually easy to reduce manually with firm, constant pressure. Treatment consists of vigorous treatment of the constipation. Also, instruct the parent regarding reduction, since repeat episodes of prolapse are likely. Sedation of the patient may allow an otherwise difficult reduction. If the pink mucosa becomes swollen and discolored, obtain surgical consultation to determine if bowel resection is necessary.

If recurrent episodes of rectal prolapse continue for 6 months despite treatment of the constipation, refer the patient to a gastroenterologist for consideration of perirectal injection of sclerosing agents.

RECTAL FOREIGN BODIES

Rectal foreign bodies are introduced through the anus in innocent childhood play, child abuse, or by accident. A wide variety of foreign bodies including thermometers, enema catheters, marbles, and toys are used. Foreign bodies can usually be palpated; however, anteriorposterior and lateral radiographs are sometimes useful to determine the foreign body's shape, size, and position. Extraction is often difficult and painful. Many blunt, small foreign bodies will pass with stooling and therefore require only reassurance and referral to a gastroenterologist or primary care physician for watchful follow-up.

If extraction is required emergently, consult a gastroenterologist. If rectal perforation is suspected in a child with severe pain, indicative physical or radiographic findings, or systemic toxicity, consult a surgeon; operative intervention may be necessary. Extraction is usually performed by rigid proctosigmoidoscopy under general anesthesia, which relaxes the anal sphincter. The child is placed in a lithotomy position, the anus is gently dilated, and the foreign body is then extracted. This procedure is best performed by experienced personnel. Proctosigmoidoscopy is necessary after extraction to search for retained objects or rectal injury.

Bibliography ■

Motson RW, Clifton MA: Pathogenesis and treatment of anal fissure. In: Henry MM, Swash M, eds: *Coloproctology and the pelvic floor: Pathophysiology and management.* Boston: Butterworths, 1985, pp. 340–349.

Ramanujam P, Prasad ML, Abcarian H: Perianal abscesses and fistulas: A study of 1,023 patients. *Dis Colon Rectum* 1984; 27:593.

Smith LE, Henrichs D, McCullah RD: Prospective studies on the etiology and treatment of pruritus ani. *Dis Colon Rectum* 1982; 25:358.

107 Gynecologic Disorders

Richard L. Sweet and Daniel V. Landers

Vulvovaginitis ■

Vulvovaginitis, an inflammatory disease of the vulva or vagina, is the most common gynecologic lesion in children. The causes are multiple and the exact etiology should be determined before beginning therapy. In the premenarchal child, vulvovaginitis can be caused by a variety of bacterial, protozoal, mycotic, viral, physical, chemical, and allergenic agents.

CLINICAL FINDINGS

Take a careful history, including genital, urinary, and gastrointestinal symptoms. Consider and address the possibility of sexual abuse.

Examining the genitalia is crucial for determining the etiology. Inspection of vaginal mucosa and the cervix is mandatory in the evaluating a genital discharge. The gynecologic examination includes inspecting the perineal skin, anus, vulva, urethral meatus, vulvar skin, and hymen. Vaginoscopy or a nasal speculum examination will determine the extent of infection, will allow specimens to be taken, and will exclude the presence of foreign bodies, parasites, and neoplasms.

The steps in the pediatric gynecologic examination are:

1. Inspection and palpation of the vulva
2. Bimanual recto-abdominal examination
3. Separating the labia and depressing the perineum downward, which allows visualization directly into the vagina if the hymeneal opening is large enough
4. Vaginoscopy or, if it does not suffice, nasal speculum examination

Most examinations can be done without anesthesia, but they require patience and gentleness. It is better to do an examination under anesthesia than to force an examination and hurt the child physically or emotionally.

The symptoms of vulvovaginitis may vary from minor discomfort to relatively intense perineal pruritus and burning accompanied by discharge. The discharge may be profuse and purulent or scanty and serous. The mother may note discharge on her daughter's underwear. The type of discharge is seldom of diagnostic significance, except for:

1. Blood-tinged, foul-smelling discharge associated with a foreign body
2. Curdy white discharge characteristic of *Candida albicans*
3. Serosanguineous discharge created by a vaginal or cervical neoplasm

A positive diagnosis is made by examining vaginal secretions (obtained by aspirating secretions with an eye dropper and 4 to 5 cm of intravenous tubing attached) or by vaginoscopy.

Ancillary Data

Vaginal aspirate can be used for:

1. Bacterial smears and/or cultures
2. Sexually transmitted disease (STD) cultures, including *Chlamydia trachomatis* and *Neisseria gonorrhoeae*
3. 10% KOH slide
4. Wet mount (saline suspension)
5. pH measurement
6. KOH ''sniff'' test for amines

On the basis of vaginal aspirate smears, treatment can be directed along specific lines.

TREATMENT

Nonspecific Vulvovaginitis

In premenarchal girls, nonspecific vulvovaginitis accounts for 75% of all the cases. It is considered to be secondary to poor perineal hygiene, including vulvar and vaginal contamination with feces. A mixture of organisms is present; no one organism predominates. A smear reveals numerous white blood cells and bacteria. KOH and saline suspensions are negative for specific agents. Cultures reveal *Escherichia coli,* streptococci, and staphylococci.

A crucial part of treatment is the institution of good perineal hygiene. Educate mothers regarding wiping from vagina toward anus. Recommend daily warm sitz baths and cleansing of child's perineum and vulva with soap and water after each bowel movement.

Treat locally with intravaginal medication:

1. The preferred therapy is urethral suppositories containing nitrofurazone (Furacin). Instruct the mother to insert half of the suppository into her child's vagina nightly for 14 days, or
2. Prescribe the vaginal suppository Vagisec nightly for 14 days.
3. Sulfabenzamide (Sultrin) cream twice a day may be prescribed for refractory infections.

Children with persistent infections usually have failed to practice good perineal hygiene, have intestinal parasites, or have repeatedly inserted foreign bodies into the vagina.

1. Pinworm infestations are responsible for many intractable vaginal infections. The worms migrate from the anus into the vagina, carrying coliform bacteria with them. The parasite must be eradicated and the vaginitis must be treated as above.
2. Most foreign bodies are paper and cloth and do not show up on x-ray. Vaginoscopy or a speculum examination is essential to exclude a foreign body as a cause of recurrent vaginitis. Treatment consists of removing the foreign body and local intravaginal medication as described above.

Monilial Vaginitis

Monilial vaginitis is usually seen in an estrogenic vagina and thus most often occurs in postmenarchal patients. It does, however, occur in young children, especially following the use of broad-spectrum antibiotics. The diagnosis is determined by the presence of hyphae characteristic of *C. albicans* on a KOH smear.

Local therapy consists of gentle cleansing of the vulva and the application of nystatin cream twice a day for 14 days. Insert a nystatin suspension in the vagina every night for 2 weeks. Give a suspension of nystatin orally in small children.

Treat postmenarchal patients with:

1. Nystatin (Mycostatin) suppositories vaginally twice a day for 14 days, or
2. Miconazole (Monistat) cream applied at bedtime for 7 days, or

3. Clotrimazole (Gyne-Lotrimin) cream applied at bedtime for 7 days

Trichomonas Vaginitis

Trichomonas vaginitis, most commonly seen in the postmenarchal group, often results from sexual transmission and is thus considered indicative of child abuse. The diagnosis is suggested by a frothy, yellow-green exudate or petechiae on the cervix and is confirmed by the presence of a motile protozoan parasite, *Trichomonas vaginalis,* in a saline suspension.

Treat with metronidazole (Flagyl):

1. Premenarchal: 35–50 mg/kg/24 hr divided into three doses for 10 days
2. Postmenarchal: 2 g orally as a single dose; also treat sexual partner(s)
3. Alternate regimen: 250 mg three times a day for 10 days

Bacterial Vaginosis (*Gardnerella vaginalis*)

Patients present with a copious discharge and acutely inflamed external genitalia. Diagnosis is based on the presence of:

1. pH above 4.5
2. Homogeneous adherent discharge
3. Clue cells (a squamous epithelial cell covered with gram-negative coccobacilli)
4. A release of amine odor with addition of KOH to discharge

Treatment consists of:

1. Metronidazole: in adolescents, 250 mg PO three times a day for 7 days; in premenarchal girls, 25 mg/kg/day in three divided doses
2. Ampicillin 500 mg PO four times a day for 7 days
3. Treatment of male partners is controversial but may be indicated for recurrent cases; use either of the above regimens.

Streptococcal Vaginitis

Streptococcus pyogenes can be cultured from girls with prepubertal vaginal discharges, especially following scarlet fever. The organism may cause genital pain or pruritus as well as discharge. Diagnosis is by positive culture. Penicillin (25–50 mg/kg/day PO in four divided doses for 10 days) is the treatment of choice. Alternatively, oral erythromycin (40 mg/kg/day in four divided doses for 10 days).

Vaginal Obstruction ■

ETIOLOGY AND PATHOPHYSIOLOGY

Obstruction of the physiologic outlet for genital secretions and menstrual blood may present in infancy with vaginal distention from mucus secretion, or later following menarche with distention from menstrual blood. The etiology of vaginal distention with mucus, watery secretions, or blood (mucocolpos, hydrocolpos, hematocolpos) commonly involves congenital anomalies such as imperforate hymen and transverse vaginal septum (vaginal atresia).

CLINICAL FINDINGS

Symptoms in infancy may include a lower abdominal mass, difficulty with urination, and a visible bulging membrane at the introitus. In puberty, the presenting complaint is usually primary amenorrhea or lower abdominal pain with a bluish bulging membrane at the introitus. Acute urinary retention can occur as a result of vaginal outflow obstruction. Rarely, this condition can lead to respiratory embarrassment in infancy.

TREATMENT

Imperforate hymen is treated by surgically creating adequate outflow through the introitus. Patients with congenital vaginal obstruction due to transverse vaginal septae may require more extensive surgical correction. Infants and children with asymptomatic vaginal outflow obstruction can be treated electively after a gynecologic referral.

Acute Pelvic Pain ■

ETIOLOGY AND PATHOPHYSIOLOGY

In the premenarchal group, appendicitis and mesenteric adenitis are the predominant causes. Occasionally, an ovarian cyst will present in young children with acute pain, especially if there is torsion of the cyst pedicle.

Adolescent girls present a dilemma in differential diagnosis. The major categories to consider in this group are appendicitis, salpingo-oophoritis, ruptured ectopic pregnancy, and ruptured or bleeding ovarian cysts.

CLINICAL FINDINGS

Salpingo-oophoritis

Salpingo-oophoritis presents as bilateral lower abdominal pain usually beginning at the end of or just after a menstrual period, if sexually transmitted organisms such as *C. trachomatis* or *N. gonorrhoeae* are involved. Typically, pain has been present 48 to 72 hours and has progressively worsened. If gastrointestinal symptoms such as nausea and vomiting are present, they are minimal and occur late in the disease process. A history of fever and chills may be present, but is not an absolute criteria. Forty percent of cases are afebrile.

The etiology is polymicrobic:

1. *N. gonorrhoeae,* 25% to 50%
2. *C. trachomatis,* 20% to 30%
3. *Mycoplasma hominis,* 5% to 10%
4. Mixed anaerobes and facultative bacteria, 25% to 50%

Examination reveals bilateral lower abdominal tenderness and rebound. On pelvic examination, cervical motion tenderness and adnexal tenderness are present. A purulent cervical discharge may be noted.

To diagnose salpingo-oophoritis, all three of the following must be present:

1. Lower abdominal pain and direct tenderness
2. Cervical motion tenderness
3. Adnexal tenderness

In addition, at least one of the following must be present:

1. Fever (temperature above 100.4°F)
2. Leukocytosis (WBC above 10,500)
3. Culdocentesis yielding a fluid that on Gram's stain has WBC or bacteria
4. Pelvic inflammatory mass noted on exam or with sonography
5. Cervical Gram's stain with intracellular gram-negative diplococci
6. More than 10 WBC per high-power field on cervical Gram's stain

Ruptured Ectopic Pregnancy

Consider a patient in a reproductive age group presenting with abdominal pain, amenorrhea, and abnormal uterine bleeding to have a ruptured ectopic pregnancy until proven otherwise.

Pain is acute and sharp. It begins unilaterally, but rapidly becomes diffuse in lower abdominal pain. In 90% of cases, patients are late for their menstrual period, but 10% of ruptured ectopics occur prior to the date of expected menses.

Early signs and symptoms of pregnancy may be present. A pregnancy test may or may not be positive, but a negative pregnancy test does not exclude a diagnosis of ectopic pregnancy. The white blood cell count is normal.

Hypovolemic shock may be present if severe intra-abdominal bleeding has occurred. Orthostatic hypotension may be an early sign of impending shock. The abdomen is tender and rebound is present. A pelvic examination reveals diffuse pelvic tenderness and cervical motion tenderness. A mass is palpable in the adnexal area in only one third of patients and is not an absolute criteria for the diagnosis.

The diagnosis is confirmed by obtaining nonclotting blood from the abdominal cavity via culdocentesis. Perform culdocentesis with a 20- or 18-gauge spinal needle attached to a 10-ml syringe. Place a tenaculum on the posterior lip of the cervix for traction and insert the needle into the peritoneal cavity via the cul de sac. If a positive diagnosis is strongly suspected and culdocentesis is inconclusive, diagnostic laparoscopy is indicated.

Ruptured or Bleeding Ovarian Cysts; Torsion of Ovarian Cysts

Pain begins unilaterally in one of the lower abdominal quadrants with radiation toward the groin and anterior thigh; eventually, pain becomes diffuse and involves the entire lower abdomen. In children, the pain is periumbilical. Unless the cyst has twisted on its pedicle, gastrointestinal symptoms are mild. The patient is usually afebrile and the blood count is within normal limits. If torsion has produced infarction and necrosis, fever and leukocytosis may be present.

Examination reveals moderate lower abdominal tenderness and rebound. A pelvic examination discloses minimal cervical motion tenderness, but it is not as severe as in salpingitis or ectopic pregnancy. Bimanual examination reveals a cystic adnexal mass in most cases; following rupture, no mass may be palpable.

Culdocentesis reveals clear straw-colored fluid with ruptured cysts. Bleeding ovarian cysts result in intra-abdominal hemorrhage, and a culdocentesis yields nonclotting blood similar to that seen with an ectopic pregnancy. Torsion of an ovarian cyst is associated with a negative culdocentesis.

TREATMENT

Salpingo-oophoritis

Obtain an endocervical culture for *N. gonorrhoeae* and *C. trachomatis*. A Gram's stain revealing gram-negative intracellular diplococci is suggestive of gonorrhea, but is not conclusive. Antibiotic therapy is the keystone of treatment.

For outpatient treatment, give cefoxitin 2 g IM *or* ceftriaxone 250 mg IM; *or* amoxicillin 3 g PO *or* ampicillin 3.5 g PO; *or* aqueous procaine penicillin G 4.8 million units IM at two sites. Give probenecid 1 g PO with each of these alternative antimicrobials.

In-hospital treatment with parenteral antibiotics is indicated if an abscess is suspected, if the patient cannot take oral medications, if the patient's temperature is higher than 38.5°C, and if the patient does not respond to outpatient treatment in 24 hours. Consider admitting all young patients with salpingo-oophoritis for treatment, especially adolescents. Pelvic rest is indicated until infection has cleared.

Follow parenteral treatment with doxycycline 100 mg PO twice a day for 10 to 14 days (in adolescents, tetracycline HCl 500 mg PO four times a day can be used). In areas endemic for penicillinase-producing N. gonorrhoeae (PPNG) (>1%), use ceftriaxone.

Acute Appendicitis

See Chapter 40.

Ruptured Ectopic Pregnancy

A culdocentesis positive for nonclotting blood is an acute surgical emergency and requires immediate surgical exploration to identify the source of hemorrhage and to secure hemostasis. Obtain emergent gynecologic consultation. Transfusion is often necessary to compensate for the massive (often 1000–1500 ml) intra-abdominal hemorrhage.

Ruptured or Bleeding Ovarian Cysts; Torsion of Ovarian Cysts

A ruptured ovarian cyst most commonly occurs in the postmenarchal age group and is due to a persistent corpus luteum cyst.

If culdocentesis reveals typical clear straw-colored fluid, observation for 24 hours is indicated. Patients usually respond within 6 hours with decrease in pain and tenderness. The surgeon must make sure no intra-abdominal hemorrhage has occurred by monitoring vital signs frequently and by performing serial hematocrits.

If ruptured cysts are diagnosed at the time of the laparoscopy or exploratory laparotomy and no bleeding is present, no specific treatment is indicated. If there is any suggestion that the ovarian cyst is more than a simple functional cyst, histologic examination of the cyst is mandatory.

If laparoscopy or exploratory laparotomy reveals significant bleeding at the site of the rupture of an ovarian cyst, surgical intervention to secure hemostasis is indicated.

Hemorrhage secondary to the rupture of a cyst may be massive and similar to that seen in ruptured ectopics. Bleeding in such instances is controlled surgically.

Ovarian Neoplasms

Although ovarian cysts are rare in children and adolescents, they have a higher incidence of malignancy (about 33%) than seen in adult ovarian neoplasms. The differential diagnosis of an abdominal-pelvic mass and pain in children must include neuroblastoma, Wilms' tumor, and polycystic kidneys. A radiologic examination of the abdomen is useful and may reveal tumor calcification in dermoid cysts. A sonogram can differentiate between solid and cystic lesions.

Early diagnosis by exploratory laparotomy is crucial to the treatment of ovarian neoplasms. The most common childhood ovarian neoplasms include germ-cell tumors (such as teratomas and dysgerminomas) and sex cord tumors (such as granulosa-cell tumors).

Toxic Shock Syndrome ■

ETIOLOGY AND PATHOPHYSIOLOGY

Toxic shock syndrome (TSS) is an acute febrile syndrome with diffuse, desquamating erythroderma and mucous membrane hyperemia, hypotension, and multiple-organ involvement.

The large majority of cases occur in menstruating women, especially in those using tampons, particularly highly absorbent brands. The highest risk group is women ages 15 to 19. Nonmenstrual cases occur in women, men, and children, almost always in association with a localized infection with *Staphylococcus aureus*. *S. aureus* strains producing a unique pyrogenic exotoxin-C or enterotoxin-F are associated with TSS.

CLINICAL FINDINGS

TSS presents with the sudden onset of fever, vomiting, diarrhea, and myalgia, followed by the development of hypotension, syncope, or dizziness. An erythematous, sunburn-like rash occurs that in survivors desquamates after 10 to 14 days. There may be mucosal involvement such as nonpurulent conjunctivitis, pharyngitis, or vaginitis. Clinical laboratory evidence of multi-organ disease is present. Table 107-1 shows the Center for Disease Control's criteria for diagnosing TSS.

TABLE 107–1. *Centers for Disease Control Established Criteria for Diagnosing TSS*

Temperature >102°F
Hypotension, syncope, or dizziness
Rash, with subsequent desquamation in survivors
Involvement of 3 or more of the following organ systems:
   Gastrointestinal (vomiting or diarrhea)
   Muscular (severe myalgias or CPK ≥ a five-fold increase)
   Mucous membranes (vaginal, oropharyngeal, or conjunctival hyperemia)
   Renal insufficiency
   Hepatic involvement
   Hematologic (thrombocytopenia, DIC)
   CNS
Negative results on:
   Blood, throat, and CSF cultures (but blood can be positive for *S. aureus*)
   Serologic tests for Rocky Mountain spotted fever, leptospirosis, and rubeola

TREATMENT

A high index of suspicion is necessary for early diagnosis. Vaginal examination and removal of the tampon are required, with cervical and vaginal cultures for *S. aureus*. Institute aggressive and adequate volume replacement in addition to a beta-lactamase-resistant antistaphylococcal antibiotic (nafcillin or oxacillin 9–10 g/day).

PREVENTION

A woman who has had TSS should not use tampons. To decrease risk, woman should not use high-absorbency tampons. Tampons should be inserted with an inserter rather than with fingers, where possible.

Bibliography ■

Centers for Disease Control: 1985 STD treatment guidelines. *MMWR* 1985; 34:755.

Davis JP et al: Toxic shock syndrome: Epidemiologic features, recurrence, risk factors and prevention. *N Engl J Med* 1980; 303:1429.

Paradise JE: Pediatric and adolescent gynecology. In: Kleisher G, Ludwig S, eds: *Textbook of Pediatric Emergency Medicine*, 2nd ed. Baltimore: Williams & Wilkins, 1988.

Shafer MB, Irwin CL, Sweet RL: Acute salpingitis in the adolescent female. *J Pediatr* 1982; 100:339.

Spiegal CA et al: Anaerobic bacteria in nonspecific vaginitis. *N Engl J Med* 1980; 303:601.

Sweet RL, Gibbs R: *Infectious Disease of the Female Genital Tract*. Baltimore: Williams & Wilkins, 1985.

108 Hematologic Emergencies

William C. Mentzer

Anemia is often first encountered in the emergency department setting. Useful information from the patient or parents and pertinent physical findings are listed in Tables 108-1 and 108-2. Laboratory studies (complete blood count, reticulocyte count, review of red cell morphology at a minimum) are essential for proper evaluation. An approach to the diagnosis of anemia is presented in Table 108-3.

A common feature of management is the use of blood transfusions (see Chapter 136). Specific therapies for individual anemias are discussed later in the chapter. For hypovolemia and acute blood-loss anemia, see Chapter 19.

The decision to transfuse a chronically anemic patient depends not only on the hemoglobin level, but also on the adequacy of oxygen transport (as determined by skin color, pulse rate, exercise tolerance, and the presence or absence of incipient or frank heart failure) and the risk of further accentuation of anemia (e.g., from hemolysis or blood loss). If anemia has developed slowly, patients can often tolerate hemoglobin levels of 4 to 5 g/dL remarkably well, and they may not need transfusion if other effective therapy (e.g., iron, vitamin B_{12}, or folate) is available. Severely anemic patients in borderline or frank cardiac failure cannot tolerate sudden increases in blood volume; slow administration (less than 2 ml/kg/hr) of packed red cells is usually safe. If a diuretic (furosemide, 1 mg/kg/body weight IV) is given prior to transfusion, the risk of circulatory overload is minimized. If rapid repair of anemia is essential in the patient with cardiac failure, partial exchange transfusion will avoid the changes in blood volume associated with simple infusion.

Inadequate Erythrocyte Production ■

Bone marrow failure states (Table 108-4) often present with severe anemia requiring immediate assessment and treatment. Obtain a complete blood count and differential to determine the number of cell lines affected. A bone-marrow examination is almost always indicated, particularly to distinguish malignant disorders from benign. Since severe bone-marrow failure is often treated by bone-marrow transplantation, minimize supportive transfusions to avoid alloimmunization and exclude family members (who may be prospective marrow donors) as red cell or platelet donors. If a transplant is imminent, use only cytomegalovirus-negative irradiated blood products (unless the donor is known to be CMV positive). Other aspects of management vary depending on the diagnosis.

Diamond Blackfan syndrome (DBS) presents in infancy, usually prior to 1 year of age. Macrocytic or normocytic anemia, reticulocytopenia, and erythroblastopenia are found. Corticosteroid therapy (prednisone 2 mg/kg/day initially, then tapered to find the lowest effective dose) is effective in most patients.

Transient erythroblastopenia of childhood (TEC) generally occurs in somewhat older infants and children than does DBS. As in DBS, anemia, reticulocytopenia, and erythroblastopenia are present. Unlike DBS, at diagnosis the MCV is low-normal and hemoglobin F levels are not elevated (but during recovery these values may be above normal). Spontaneous recovery in 1 to 2 months is the rule. Corticosteroids are of no benefit and should not be used.

Isolated *neutropenia* requires careful evaluation, since treatment of the underlying cause (Table 108-4) is the most effective therapy in most instances. In autoimmune neutropenia, corticosteroids or high-dose intravenous gamma globulin therapy may raise the neutrophil count. Severely neutropenic patients (ANC less than 500/µL) with fever require comprehensive evaluation for sepsis and broad-spectrum antibiotic therapy (see Chapter 109).

Thrombocytopenia is discussed in Chapter 19.

Congenital aplastic anemia (Fanconi's anemia) is a slowly developing pancytopenia that usually becomes clinically apparent at about 8 to 10 years of age. The diagnosis is suggested by the presence of one or more associated non-hematologic congenital anomalies (radial-side skeletal anomalies of the forearm and hand, skin hyperpigmentation, microsomy, microcephaly, hypogenitalia, renal anomalies, etc.) and is confirmed by chromosome analysis revealing the characteristic breaks, exchanges, and endoreduplications. Management consists of supportive care, androgens, and consideration of bone-marrow transplantation if a compatible donor is available.

Acquired aplastic anemia may follow infections or exposure to drugs or toxins, or it may be idiopathic. Removal of the underlying cause, if possible, is an important initial step in management. Mild aplastic anemia may only require supportive care until recovery occurs. Severe aplastic anemia is defined as the presence of at least two of the following: platelet count less than 20,000/μL, granulocyte count less than 500/μL, corrected reticulocyte count less than 1%. It is often fatal and more aggressive treatment is warranted. Bone-marrow transplantation is recommended if a compatible donor is available; if not, antithymocyte globulin (ATG) or antilymphocyte globulin (ALG) therapy is an effective alternative.

Decreased Erythropoietin Production ■

Chronic renal disease and prematurity are two settings in which anemia may be the result of inadequate erythropoietin production. Treatment with recombinant erythropoietin is effective in the former condition and is under evaluation in the latter. Red cell transfusions are used in both.

Disordered Erythrocyte Maturation ■

NUTRITIONAL ANEMIAS

These anemias may be severe, but because they develop slowly they are often surprisingly well tolerated. Iron deficiency is relatively common, while folate deficiency is rare and B_{12} deficiency exceedingly rare in children. Suspect a nutritional anemia when either microcytosis (iron deficiency) or macrocytosis (B_{12}, folate deficiency) is present. Specific assay of the serum concentration of the appropriate nutrient (Fe, B_{12}, folate) establishes the diagnosis. Search for the underlying cause (*i.e.*, bleeding or inadequate intake of iron in the case of iron deficiency).

Treatment consists of providing adequate amounts of the deficient nutrient. Oral folic acid, 1 mg/day, will produce a prompt hematologic response; larger doses may be required if malabsorption is present. Because malabsorption is commonly the basis for B_{12}

TABLE 108–1. *Questions to Ask When a Child Has Anemia*

Is There a History of:
 Bleeding
 Antecedent acute or chronic illness, particularly infection
 Exposure to drugs or toxins
 Jaundice, gallstones, abdominal pain
 Travel outside the United States
 Diet inadequate in iron, folic acid, or vitamin B_{12}

Is There a Family History of:
 Anemia
 Gallstones
 Splenectomy
 Bleeding disorder

deficiency, this nutrient is often given parenterally (50–1000 μg/month IM). The rare infant who develops B_{12} deficiency as a result of a vegan diet, however, will respond to oral B_{12} therapy.

Oral ferrous sulfate (3 mg iron/kg/day in 2–3 divided doses) is the standard treatment for iron deficiency. If given with meals, iron absorption will be diminished but there is less chance of uncomfortable gastrointestinal side effects.

When the appropriate nutrient therapy is given, a reticulocyte response will occur in 3–7 days and the hemoglobin will begin to rise shortly thereafter.

Blood Loss Anemias ■

See Chapter 19.

Hemolytic Anemias ■

Patients may seek emergency care for acute hemolysis or for complications associated with a chronic hemolytic state. The latter include:

1. Symptoms relating to bilirubin gallstones, formed as a consequence of longstanding hemolysis

TABLE 108–2. *Physical Findings to Look for in the Anemic Child*

Jaundice
Splenomegaly
Signs of infection
Congenital anomalies, particularly of the skeleton
Petechiae, purpura
Compromised cardiovascular function

TABLE 108-3. *Classification of Anemias*

Condition	MCV	Red Cell Morphology
Inadequate Red Cell Production (reticulocyte count low)		
Bone marrow failure syndromes	Normal to high	Normal, ovalocytes
Decreased erythropoietin production	Normal	Normal
Disordered Erythrocyte Maturation (reticulocyte count usually low)		
Iron deficiency	Low	Hypochromia
Folate or B_{12} deficiency	High	Normal, occ. fragmented RBC
Dyserythropoietic anemias	High	Abnormal
Blood Loss (reticulocyte count normal or elevated)		
Acute	Normal	Normal
Chronic	Normal to high	Normal
Chronic with 2° iron deficiency	Normal to low	Hypochromia
Hemolysis (reticulocyte count elevated)		
Extracorpuscular	Low to high	Abnormal
Membrane disorders	Low to high	Abnormal
Hemoglobinopathies	Low to high	Abnormal
Metabolic disorders	Normal to high	Normal (usually)

2. Severe anemia due to transient, infection-associated bone marrow suppression (an "aplastic crisis"). Parvovirus infection is a common cause. The reticulocyte count is low. Because the red-cell life span is short, anemia may develop rapidly (in a few days) and red cell tranfusions may be necessary.

TABLE 108-4. *Bone Marrow Failure States*

Erythroblastopenia
  Congenital (Diamond-Blackfan syndrome)
  Acquired (transient erythroblastopenia of childhood, pure red cell aplasia)

Neutropenia
  Congenital (Kostmann's syndrome, etc.)
  Acquired (immune, drugs, infections, malignancy)

Thrombocytopenia
  Congenital (*e.g.,* absent RADII syndrome)
  Acquired

Pancytopenia (aplastic anemia)
  Congenital (Fanconi's anemia, Schwachman's syndrome, etc.)
  Acquired (drugs, infection, idiopathic)

3. An acute exacerbation of hemolysis (a "hemolytic crisis"), occurring during infections and probably due to acute splenomegaly, reticuloendothelial system hyperactivity, and/or in susceptible individuals (e.g., G6PD deficiency) oxidant stress. Treatment of an acute hemolytic crisis consists of removal of the initiating agent, if identified; transfusion with packed red cells; and management of hemoglobinuria so as to prevent acute renal failure. If hemoglobinuria is present, initiate an osmotic diuresis with 20% mannitol (2.5 ml/kg IV, given over 15 minutes); maintain by administration of adequate intravenous fluids and a diuretic such as furosemide (1 mg/kg IV for children) until the urine is clear. Despite these measures, renal failure may ensue and require treatment by dialysis and fluid restriction.

EXTRACORPUSCULAR CAUSES OF HEMOLYSIS

Changes in the environment of the red cell may cause hemolysis (Table 108-5). In most cases, management consists of supportive care with red cell transfusions and elimination of the underlying cause (*i.e.,* treatment of infections with antibiotics).

TABLE 108–5. *Extracorpuscular Causes of Hemolysis*

Chemical injury to RBC: Oxidants (chlorates, dapsone, salicylazosulfidine, naphthalene, hyperbaric oxygen), heavy metals (lead, copper)
Hypersplenism
Hypophosphatemia
Immune: Autoimmune hemolytic anemias, isoimmune hemolytic anemia of the newborn, transfusion reactions
Infections: Bacterial (influenza, bartonella, clostridial species, etc.), parasitic (malaria)
Insect and snake venoms
Physical injury to RBC: Microangiopathic hemolytic anemia (DIC, hemolytic uremic syndrome, hemangioma), macroangiopathic hemolytic anemia (artificial heart valves), March hemoglobinuria, heat, inadvertent intravenous administration of distilled water
Vitamin E deficiency

IMMUNE HEMOLYTIC ANEMIAS

Immune hemolytic anemias, listed in Table 108-6, occur when an auto-antibody (or alloantibody) binds to target red cells, with or without complement, and causes hemolysis, either intravascular (complement-mediated) or as a result of reticuloendothelial sequestration. They may be idiopathic or secondary to underlying disorders, the most common of which are immunodeficiency states, autoimmune diseases, or malignancies. Spherocytes and erythrophagocytosis (warm AIHA) or red cell agglutination (cold AIHA) suggest the diagnosis, but demonstration of IgG or complement respectively on affected red cells (Coombs test) is required for confirmation. Treatment differs according to the type of AIHA found.

With *warm antibody AIHA*, hemolysis may be rapid and the ensuing anemia life-threatening. Provide immediate treatment with prednisone (2 mg/kg/day) or an equivalent injectable corticosteroid; higher prednisone doses (up to 10 mg/kg/day) may be effective if the standard dose is not. Continue treatment until the anemia has been corrected and hemolysis has subsided.

Transfusion of packed red cells may be required while awaiting a prednisone response, if anemia is severe. Fully crossmatched blood will probably not be available, as the auto-antibody is generally reactive with all donor red cells. Choose the least incompatible units for administration. When giving donor red cells, use the least amount necessary to support the patient, as donor red cell survival will be no better than autologous red cell survival. This practice will minimize hemoglobinuria and the resulting possibility of acute renal failure.

Splenectomy may be indicated if the response to corticosteroids does not occur or is transient. Immunosuppressive agents such as cyclophosphamide or azothioprine may be tried as an alternative to splenectomy.

Cold hemagglutinin AIHA is most commonly seen in association with infections (Mycoplasma pneumonia, infectious mononucleosis) or lymphoreticular malignancies. Treatment of the underlying condition and avoidance of exposure to cold are generally sufficient to control hemolysis. If packed red cell transfusions are required, warm the blood before administration. Unlike warm AIHA, corticosteroids and splenectomy are of little or no therapeutic value.

Paroxysmal cold hemoglobinuria (PCH) is characterized by the sudden appearance of red-brown urine and anemia following exposure to low temperatures. It usually occurs during or after an acute infection, commonly of viral origin, but it may be idiopathic. The course is brief (generally 1–2 weeks) and recurrences are rare. A complement-binding IgG (Donath-Landsteiner) antibody with anti-P specificity is found in the serum of affected children.

Drug-associated AIHA: Several drugs may induce antibody formation. When the drug/antibody complex or, at times, the antibody alone binds to red cells, hemolysis ensues. Drugs implicated include methyldopa, chlorpromazine, ibuprofen, L-dopa, mefenamic acid, phenacetin, and procainamide. Cessation of drug administration terminates AIHA; corticosteroid therapy may be beneficial in severe cases.

Paroxysmal nocturnal hemoglobinuria (PNH), an acquired clonal disorder of hematopoietic cells, is suggested by acute or chronic intravascular hemolysis resulting in hemoglobinuria. PNH red cells are abnormally susceptible to the lytic action of complement, as can be detected *in vitro* by the Ham's or sucrose hemolysis tests used to diagnose the disorder. The white cell and platelets count may be subnormal. Prednisone (1–2 mg/kg/day) or androgens may help reduce the rate of hemolysis. If transfusion is nec-

TABLE 108–6. *Immune Hemolytic Anemias*

Autoimmune hemolytic anemias (AIHA):
  Warm antibody (1gG-mediated) AIHA
  Cold hemagglutinin (1gM-mediated) AIHA
  Paroxysmal cold hemoglobinuria
  Drug-induced AIHA
Paroxysmal nocturnal hemoglobinuria
Alloimmune hemolytic anemias:
  Passive transfer of antibody
  Active immunization

TABLE 108–7. *Hereditary Erythrocyte Membrane Disorders*

Disorder	Inheritance	Severity of Hemolysis	Osmotic Fragility
Spherocytosis	Dominant	Mild to severe	Increased
Elliptocytosis	Dominant	Mild to severe	Normal or increased
Poikilocytosis	?	Severe	Increased
Stomatocytosis	Dominant or ?	Moderate to severe	Increased
Xerocytosis	Dominant	Minimal to severe	Decreased

essary, use washed red cells to minimize exposure to complement (and perhaps other factors) in donor plasma.

Alloimmune hemolytic anemias: Passive transfer of maternal antibody from mothers affected with warm antibody AIHA may produce hemolytic anemia in their infants (Table 108-7). Isoimmune sensitization due to blood group incompatibility between mother and infant may have a similar result (ABO or Rh incompatibility). Finally, transfusion of incompatible blood may sensitize the recipient (see Chapter 136).

Sickle Hemoglobinopathies ■

The clinical features of sickle-cell disease are presented in Table 108-8. If the diagnosis of sickle-cell disease is suspected but not established, sickle screening tests (e.g., a solubility test or a sodium-metabisulfite sickling preparation) will rapidly confirm the presence of sickle hemoglobin. Hemoglobin electrophoresis is mandatory for ascertaining the precise nature of the hemoglobinopathy.

Clinical problems that bring the child with sickle-cell disease to the ED include vaso-occlusive events, episodes of profound anemia, and sudden overwhelming bacterial infections.

VASO-OCCLUSIVE EVENTS

Vaso-occlusive events are associated with severe local pain, fever, leukocytosis, and/or impaired organ function. They may mimic other emergency conditions. A major problem is the differentiation of infarction from infection. High fever (greater than 102°F), a strikingly elevated white blood count (greater than 20,000/μL), an absolute band count greater than 1,000/μL, an erythrocyte-sedimentation rate greater than 20 mm/hr, elevated leukocyte alkaline phosphatase, and elevated serum α-hydroxybutyrate levels point to infection. Compare laboratory results to baseline values obtained during crisis-free intervals.

Abdominal pain may suggest appendicitis, cholecystitis, or other surgical emergencies. The presence of bowel sounds favors the diagnosis of sickle-cell crisis. Appendicitis appears to be uncommon in sickle-cell anemia. Fever and leukocytosis occur in both sickle-cell crisis and in appendicitis. If the fever or WBC is unusually high sepsis, perhaps intra-abdominal, is suggested.

TABLE 108–8. *Clinical Features of Common Sickling Variants*

	HB (gm/100 ml)	MCV (fl)	Reticulocytes (%)	HB Electrophoresis	Clinical Severity
Sickle-cell Anemia	7.8 ± 1.2	99 ± 10	10.3 ± 4	S.F. (2%–20%), A_2	Moderate to severe
SC Disease	11.7 ± 1.7	79.3 ± 6.6	3.1 ± 1.5	S, C	Mild to severe
Sickle-β^0-thalassemia	8.1 ± 1.1	69.8 ± 7.5	8.6 ± 3.7	S, F, A_2 ($\uparrow$)	Moderate to severe
Sickle-β^+-thalassemia	10.7 ± 1.2	72 ± 6.6	3.2 ± 1.9	S, A (10%–30%), F, A_2 ($\uparrow$)	Mild to severe
Sickle Trait	NL	NL	NL	S (25%–40%), A, A_2	Usually no symptoms

(Serjeant GR, Serjeant BE: A comparison of erythrocyte characteristics in sickle-cell syndromes in Jamaica. *Brit J Haematol* 1972;23:205.)

Vaso-occlusive events are rare in infants under 2 to 3 months of age. The hand-foot syndrome (painful, warm swelling of one or more hands or feet) is a common initial vaso-occlusive episode in young children.

Bone pain is usually due to local infarction of the bone marrow. Aseptic necrosis may result from infarcts in areas with poor collateral circulation (head of humerus or femur). The incidence of osteomyelitis is increased, and differentiating osteomyelitis from bone infarct is often difficult. X-ray and radionuclide scans are of little or no assistance. When high fever, chills, and toxicity suggest osteomyelitis, consider bone aspiration.

Joint pain (migratory, recurrent, or constant) may occur and may be associated with swelling and limitation of motion, simulating rheumatoid arthritis or rheumatic fever.

Episodes of hyperbilirubinemia (total bilirubin may reach or exceed 50 mg/dL) may result from cholelithiasis with obstruction of the common bile duct, sickling-induced multiple micro-infarcts of the liver, viral hepatitis, or hemolytic crisis.

Splenic infarcts are a frequent source of abdominal pain in the child. Recurrent infarcts lead to progressive atrophy and fibrosis (autosplenectomy) of the spleen.

Neurologic symptoms, such as persistent headache, visual or auditory disturbances, dizziness, coma, convulsions, facial nerve palsies, changes in personality, and paresthesias may occur singly or in combination when a vaso-occlusive crisis involves the nervous system. Stroke is more commonly due to large vessel thrombosis in children and to subarachnoid hemorrhage in adults. CT or MRI imaging is helpful in diagnosis. Do angiographic studies of the cerebral vessels after partial exchange transfusion; pay careful attention to adequate hydration and oxygenation.

Pulmonary signs and symptoms (coughing, chest pain, shortness of breath, and tachypnea) may be due to pulmonary infarcts or infection, or to a combination of the two. Measurement of arterial blood gases or pulse oximetry is helpful since pulmonary sickling is one setting in which oxygen therapy may be valuable.

Traumatic hyphema may be followed by sickling of red cells in the anterior chamber, causing increased intraocular pressure (secondary glaucoma) and eventually occlusion of the central retinal artery and blindness.

Other problems associated with vaso-occlusion include priapism, hematuria, retinopathy, and leg ulcers.

Patients with sickle-hemoglobin variants (SC disease, SD disease, S-β-thalassemia), though less prone to vaso-occlusive crisis, may exhibit any of the symptoms listed above.

Treatment

Specific drug therapy to prevent or arrest painful sickle crisis is not yet available. Therapy is aimed at alleviating pain and minimizing conditions that favor sickling:

1. *Oxygenation.* Episodes of infarction are probably not influenced by supplemental oxygen therapy unless hypoxemia is present. Obtain arterial blood gas measurements or pulse oximetry before giving oxygen. Prolonged (24 hours or more) use of high-oxygen environments may produce transient erythroid hypoplasia in the bone marrow and should be discouraged.

2. *Hydration.* Dehydration, which promotes the sickling process, is a frequent occurrence (owing to the hyposthenuria found in most patients with sickle-cell disease). Pain associated with vaso-occlusive crisis may lead to a reduction in voluntary water intake, while fever, which commonly accompanies such crises, increases insensible water loss.

   Immediate hydration with 3 ml/kg body weight/hr using 5% dextrose plus one fourth normal saline and bicarbonate (see below) will often provide considerable symptomatic relief within several hours. Subsequently, keep a complete record of fluid intake and loss and calculate adequate replacement therapy on the basis of observed losses. Weigh the patient daily.

   Serum sodium is of particular value in monitoring therapy. Monitor serum sodium closely to avoid hyponatremia, as patients in crises may sustain urinary sodium losses of 6 to 11 mEq/kg/day.

3. *Acid-base balance.* Obtain serum bicarbonate and blood pH immediately. Correct acidosis with intravenous bicarbonate (dose may be calculated from the serum bicarbonate or approximated by using 3 mEq/kg/12 hr).

4. *Analgesia.* Pain is a genuine and often severe component of vaso-occlusive crisis. Useful analgesics for mild pain include acetaminophen 5–10 mg/kg/4 hr PO (or acetylsalicylic acid 10 mg/kg/4 hr PO) and codeine 0.5 mg/kg/4 hr PO. More potent analgesics such as morphine sulfate (0.1–0.15 mg/kg/2–4 hr SC) or meperidine (1 mg/kg/3–4 hr IM) may be required. Give these on a regular schedule (not prn) in sufficient dosages to alleviate pain. Have the patient quantitate the degree of pain (for example, on a scale of 1 to 10) to optimize dosing. The risk of addiction to nar-

cotics is minimal if the course of therapy is brief and carried out in the hospital, not at home.

Agents that quell anxiety can often be useful adjuncts to analgesics in the treatment of pain (the oral dose of hydroxyzine is 0.5 mg/kg/6 hr). As these agents may potentiate the action of narcotics, use lower doses of both agents when they are used together.

5. *Blood transfusion* is an important aspect of therapy. Life-threatening vaso-occlusive episodes (e.g., cerebral sickling) may often be terminated or prevented by partial exchange transfusion, in which 50% or more of the patient's sickle cells are replaced by normal (HbA) red cells. A general guide for partial exchange transfusions, is shown in Table 108-9. Quantitation by densiometry (following hemoglobin electrophoresis) will verify that the desired concentration of hemoglobin S has been achieved. To avoid errors in monitoring the effectiveness of the transfusion, screen each unit of blood for the presence of sickle hemoglobin (using solubility tests or a sickle preparation) prior to use. Units from donors with sickle trait, which should not be used for exchange transfusion of sickle-cell anemia patients, will be identified by this procedure.

The usual hazards associated with transfusion limit the use of partial exchange transfusion to the following circumstances:
a. Termination or prevention of prolonged, severe, or life-threatening vaso-occlusive episodes (e.g., cerebral sickling, pulmonary sickling, priapism)
b. Preparation of the patient for surgery if there is to be prolonged anesthesia, the possibility of hypoxemia, or temporary underperfusion of a particular region as a consequence of the surgical procedure
c. Treatment of severe anemic crises

ANEMIC CRISES

A dramatic, swift decline in hemoglobin levels is associated with:

1. Sudden splenic sequestration of sickled erythrocytes that may produce massive splenic enlargement, severe anemia, shock, and death: such episodes occur in early childhood, prior to autoinfarction of the spleen, and are one of the two most common causes of death in young sickle-cell patients.
2. Transient bone marrow aplasia following parvovirus and other infections: A low reticulocyte count is characteristic.
3. Hemolysis due to G6PD deficiency, transfusion reactions, or other causes not directly related to sickle hemoglobin: reticulocytosis and jaundice are prominent findings.
4. Megaloblastic anemia due to depletion of folate stores by accelerated erythropoiesis: severe anemia is uncommon unless generalized malnutrition is also present and the anemia develops gradually, not rapidly.

Immediate transfusion of packed red cells is indicated for severe anemic crises (to be considered whenever the hemoglobin falls below 6 g/100 ml). Transfusion of 10 ml packed red cells/kg body weight over 3 to 4 hours is safe and will raise the hematocrit by approximately 10 points. An enlarging spleen accompanied by a falling hemoglobin level (splenic

TABLE 108–9.   *Procedure for Partial Exchange Transfusion**

Degree of Anemia	Procedure	Product Used	Volume†
Severe (Hct < 19%)	Exchange transfusion	Packed RBCs (Hct 70%)	0.04 × body weight
Moderate (Hct 20–33%)	1. Exchange transfusion, *then immediately*	Packed RBCs	0.04 × body weight
	2. Exchange transfusion	Whole blood (Hct 40%)	0.03 × body weight
Minimal (Hct > 33%)	1. Phlebotomy, *then*		0.08 × body weight
	2. Infusion (IV), *then*	Normal saline	0.008 × body weight
	3. Exchange transfusion, *then*	Packed RBCs (Hct 70%)	0.04 × body weight
	4. Exchange transfusion	Whole blood (Hct 40%)	0.04 × body weight

HCT = hematocrit RBCs = red blood cells
* Table is from Reference 3, which summarizes recommendations made in Reference 1.
† Body weight in kilograms, volume in liters

sequestration crisis) is a particularly dangerous situation, because the child may die within hours unless transfused. Evidence of bone-marrow hypoplasia (reticulocyte count under 2%) is an indication for transfusion whenever hemoglobin levels fall substantially below values usual for the patient because the short life span of sickle cells will soon produce severe anemia in the absence of adequate erythropoiesis. If congestive heart failure accompanies severe anemia, partial exchange transfusion rather than simple transfusion may prevent aggravation of cardiac failure due to volume overload.

SUSCEPTIBILITY TO INFECTION

Susceptibility to infection is increased. Pneumococcal (and to a lesser extent *Haemophilus influenzae*) septicemia is particularly prevalent, and death may occur within just a few hours of onset. Splenic hypofunction and diminished opsonization of pneumococci by serum from sickle-cell patients have been identified as factors increasing susceptibility to infection. Necrotic areas of infarcted bone marrow may become foci of infection, perhaps explaining the increased incidence of osteomyelitis (particularly *Salmonella*) also characteristic of sickle-cell disease. Mycoplasma pneumonia may follow an unusually severe course in sickle-cell disease.

Because overwhelming infection is rapidly fatal, treatment must be prompt and, at times, anticipatory. In young children presenting with sudden high fever (greater than 102°F), particularly those without localizing signs of infection, obtain blood cultures, treat immediately with an intravenous antibiotic, and hospitalize the child. The same policy is often indicated in older children. In view of the reported increased incidence of *H. influenzae* infections in patients with sickle-cell anemia, many physicians use intravenous ampicillin (200–250 mg/kg/24 hrs). If ampicillin-resistant organisms are prevalent in the community, other antibiotics, such as cefuroxime (100 mg/kg/24 hrs) will provide more effective coverage.

In older children and in cases where fever is of several days duration or is accompanied by physical signs (such as rash) that indicate that infection is not of bacterial origin, immediate intravenous antibiotic therapy may not be appropriate. In such circumstances, give antibiotics orally if they are indicated.

Immunization with polyvalent pneumococcal polysaccharide vaccine 23 (0.5 ml SC) helps prevent overwhelming pneumococcal sepsis in children over 2 years of age who have sickle-cell disease. Give the *H. influenzae b* conjugate vaccine (0.5 ml SC) to all infants with sickle-cell disease at 18 months of age.

Keep all children with sickle-cell disease under 6 years of age on daily prophylactic penicillin VK, which has been proven to be effective in preventing or ameliorating pneumococcal sepsis. Children under 3 years old receive 125 mg b.i.d., those over 3 years old 250 mg b.i.d.

SICKLE TRAIT

The *sickle trait* is asymptomatic in most individuals, but examination of the urine may reveal hematuria, a consequence of renal microinfarcts. Traumatic hyphema may produce increased intraocular pressure. Rarely, under appropriate circumstances (e.g., hypoxia associated with high-altitude flying), vaso-occlusive episodes are said to occur in sickle trait.

Other Hemoglobinopathies ∎

THALASSEMIAS

Alpha Thalassemia

Four clinical syndromes are recognized (Table 108-10). Severe exacerbations of hemolytic anemia may occur in hemoglobin H disease, particularly during infections. The spleen is commonly enlarged during these episodes. Transfusion with packed red cells may be urgently required as the hemoglobin level can fall rapidly. If transfusion is withheld, monitor hemoglobin and hematocrit daily until the pace of hemolysis is ascertained. Hemoglobin H is unstable when exposed to oxidants, so avoid drugs that cause hemolysis in G6PD deficiency (Table 108-12. Consider the diagnosis of hemoglobin H disease if microcytosis and the customary abnormalities of red cell morphology (target cells, elliptocytes, poikilocytes) are encountered, particularly in ethnic groups (Southeast Asians, Chinese, Mediterraneans) in which alpha thalassemia is common. Confirmatory tests for hemoglobin H disease include hemoglobin electrophoresis and a brilliant cresyl blue inclusion body preparation.

Beta Thalassemia

Heterozygous β-thalassemia is characterized by microcytosis and minimal or no anemia.

Homozygous (or compound heterozygous) β-thalassemia is usually first detected in infancy when an increasingly severe microcytic anemia unresponsive to iron is discovered. Hemoglobin electrophoresis reveals persistence of hemoglobin F and little or no hemoglobin A. Refer these infants to a hematologist so that a regular transfusion program and, later, an iron chelation program can be initiated.

Thalassemics receiving chronic transfusions inevitably accumulate toxic amounts of iron. Older chil-

TABLE 108–10. *The Alpha Thalassemia Syndromes*

Syndrome	α-Globin Genes Deleted	Clinical Features	Laboratory Features
Silent carrier	1	None	None
α-Thalassemia trait	2	None	Microcytosis, mild or no anemia
Hemoglobin H disease	3	Moderate hemolytic anemia with or without splenomegaly	Microcytosis, hemoglobin 8–10 g/dL, reticulocytosis, hemoglobin H (2–40%)
Homozygous α-thalassemia	4	Hydrops fetalis (stillborn)	Hemoglobin 3–10 g/dL, >50% hemoglobin Barts

dren or adolescents may require emergent treatment for manifestations of hemosiderosis, which include cardiac arrhythmias, intractable heart failure, diabetes mellitus, hypoparathyroidism, and other endocrinopathies. These complications can be delayed or avoided by daily treatment with subcutaneous desferrioxamine (20–60 mg/kg/day) delivered by infusion pump over 8–12 hours.

Other complications of chronic transfusion therapy include transmission of viral infections (human immunodeficiency virus, cytomegalovirus, Epstein-Barr virus, hepatitis virus, etc.) and alloimmunization. To avoid febrile transfusion reactions, many thalassemics require premedication with acetaminophen and diphenhydramine and the use of washed, filtered, or frozen packed red cells. The presence of minor blood group incompatibilities gradually shortens the life span of transfused red cells in repeatedly transfused children. Splenectomy restores the life span of these cells to normal or near normal, usually at around the age of 10. The risk of overwhelming bacterial infection post-splenectomy is similar to or even greater than that seen in other splenectomized children and mandates the use of daily oral penicillin prophylaxis

(250 mg b.i.d.) and immunization with the pneumococcal vaccine.

Children with milder forms of thalassemia (β-thalassemia intermedia) do not require regular transfusion if their baseline hemoglobin level is 8 g/dL or higher. At slightly lower hemoglobin levels, however, the benefits of regular transfusions outweigh the risks.

Disorders of Erythrocyte Metabolism ■

Inherited defects in erythrocyte enzymes involved in glucose or nucleotide metabolism may be associated with hemolytic anemia (Table 108-11). These disorders are usually suspected and diagnosed only after other causes of hemolysis have been excluded, as they have few specific identifying features other than hemolysis itself. Red cell morphology is usually normal. Definitive diagnosis requires assay of the activity of the defective enzymes. In the ED, these individuals usually present with symptoms relating to bilirubin gallstones or with severe anemia due either to tran-

TABLE 108–11. *Most Common Erythrocyte Enzymopathies*

Defective Enzyme	Frequency	Inheritance	Clinical Features
Pentose Phosphate Pathway			
Glucose 6-phosphate dehydrogenase	Common	Sex-linked	Episodic hemolysis, CNSHA (rare)
Embden-Meyerhoff Pathway			
Pyruvate kinase	Rare	Recessive	CNSHA, leg ulcers
Glucose phosphate isomerase	Rare	Recessive	CNSHA (rare)
Nucleotide Metabolism			
Pyrimidine-5^1-nucleotide	Rare	Recessive	CNSHA, basophilic stippling

CNSHA = chronic non-spherocytic hemolytic anemia

TABLE 108–12. *Drugs and Chemicals That Produce Clinically Significant Hemolytic Anemias in G6-PD Deficiency*

Acetanilid	Primaquine
Methylene blue	Sulfacetamide
Nalidixic acid (NegGram)	Sulfamethoxazole
Nephthalene	(Gantanol)
Niridazole (Ambilhar)	Sulfanilamide
Nitrofurantoin (Furadantin)	Sulfapyridine
Pamaquine	Thiazolesulfone
Pentaquine	Toluidine blue
Phenylhydrazine	Trinitrotoluene (TNT)

(Beutler E: *Hemolytic Anemia in Disorders of Red Cell Metabolism.* New York. Plenum, 1978)

sient, infection-associated bone marrow suppression, or to exposure to oxidant agents or to infection. The latter complication is the hallmark of G6PD deficiency and, perhaps, other disorders of the pentose phosphate pathway but is rare to nonexistent in disorders of other pathways. Agents that induce hemolysis in G6PD deficiency are listed in Table 108-12.

Methemoglobinemia ■

See Chapter 83.

Bibliography ■

Brain MC, Carbone PP, eds: *Current Therapy in Hematology-Oncology 3.* Toronto, BC Decker, 1988.

Charache S, Lubin B, Reid CD, eds: *Management and Therapy of Sickle Cell Disease.* NIH Publication 84-2117, 1984.

Mentzer WC, Wagner GM, eds: *The Hereditary Hemolytic Anemias.* New York: Churchill-Livingstone, 1989.

Nathan DG, Oski FA, eds: *The Hematology of Infancy and Childhood,* 3rd ed. Philadelphia, WB Saunders, 1987.

Oski FA, Naiman JL, Stockman JA, Pearson HA: *Hematologic Problems in the Newborn,* 3rd ed. Philadelphia, WB Saunders, 1982.

109 Oncologic Disorders

Katherine K. Matthay

Many children with malignancies receive a combination of aggressive chemotherapy and radiotherapy. When emergencies arise, these children may be seen with problems that immediately threaten vital organ function or long-term quality of life. Keep in mind the overall treatment goals when initiating any therapy: knowing the diagnosis, underlying disease status, nutritional state, organ dysfunction, and previous surgery, radiotherapy, and chemotherapy is critical to any treatment decision.

This chapter will discuss the immediate management of emergencies that arise either due to the disease process itself or to complications of the treatment (such as immunosuppression or direct organ damage from the cytotoxic therapy). The physician presented with these problems must consult with an oncologist involved with the child's long-term management.

Certain oncologic emergencies are dealt with in other chapters, including bleeding (Chapter 9), seizures (Chapter 26), infections in the compromised host (Chapter 124), pain (Chapter 39), and death (Chapter 127).

Respiratory Distress ■

ETIOLOGY AND PATHOPHYSIOLOGY

Respiratory distress may be a direct result of tumor involvement or only indirectly related to the tumor as a consequence of cytotoxic therapy (Table 109-1). A mass growing in the anterior mediastinum may occlude or invade the thin-walled superior vena cava (SVC) and cause venous hypertension and airway compression. Most (85%) cases of SVC compression are caused by malignancy, in children usually leukemia or lymphoma (70%) but rarely a neuroblastoma, sarcoma, primary germ-cell tumor, or a metastatic tumor. Tumor progression may also involve the lung parenchyma, seen with leukemia with hyper-

leukocytosis, lymphomas, and with extensive metastases from solid tumors. Malignant pleural or pericardial effusions may occur with any of the above cancers.

CLINICAL FINDINGS

Superior Vena Cava Syndrome

Respiratory symptoms due to airway compression by the mass include dyspnea, cough, hoarseness, and stridor. Venous hypertension manifests as facial, neck, and upper extremity edema, distended neck veins, and tortuous chest wall collateral veins. Decreased venous drainage may lead to increased intracranial pressure, with headache, stupor, coma, and seizures. Death may occur from cerebral edema, airway obstruction, or cardiac complications.

Parenchymal Infiltrates

The clinical presentation of pneumonitis or parenchymal tumor is similar to pulmonary infiltrates of any cause: tachypnea, rales, and possibly fever. Differential diagnosis depends on a careful history of prior pulmonary toxic therapy (Table 109-2), prior antibiotics, underlying diagnosis, and disease status. Radiation pneumonitis may often be distinguished because the infiltrates will stop abruptly at the edge of the radiation portal.

Miscellaneous

The diagnosis of the remaining causes of respiratory distress (Table 109-1) is clear from the history and physical examination, such as acute bronchospasm seen with *anaphylaxis* to certain chemotherapeutic agents, most commonly with L-asparaginase, teniposide (VM-26), and bleomycin. *Pleural effusion* and

TABLE 109–1. *Causes of Respiratory Distress in a Child With Cancer*

Tumor Progression
Airway compression
Superior vena cava syndrome
Pulmonary parenchymal tumor infiltration
Pleural effusion
Pneumothorax
Cardiac tamponade

Treatment Related
Anaphylaxis with bronchospasm
Circulatory overload
Pneumonitis:
    Infections—bacterial, viral, fungal, parasitic
    Toxic—Radiation, chemotherapy
Pulmonary embolus

TABLE 109–2. *Cytotoxic Agents Causing Pulmonary Infiltrates*

Radiation therapy
Bleomycin
Methotrexate
Busulfan
Cyclophosphamide
Nitrosoureas

pneumothorax may be diagnosed by the unilateral absence of breath sounds and by the chest x-ray. Neoplastic *cardiac tamponade,* rare in children, manifests with the usual signs of tamponade including low blood pressure, decreased pulse pressure, engorged neck veins, and peripheral cyanosis. *Pulmonary embolus* generally causes acute chest pain and dyspnea and may arise from deep venous thrombosis.

DIAGNOSIS AND TREATMENT

For an overview, see Figure 109-1. The clinical diagnosis is made from the signs listed above. In addition, obtain a complete blood count, arterial blood gas measurements, and a chest x-ray. The chest x-ray differentiates mass lesions from parenchymal, pleural, or pericardial involvement. For mass lesions, a chest CT scan provides more accurate definition and localization of the mass. Although it is desirable to establish a tissue diagnosis before instituting treatment, this must be done quickly and without undue risk to the patient in respiratory distress. Give oxygen in the ED while awaiting diagnostic tests; obtain immediate oncologist consultation.

Superior Vena Cava Syndrome

Since lymphoma/leukemia is the most common cause of SVC compression in childhood, obtain a complete blood count, differential, platelet count, and bone-marrow aspiration. If these are nondiagnostic, a superficial node biopsy under local anesthesia may be required. Biopsy of the mediastinal mass itself is often dangerous because of hemorrhage and respiratory compromise, aggravated by placing the patient in the supine position. Diagnostic efforts should not delay prompt consultation and treatment, outlined in Table 109-3. If treatment is necessary to relieve symptoms before biopsy, the oncologist will limit the radiation field and do the biopsy outside the area of maximal irradiation.

Parenchymal Infiltrates

When infection is the most likely etiology, as suggested by prior treatment, recent onset, and immunosuppression or neutropenia, obtain appropriate cultures including blood and bronchial washings or open lung biopsy. Suspect viral, fungal, and parasitic pathogens (*Pneumocystis carinii*), in addition to bacteria. If bronchial washing or open lung biopsy is delayed, initiate broad-spectrum antibiotic coverage with additional coverage for fungus (amphotericin B), pneumocystis (trimethoprim/sulfamethoxazole), and herpes or varicella (acyclovir), if clinically indicated.

For radiation and some chemotherapy-induced pneumonitis, steroids are of value, usually in a standard dose of prednisone 2–3 mg/kg/day. With infiltrates from tumor progression such as leukemia/lymphoma or advanced metastases, the treatment is specific chemotherapy or radiation. Diffuse infiltrates resulting from circulatory overload are not uncommon in oncology patients, who often require blood transfusions because of the need for vigorous hydration to prevent renal damage with chemotherapeutic agents such as cisplatin and methotrexate. The treatment is oxygen, diuresis, and fluid restriction.

Pleural Effusion and Pericardial Tamponade

Pleural effusion may be the result of malignancy or fluid overload. When respiratory distress is present, perform diagnostic and therapeutic thoracentesis (see Chapter 139) in the ED. Infuse intravenous fluids (see Chapter 8) for hypotension. Send specimens for cultures and Gram's stains, as well as cell count, cytology, appropriate immunologic markers (lym-

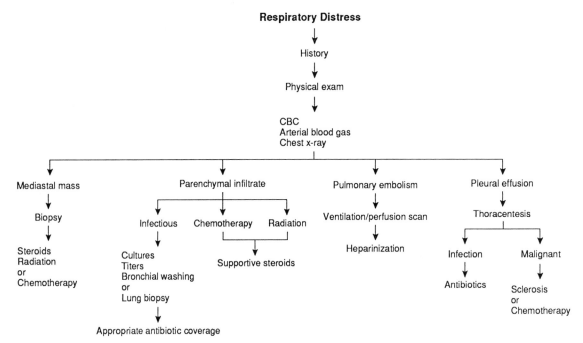

Respiratory Distress

Management of respiratory distress.

FIGURE 109–1. Management of respiratory distress.

phoma), protein, and LDH. When the effusion is malignant, refer the patient for appropriate chemotherapy or, in the case of refractory disease, for instillation of a sclerosing agent such as tetracycline (500–1000 mg in 20 ml 0.9% saline) after drainage of the pleural space. For pericardial tamponade, remove the fluid under echocardiographic guidance (see Chapter 139). Definitive later treatment might be chemotherapy, a surgical window, or tetracycline sclerosis.

TABLE 109–3. *Treatment of Superior Vena Cava Syndrome*

1. Prompt irradiation is the main emergency treatment (200–400 cGy/day).
2. Glucocorticoids (dexamethasone 4 mg/m² every 6 hr) before and during irradiation
3. Monitor uric acid level before and during therapy because of possible rapid tumor lysis. (Treat as in section on hyperleukocytosis.)
4. Head elevation, diuretics, and chemotherapy when appropriate

Pulmonary Embolus

Establish definitive diagnosis by a ventilation/perfusion scan. Use anticoagulation if no contraindications are present.

Neurologic Emergencies ■

SPINAL CORD COMPRESSION

Etiology and Pathophysiology

Spinal cord or cauda equina compression from tumor is usually extramedullary. It may reach the cord through an artery, vein, direct extension from an involved vertebra, or, most commonly in children, through a neural foramen from a retroperitoneal or paraspinal tumor. Early diagnosis and treatment are mandatory to avoid irreversible neurologic impairment (Table 109-4).

Spinal cord compression syndrome in oncology patients usually is due to a direct effect of tumor, but consider possible nonmalignant causes: radiation myelopathy, infection with transverse myelitis, cord stroke, hematoma, and extradural abscess.

TABLE 109–4. *Differential Diagnosis of Malignant Spinal Cord Compression in Childhood*

Primary tumors
  Neuroblastoma
  Rhabdomyosarcoma
  Lymphoma
  Germ cell tumor
Any metastatic tumor causing extradural compression
Malignant intramedullary cord compression
  Medulloblastoma
  Parameningeal sarcoma

Clinical Findings

The most common symptom is pain, either local or radicular. It is only later that the more obvious and sometimes irreversible neurologic signs may develop, such as weakness or sphincter loss (Table 109-5).

Diagnosis

Plain x-rays and bone scans may be helpful in defining vertebral involvement. For localization and definition of the cord compression and the tumor mass, metrizamide myelography with computed tomography (CT) is most helpful. A cisternal or cervical injection may be necessary to define the upper limits if the block is complete. An alternative to myelography is magnetic resonance imaging (MRI), which is particularly sensitive when gadolinium contrast is used for tumor enhancement. Submit cerebrospinal fluid obtained at myelography for cytologic analysis and glucose and protein levels. An oncologist will perform a biopsy promptly for diagnosis, but do not delay therapy while awaiting the result.

Treatment

To avoid irreversible neurologic damage, initiate therapy as soon as possible (within hours) (Table 109-6) after oncologic consultation. Radiation therapy is the usual approach, although in a very radioresistant tumor, surgical decompression might be appropriate. Chemotherapy alone is a third alternative, but still controversial.

INCREASED INTRACRANIAL PRESSURE (ICP)

Etiology

Malignant causes of increased ICP in children include primary brain tumors, central nervous system (CNS)

TABLE 109–5. *Signs and Symptoms of Spinal Cord Compression*

Pain
Paresthesia
Gait disturbance
Paraparesis
Extensor-plantar reflex
Sensory impairment
Sphincter loss

leukemia, and metastatic tumors. Do not overlook acute hemorrhage and opportunistic infections as alternative causes in the oncology patient.

Clinical Findings

The clinical symptoms and signs will be referable to the site and severity of the lesion, as in any cause of ICP. In all patients except those with known leukemia, CT with contrast or MRI is the safest and most informative test. Avoid lumbar puncture because of the risk of herniation. In the patient with known leukemia, CNS leukemia is by far the most likely diagnosis. However, since mass lesions would not be present unless infection with abscess is suspected, lumbar puncture with cell count and cytocentrifuge preparation of CSF to detect blast cells is usually a safe and effective test.

Treatment

See Figure 109-2. For mass lesions, an emergency ventriculo-peritoneal shunt may be required to prevent herniation. Consult an oncologist emergently so that corticosteroids and radiation therapy can be initiated promptly. For leukemia, methotrexate (6 mg, age 0–1 year; 8 mg, age 1–2 years; 10 mg, age

TABLE 109–6. *Treatment of Malignant Spinal Cord Compression*

1. Immediate radiation therapy (200–400 cGy/day) to site of cord compression
2. Give corticosteroids immediately and during the first several days of radiation (dexamethasone 50 mg/m² IV bolus, then 10 mg/m² every 6 hr)
3. Decompression laminectomy if the tumor is known to be radioresistant or if it is necessary for tissue diagnosis
4. The functional outcome is usually better if laminectomy can be avoided before radiation

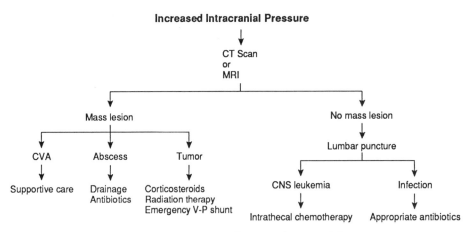

Increased Intracranial Pressure

FIGURE 109-2. Management of increased intracranial pressure.

2–3 years; 12 mg, >3 years) administered intrathecally in a preservative-free, isotonic solution will usually result in some response within a few days. Corticosteroids may help initially to relieve symptoms. Radiation therapy is usually deferred for several weeks.

Cerebrovascular Accident (CVA) ■

ETIOLOGY AND PATHOGENESIS

Cerebrovascular compromise may develop due to metastatic or local spread of tumor, including hyperleukocytosis in leukemia. Strokes are often treatment-related, due to chemotherapy (methotrexate or L-asparaginase), radiation, coagulation abnormalities (disseminated intravascular coagulation [DIC] or low platelets), or CNS infections.

CLINICAL FINDINGS

The child with a CVA usually presents with the abrupt onset of defective motor function or speech, often with seizures. Coma or obtundation may occur if a major area or the brain stem is involved.

DIAGNOSIS AND TREATMENT

Obtain a complete blood count and coagulation studies (platelet count, prothrombin, partial thromboplastin time, fibrinogen, fibrin degradation products, antithrombin III). After stabilization and oncologist consultation, perform a CT scan with and without contrast. If there is no mass lesion, perform a lumbar puncture to rule out infection or meningeal malignant disease.

The management for CVA is supportive, unless it is due to progression of malignant disease, in which case specific antineoplastic therapy is indicated.

Hyperleukocytosis in Acute Leukemia ■

ETIOLOGY AND PATHOPHYSIOLOGY

See Table 109-7. The presence of more than 100,000/μL blast cells in the peripheral blood of patients with acute leukemia (10% of acute lymphoblastic leukemia [ALL], up to 20% of acute nonlymphoblastic leukemia [ANLL]) has often been the cause of fatal complications due to hyperviscosity and/or metabolic derangements.

Leukostasis in the brain as a result of increased viscosity may cause fatal intracranial hemorrhage by leading to blast cell aggregates or microthrombi in the small capillaries. Leukostasis in the lungs may produce pulmonary edema, especially in ANLL. A syndrome of hyperuricemia, hyperkalemia, hyperphosphatemia, and hypocalcemia occurs with rapid tumor lysis and release of intracellular constituents in patients with hyperleukocytosis, most commonly in ALL. The hyperuricemia may lead to uric acid nephropathy with renal failure. Hyperleukocytosis may also be associated with DIC, especially in acute promyelocytic leukemia, where thrombogenic materials may be released from blast cells.

CLINICAL FINDINGS

Patients have the usual signs of leukemia (pallor, petechiae, and fever) and in addition may have massive

TABLE 109–7. Complications of Hyperleukocytosis

Coagulation
Thrombocytopenia
Disseminated intravascular coagulation

Metabolic
Hyperuricemia
Hyperkalemia
Hyperphosphatemia/hypocalcemia

Respiratory
Pulmonary edema from blast cell aggregates in lung
Superior vena cava syndrome from mediastinal mass

Central Nervous System
CNS leukostasis with lethargy, dizziness, headache
CNS hemorrhage

lymphadenopathy or organomegaly. If CNS leukostasis is present, symptoms of hyperviscosity may occur with lethargy, dizziness, and headache. Dyspnea indicates pulmonary involvement or mediastinal mass. Generalized bleeding can occur with DIC.

DIAGNOSIS AND TREATMENT

A peripheral blood smear suggests the diagnosis, but the definitive diagnostic procedure is a bone-marrow aspiration. Institute supportive therapy immediately after oncologist consultation, without waiting for the bone-marrow study. Additional laboratory studies include leukocyte count, hemoglobin, platelet count, uric acid, K^+, PO_4, BUN, creatinine, Ca^{++}, and urinalysis. Obtain a chest x-ray to detect mediastinal lymphadenopathy and pulmonary disease. An abdominal flat plate and/or ultrasound can help estimate kidney size.

Immediate intervention is recommended for patients with a blast count above 100,000/μL. Avoid further increasing blood viscosity with nonessential transfusions. Do not raise hemoglobin above 8 g/dL. Cranial radiation (400 cGy, entire brain) may help prevent intracranial hemorrhage, although prompt cytoreductive measures are more important. Leukophoresis or exchange transfusion can be used to lower the white count before initiating chemotherapy. It will decrease the risk of electrolyte abnormalities with treatment, although the effect on survival is not proven. Leukemic infiltration causing enlarged kidneys and decreased urine output can be reversed with immediate radiation (400 cGy to start).

Treat hyperuricemia and metabolic problems as in Table 109-8 and Chapter 102. In severe cases, hemodialysis may be necessary to bring the uric acid and potassium into a near-normal range so that che-

motherapy can be safely initiated. Treat electrolyte abnormalities with replacement, binders, or dialysis when appropriate. Treat intravascular consumptive coagulopathy with heparin infusion (10–25 U/kg/hr) and platelet or plasma support as needed.

Treatment-Related Emergencies ■

The acute problems related to chemotherapy and radiation that may bring the patient to the ED are *congestive heart failure, renal failure, ileus,* or *syndrome of inappropriate antidiuretic hormone (SIADH)*. CVA, pneumonitis, and anaphylaxis have been discussed above, while infection in the immunocompromised host is discussed in Chapter 124.

PATHOPHYSIOLOGY

Most cancer treatments in current use are designed to arrest growth and to kill rapidly proliferating tumor cells. They will inevitably damage a portion of normal cells, resulting in unwanted toxicity. Since supportive treatments for the various organ toxicities are covered in other sections of this book, only the pertinent clinical features, the usual offending drugs, and the unique features of treatment will be discussed here. *Early oncologist consultation is imperative.*

CLINICAL FINDINGS AND TREATMENT

Congestive Heart Failure

Congestive heart failure is usually due to the anthracyclines (such as Adriamycin and daunomycin) and may be either insidious or rapidly progressive. It may be elicited unexpectedly after a fluid challenge accompanying chemotherapy or a transfusion. It is often

TABLE 109–8. Management of Hyperleukocytosis With Tumor Lysis

Hydration: 3000 ml/m^2/d
Alkalinization: NaHCO$_3$ (150 mEq/m^2/d to keep urine pH 7–7.5)
Allopurinol: 300 mg/m^2/d
Monitor: electrolytes, Ca^{++}, PO$_4$, uric acid, BUN, creatinine, urinalysis, urine output
Dialyze for K$^+$ > 7 mEq/L, severe volume overload with decreased urine output, hypertension unresponsive to medical management, rising uric acid > 12 despite above measures, symptomatic hypocalcemia

irreversible and dose related (more likely to occur in patients who have received a total dosage greater than 450 mg/m², or who have received a lesser dose in the presence of pre-existing heart disease, or mediastinal irradiation). Treatment is supportive, with fluid restriction, diuretics, digoxin, and afterload reducers.

Renal Failure

Acute renal failure may occur following high-dose methotrexate, as a result of intratubular precipitation, or cisplatin, which can cause acute tubular necrosis. Predisposing or aggravating factors include other nephrotoxic agents often used in oncology patients, such as radiation or aminoglycoside antibiotics. Treatment for methotrexate-induced renal failure includes a high-dose citrovorum factor to prevent systemic toxicity (100 mg/m² q 3 hr IV) as well as alkalinization (NaHCO₃) and hydration to improve excretion. For cisplatin, vigorous diuresis with mannitol, furosemide, and intravenous fluids may prevent irreversible damage.

Adynamic Ileus

Ileus may result from vincristine, due to its toxicity to the autonomic nervous system. Treatment is supportive with intravenous fluids and tube decompression until recovery.

SIADH

The diagnosis of SIADH rests on a urine osmolality inappropriately high for the serum osmolality. Adrenal, thyroid, and renal disease must be ruled out, as well as hypotonic dehydration. SIADH may occur following vincristine, even several days later, with resulting fluid retention, hyponatremia, and seizures. A transient SIADH-like syndrome also occurs after intravenous cyclophosphamide (onset, 4–12 hours) but is due to direct renal impairment of water excretion rather than a central effect. Exclude CNS disease and lung disease as other possible causes.

The treatment is fluid restriction unless the hyponatremia is severe and accompanied by seizures, in which case a combination of furosemide with hypertonic (3%) saline infusion can rapidly correct the serum sodium.

Bone-Marrow Suppression

Bone-marrow suppression may be caused by radiation or chemotherapy with resulting serious anemia, thrombocytopenia, or neutropenia. Treat anemia and thrombocytopenia by component transfusions (see Chapter 136). It is advisable to irradiate all blood products (3000 cGy) prior to administration to prevent graft-versus-host reaction in the immunocompromised oncology patient. Consider neutropenia with fever an emergency requiring immediate cultures and antibiotics for possible sepsis in the immunocompromised patient. Any child with an absolute neutrophil count below 500/μL (total white blood count × percentage neutrophils) and a fever above 38°C requires blood and urine cultures as well as appropriate special cultures (because meningitis is very rare in neutropenic patients, routine lumbar puncture is not indicated). Obtain a chest x-ray if any clinical indication is present. Initiate broad-spectrum antibiotics promptly; include coverage for *Staphylococcus* and *Pseudomonas* (*i.e.*, a cephalosporin, ticarcillin, and aminoglycoside) (see Chapter 124).

Bibliography ■

Hathorn JW, Pizzo PA: Infectious complications in the pediatric cancer patient. In: Pizzo PA, Poplack DG, eds: *Principles and Practice of Pediatric Oncology*. Philadelphia: JB Lippincott, 1989.

Issa PY, Brihi ER, Junin Y, Slim MS: Superior vena cava syndrome in childhood. Report of 10 cases and review of the literature. *Pediatrics* 1983; 71:337–341.

Lange B, D'Angio G, Ross AJ, et al: Oncologic emergencies. In: Pizzo PA, Poplack DG, eds: *Principles and Practice of Pediatric Oncology*. Philadelphia: JB Lippincott, 1989.

Lewis DW, Packer RJ, Raney B, et al: Incidence, presentation and outcome of spinal cord disease in children with systemic cancer. *Pediatrics* 1986; 78:438–443.

Matthay KK: Oncologic and hematologic problems in the pediatric intensive care unit. In: Vincent JL, ed: *Update in Intensive Care and Emergency Medicine*. New York: Springer-Verlag, 1987.

Maurer HS, Steinherz PG, Gaynon PS, et al: The effect of initial management of hyperleukocytosis on early complications and outcome of children with acute lymphoblastic leukemia. *J Clin Oncol* 1988; 6:1425–1432.

Packer RJ, Rorke LB, Lange BL, et al: Cerebrovascular accidents in children with cancer. *Pediatrics* 1985; 76:494–201.

Priest JR, Ramsay NK, Latchau RE, et al: Thrombotic and hemorrhagic strokes complicating early therapy for childhood acute lymphoblastic leukemia. *Cancer* 1980; 46:1548.

Yarbro J, Bornstein R: *Oncologic Emergencies*. New York: Grune & Stratton, 1981.

110 Neurologic Disorders

Donna M. Ferriero

A number of pediatric neurologic disorders present in the ED setting; the most common are *acute ataxia, acute ascending polyneuropathy* (*Guillain-Barré*), *stroke,* and *alternating hemiplegia of childhood.* This chapter addresses the age-association of these entities, their clinical findings, mode of onset, and ED treatment and disposition.

Acute Ataxia ■

The cardinal feature of acute cerebellar ataxia, a syndrome occurring in childhood, is the *acute* onset of ataxia of gait without evidence of intoxication, tumor, abscess, polyneuritis, meningitis, or metabolic, familial, or degenerative diseases (Table 110-1). The mean age at presentation is 5 years. Many children will have varicella, Epstein-Barr virus, mononucleosis, or a viral disease of unknown origin. Associated physical findings include dysmetria, nystagmus, hypertonia, hypotonia, cranial nerve palsy, and hemiparesis. The CSF may be abnormal with pleocytosis and elevated protein content. The IgG index may be elevated, along with a documented rise in viral serology.

DIAGNOSIS

1. Perform a fundoscopic examination to rule out papilledema caused by increased intracranial pressure from subtentorial mass lesion (cerebellar astrocytoma, medulloblastoma, brain stem glioma).
2. Test the gait to ensure that weakness is not a cause of ataxia.
3. Obtain serum and urine drug screens to rule out intoxication.
4. Obtain complete blood count and platelet count, liver function tests (LFTs), ammonia, and bilirubin to look for signs of systemic disease (especially hepatic involvement).
5. Obtain a CT scan of the brain to look for mass lesion.
6. Perform a lumbar puncture to rule out acute CNS infection.

TREATMENT AND DISPOSITION

The treatment of acute ataxia is usually supportive. Neurologist consultation is helpful. Hospital admission may be necessary for intravenous management of fluid and electrolyte status if significant vomiting has occurred. In extreme cases of postinfectious cerebellitis, steroid therapy may help. If a mass lesion is present, obtain immediate neurosurgical consultation.

Guillain-Barré Syndrome (GBS) ■

Acute ascending polyradiculoneuropathy can present at any age and is probably a disease of toxic or infectious origin. It can follow or be associated with coxsackie, measles, mycoplasma, campylobacter, Epstein-Barr, and echoviruses infection, and can also follow immunizations or surgery. It is an *acute* monophasic illness that produces weakness of the limbs.

CLINICAL FINDINGS

The clinical features of GBS are listed in Table 110-2, the differential diagnosis in Table 110-3. The occurrence of a *purely sensory* syndrome rules out the diagnosis. Brain stem encephalitis (BSE) may be a central variant of peripheral GBS. Table 110-4 compares the features of these disorders.

TREATMENT AND DISPOSITION

Admit all patients with ascending paralysis. Frequent monitoring of vital signs and neurological function is mandatory. If a decline in pulmonary function is evident, transfer patients to the ICU or to a regional pediatric critical care center for constant observation or intubation and pulmonary support.

Treatment consists of plasmapheresis for those patients with decreasing forced vital capacity. In patients unable to cooperate with PFTs (pulmonary function tests), evidence of declining respiratory function us-

TABLE 110–1. *Differential Diagnosis of Acute Ataxia*

Acute cerebellar ataxia
Posterior fossa tumors
Brain abscess
Cerebellar hemorrhage from ruptured AVM
Head injury
Encephalitis
Neuroblastoma (remote effect)
Intoxications
    Drugs (ethanol, anticonvulsants, phenothiazines,
      sedatives, bromides)
    Animal venoms (puffer fish, shellfish)
    Insecticides (DDT, lindane, thallium)
    Heavy metals (methyl mercury, lead)
Developmental anomalies of posterior fossa
Heredodegenerative diseases (Friedreich's
    spinocerebellar degeneration)
Ataxia-telangiectasia
Intermittent ataxias (Hartnup's disease)

ing transcutaneous PO_2 electrodes will suffice, although any rapidly decompensating patient may benefit from plasma exchange. Rapid decompensation is possible at any time in the initial course. Avoid steroids, which have proven to be of no benefit.

Stroke ■

Strokes are uncommon in childhood, with an average yearly incidence of about 2.5 cases per 100,000 children (excluding neonatal cerebrovascular disease). Children with stroke may present acutely or may have

TABLE 110–2. *Guillain-Barré Syndrome: Diagnostic Features*

Required Features
  Progressive weakness of more than one limb
  Areflexia

Strongly Supportive Features
  Progression over days to weeks
  Relative symmetry
  Mild sensory signs
  Cranial nerve weakness
  Recovery after 2 to 4 weeks
  Autonomic dysfunction
  Absence of fever at onset
  Elevated CSF protein after the first week; WBC counts
    of 10 or fewer monocytes/μL
  Nerve conduction slowing or block or prolonged F
    waves

TABLE 110–3. *Differential Diagnosis of Guillain-Barré Syndrome*

Poliomyelitis
Botulism
Hysterical paralysis
Toxic neuropathy (hexacarbon abuse)
Porphyria
Diphtheria
Lead intoxication
Tick paralysis

a protracted course. The basic principles underlying stroke in children are the same as those for adults, and thus strokes can be classified by the vascular mechanism: thrombotic, embolic, hemorrhagic, or pseudovascular (see Table 110-5).

CLINICAL FINDINGS AND ANCILLARY DATA

The presenting signs and symptoms are sometimes helpful in discerning the etiology. Patients with thrombosis can present with headache, focal neurologic deficits, and obtundation. With intracranial hemorrhage, patients usually complain of headache and show nuchal rigidity. Patients with embolic strokes often present with focal seizures.

The general physical examination may give clues to the diagnosis. Cardiac murmurs, hepatosplenomegaly, and lung disease can signal undiagnosed congenital cardiac disease. Examine the skin for hemangiomas (Sturge-Weber, Osler-Weber-Rendu, and von Hippel Lindau) and café-au-lait spots (neurofibromatosis). The presence of intracranial bruits,

TABLE 110–4. *Guillain-Barré vs Brain Stem Encephalitis*

	Guillain-Barré Syndrome	Brain Stem Encephalitis
Cranial Neuropathies	+	+++
Ophthalmoplegia	±	++
Gaze abnormalities	−	+
Drowsiness	−	+
Ataxia	−	++
Reflexes	−	±
NCV	Block; F wave prolonged	Normal
Progression	Caudorostral	Rostrocaudal

even though common in normal children under age 6, can, when asymmetric, signify the increased cerebral blood flow of an arteriovenous malformation.

Magnetic resonance imaging (MRI), when available, is the single most useful test due to its sensitivity for vascular malformations as well as the early edema associated with stroke. However, first perform a noncontrast CT scan emergently to rule out intracranial hemorrhage and mass lesion. Cerebral angiography remains the most important tool for outlining vascular anatomy, especially if Moya-Moya or dissection of the carotid artery is suspected.

Before performing angiography, exclude *homocystinuria* with a urine nitroprusside test, since already fragile vessels can be further damaged if these patients are subjected to angiography.

Appropriate screening laboratory values include complete blood count and platelet count, prothrombin time, partial thromboplastin time, liver and kidney panel, cholesterol and triglycerides, erythrocyte sedimentation rate, and antinuclear antibodies (for vasculitis). If a blood dyscrasia is suspected (as in cases of venous thrombosis), obtain factor assays, plasminogen, fibrinogen, and antithrombin III levels, protein C and S levels, and thrombin time.

TREATMENT AND DISPOSITION

The appropriate management of a patient with stroke involves first the proper evaluation of cause, then neurologist consultation. Admit the child to a constant observation room for frequent neurologic monitoring over the first 24 to 48 hours. Keep the patient calm. If hemorrhage is ascertained as a cause, obtain prompt neurosurgical consultation.

Do not lower blood pressure, (unless in malignant ranges) with vasodilator agents, since the hemodynamic mechanisms responsible for hypertension are usually compensatory. Reducing blood pressure could result in further neurologic deficit. If a stroke is in evolution or is thought to be embolic, consider anticoagulation with heparin.

Alternating Hemiplegia of Childhood ■

In alternating hemiplegia, transient attacks of hemiplegia alternately involve both sides of the body. Onset is always before 18 months of age and usually before 6 months. The attacks fluctuate in intensity and are interrupted by sleep. Other paroxysmal phenomena such as choreoathetosis, tonic fits, or dys-

TABLE 110–5. *Cerebrovascular Disorders in Children and Adolescents*

Thrombotic Arterial/Venous
  Trauma (oral, cervical)
  Positional (hypertension)
  Dehydration
  Hematologic (sickle-cell anemia, disseminated
    intravascular coagulation, etc.)
  Infection (meningitis, mastoiditis)
  Vasculitis
  Atherosclerotic/hyperlipidemia
  Cancer/chemotherapy/radiation
  Neurocutaneous disorders
  Migraine
  Structural (fibromuscular hyperplasia)

Embolic
  Congenital heart disease/surgery
  Endocarditis
  Pulmonary disease
  Atrial myxoma/rhabdomyoma
  Air/fat
  Mitral valve prolapse

Hemorrhagic
  Coagulation disorders
  Blood dyscrasias
  Street drugs
  Arteriovenous malformations
  Aneurysms

Pseudovascular Disorders
  Focal encephalitis
  Brain abscess
  Trauma
  Epilepsy
  Post-immunization/infectious
  Demyelinating
  Tumor (primary or metastatic)

(Rothner AD, Cruse RP: Cerebrovascular disease in children and adolescents. *Intl Pediatr* 1987;2:124–128)

tonia can occur with the episodes, and the course is progressive.

Bibliography ■

Asbury AK: Diagnostic considerations in Guillain-Barré syndrome. *Ann Neurol* 1981; 9:1–5.

Dreyfuss PM, Oshtory M, Gardne ED, et al: Cerebellar ataxia. *West J Med* 1978; 128:499–511.

Golden GS: Stroke syndromes in childhood. *Neurol Clin North Am* 1985; 3:59–75.

Koch TK, Berg BO: Ataxia of childhood. In: Berg BO, ed: *Child Neurology: A Clinical Manual.* Greenbrae, CA: Jones Medical Publications, 1984.

Rothner AD, Cruse RP: Cerebrovascular disease in children and adolescents. *Intl Pediatr* 1987; 2:124–128.

111 Renal Disorders

Anthony A. Portale

Acute Renal Failure ■

Acute renal failure (ARF) is characterized by a sudden decrease in renal function sufficient to cause retention of nitrogenous wastes, usually measured as an increase in blood urea nitrogen (BUN) and serum creatinine concentrations. When ARF is due to hypovolemia or shock, oliguria usually occurs; when it is due to toxic or inflammatory injury to the kidney, urine output may be normal. ARF caused by ischemic or toxic injury to the nephron is referred to as acute tubular necrosis (ATN).

ETIOLOGY

Common causes of ARF are listed in Table 111-1. ARF can occur when there is inadequate perfusion of the kidneys, such as with severe dehydration, hemorrhage, or shock (prerenal causes). Prompt restoration of circulating blood volume may reverse oliguria and azotemia in such cases, but prolonged renal hypoperfusion can lead to established renal failure. Intrinsic renal causes of ARF are nephrotoxic, inflammatory, or renovascular disorders, and postrenal causes are obstructive lesions of the urinary tract. In the neonate, ARF can be due to congenital renal abnormalities such as multicystic dysplasia, hypoplasia, agenesis, polycystic kidneys, or obstructive lesions such as posterior urethral valves.

CLINICAL FINDINGS

The *history* provides clues as to the underlying cause of ARF. A prerenal cause is suggested by a history of severe vomiting and diarrhea, hemorrhage, shock due to cardiac arrest, sepsis, or anaphylaxis, or hypovolemia due to severe nephrotic syndrome, diabetic ketoacidosis, or burns. Patients with pre-existing chronic renal insufficiency, polycystic kidneys, or diabetes insipidus may be more susceptible to prerenal ARF and to nephrotoxic renal injury.

An intrinsic renal cause is suggested by a history of exposure to nephrotoxins such as aminoglyco

sides, amphotericin B, radiocontrast agents, drugs that can cause tubulointerstitial nephritis such as the penicillins, or, in patients with cardiac dysfunction, drugs that reduce renal blood flow such as indomethacin. A history of gross hematuria suggests acute glomerulonephritis; bloody diarrhea, oliguria, and pallor suggest hemolytic uremic syndrome.

Obstructive disorders are suggested by a history of abdominal or flank pain, dysuria or urinary tract infection, poor urinary stream, passage of renal stones, prior administration of anticancer chemotherapeutic agents, renal tubular acidosis, or instrumentation of the urinary tract.

The *physical examination* may reflect the underlying cause and should focus on assessing the patient's state of hydration. Hypovolemia is revealed by sunken eyes, decreased skin turgor, tachycardia, and orthostatic hypotension; volume overload is revealed by periorbital or pedal edema, hypertension, or congestive heart failure. Enlarged kidneys suggest hydronephrosis, polycystic disease, or renal vein thrombosis; a palpable bladder suggests urethral obstruction.

ANCILLARY DATA

The following measurements are essential for evaluation: complete blood count, serum concentrations of sodium, potassium, chloride, carbon dioxide content, BUN, creatinine, calcium, phosphorus, total protein, and albumin. Obtain urine for urinalysis, culture, and measurement of osmolality and concentrations of sodium and creatinine as soon as possible, and before giving diuretics. Measure serum complement, ANA levels, and ASO titer when acute glomerulonephritis is suspected.

Oliguria is defined as urine output in children of less than 0.8 ml/100 kcal/hr, in infants of less than 1 ml/kg/hr, and in adolescents and adults of less than 400 ml/day. In oliguric patients, the urinary composition is a valuable aid in distinguishing established intrinsic renal failure from prerenal azotemia (Table 111-2); the latter is potentially reversible

TABLE 111–1. *Causes of Acute Renal Failure in Children*

Pre-Renal	Intrinsic-Renal	Post-Renal
Hypovolemia	Nephrotoxins	Ureteral obstruction
Severe dehydration	Aminoglycosides, cephalosporins, amphotericin	Calculi, clot, tumor
Hemorrhage (surgical	B	Ureteropelvic junction,
traumatic, obstetrical)	Radiocontrast agents	Ureterovesical
Burns	Heavy metals	junction
Diabetic ketoacidosis	Organic solvents, pesticides	Urethral obstruction
Hypotension/hypoperfusion	Myoglobin (crush syndrome)	Posterior urethral valves
Shock (cardiogenic, septic,	Parenchymal disorders	Diverticulum, stricture
anaphylactic)	Acute glomerulonephritis	Ureterocele
Cardiac surgery	Hemolytic uremic syndrome	Hydrocolpos
Severe nephrotic	Systemic vasculitis	Tumor
syndrome, hepatic	(Henoch-Schonlein nephritis, systemic lupus	
cirrhosis	erythematosus, polyarteritis)	
Hepatorenal syndrome	Acute interstitial nephritis (bacterial); allergic	
	(methicillin, penicillin, cephalosporins,	
	trimethoprim-sulfa)	
	Tubular obstruction (uric acid, oxalic acid)	
	Acute tubular necrosis (prolonged ischemia)	
	Vascular disorders	
	Renal artery thrombosis, embolism	
	Renal vein thrombosis	
	Indomethacin	

with prompt restoration of extracellular fluid (ECF) volume. All patients with unexplained acute renal failure require an immediate renal ultrasound to rule out urinary tract obstruction. Chest x-ray and electrocardiogram are indicated when volume overload or hyperkalemia is present.

TREATMENT

The objectives of initial management are assessment of intravascular volume status, treatment of life-threatening complications, and diagnosis of acute urinary tract obstruction. Initiate diagnostic evalua-

TABLE 111–2. *Laboratory Findings in Acute Renal Failure*

Test	Pre-Renal	Intrinsic-Renal	Post-Renal
Ultrasound	Normal	Normal/increased size or echogenicity	Dilated pelvis, ureter, bladder
Urine osmolality (mOsm/kg)	>500	<350	Urinary indices not helpful
Urine/plasma creatinine	>14:1	<14:1	
Urine sodium (mEq/L)	<20	>30	
Fractional excretion of sodium (%)*	<1	>2	
	<2.5 in neonates	>2.5 in neonates	
Urinary sediment	Minimal findings	Trace to 2+ protein	Unremarkable WBC with infection
	Few granular casts	Few WBC, RBC	
		Brown granular casts	
		Tubular epithelial cells	

* Fractional excretion of sodium (%) = $\dfrac{U_{Na}\ (mEq/L)}{U_{creat}\ (mEq/L)} \times \dfrac{S_{creat}\ (mg/dL)}{S_{Na}\ (mg/dL)} \times 100$

tion, although diagnosis of the underlying cause may not be possible in the acute setting. Obtain nephrology consultation.

For patients with oliguria and signs of ECF volume depletion, give isotonic fluid (0.9% sodium chloride or Ringer's lactate) intravenously, 10 to 20 ml/kg over 15 to 30 minutes, or colloid or blood, until skin turgor, pulse, blood pressure, and central venous pressure (CVP) are normal. If urine output increases, a prerenal cause of ARF is likely. If oliguria persists, give furosemide (Lasix) 1 to 2 mg/kg intravenously, or mannitol 0.5 to 1 g/kg intravenously over 15 to 30 minutes, the latter only when volume overload is absent and with careful monitoring of cardiopulmonary status and blood pressure.

If urine output increases (positive response is urine output of 5 to 10 ml/kg over 1–3 hours), continue efforts to maintain diuresis. If oliguria still persists, then renal failure is established and fluid should be restricted to insensible water loss (estimated at 35 ml/100 kcal/day).

Patients with ARF due to intrarenal obstruction by uric acid crystals (tumor lysis syndrome) may benefit from a sustained mannitol-induced diuresis, achieved by infusing a solution of 3% mannitol in 0.25% saline at a rate equal to that of urine output.

Acute life-threatening complications of ARF that require immediate treatment are severe ECF volume overload with congestive heart failure, pulmonary edema (Chapter 9), severe hypertension (Chapter 11), and severe hyperkalemia (Chapter 102).

Urgent dialysis, either peritoneal or hemodialysis, is required for children who fail to respond to initial treatment of the above complications.

DISPOSITION

After initial stabilization, children with ARF require inpatient evaluation and treatment in consultation with a nephrologist. Frequent monitoring of blood pressure, cardiovascular status, urine output, and meticulous fluid and electrolyte management are essential components of care. Admit children with ECF volume overload, hypertension, or electrolyte abnormalities to a pediatric critical care unit or transfer to a pediatric critical care center; less ill patients may often be managed on a pediatric ward.

Acute Glomerulonephritis ■

Acute glomerulonephritis or acute nephritic syndrome is a clinical state characterized by the sudden onset of gross or microscopic hematuria, edema, oliguria, and hypertension. Mild to moderate proteinuria and azotemia are most common, although some pa-

tients may develop nephrotic syndrome, severe azotemia, or acute renal failure. The clinical findings reflect an acute inflammatory process, presumably of immunologic origin, that affects principally the glomerulus. The disorder usually occurs after infection with a variety of bacteria or viruses, or it may occur as part of a systemic disease.

CLINICAL FINDINGS

The most commonly recognized clinical picture appears in school-age children following infection with the group A beta-hemolytic streptococcus (poststreptococcal acute glomerulonephritis [PSAGN]). The typical case is a child who suddenly develops edema and dark urine and is hypertensive when first evaluated. The history reveals a pharyngitis or skin infection that occurred 1 to 2 weeks, or 3 to 6 weeks, earlier, respectively. Serologic evaluation reveals recent streptococcal infection and a reduction in the serum complement level. The clinical course is characterized by resolution of the acute signs and symptoms within 1 to 3 weeks and apparent resolution of the disease within 6 to 12 months. Most children recover completely; fewer than 5% of cases progress to chronic renal insufficiency.

ANCILLARY DATA

1. Urinalysis: Microscopic hematuria or grossly bloody (brown, tea-colored, smoky) urine is present in almost all affected patients, and red blood cell casts in 60% to 80%. Proteinuria is moderate, rarely more than 2 $g/m^2/day$. White blood cells and granular casts are common. The urine is concentrated and contains little sodium.

2. Anemia: Moderate anemia is common in the early phase and parallels the degree of volume expansion, suggesting that the cause of the anemia is mainly dilutional.

3. Azotemia: Serum BUN and creatinine levels are increased in patients with moderate and severe disease. When severe, oliguric acute renal failure may occur, with severe azotemia, hyperkalemia, hyperphosphatemia, and metabolic acidosis.

4. Serology: The ASO titer increases significantly in most patients after streptococcal pharyngitis; the increase after streptococcal pyoderma is poor, and antibiotic treatment may prevent the rise in some patients. The anti-DNase B and antihyaluronidase titers are more sensitive indicators of recent infection. Serum total complement (CH50) and C3 levels decrease in 80% to 90% of patients within the first 2 weeks and return to normal within 4 to 8 weeks.

TREATMENT AND DISPOSITION

Hospitalize patients with signs of ECF volume expansion (*i.e.*, peripheral edema, pulmonary edema, and hypertension) or with acute renal failure, preferably in a pediatric critical unit, and obtain nephrology consultation. Transfer to a pediatric critical care center may be necessary. Patients with milder disease can be managed as outpatients but require close follow-up of renal and electrolyte status, blood pressure, and ECF volume status.

1. *Fluid overload and edema:* Restrict sodium and fluids in patients with oliguria. If edema or circulatory congestion is present, give furosemide 1 to 3 mg/kg/day orally or intravenously in divided doses. Progressive circulatory congestion can give rise to dyspnea, cough, and pulmonary edema, the latter requiring urgent dialysis.
2. *Hypertension:* Hypertension is due largely to retention of sodium and water, and if severe may be associated with CNS signs such as headaches, vomiting, confusion, somnolence, and seizures. Treatment of hypertension is discussed in Chapter 11.
3. *Antibiotics:* Antibiotic treatment of the infecting organism is appropriate but is unlikely to affect the clinical course of the nephritis.
4. *Oliguric acute renal failure* develops in about 10% of hospitalized patients. Management of ARF is discussed in the preceding section.

Nephrotic Syndrome ■

The nephrotic syndrome is a clinical state characterized by severe proteinuria and hypoalbuminemia, usually accompanied by edema and hypercholesterolemia and sometimes accompanied by hematuria, hypertension, and azotemia. The nephrotic syndrome may be associated with a variety of histopathologic diseases that principally affect the kidney (primary nephrotic syndrome) or in which the kidney is involved as part of a systemic disease (secondary nephrotic syndrome) (Table 111-3).

ETIOLOGY AND PATHOPHYSIOLOGY

The primary nephrotic syndrome is chiefly a disease of children, and minimal change nephrotic syndrome (MCNS) is the most common cause, accounting for 80% to 85% of cases in children, as compared with 15% to 20% of cases in adults.

Increased permeability of the glomerular capillary wall to plasma proteins, principally serum albumin, gives rise to a reduction in colloid oncotic pressure and the movement of fluid from the vascular to the interstitial space. The resultant decrease in effective blood volume stimulates the secretion of renin-angiotensin-aldosterone and vasopressin, which results in renal retention of sodium and water and the development of edema.

TABLE 111–3. *Causes of the Nephrotic Syndrome in Children*

Primary
  Minimal change nephrotic syndrome (lipoid nephrosis, nil disease)
  Focal glomerular sclerosis
  Mesangial proliferative glomerulonephritis
  Membranoproliferative glomerulonephritis
  Congenital nephrotic syndrome (age <3 months)
Secondary
  Acute glomerulonephritis
  Systemic vasculitis (systemic lupus erythematosus, Henoch-Schönlein nephritis)
  Hemolytic uremic syndrome
  Infections (malaria, syphilis, hepatitis B)
  Lymphoma, carcinoma
  Sickle-cell disease
  Toxins/drugs (bee sting, poison oak, mercury, gold)

CLINICAL FINDINGS

Most children with MCNS are between 2 and 6 years of age. The most common clinical presentation is the appearance of edema, usually of the face and periorbital area in the morning and of the ankles and legs later in the day. The onset of edema is often preceded by pharyngitis or upper respiratory tract infection. Progressive, severe edema can give rise to anasarca and abdominal distention, umbilical or inguinal hernia, pleural effusion, and respiratory distress. Blood pressure in children with MCNS is usually normal, but it may be increased in those with other causes. Relapses occur in 50% of affected children.

ANCILLARY DATA

1. Urine protein excretion is more than 1 g/m²/day; excretion rates of more than 5 g/day are common in young children. Albumin is the principal urinary protein in MCNS.
2. Hypoalbuminemia (less than 2.5 g/dL) is characteristic. Serum levels of alpha-1 globulin are decreased; levels of alpha-2 globulins, beta globulins, and fibrinogen show a relative or absolute increase.
3. Serum levels of cholesterol, triglycerides, and total lipids are increased, reflecting both increased production and decreased clearance of lipid. Cholesterol levels vary inversely with serum albumin levels.

4. The urine contains hyaline and granular casts, free lipid, cholesterol-containing bodies, and fatty casts. Microscopic hematuria is present in 25% of children with MCNS; gross hematuria or red blood cell casts suggests other glomerular diseases.

5. Serum BUN and creatinine levels are mildly increased in 25% of children with MCNS, reflecting reduced intravascular volume; the levels normalize with onset of diuresis. Persistent or worsening azotemia suggests other glomerular diseases.

6. Serum complement levels are normal; a decrease suggests membranoproliferative glomerulonephritis or systemic lupus erythematosus. Decreased serum levels of Factor B and IgG may contribute to increased susceptibility to infection, decreased serum antithrombin III and plasminogen to increased risk of thrombosis.

COMPLICATIONS

Nephrotic children are at increased risk of serious bacterial infection (*S. pneumoniae, E. coli, H. influenzae*), including septicemia, spontaneous peritonitis, urinary tract infection, and cellulitis. Promptly evaluate children with fever, abdominal pain, dysuria, etc. and initiate appropriate antibiotic therapy as indicated. The risk of deep venous and renal vein thrombosis is increased in nephrotic patients, due to their hypercoagulable state.

TREATMENT AND DISPOSITION

Hospitalize nephrotic children with anasarca, respiratory distress, hypertension, infection, or those requiring intravenous therapy. Otherwise, most diagnostic and therapeutic maneuvers can be accomplished on an outpatient basis, with close clinical follow-up.

1. *General measures:* Monitor body weight, fluid intake and urine output, blood pressure, and renal function closely. Bed rest is of unproven value. Restrict vigorous activity in severely edematous patients.

2. *Diet:* Restrict sodium intake; otherwise, provide nutrition appropriate for the child's age.

3. *Diuretics:* In patients with severe incapacitating edema, pleural effusion, marked ascites, respiratory distress, or cellulitis, rapid diuresis can be induced by giving salt-poor human albumin 1 g/kg/dose intravenously over 1 hour, followed by furosemide 1 mg/kg/dose intravenously, with careful in-hospital monitoring for hypertension and signs of pulmonary edema. In less edematous patients, oral diuretics may be used cautiously while awaiting induction of diuresis with prednisone (see below).

Give hydrochlorothiazide 1 mg/kg/day given q 12 hr orally, or furosemide (Lasix) 1 to 2 mg/kg/day given q 12 hr orally, with careful monitoring of blood pressure, renal function, and electrolyte status. Avoid large intravenous doses of diuretics or paracentesis because of the risk of depletion of intravascular volume.

4. *Corticosteroids:* Treat children with the typical clinical features of MCNS with prednisone. Consult a nephrologist before treating atypical patients.

5. *Immunosuppressive drugs:* Consult a nephrologist for children who have more than two relapses within 6 months of diagnosis (frequent relapser), who relapse as the prednisone dosage is being decreased (steroid dependence), or who fail to respond to 8 weeks of prednisone therapy (steroid resistance). For such children, and when signs of serious steroid toxicity are present (*i.e.*, growth failure, obesity, hypertension, striae), consider giving cyclophosphamide. A renal biopsy is generally performed prior to beginning this therapy.

6. *Vaccination with the pneumococcal vaccine* is advised when patients are in remission and are not receiving steroid or immunosuppressive drugs.

Hemolytic Uremic Syndrome ■

Hemolytic uremic syndrome (HUS) is characterized by the acute onset of microangiopathic hemolytic anemia, thrombocytopenia, and acute nephropathy, the latter usually manifested as gross or microscopic hematuria, proteinuria, oliguria, and azotemia. The etiology is unknown, although the likely initial pathogenic event is injury to the endothelial cells of the renal vasculature, probably caused by bacterial toxins. Many cases in North America are preceded by enteric infection with verotoxin-producing *E. coli*.

CLINICAL FINDINGS

Classic HUS affects principally infants and young children (average age is about 3 years in North America). A gastrointestinal prodrome of abdominal pain, vomiting, and diarrhea, often bloody, is most common; gastrointestinal symptoms may be severe and mimic acute appendicitis, toxic megacolon, or intussusception. In some children, the prodrome is that of an upper respiratory tract infection. The spectrum of renal disease is variable, ranging from hematuria with red blood cell casts, proteinuria, and mild azotemia, to oliguric acute renal failure that persists for days to weeks. Physical examination may reveal fever, pallor, edema or dehydration, petechiae, ecchymoses, and hypertension, the latter often severe.

CNS abnormalities occur in 40% to 50% of affected children and include irritability, lethargy, confusion, seizures, cortical blindness, hemiparesis, decerebrate posturing, and coma. Less commonly, patients may have jaundice, hepatomegaly and hepatitis, pancreatic involvement with insulin-dependent diabetes mellitus, or involvement of the pericardium, myocardium, or lung.

ANCILLARY DATA

1. Hematologic: Hemolysis usually occurs rapidly and often is severe, with hemoglobin values being as low as 4 mg/dL, presumably due to microangiopathic physical destruction of red blood cells; direct toxic damage to red cell membranes may also play a role. The peripheral blood smear reveals shistocytes and helmet and burr cells. The direct and indirect Coombs tests are usually negative. The white blood cell count is usually increased, up to 20,000 to 30,000.
2. Thrombocytopenia: Mild to severe thrombocytopenia is present in nearly every patient. Platelet survival time is shortened by 50% to 80%.
3. Renal: The urine contains red blood cells, red cell casts, and moderate protein; the nephrotic syndrome is rare. Serum levels of BUN and creatinine are mildly to severely increased. Hyperkalemia, acidosis, hypocalcemia, and hyperphosphatemia are common in patients with severe renal involvement.

TREATMENT AND DISPOSITION

Hospitalize children for initial diagnosis and for careful monitoring of urine output, ECF volume status, blood pressure, and renal, electrolyte, and hematologic status. Patients with mild nonoliguric disease can be managed with restriction of fluids and sodium, correction of metabolic acidosis, and transfusion of blood if necessary. Patients with severe disease are often anuric and hypertensive, and may have CNS involvement including seizures. Meticulous, comprehensive supportive therapy, preferably in a pediatric critical care setting, is important to avoid serious morbidity in such patients. Consult a nephrologist or hematologist.

1. The treatment of fluid and electrolyte abnormalities, azotemia, and hypertension is similar to that described earlier for acute renal failure. Because of red cell hemolysis, hyperkalemia may develop rapidly and may be severe; thus, frequent monitoring of the serum potassium concentration is necessary.
2. Because hemolysis can be rapid, frequent monitoring of the hemoglobin and hematocrit is re-

quired. Transfuse only patients with severe anemia (hematocrit less than 16–20%) or when tachycardia, gallop rhythm, or hypoxia is attributed to the anemia. Transfusion can precipitate pulmonary edema or can greatly exacerbate hypertension in fluid-overloaded patients. Transfuse packed red cells, 5 to 10 ml/kg, over 2 to 4 hours with frequent monitoring of blood pressure and cardiovascular status.
3. Thrombocytopenia, unless unusually severe or associated with active bleeding, rarely requires specific management.
4. Treatment of seizures is discussed in Chapter 26.
5. Nutrition: Initiate enteral nutrition as soon as vomiting and diarrhea have resolved. Consider central intravenous alimentation for patients with protracted or severe colitis to avoid prolonged periods of undernutrition.

PROGNOSIS

More than 85% of children with classic HUS in the United States recover completely with supportive care. Patients with prolonged anuria (longer than 3 weeks) have a 50% incidence of chronic renal insufficiency. The reported mortality is 5% to 10%.

Bibliography ■

Brezis M, Rosen S, Epstein FH: Acute renal failure. In: Brenner BM, Rector FC, eds: *The Kidney*, 3rd ed. Philadelphia: WB Saunders, 1986.

Dodge WF, Spargo BH, Travis LB, et al: Poststreptococcal glomerulonephritis: A prospective study in children. *N Engl J Med* 1972; 286:273.

Feld LG, Springate JE, Fildes RD: Acute renal failure. I. Pathophysiology and diagnosis. *J Pediatrics* 1986; 109: 401.

Fildes RD, Springate JE, Feld LG: Acute renal failure. II. Management of suspected and established disease. *J Pediatrics* 1986; 109:567.

Fong JSC, de Chadarevian JP, Kaplan BS: Hemolytic uremic syndrome: Current concepts and management. *Pediatr Clin North Am* 1982; 29:835.

Grupe WE: Primary nephrotic syndrome in children. *Adv Pediatr* 1979; 26;163.

Nissenson AR, Baraff LJ, Fine RN, Knutson DW: Poststreptococcal glomerulonephritis: Fact and controversy. *Ann Int Med* 1979; 91:76.

Rodriguez-Iturbe B, Garcia F: Acute glomerulonephritis. In: Holliday MA, Barratt TM, Vernier RR, eds: *Pediatric Nephrology*, 2nd ed. Baltimore: Williams & Wilkins, 1987.

Siegler RL: Management of hemolytic uremic syndrome. *J Pediatr* 1988; 112:1014.

Vernier RL: Primary nephrotic syndrome. In: Holliday MA, Barratt TM, Vernier RR, eds: *Pediatric Nephrology*, 2nd ed. Baltimore: Williams & Wilkins, 1987.

112 Urologic Disorders

Jack W. McAninch

Paraphimosis ■

This condition occurs when the foreskin of an uncircumcised child is retracted over the glans penis and cannot be returned to its usual position.

CLINICAL FINDINGS

A tight constricting ring of skin will usually be noted at the base of the glans in the coronal sulcus, and marked distal edema will soon follow. The patient experiences extreme pain. A bluish discoloration of the glans penis may be apparent secondary to decreased blood flow from the severe edema. The patient may have difficulty voiding, although this is an inconsistent finding.

TREATMENT AND DISPOSITION

No laboratory studies are necessary to establish the diagnosis. Return the foreskin to its normal position after achieving appropriate sedation (see Chapter 39). Gentle, firm, continuous digital pressure to the glans will force out the edema fluid. Once it has returned to near-normal size, the constricting ring of skin will slide forward. Should this technique be unsuccessful, consult a urologist.

Next, slit the dorsal aspect of the constricting ring immediately under either local or general anesthesia. After healing is complete, the urologist must perform circumcision.

COMPLICATIONS

If the condition is ignored or diagnosis delayed, ischemic tissue necrosis may occur distal to the constricting ring. This could result in partial tissue loss.

Balanoposthitis ■

Infection under the foreskin usually occurs in boys with severe phimosis who have poor hygiene. Oc-
casionally, the foreskin may adhere to the glans penis, which prevents drainage of subcoronal glands and promotes accumulation of smegma. These pre-existing conditions usually allow gram-negative or gram-positive pathogens to initiate an infectious process underneath the foreskin.

CLINICAL FINDINGS

Pain, erythema, and purulent drainage are common. The foreskin cannot usually be retracted sufficiently to visualize the urethral meatus or glans penis. Inguinal lymph nodes may be enlarged or tender.

ANCILLARY DATA

A culture from underneath the foreskin will detect the offending organisms, which generally are gram-negative Enterobacteriaceae.

TREATMENT AND DISPOSITION

Warm sitz baths twice daily are helpful. The parent should retract the boy's foreskin as far as comfortably possible while he is in the bath and cleanse the area gently with soap. Oral antibiotics may be necessary in severe cases. Refer the patient to a urologist for circumcision after the infection has cleared.

Constricting Foreign Bodies ■

Constricting foreign bodies such as hair, fine string (dental floss), or occasionally rubber bands surrounding the base of the penis can cause massive edema and soft-tissue damage.

CLINICAL FINDINGS

Frequently this edema develops over several hours or days, and its extent may easily conceal the offending foreign body. Careful inspection of the area just proximal to the edema will reveal the constricting agent, which then can be removed. Superficial skin necrosis and secondary infection may be evident if diagnosis and treatment have been delayed.

TREATMENT AND DISPOSITION

The edema generally resolves promptly with release of the constriction. Large constricting objects (toys, bolts, steel rings) must be removed with appropriate cutting tools. This procedure may require urologist involvement. Observe closely the areas of skin with a compromised blood supply; debride those that are not viable. Refer the patient to a urologist if complications exist, or to the primary physician for routine follow-up.

Priapism ■

Priapism is a persistent, painful erection unrelated to sexual desire. In children it is a manifestation of underlying systemic disease, most commonly sickle-cell disease or trait and leukemia.

CLINICAL FINDINGS

The penis is very tense, firm, and tender to palpation. The child usually voids without difficulty.

ANCILLARY DATA

Patients require careful hematologic evaluation for leukemic cells. Screen for sickle-cell disease or trait by hemoglobin electrophoresis.

TREATMENT AND DISPOSITION

Early management (within the first 6 hours) includes sedation and ice packs. Hyperbaric oxygen chambers and blood transfusions have been beneficial in patients with sickle-cell disease.

If priapism persists more than 6 hours, surgical management is imperative. Obtain urologist consultation; usually, drainage of the accumulated blood in the erectile tissue and creation of a shunt between the corpus cavernosum and corpus spongiosum is necessary. A biopsy needle or a surgical scalpel is adequate to establish the shunt opening. Observe the patient closely to prevent recurrence.

COMPLICATIONS

Recurrence is often seen in patients with sickle-cell disease or trait or leukemia. Once priapism has developed with one of these disease processes, expect recurrence.

Hematuria ■

The sudden onset of gross hematuria is distressing to parents and the patient. It can occur in neonates as well as in older children. A careful medical history will aid in determining the cause.

ETIOLOGY AND PATHOPHYSIOLOGY

Gross hematuria in the neonate is an emergency. The child may be asymptomatic, but suspect a major underlying pathologic condition. Some of these conditions may be lethal if not properly diagnosed and treated (*e.g.*, renal artery thrombosis, renal vein thrombosis, and renal cortical necrosis). Other causes of hematuria in the neonate are obstructive uropathy, polycystic renal disease, sponge kidney, Wilms' tumor, neonatal glomerulonephritis, hemorrhagic disorders, and birth trauma.

Gross hematuria in the older child is most often due to acute poststreptococcal glomerulonephritis, which has its peak incidence at 3 to 8 years of age. This is characterized by proteinuria, hypertension, and hematuria (see Chapter 111). A variety of other types of glomerulonephritis, less commonly seen, may also cause hematuria, including systemic lupus erythematosus, periarteritis nodosa, anaphylactoid purpura, Goodpasture's syndrome, and subacute bacterial endocarditis.

Urinary tract infections may cause gross hematuria and are often associated with symptoms of bladder infection or pyelonephritis. Consider congenital obstructive uropathy (*e.g.*, ureteropelvic junction obstruction, urethral valves, and ureterovesical junction obstruction) in such patients. These children are often asymptomatic because of the longstanding nature of the obstruction and present only with intermittent hematuria. Calculi are rare in children and are more often associated with microscopic hematuria.

CLINICAL FINDINGS

A careful history is most important in determining the site of bleeding. Spotting of blood on the diapers or underwear in the initial portion of the urinary stream suggests urethral abnormalities. Hematuria at the end of the stream suggests prostatic or bladder abnormalities. Hematuria throughout the stream (total gross hematuria) implicates the bladder, urethra, or kidneys as a possible source. If dysuria is present, infection is most often the cause. If abdominal examination reveals a palpable mass, obstructive uropathy or a solid tumor is likely.

ANCILLARY DATA

Obtain urine of children with gross hematuria for urinalysis and culture and sensitivity testing. Also send blood specimens for complete blood count, creatinine and BUN, serum complement, and anti-streptolysin O titer. Abdominal sonography, radio-nucleotide renal scanning, excretory urography, and computed tomography will differentiate among etiologies for gross hematuria. An excretory voiding cystourethrogram with the excretory urogram will provide additional key information regarding the bladder and urethra while avoiding urethral catheterization. Cystoscopy may be indicated to investigate an abnormality noted on another study, but is not routinely warranted for the child with hematuria.

TREATMENT AND DISPOSITION

Treatment of gross hematuria depends on the cause. Total gross hematuria warrants hospitalization and immediate urologic consultation to initiate the evaluation.

Bibliography ■

Govan DE, Fair WR, Friedland GW, Filly RA: Urinary tract infections in children. III. Treatment of ureterovesical reflux. *West J Med* 1974; 121:382

Smellie J, Edwards D, Hunter N, et al: Vesico-ureteric reflux and renal scarring. *Kidney Int* 1975; 8:S65–S72.

Walther PC, Kaplan G: Cystoscopy in children. Indications for its use in common urologic problems. *J Urol* 1979; 122:717.

XI
Infectious Diseases

113 Septicemia

Moses Grossman

Septicemia is an infection characterized by a positive blood culture. It may or may not be associated with a focal infection such as pneumonia or meningitis or with endotoxic shock; when the complication of endotoxic shock develops, the illness becomes considerably more severe with a significant mortality.

Occult bacteremia in a young febrile child is discussed in Chapter 24. Sepsis in immunocompromised children is discussed in Chapter 124.

Etiology and Pathophysiology ■

The most common microorganisms causing bacteremia in children are listed in Table 113-1. Immunocompromised children and those with indwelling lines are particularly prone to develop bacteremia. The ability of bacteria, many of them normal inhabitants of the nasopharynx and gastrointestinal tract, to invade the blood stream is usually the result of an interplay between inherent invasive properties of the bacteria (pathogenicity) and host defenses. Some gram-negative organisms (*e.g., Salmonella typhosa*) will often produce bacteremia in normal hosts; others seldom do so (*e.g., Pseudomonas aeruginosa*), and then only when host defenses have been compromised. One of the results of bacteremia is that the organism is disseminated throughout the body and may produce localized infection in different organs (*e.g.*, abscesses, arthritis, meningitis) depending on the bacteria.

Another life-threatening complication of bacteremia particularly due to Enterobacteriaceae and *Neisseria meningitidis* is *endotoxic shock*. Endotoxin present in these and other organisms is a very complex lipopolysaccharide. Bacteria, endotoxin, or some interaction between bacteria and leukocytes activate the prekallikrein-kallikrein system. This results in the release of bradykinin and many other vasoactive components and activation of the complement cascade. A complex and multiorgan physiologic response results with peripheral vasodilata-tion, decreased peripheral resistance, pooling of blood peripherally, and decreased return of venous blood to the heart. The accompanying shock is known as *distributive shock*, abnormal distribution of blood volume (as opposed to inadequate blood volume) leading to poor tissue perfusion and oxygenation (see Chapter 8).

Metabolic complications of endotoxic shock include hypoglycemia, liver dysfunction, acute renal failure, shock lung, and CNS dysfunction. Disseminated intravascular clotting (DIC) may also occur. Unless promptly reversed, this sequence of events may culminate in multiple organ failure and death.

Clinical Findings ■

In young children, so-called "occult" bacteremia may present with a single clinical manifestation of high fever and no localizing findings (Chapter 24). Bacteremia may also be a concomitant finding in some well-known clinical entities such as pneumonia (Chapter 116), periorbital cellulitis (Chapter 117), urinary tract infection (Chapter 122), and typhoid fever.

Meningococcemia is a clinical entity in which *N. meningitidis*, a relatively common colonizer of the nasopharynx, gains access to the bloodstream. The resultant clinical illness is characterized by high fever, a petechial rash, and rapid progression leading to shock, DIC, and at times death. Coexisting meningococcal meningitis may or may not be present. Timely intervention is life-saving.

In most instances *septicemia* represents an unexpected spread of an infection to the bloodstream. The history must review organ systems where the initial infection might have occurred, especially the skin, urinary tract, and gastrointestinal tract. The history must also address issues of host susceptibility, such as sickle-cell disease, splenectomy, neutropenia, recent manipulative procedures (*e.g.*, dental work), or the presence of indwelling foreign bodies (*e.g.*, catheters). Toxic shock syndrome (Chapter 107) caused by a staphylococcal toxin resembles septicemia. Septicemia is often heralded by fever, chills, nausea, and diarrhea, and sometimes by altered mental status.

Physical Examination ■

Concentrate on early signs of shock (see Chapter 8) and signs of DIC (see Chapter 19) and look for clues to possible etiology. Vital signs, mental status, and skin condition (cool, warm, capillary refill, presence of petechiae and purpura) are of the utmost importance. Carefully examine the heart, lungs, and abdomen to ascertain the child's cardiopulmonary status; a thorough assessment may yield clues to the original sites for bacteremia. Examine for signs of meningeal irritation (stiff neck; Kernig's and Brudzinski's signs); meningitis often coexists in children with bacteremia.

Ancillary Findings ■

A white blood cell count and differential will provide both diagnostic and prognostic clues (very low PMN count signifies poor prognosis). A urinalysis and urine culture are important; a blood culture prior to antimicrobial therapy and cultures of all sites suspicious for the initial infection (wound sites, pustules, indwelling catheters) may lead to a microbiologic diagnosis. *Do a lumbar puncture whenever in doubt.* The laboratory evidence of DIC is thrombocytopenia, prolonged prothrombin and partial thromboplastin times, and the presence of split fibrin products.

Obtain early clues to the specific bacterial etiology with gram stains of pus, urinary sediment, sputum, and tracheal secretion when pertinent. Latex agglutination studies of bacterial products in the urine or other body fluids may provide invaluable information. Latex agglutination is available for polysaccharide capsules of *Haemophilus influenzae* type b, *Streptococcus pneumoniae*, and *Escherichia coli* type K1.

Treatment ■

SELECTION OF ANTIMICROBIAL AGENTS

Treat bloodstream infection *promptly* with intravenous bactericidal drugs: the object is to arrest further spread of the infection and to prevent septic shock. Chapter 24 describes the selection of antimicrobials to treat the occult bacteremia in a febrile young child. Chapter 124 describes the management of the immunocompromised child.

When the etiology of bacteremia is known at the

TABLE 113–1.	*Microorganisms Causing Bacteremia in Children Beyond the Newborn Period*

In Normal Children

Streptococcus pneumoniae	Association: Complement deficiency, sickle-cell disease, immunodeficiency, skin infections
Haemophilus influenzae type b	
Neisseria meningitides	
Salmonella species	
Staphylococcus aureus	

In Children With Heart Disease (Endocarditis)
Streptococcus viridans
Staph aureus
Staph epidermidis

In Immunocompromised Children
All of the above
Enterobacteriaceae
Pseudomonas species
Fungi

initiation of therapy, select an antimicrobial agent to which the bacteria are most likely to be sensitive (from literature and local experience) and that covers subsets of bacterial population as well (*e.g.*, beta-lactamase-producing strains). When the bacterial etiology is unknown and treatment is presumptive, cover the *most likely* and the *most serious* possibilities. Third-generation cephalosporins will usually provide such coverage for most but not all such settings. Ceftriaxone (100 mg/kg/24h divided into two doses) or cefotaxime (150 mg/kg divided into three doses) or cefuroxime, a second-generation cephalosporin (150 mg/kg/day divided into 3 doses), and several other cephalosporins will provide such coverage. For methicillin-resistant staphylococci, vancomycin (40–60 mg/kg/day) is the only suitable drug.

Enterococcal sepsis requires a combination of a penicillin or ampicillin and an aminoglycoside (*e.g.*, gentamicin). *P. aeruginosa*, seen almost exclusively in immunocompromised children as a nosocomial infection, calls for a combination of an aminoglycoside and an extended penicillin (*e.g.*, piperacillin) until sensitivities are available. Ceftazidime could provide alternative treatment (see Table 113-2).

Consider whether there is a collection of pus serving as a continual reservoir for bacteremia. Surgical drainage is imperative in this setting.

The treatment of shock is discussed in Chapter 8, the treatment of DIC in Chapter 19. Consult a pediatric hematologist for assistance with management of DIC.

See Chapter 8 for the treatment of shock other than antimicrobial selection.

TABLE 113-2. *Antimicrobial Therapy of Septicemia*

Clinical Setting and *Etiologic Organism*	*Antimicrobial* (see Chapter 143 for dosing)
Organism known	Suitable bactericidal antimicrobial
Strep pneumoniae, Haemophilus influenzae, suspected Group A streptococci	Cefuroxime, cefataxime, or ceftriaxone
Staph aureus (community acquired)	Nafcillin or cefazolin
Staph aureus (hospital acquired)	Vancomycin
Unknown, gram-negative organism suspected	Cefuroxime or cefataxime or ceftriaxone
Enterococci	Penicillin or ampicillin + gentamicin
Pseudomonas	Piperacillin + gentamicin or ceftazidime

Disposition ■

Hospitalize all children with known or strongly suspected septicemia and treat with parenteral antimicrobials presumptively based on history, physical assessment, and ancillary studies. Monitor carefully for signs of septic shock; treated early, this is a reversible condition, but late treatment is associated with a high mortality.

Bibliography ■

Havens PL, Garland JS, Brook MM, et al: Trends in mortality in children hospitalized with meningococcal infection, 1957–1987. *Pediatr Infect Dis J* 1989; 8:8.

McCartney AC, Banks JG, Clements GB, et al: Endotoxemia in septic shock: Clinical and post-mortem correlation. *Intensive Care Med* 1983; 9:117.

Root RK, Sande MA: *Septic Shock.* New York: Churchill-Livingstone, 1985.

Rubin LG, Moxon ER: Pathogenesis of blood stream invasion with *Haemophilus influenzae* type b. *Infect Immun* 1983; 41:280.

Wong KV, Hitchcock W, Mason WH: Meningococcal Infection in children: A review of 100 cases. *Pediatr Infect Dis J* 1989; 8:224.

114 Meningitis

Jay H. Tureen

Meningitis is an inflammatory disorder of the central nervous system clinically characterized by alteration in level of consciousness, fever, and in many instances stiff neck. It may be caused by a variety of infectious agents, and has both acute and chronic presentations. Acute bacterial meningitis, the most worrisome condition, occurs at a frequency of 300/100,000 live births in the newborn period and 5/100,000 patients per year from 1 month to 4 years of age.

Etiology and Pathophysiology ■

Meningitis may be caused by bacterial, viral, fungal, mycobacterial, spirochetal, and protozoan pathogens (Table 114-1). Acute meningitis is usually due to either bacterial or viral agents, whereas chronic meningitis is more likely due to the other types of infecting organisms. The critical pathophysiologic event is introduction of pathogenic organisms into the subarachnoid space. This occurs most commonly by hematogenous seeding through the choroid plexus, although direct extension from a contiguous infected focus (otitis media, sinusitis, mastoiditis) or through a break in normal anatomic barriers (skull fracture, postoperative, or congenital defect) may also occur.

Clinical Findings ■

Clinical findings may be nonspecific, especially in the child under 18 months. In this age group, the only symptoms may be irritability, fever, poor feeding, lethargy, and high-pitched crying. In the older child, complaints are more specific and include headache, stiff neck, photophobia, and fever. Signs and symptoms in the newborn may include abdominal distention, feeding intolerance, and hypothermia.

Cardinal physical features of purulent meningitis include fever, alteration in level of consciousness, and stiff neck. Brudzinski's or Kernig's signs may be present in the absence of frank neck stiffness and suggest meningeal irritation. Brudzinski's sign is flexion of the knee as the examiner rapidly flexes the child's neck. Kernig's sign is posterior thigh and knee pain as the examiner extends the child's knee, with the hip at a 90-degree flexion. *Infants under 18 months of age may not manifest any signs of meningeal irritation.* Bulging fontanelle is a late physical finding.

Other important historical points or physical findings are noted in Table 114-2. Prompt recognition of worrisome signs and symptoms is essential for early diagnosis and institution of appropriate supportive and antimicrobial therapy, which are imperative in improving survival and reducing sequelae.

Differential diagnosis includes meningitis due to other pathogens, or other pyogenic causes of CNS infection (brain, epidural abscess, subdural empyema). Noninfectious causes that may present with similar symptoms include subarachnoid hemorrhage, carcinomatous meningitis, and meningitis due to autoimmune disease.

Ancillary Data ■

Diagnosis is established by cerebrospinal fluid (CSF) analysis and culture (Table 114-3). Antigen detection tests (latex particle agglutination [LPA], counterimmunoelectrophoresis [CIE]) are useful for rapid identification of certain pathogens (*Haemophilus influenzae* type b, Group B streptococcus, *Streptococcus pneumoniae,* certain meningococci). They are particularly valuable when prior oral antibiotic therapy may render the culture negative. Blood culture is positive in about 75% of cases.

Never delay lumbar puncture (LP) unless there are focal neurologic signs suggesting a space-occupying lesion (abscess, subarachnoid hemorrhage). In this

TABLE 114-1. *Etiologic Agents of Meningitis by Age Group*

Patient	Organism	
	Purulent Meningitis	Aseptic Meningitis
Neonate (0–28 days)	Group B streptococcus, *E. coli,* other gram-negative enterics, *Listeria*	Enterovirus, *Candida albicans*
Infant (1–3 mo)	Group B streptococcus, *E. coli, Listeria, Haemophilus influenzae, Streptococcus pneumoniae, Neisseria meningiditis*	Enterovirus
Infant—child (3 mo–6 yr)	*Haemophilus influenzae, Streptococcus pneumoniae, Neisseria meningiditis*	Enterovirus, mumps, *M. tuberculosis,* cryptococcus, coccidioidomycosis
Older child	*Streptococcus pneumoniae, Neisseria meningiditis*	Enterovirus, mumps, *M. tuberculosis,* cryptococcus, coccidioidomycosis, leptospirosis, Lyme disease

situation, obtain an emergency head CT scan and a blood culture, then initiate antibiotics appropriate to the patient's age and likely pathogens. If the CT does not show a mass lesion or bleeding, perform an LP, with antigen detection tests to augment the Gram's stain and culture.

Other important diagnostic studies include:

1. CSF exam for culture, cell count, glucose, protein, and Gram's stain; measure opening pressure with a manometer
2. CSF for LPA or CIE if above studies are suggestive of meningitis but not diagnostic of etiology, or if prior antibiotics have been taken
3. Blood culture
4. Serum glucose and electrolytes

TABLE 114-2. *Signs and Symptoms of Meningitis*

Fever (95%)
Alteration in level of consciousness (95–100%)
 Irritability (60–75%)
 Lethargy (15–20%)
 Somnolence (5%)
 Coma (1%)
Stiff neck, positive Kernig or Brudzinski sign
 >18 months—usually present
 <18 months—variably present
Headache
Vomiting
Bulging fontanelle
Generalized seizures
Focal neurologic signs
 Cranial nerve palsy (sixth nerve is most common)
 Focal seizure
 Hemiparesis or hemiplegia

Treatment ■

To optimize outcome, comprehensive care for the patient with bacterial meningitis must include prompt diagnosis, appropriate supportive measures, administration of age-appropriate, empiric antibiotics, and anticipatory management of the common complications.

SUPPORTIVE MEASURES

Assess level of consciousness. If the patient is comatose or severely neurologically depressed with impaired gag reflex, consider elective intubation for airway protection.

Assess status of circulation by blood pressure, capillary refill, and orthostatic blood pressure measurement. This is an important clinical consideration, as patients may be hypovolemic due to poor intake or vomiting, or as a consequence of endotoxemia (meningococcal or gram-negative enteric infection). Conversely, if inappropriate secretion of antidiuretic hormone (SIADH) is present, patients may be unable to excrete a water load and may become fluid-overloaded in response to too-vigorous fluid administration. Figure 114-1 presents an algorithm for assessment and treatment of varying levels of hydration in patients with meningitis.

ANTIMICROBIAL TREATMENT

Choose antibiotics empirically based on the patient's age and the likely pathogens (Table 114-4). A conclusive Gram's stain interpreted by a trained clinician or microbiologist may be an indication to modify treatment prior to culture and sensitivity results, but

TABLE 114–3. *CSF Findings in Diseases of the Central Nervous System*

Diagnosis	WBC (%PMN)	Glucose (% serum) (mg/dl)	Protein (mg/dl)	Gram's stain	Intracranial pressure (mm H$_2$O)
Normal	<6 (0)	>40 (>50)	<35	negative	<180
Bacterial meningitis	200–10,000 (80–100)	<40 (<50)	100–500	positive	>200
Partially treated	200–10,000 (40–100)	same as above		Positive or negative	>200
Viral	25–1000 (<50)	>40 (>50)	50–100	negative	<180
Mycobacterial	50–1000 (<50)	<40	50–300	negative	>200
Fungal	50–1000 (<50)	<40	50–300	negative	>200
Brain abscess	50–200 (<50)	>40 (>50)	50–100	negative	>200
Subarachnoid hemorrhage	bloody	<40	50–100	negative	>200

because errors in interpretation occur up to 10% of the time, this must be done with caution. Select bactericidal antibiotics that achieve a CSF concentration 10 times the minimal bactericidal concentration for the pathogen.

Dexamethasone

A recent clinical study demonstrated a significant reduction in hearing impairment in infants with bacterial meningitis who were given a short course of dexamethasone with the initial dose of antibiotic. While this therapy has not been critically evaluated in neonates or older children, it may be a useful adjunct for the infant or toddler with bacterial meningitis. Give dexamethasone 0.6 mg/kg/day, divided

q 6 hours, for 4 days, with the first dose given in the ED when antibiotic therapy is initiated.

Complications ■

Complications may be acute (likely to be present on admission or occurring within the first few days of hospitalization) or long term (likely to be permanent or take months to resolve).

ACUTE PROBLEMS

1. Seizures (25%): Of little prognostic significance if nonfocal, occurring within 24 hours of admission, and easy to control with anticonvulsants
2. SIADH (30%)

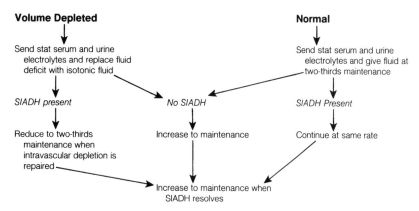

FIGURE 114–1. Clinical assessment of volume status in meningitis.

TABLE 114–4. *Empiric Antibiotics in Purulent Meningitis*

Patient	Antibiotic	Dose mg/kg/day	Emergency Dose mg/kg
Neonates (0–28 day)	Ampicillin **plus**	200	50
	Aminoglycoside or	7.5	2.5
	Cefotaxime*	200	50
Infants (1–3 mo)	Ampicillin **plus**	300	75
	Cefotaxime or	200	50
	Ceftriaxone	100	50
Infant—child (3 mo–6 yr)	Cefotaxime or	200	50
	Ceftriaxone	100	50
	or		
	Ampicillin **plus**	300	75
	Chloramphenicol	100	25
Older child—adult (>6 yr)	Penicillin G	300,000 units	50,000 units

* Cefotaxime is indicated in meningitis due to gram-negative organisms because of poor penetration of ominoglycocides into CSF.

3. Brain stem herniation due to increased intracranial pressure
4. Infarction, either arterial or venous
5. Brain edema
6. Subdural effusion or empyema
7. Abscess

LONG-TERM SEQUELAE

1. Seizure disorder
2. Hydrocephalus
3. Deafness
4. Weakness or paralysis
5. Cranial nerve palsy
6. Brain damage

Disposition ■

All cases of pyogenic meningitis require hospitalization. Patients with viral meningitis may need hospitalization for supportive care such as intravenous fluid administration or pain management. Arrange rifampin prophylaxis for family, household, and day-care center contacts of patients with *H. influenzae* or meningococcal meningitis. Give rifampin to the patient as well to minimize the chance for secondary cases.

Bibliography ■

Barson WJ, Miller MA, Brady MT, et al: Prospective comparative trial of ceftriaxone vs. conventional therapy for treatment of bacterial meningitis in children. *Pediatr Infect Dis J* 1985; 4:362.

Dodge PR, Swartz MN: Bacterial meningitis: A review of selected aspects. *N Engl J Med* 1965; 272:954.

Feigin RD: Bacterial meningitis in the newborn infant. *Clin Perinatol* 1977;4:103.

Klein JO, Feigin RD, McCracken GH Jr: Report of the task force on diagnosis and management of meningitis. *Pediatrics* 1986; 78:959.

Lebel MM, Freij BJ, Syrogiannopoulos GA, et al: Dexamethasone therapy for bacterial meningitis: Results of two double-blind, placebo-controlled trials. *N Engl J Med* 1988; 319:964.

McCracken GH: Management of bacterial meningitis in infants and children. Current status and future prospects. *Am J Med* 1984; 76:215.

Odio CM, Faingezicht I, Salas JL, et al: Cefotaxime vs. conventional therapy for the treatment of bacterial meningitis in infants and children. *Pediatr Infect Dis J* 1986; 5:402.

Sande MA: Antibiotic therapy of bacterial meningitis: Lessons we've learned. *Am J Med* 1981; 71:507.

Sell SH: Long-term sequelae of bacterial meningitis in children. *Pediatr Infect Dis J* 1983; 2:90.

115 Upper Airway Infections

Moses Grossman

Infections involving the upper airway usually result in edema of the mucous membranes and varying degrees of inflammation of the underlying tissues. In an infant or young child, a small amount of swelling may occlude the airway, so even mild infections of the upper airway are potentially dangerous. *The paramount consideration is the patency of the airway.* Good initial assessment, repeated assessments, and careful follow-up are essential to avoid a life-threatening emergency. Most children with croup suffer from a viral infection, but the minority with epiglottitis or bacterial tracheitis must be identified early so that their airways can be secured.

Croup ■

Croup (laryngotracheobronchitis) is an infection of the upper airway that always involves the larynx and usually involves the subglottic area, the trachea, and bronchi as well. It can be caused by several respiratory viruses but most commonly is caused by parainfluenza viruses.

ETIOLOGY AND PATHOPHYSIOLOGY

Croup usually occurs in children between 6 months and 4 years of age, rarely thereafter. The infection produces edema in the subglottic area and compresses the airway.

The parainfluenza virus often affects other parts of the respiratory mucosa; thus, it is not uncommon to find coryza, otitis, or conjunctivitis along with the laryngotracheobronchitis.

Viral croup must be differentiated from other causes of upper airway obstruction (see Chapter 13). The most important of these is epiglottitis (see Table 115-1). Patients with epiglottitis are often older, have a more abrupt onset, are more febrile, more toxic, and may exhibit drooling or complain of pain on swallowing.

CLINICAL FINDINGS

Usually, onset is gradual with runny nose, cough, hoarseness, "seal bark," and an inspiratory whoop. Low-grade fever may be present. Suprasternal and xiphoid retractions occur, and the use of accessory muscles of respiration is notable.

As croup progresses and the airway becomes more jeopardized, signs of anoxia appear: rising pulse rate, restlessness, increased retractions, and cyanosis. A chest film often reveals the "steeple sign" of upper laryngeal narrowing (Fig. 115-1).

TREATMENT

1. If epiglottitis is suspected, a lateral film of the neck is helpful. See the section below for precautions.
2. If still in doubt, direct visualization of the epiglottis may be indicated. (This should be performed in the operating room.)
3. Close, repeated evaluations of the clinical picture are invaluable. A "respiratory score sheet," plotting periodic observations of pulse rate, respiratory rate, and retractions on the same sheet, is very helpful.
4. Blood gas determinations or pulse oximetry are of little value in the earlier stage of this disease; later, hypoxia is common.
5. Give steam, particularly cold steam, for symptomatic relief. In a hospital setting, a croupette with an effective nebulizer is best.
6. Provide hydration by intravenous fluids, if necessary.
7. Do not disturb the child. Make the child as comfortable as possible.
8. Do not sedate the child. Severe restlessness may indicate anoxia.
9. Corticosteroids have not been shown to be of value in controlled trials, but many physicians treat empirically in cases of very severe croup (0.3

TABLE 115-1. *Differential Diagnosis of Epiglottitis and Viral Croup*

	Epiglottitis	Viral Croup
Age	1–6 years Rare in adults	3 months–3 years
Etiology	*H. influenzae* type B (rare Gr A BHS)	Viral (parainfluenza)
Onset	Abrupt	Gradual
Duration of illness before hospital	Several hours	1–2 days
Presenting complaints	High fever, muffled guttural voice, dyspnea, dysphagia, drooling	Fever, barking cough, hoarseness, inspiratory stridor
Physical exam	Diminished breath sounds, inspiratory rhonchi, pallor	Diminished breath sounds, inspiratory rales
Laryngeal findings	Cherry-red epiglottis	Edema vocal cords, decreased subglottic area
Leukocytosis	Marked	Moderate
Clinical course	Rapidly progressive abrupt obstruction; medical emergency	Self-limited; may last 1 week
Bacterial complications	Other organs may be seeded	Rare
Treatment	Establish airway. Initiate antimicrobial therapy (cefuroxime, cefataxime, or ceftriaxone).	Humidification, support, racemic epinephrine with IPPB, steroids

mg/kg of dexamethasone initially and repeated in 2 hours).

10. If the illness is severe, immediately consult the appropriate specialists, including an anesthesiol-

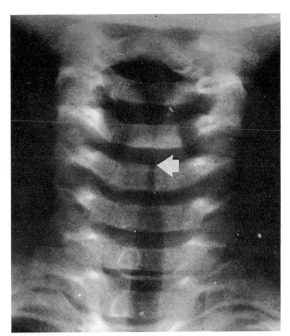

FIGURE 115-1. Anterioposterior view of the neck demonstrates narrowing of the subglottic airway (*arrow*) indicative of edema seen with croup.

ogist and an otolaryngologist to ensure airway protection.

11. Ensure that a laryngoscope and an appropriately sized endotracheal tube are readily available in case of emergency.

12. Parainfluenza virus is *in vitro* susceptible to ribavirin, but the efficacy of this drug in the treatment of croup has not been demonstrated.

DISPOSITION

Hospitalize moderately severe and severe cases of croup. Anticipate that the child's condition will worsen during the evening and night hours. Any child with croup severe enough to receive corticosteroids belongs in the hospital.

Provide the parents with discharge instructions for children going home. Make sure they know how to secure urgent medical care if the child gets worse. Discuss how to administer steam in the home (rent a good vaporizer; ensure the child does not sustain a burn). Ensure follow-up with the primary care provider (by telephone or visit, as indicated by the child's condition).

Epiglottitis ■

Epiglottitis is a bacterial infection of the epiglottis that produces a greatly enlarged, "cherry red" epiglottis that may obstruct the airway. The offending agent is most commonly *Haemophilus influenzae* type b.

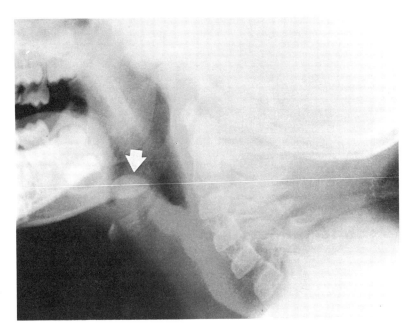

FIGURE 115–2. Epiglottitis. Lateral view of the neck demonstrates a markedly enlarged epiglottis (*arrow*) characteristic of epiglottitis. See normal film for comparison.

CLINICAL FINDINGS

The child may be of any age, but most commonly is 3 to 7 years old (older than in the case of viral croup) (see Table 115-1). The onset is abrupt, with high fever, hoarseness, and cough. Drooling is often present. Pain on swallowing is a prominent symptom. The child usually appears ill and toxic. The classical position is to thrust the chest forward and hyperextend the neck to improve the airway.

There may be leukocytosis with an increase in younger polymorphonuclear cells (left shift). The lateral neck radiograph shows a wide rounded configuration of the inflamed epiglottitis ("thumb sign") (Fig. 115-2) as opposed to the slender normal epiglottis (Fig. 115-3).

TREATMENT

1. Suspected epiglottitis is an emergency, since the child could experience an acute loss of airway patency. Do not attempt throat examination or laryngoscopy until the patient is in the operating room.
2. Obtain a lateral film of the neck if the diagnosis is unclear. An experienced physician with a laryngoscope and endotracheal tubes should accompany the child to the x-ray department.
3. If the clinical presentation is very suggestive of epiglottitis, the radiologic examination is best omitted; proceed to a direct examination of the epiglottis in the operating room.

4. Many authorities believe that if the diagnosis of epiglottitis (large "cherry red" epiglottis) is made, prophylactic intubation is usually indicated. More than half of all children will require intubation or

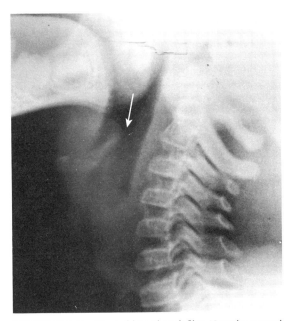

FIGURE 115–3. Normal lateral neck film. Note the normal slender epiglottis (*arrow*).

a tracheostomy, and there is some advantage in performing this procedure electively. We recommend this approach. We also recommend intubation over tracheostomy, but each physician and his/her consultants will have to make these decisions.

5. Obtain cultures of the epiglottis as well as blood cultures.
6. Intravenous fluid maintenance is essential.
7. Institute specific antimicrobial therapy directed against *H. influenzae.* Intravenous cefuroxime, cefotaxime, or ceftriaxone are the antimicrobials of choice.
8. Cold steam may make the patient more comfortable.
9. Epiglottitis is a manifestation of invasive *H. influenzae* disease. Thus, treat the patient and all household members with rifampin 20 mg/kg once daily for 4 days as prophylaxis. This is unnecessary if there are no children younger than 4 years in the household. If the child attends a day-care center or nursery school, notify the institution of the infection so that prophylactic therapy might be considered.

Bacterial Tracheitis ■

This is an important cause of severe upper respiratory obstruction. It generally occurs in children younger than 3 years and is caused by a number of bacterial pathogens, principally *Staphylococcus aureus.* Beginning as a case that resembles croup, the child rapidly becomes much sicker, more febrile, and more toxic, and develops more of a leukocytosis. The tracheal mucosa often sloughs, forming thick mucopurulent secretions that the child cannot bring up. Radiologic imaging may be helpful, but ultimately the diagnosis depends on direct visualization of the trachea.

TREATMENT

1. Hospitalize the child and administer intravenous fluids.

2. Monitor cardiopulmonary status closely.
3. When the diagnosis of bacterial tracheitis is made, intubate the child to protect the airway.
4. Provide high-flow oxygen.
5. Obtain bacterial cultures of the tracheal secretions.
6. Initiate intravenous antimicrobial therapy. Use broad antimicrobial coverage initially (cefuroxime or nafcillin and ampicillin), but the principal target is *S. aureus.*

Laryngeal Diphtheria ■

This form of diphtheria, uncommon in the United States today (see Chapter 123), may be seen in unimmunized individuals. Involvement of the larynx may occur in conjunction with pharyngeal diphtheria, in which case the visible confluent exudate suggests the diagnosis. When laryngeal diphtheria alone is present, the child's marked toxicity will help rule out viral croup. Direct inspection of the larynx in the operating room will reveal the exudate and usually suggest the diagnosis.

Management includes immediate intubation, administration of diphtheria antitoxin and an antimicrobial agent (penicillin or erythromycin).

Bibliography ■

Battaglia JD. Severe croup: The child with fever and upper airway obstruction. *Pediatr in Rev* 1986; 7:227–233.

Butt W, Walker C, et al: Acute epiglottitis: A different approach to management. *Crit Care Med* 1988; 16:43.

Crysdale WS, Sendi K: Evolution in the management of acute epiglottitis: A 10-year experience with 242 children. *J Anesthesiol Clin* 1988; 26:32–38.

Edwards KM, Dundin MC, Altemeier WH: Bacterial tracheitis as a complication of viral croup. *Pediatr Infect Dis J* 1983; 2:390–391.

Lockhart CH, Battaglia SD: Croup (laryngotracheal bronchitis) and epiglottitis. *Pediatr Ann* 1977; 6:262–269.

Tunneson WW Jr, Feinstein HR: The steroid-croup controversy: An analytic review of methodological problems. *J Pediatr* 1980; 96:751–756.

Bronchiolitis and pneumonia are common infections of childhood. Most pneumonias in young children are viral; in later years, bacterial and mycoplasma pneumonias become more frequent. Any pneumonia can be so extensive that it interferes with blood oxygenation or exhausts ventilation, thus becoming an emergency (see Chapter 7). Bacterial pneumonias generally run a more rapid and more virulent course. Pneumococcal pneumonia, the most common of the bacterial pneumonias, may progress very rapidly and may require urgent antimicrobial therapy. This chapter will deal with three of the most immediately life-threatening infections: bronchiolitis, pneumonia, and empyema.

Bronchiolitis ■

Bronchiolitis is an inflammatory reaction of the bronchioles, producing expiratory obstruction and air-trapping.

ETIOLOGY AND PATHOGENESIS

The infection is almost always viral in etiology; the most common agent is the respiratory syncytial virus (RSV). In a young infant, it is difficult to differentiate bronchiolitis from bronchial asthma.

Inflammation and obstruction at the level of the bronchiole produce air trapping, interfere with gas exchange, and produce shifting atelectasis, resulting in hypoxemia and CO_2 retention. RSV-induced bronchiolitis causes apneic spells in young infants (under 2 months), probably as a result of hypoxemia.

Reassess the clinical situation periodically, following the respiratory rate, heart rate, air exchange, severity of retractions, CO_2 retention, degree of arterial oxygenation, and level of fatigue.

CLINICAL FINDINGS

1. Low-grade fever
2. Tachypnea
3. Tachycardia
4. Intercostal retractions
5. Expiratory wheezing
6. Palpable and depressed liver edge because the diaphragm is depressed
7. Other manifestations of viral infection such as conjunctivitis, otitis, and pneumonia

ANCILLARY DATA

The chest film shows air-trapping, changing patterns of atelectasis, and depressed diaphragm. Blood gas measurements determine the degree of oxygen saturation and CO_2 retention. RSV may be demonstrated in the nasopharynx either by culture or by direct immunofluorescence.

DIFFERENTIAL DIAGNOSIS

Do not confuse lower airway obstruction with upper airway obstruction. The clinical picture for each is distinctive (see Table 116-1). The principal differential diagnosis is between bronchiolitis, bronchial asthma, and foreign body aspiration.

TREATMENT

1. Assess the child carefully to determine urgency of immediate care as well as disposition. Respiratory rate, heart rate, and degree of oxygen saturation and CO_2 retention are the key indicators.
2. Monitor all infants younger than 2 months to detect apneic spells.
3. Provide humidified oxygen for infants who are clinically very ill or those who show hypoxia.
4. Give intravenous maintenance fluids to infants who are dehydrated or whose respiratory distress interferes with sucking.
5. The child will often be comfortable in a semi-sitting position with the neck hyperextended to decrease airway resistance.
6. Try a treatment of nebulized albuterol for symptomatic relief; continue these treatments if they help the baby.

537

TABLE 116–1. *Differential Diagnosis of Bronchiolitis*

Pathology	Distinguishing Features
Bronchiolitis	Infant younger than 2 years; low-grade fever, tachypnea, expiratory wheeze, intercostal retractions, other manifestations of viral URI
Bronchial asthma	Family history of allergy, eosinophilia, nasal allergy; response to epinephrine; previous episodes
Foreign body	Sudden onset; afebrile, no sign of viral infection; wheeze, other chest findings, and chest film show lateralized findings
Upper airway obstruction	Stridor; suprasternal retraction; no wheeze, no air-trapping on film

7. Follow all moderately or severely ill children with periodic pulse oximetry.
8. Consider antiviral therapy (nebulized ribavirin) for infants who are positive for RSV *and* are either seriously ill or have an underlying cardiopulmonary disorder.

DISPOSITION

Hospitalize infants younger than 2 months and those who need oxygen or intravenous fluids. Babies who show signs of respiratory failure (PCO_2 of more than 65 torr or exhaustion) should be admitted to intensive care.

Refer mildly ill infants for careful follow-up in the ambulatory setting. These infants need to be seen frequently to determine that they are ventilating and oxygenating safely.

Pneumonia ■

Pneumonia is the infection of a lung or portion of a lung by a microorganism and the resultant tissue response to the infection.

ETIOLOGY AND PATHOPHYSIOLOGY

See Table 116-2. Most childhood pneumonias are of viral, bacterial, or mycoplasmal origin; viral pneumonias are more common in younger children. The viral infection almost always involves some portion of the respiratory mucosa along with the alveoli. Thus, an infant or toddler with viral pneumonia will usually also have some otitis, pharyngitis, or rhinitis. The most common viruses are RSV, parainfluenza viruses, and adenoviruses.

Chlamydial pneumonia occurs in the first 4 months of life and is characterized by lack of fever and a paroxysmal cough.

The most common bacterial pneumonia is due to *Streptococcus pneumoniae*; the most severe bacterial pneumonia is due to *Staphylococcus aureus*. After age 6 years, the most common pneumonia is due to *Mycoplasma*. It is often characterized by familial spread.

Children seldom bring up sputum; therefore, sputum Gram's stains are seldom useful. The nasopharyngeal flora, on the other hand, does not reflect microbiology in the lung.

CLINICAL FINDINGS

1. Fever
2. Cough
3. Tachypnea
4. Dyspnea, dilation of nasal alae, flaring, grunting, and use of accessory muscles of respiration (retracting)
5. Abdominal pain or ileus
6. Radiologic evidence of pneumonia

TREATMENT

1. Give oxygen if hypoxia is present.
2. Begin antimicrobial therapy to cover the most likely bacterial etiology. Children being sent home will need oral medication; those admitted will need early intravenous therapy (see Table 116-3).
3. A child who is having serious difficulty with taking oral medication (vomiting, poor parental compliance) could be treated with ceftriaxone (IM or IV) and seen again in 24 hours.
4. The only specific antiviral therapy is ribavirin for RSV.

DISPOSITION

Hospitalize infants younger than 2–3 months, those who need intravenous fluids, those with hypoxia (pO_2 less than 75 torr), an oxygen gradient of more than 30–35 mm Hg, those who are exhausted, immunocompromised patients (including those with sickle-cell disease), and those with pneumonia in two or more lobes.

Children followed on an ambulatory basis require careful attention and a scheduled follow-up visit.

Empyema ■

Empyema is the collection of pus in the pleural space.

TABLE 116–2. *Etiologic Causes of Pneumonia*

Etiology	Distinguishing Features
Bacterial	
Streptococcus pneumoniae	All ages. Most common bacterial cause. Often lobar. High WBC with left shift
Group B streptococcus	In newborn infants. Overwhelming disease
Chlamydial pneumonia	Infants 2 weeks to 4 months. Afebrile, with paroxysmal cough. Eosinophilia
Haemophilus influenzae type b	Ages 2 months to 4 years. Few distinguishing features
Staphylococcus	Very severe, rapidly progressing; frequent cause of empyema
Mycoplasma pneumoniae	Protracted severe cough, often familial. Affects children older than 8 years
Viral	
Respiratory syncytial virus	Causes bronchiolitis and pneumonia, mostly during first year of life
Parainfluenza	Causes croup and pneumonia
Adenovirus	May cause very severe pneumonia. May be accompanied by conjunctivitis
Influenza A and B	During community epidemics
Granulomatous	
Tuberculosis	Accompanied by hilar adenopathy
Coccidioidomycosis	Geographically distributed
Opportunistic	
Pneumocystis carinii	
Candida	In immunocompromised individuals
Aspergillosis	

ETIOLOGY AND PATHOPHYSIOLOGY

The presence of pus in the pleural space indicates infection with a pyogenic organism; the most common organisms are staphylococci and pneumococci. Early evacuation of the pus through a chest tube and underwater suction will prevent fibrin deposition and future limitation of lung mobility.

CLINICAL FINDINGS

1. Initial diagnosis is made by clinical findings of an area of dullness and absent breath sounds in the chest of a child who has other signs of infection and pneumonia.
2. Obtain radiographs to confirm the clinical findings. An upright and decubitus film may be helpful. Ul-

TABLE 116–3. *Antimicrobial Therapy for Bacterial Pneumonia*

Suspected Pathogen	Antibiotic*
Streptococcus pneumoniae	Penicillin
	Amoxicillin
	Ampicillin
Haemophilus influenzae	Cefuroxime
	Cefaclor
	Augmentin
Staphylococcus	Nafcillin
	Vancomycin
Chlamydia	Erythromycin
Mycoplasma pneumoniae	Erythromycin

* See Chapter 145, Emergency Drugs, for doses.

trasound examination may also confirm the presence of fluid.

3. A diagnostic pleural tap confirms the diagnosis.

TREATMENT

1. Whenever pleural fluid is present, a diagnostic tap is always indicated.
2. Examine the fluid to distinguish a transudate from an exudate (by specific gravity and protein content) and to determine the cellular elements present (lymphocytes, PMNs or abnormal cells). In empyema, the fluid is an exudate, has a specific gravity of 1.015, has a high protein content, and contains more than 20,000 PMN cells/ml.
3. Smear and cultures for infecting microorganisms should also be performed.
4. If staphylococci are found on a smear, a chest tube connected to underwater suction is indicated.
5. If enough fluid is present to cause dyspnea by limiting lung mobility, either repeated therapeutic thoracentesis or a chest tube connected to suction is indicated.
6. Specific antimicrobial management of the patient depends on the etiology of the empyema. Give nafcillin for staphylococcal pneumonia and penicillin for pneumococcal pneumonia.

DISPOSITION

Hospitalize children with acute empyema for intravenous antimicrobial therapy.

Bibliography ■

Conrad DA, Christenson JC, Waner JL, et al: Aerosolized ribavirin in treatment of respiratory syncytial virus infection in infants hospitalized during an epidemic. *Pediatr Infect Dis J* 1989; 8:152–158.

Denny FW, Clyde WA Jr: Acute lower respiratory tract infection in nonhospitalized children. *J Pediatr* 1986; 108: 635–646.

Grossman M, Klein JD, McCarthy PL, et al: Management of presumed bacterial pneumonia in ambulatory children. *Pediatr Infect Dis J* 1984; 3:497.

Hall CB, Hall WJ, Gala C: Long-term prospective study in children after respiratory syncytial virus infections. *J Pediatr* 1984; 105:358–364.

Long SS: Treatment of acute pneumonia in infants and children. *Pediatr Clin North Am* 1983; 30:297–321.

McLaughlin FJ, Goldman DA, Rosenbaum DM, et al: Empyema in children: Clinical course and long-term follow-up. *Pediatrics* 1984; 73:58–593.

Nelson JD: Pleural empyema. *Pediatr Infect Dis J* 1985; 4: 531–532.

Smith JF, Lemen RJ, Taussig LM: Mechanism of viral induced lower airway obstruction. *Pediatr Infect Dis J* 1987; 6: 837–842.

117 Sinusitis and Periorbital Cellulitis

Moses Grossman

Sinusitis ■

Sinusitis is an inflammation, usually due to an infection, of one or more of the paranasal sinuses.

ETIOLOGY AND PATHOGENESIS

Ethmoid and maxillary sinuses are present at birth; the sphenoid and frontal sinuses begin to develop at 5 or 6 years of age but become clinically important mostly after puberty. The sinuses are lined with ciliated columnar epithelium. The cilia normally keep the paranasal sinuses free of bacteria and keep the mucus moving toward the ostia and the nose. Immunoglobins contained in the mucus are also important in keeping the sinuses bacteria-free. Damage to the cilia or the mucus will result in the entrance of bacteria; mucosal swelling obstructing the ostia will further encourage bacterial proliferation and will result in purulent sinusitis. The most common predisposing factors are first, a viral upper respiratory infection and second, respiratory allergy. The bacterial organisms that invade the sinuses are essentially inhabitants of the nasopharynx, flora that are also the common pathogens in otitis media. The most important microorganisms are listed in Table 117-1.

CLINICAL FINDINGS

Younger children with sinusitis typically present with an upper respiratory infection that will not go away, nasal discharge (particularly a purulent discharge), and a persistent cough, especially during the day. The major historical and physical findings of sinusitis are listed in Table 117-2. Pain from sinusitis may be directly over the involved sinus or referred: maxillary sinusitis causes pain of the teeth, cheek, or ear; frontal sinusitis, the forehead; ethmoid sinusitis, the retro-orbital area; sphenoid sinusitis, the parietal or occipital areas.

ANCILLARY FINDINGS

The diagnostic gold standard for sinusitis is the aspiration of pus from a sinus, but this procedure is frightening for children and seldom necessary in this age group. Transillumination of maxillary and frontal sinuses is helpful *only* if normal or completely opacified.

The usual diagnostic approach is radiologic. Finding air-fluid levels, total opacification of sinus cavities, or thickened mucosa suggests the radiologic diagnosis of sinusitis.

Ultrasonographic diagnosis of sinus infections, is not completely established in pediatrics. It is most useful in differentiating mucosal thickening from sinus secretions.

DIAGNOSIS

The diagnosis can be made clinically and confirmed by radiographs or by response to a trial of antimicrobial therapy. Be careful not to overlook an important predisposing condition such as allergy or cystic fibrosis; treatment may need to be directed at the underlying illness as well as the sinusitis.

COMPLICATIONS

Epidural abscess is an infrequent but very serious complication of frontal sinusitis. Periorbital cellulitis may occur by direct extension from the sinuses.

TREATMENT AND DISPOSITION

Sinusitis can be treated on an ambulatory basis, although children with serious complications such as epidural abscess will require hospitalization.

The essence of therapy is the use of suitable antimicrobial agents. Table 117-1 shows the common etiologic microbial agents, and Table 117-3 presents the choice of antimicrobial agents. The duration of

TABLE 117–1. *Bacterial Etiology of Sinusitis*

Haemophilus influenzae*
Streptococcus pneumonia
Branhamella catarrhalis*
Anaerobes†

* 25–35% beta-lactamase-positive
† Found less commonly; usually penicillin sensitive

therapy is 10 to 14 days. Amoxicillin is the least expensive drug and is effective against the common organisms, except beta-lactamase-producing strains of *H. influenzae* and *B. catarrhalis*. Adding a clavulinate salt (Augmentin) enables the amoxicillin to be effective against these strains as well. Trimethoprim-sulfomethoxazole is not effective against group A Streptococci. However, the flora is often polymicrobial and good clinical results can be achieved by treating most (not necessarily all) of the bacteria present. In debilitated or seriously ill patients, aspiration of pus for Gram's stain and culture and for decompression may be indicated.

If allergy is an underlying predisposing factor, address that problem as best as possible to prevent recurrences.

Periorbital and Orbital Cellulitis ■

Periorbital cellulitis, the more common and less serious of these two entities, is an infection and inflammation of the soft tissues lying anterior to the orbital septum.

Orbital cellulitis occurs less commonly and is much more serious. It is an infection and inflammation of the orbit itself (posterior to the orbital septum).

TABLE 117–2. *Clinical Findings in Sinusitis*

Persistent rhinorrhea (particularly longer than 10 days
  and purulent)
Cough (particularly during the day)
Fever
Headache (usually dull, frontal) or sinus pain
Malodorous breath
Periorbital swelling
History of allergies
Posterior pharyngeal pus
Facial tenderness

TABLE 117–3. *Antimicrobial Therapy of Sinusitis*

Drug	mg/kg 24 hr	Doses per day
Amoxicillin	40–50	3–4
Amoxicillin/clavulanate (Augmentin)	40/10	3–4
Cefaclor (Ceclor)	40	3
Erythromycin/sulfisoxazole	50/150	4
Trimethoprim/sulfamethoxazole	8/40	2

PATHOPHYSIOLOGY AND ETIOLOGY

Soft tissues surrounding the eyes are prone to infection, particularly in children. The causes are multiple: proximity of the paranasal sinuses, thinness of the skin around the eyes, and frequency of eye infections all play a role. Additionally, hematogenously disseminated *H. influenzae* type b organisms are prone to infect this space in children younger than 3 or 4 years. A variety of other microorganisms may also be responsible (Table 117-4).

The orbital septum is a very important anatomic marker in these infections. Anterior to the septum there is a lot of loose tissue, a lot of space for edema and distention, and no immediately adjacent vital structures. The orbit itself, on the other hand, is a rigid, non-distensible structure. Pressure from inflammation and edema in the orbit may interfere with venous drainage of the eye itself or may compress and injure the optic nerve; the cavernous sinus is immediately adjacent and also subject to contiguous spread of infection. Orbital compression fractures breaking through the walled paranasal sinuses may

TABLE 117–4. *Microorganisms Causing Periorbital and Orbital Cellulitis Bacteria*

Haemophilus influenzae type b[1,2]
Streptococcus pneumoniae[2]
Staphylococcus aureus[3]
Streptococcus group A[3]
Anaerobes (from paranasal sinuses)[4]
Fungi (such as zygomycetes)[5]

[1] Most common cause of preseptal cellulitis in children
[2] May be associated with hematogenous spread
[3] Tends to be present when the skin is broken (trauma, insect bite)
[4] In orbital (postseptal) cellulitis
[5] In debilitated and diabetic patients

result in orbital sinusitis. Even without a history of trauma there is a strong association between sinusitis and orbital cellulitis. These factors make the infection of this space much more serious, and it is imperative to recognize it and distinguish it from preseptal infections.

CLINICAL FINDINGS

Periorbital cellulitis (preseptal) in young children usually presents with acute unilateral swelling, redness, tenderness, and often a purplish discoloration of the upper and lower eyelids. This may be accompanied by fever, irritability, chemosis, difficulty in opening the eye actively or passively, and a mucopurulent conjunctivitis. The child may appear mildly or profoundly ill. The disease is often disseminated hematogenously; thus, other manifestations of *H. influenzae* type b infection, such as meningitis, may be present.

Orbital cellulitis (postseptal) may have very similar manifestations but in addition there may be proptosis, pain on movement of the eyeball, and decreased mobility of the eyeball; vision may be decreased. It may be difficult to evaluate the eye findings fully because it is often impossible to pry the eyelids open; lid retractors may be necessary. When in doubt, seek an ophthalmology consultation.

ANCILLARY FINDINGS

The white blood cell count is often elevated with a shift to the left. Obtain a blood culture; it is often positive in younger children. Consider whether a lumbar puncture is indicated.

Radiographic examination of the paranasal sinuses may reveal infection or may reveal fractures following trauma. A computed tomography scan of the orbit is enormously helpful when orbital cellulitis (postseptal) is suspected. The scan permits a clear anatomic diagnosis, a determination of the amount of pus and swelling present, and exact delineation of the state of the paranasal sinuses, necessary information before deciding on surgical drainage.

TREATMENT AND DISPOSITION

Both periorbital and orbital cellulitis require urgent treatment.

First, make a working diagnosis of whether the infection is preseptal or postseptal. Hospitalize all children with orbital cellulitis (postseptal) for intravenous antimicrobial therapy. Hospitalize all children with periorbital cellulitis who are moderately or se-

verely ill, and those whose compliance with ambulatory therapy and follow-up cannot be ensured.

Treat all children with periorbital cellulitis with parenteral antimicrobials, at least initially. Treat the ambulatory child with a long-acting third-generation cephalosporin (ceftriaxone 100 mg/kg every 24 hours) until the overall state of the child's infection is assessed (blood culture, neighborhood structures, meningitis) and clear improvement is evident. At that time, the child can be placed on oral antimicrobial therapy (Table 117-3) using the same drugs recommended for sinusitis.

Selection of Antimicrobial Agent

For children younger than 4 years, select intravenous therapy suitable to treat *H. influenzae* type b, including beta-lactamase-producing strains and *Streptococcus pneumoniae*. These agents include third-generation cephalosporins (cefuroxime, ceftriaxone, cefotaxime, and others). For children whose infection was introduced externally (trauma, insect bites), select an agent with good antistaphylococcal potency (*e.g.*, nafcillin, cefazolin). When orbital infection results as a direct extension from paranasal sinusitis, consider covering anaerobic bacteria in addition to the rest of the nasopharyngeal flora (penicillin, clindamycin).

Surgical Consideration

In the case of orbital cellulitis, consult an ophthalmologist and an otolaryngologist. Surgical intervention such as draining an abscess, draining the paranasal sinuses, or decompression of the orbital space is often necessary for optimal results.

CAVEATS

1. Distinguish between preseptal and orbital cellulitis.
2. Watch for other sites of disseminated infection when *H. influenzae* type b is suspected (*e.g.*, meningitis, arthritis).
3. Remember the paranasal sinuses as possible sites of primary infection.
4. Ensure good follow-up.
5. Do not overlook a fungal infection of the orbit (mucormycosis), which presents in debilitated or diabetic patients. Local thrombophlebitis is a frequent clinical manifestation.

Bibliography ■

Barkin RM, Todd JK, Amer J: Periorbital cellulitis in children. *Pediatrics* 1978; 62:290.

Diagnosis and management of sinusitis in children: Proceedings of a closed conference. *Pediatr Infect Dis J* 1985; 4:S49–S81.

Israele V, Nelson JD: Periorbital and orbital cellulitis. *Pediatr Infect Dis J* 1987; 6:404.

Shapiro GG, Furukawa CT, Person WE, et al: Blinded comparison of maxillary sinus radiography and ultrasound for diagnosis of sinusitis. *J Allergy Clin Immunol* 1986; 77:59.

Simon MW, Broughton RA: Orbital cellulitis. *Clin Pediatr* 1985; 24:226.

Wald E: Sinusitis in children. *Pediatr Infect Dis J* 1988; 7: S150.

118 Soft-Tissue Infections

Moses Grossman

The skin is a very important barrier against infection. When it is breeched or disrupted through scratching, insect bites, or minor wounds and abrasions, pathogenic organisms may initiate an infection of the skin or underlying subcutaneous soft tissues and may invade lymphatic channels, causing lymphangitis and lymphadenitis.

Etiology and Pathophysiology ■

The most common bacteria causing these infections are *Staphylococcus aureus* and group A hemolytic *Streptococcus*. These bacteria are either present on the skin, inoculated when the abrasion occurs, or introduced by scratching fingers (*e.g.*, secondarily infected chicken pox). Normal resident flora of the skin (*Staphylococcus epidermidis*, micrococci, *Propionibacterium acnes*) are unlikely to cause infection in a normal host. The clinical response to infection and thus the clinical entity depends on the organism or mixture of organisms inoculated, toxin production, the site involved, and the host defenses.

In children younger than 4 years, *Haemophilus influenzae* type b plays an important role, producing cellulitis predominantly of the face and orbits (see Chapter 117). Impetigo, bullous impetigo, and ecthyma are discussed in Chapter 104.

Specific Conditions ■

ERYSIPELAS

Clinical Findings

Erysipelas is a specific form of superficial cellulitis involving the dermis and only the uppermost layer of subcutaneous tissue. Caused by group A streptococci, it is a very distinctive clinical entity: the skin is edematous, deeply erythematous, and slightly indurated with a sharp, rapidly advancing edge. It is tender to the touch and may have fluid-filled bullae.

The child is often toxic and febrile. Streptococci may be recovered by aspiration from the sharp advancing margin; however, even without Gram's stain or culture the diagnosis can be made clinically.

Treatment

Penicillin is the drug of choice. Initiate antimicrobial therapy parenterally because of the rapid spread of the infection. Hospitalize the very toxic febrile child for intravenous therapy. For most children, give an immediate dose of intramuscular procaine penicillin and then follow with a 10-day outpatient course of oral penicillin. See Chapter 145 for dosing.

FURUNCLES AND CARBUNCLES

Clinical Findings

Both infections are caused by coagulase-positive staphylococci. Furuncles develop around hair follicles and represent very superficial abscesses. Carbuncles are deeper and larger with thick abscess wall formation. They are most common in hairy areas of the body: neck, axillae, perineum, and extremities. The furuncles may spread to other areas of the body. Hematogenous dissemination is unusual but may occur and cause deep tissue abscesses and osteomyelitis. The diagnosis is clinical and can be made by inspection.

Treatment

The principles of treatment are local scrubbing, drainage if necessary, and systemic antistaphylococcal antimicrobials. Treat superficial minor furuncles with warm soaks and mild scrubbing with a washcloth to remove crusts and pus. Apply bacitracin ointment around the furuncle to protect the adjacent skin. Minor furuncles do not require antimicrobial therapy. For a more extensive involvement, prescribe a 7-to-10-day course of oral antistaphylococcal therapy (cloxacillin 50 mg/kg/day PO divided every 6 hr or cephradine/cephalexin 50 mg/kg/day PO divided every 6 hr). Deep carbuncles require incision and drainage in addition to the measures described above.

Recurrent furuncles and carbuncles, particularly when the cycle includes other household members, present a special problem. Refer these children to the primary care provider for careful counseling about sanitary practices. A workup for immunologic or white cell abnormalities may occasionally be indicated, but such abnormalities are seldom found when the infection is limited to the skin.

CELLULITIS

Clinical Findings

Cellulitis is manifested by erythema, edema, tenderness, and warmth. The skin itself is usually free of infection, although the portal of entry may be evident. Fever is often absent. Proximal lymph nodes may be enlarged and tender.

Cellulitis due to *H. influenzae* type b occurs in children younger than 4 years, usually involves some aspect of the face, and often though not always has a violaceous hue. This form of cellulitis is often associated with bacteremia. Consider this pathogen in young children, because diagnosis (including blood cultures) and treatment must be more aggressive (see Chapters 24 and 113).

Cellulitis in older children is most commonly caused by streptococci and coagulase-producing staphylococci, although any organism may produce cellulitis. For that reason, try to obtain bacterial aspirates for Gram's stain and culture from likely sites of entry, particularly in an immunocompromised host (see Chapter 124).

Treatment

The mainstay of therapy is antimicrobial. Indications for hospitalization include toxicity, impaired host defenses, poor family compliance, and inability to bear weight. Initiate empiric antimicrobial therapy intravenously for the child requiring hospitalization, orally for those who can be treated at home. The choice of drugs must include antistreptococcal and antistaphylococcal coverage (nafcillin or cefazolin intravenously, cloxacillin or cephradine/cephalexin orally).

For children younger than 4 years with cellulitis of the face, institute coverage for *H. influenzae* type b including beta-lactamase-producing strains. Initiate treatment intravenously (cefuroxime, cefotaxime, or ceftriaxone) or intramuscularly (ceftriaxone) because of the likelihood of bacteremia. Total duration of antimicrobial therapy for all forms of cellulitis is 10 days. Additional treatment measures may include elevation of the extremity and warm compresses. Occasionally cellulitis culminates in abscess formation, requiring surgical drainage.

NECROTIZING CELLULITIS AND NECROTIZING FASCIITIS

Clinical Findings

These life-threatening infections involve extensive amounts of subcutaneous tissue and fascia in fascial planes. Occasionally muscles may also be involved (pyomyositis). The infection is usually caused by synergistic action of two or more bacteria including an anaerobe (*e.g.*, microaerophilic Streptococcus) and an aerobe (usually *S. aureus* and one of the enteric group of bacterial organisms). Initially, the clinical presentation may be one of ordinary cellulitis, but the child usually becomes systemically very ill and toxic with debility, tachycardia, and fever. The local cellulitis progresses relentlessly with edema and pain. Areas of necrosis appear on the skin; blebs and bullae may present. A thin malodorous discharge may emanate from wounds. The infection progresses rapidly despite parenteral antimicrobial therapy.

Gram's stain of needle aspirate often reveals polymicrobial flora. When the clinical findings are uncertain, a frozen section of biopsied tissue may confirm the diagnosis and guide appropriate treatment.

Treatment

Effective therapy is based on early clinical recognition and early, extensive surgical debridement of infected tissues. Admit the child to the hospital. Reverse fluid and metabolic derangements. Obtain urgent surgical consultation. Start an intravenous infusion and begin broad intravenous antimicrobial therapy including coverage for anaerobes. More specific antimicrobial coverage is determined by cultures taken at surgery.

PYOMYOSITIS

Clinical Findings

Pyomyositis is the presence of pyogenic infection, almost always caused by coagulase-positive Staphylococci, within skeletal muscles. The entity is more common in the tropics and the disease is often referred to as tropical pyomyositis. The most common location is in the thigh, followed by the calf, buttocks, and other locations. Clinically, the child presents with fever and extremity pain. Eventually a mass appears, but it may be difficult to delineate because of its location within deep muscles. Once suspected, confirm the diagnosis by radioscanning with gallium 67 citrate. Needle aspiration will reveal the presence of pus.

Treatment

Surgical incision and drainage is the mainstay of therapy. Antimicrobial therapy with an antistaphylococcal agent is indicated. Start with a few days of intravenous therapy followed by 10 days of oral therapy after incision and drainage.

LYMPHANGITIS AND LYMPHADENITIS

Clinical Findings

Lymphangitis is the infection and inflammation of lymph channels. It is almost always caused by group A streptococci and appears as a red, slightly tender streak extending proximally from the focus of skin infection, usually on an extremity.

Lymphadenitis is infection and inflammation of one or more regional nodes. Almost all infections drain into regional nodes, which are often enlarged and tender. Chapter 36 discusses infection of the cervical nodes; Chapter 37 discusses involvement of preauricular nodes draining the infected eye. Inguinal and axillary lymphadenopathy and lymphadenitis may occur in pyogenic infections of the legs, perineum or rectum, or the upper extremities. Usually the cause of the large tender nodes is apparent clinically. Therapy directed at the primary site of infection will treat the lymph nodes as well. Occasionally, however, the cause of lymphadenopathy is not clear. The differential diagnosis of nonpyogenic regional lymphadenopathy is presented in Table 118-1.

TABLE 118–1. *Differential Diagnosis of Non-Pyogenic Regional Nodes*

Tuberculosis
Atypical mycobacterial infection
Cat-scratch fever
Tularemia
Plague

Treatment

Treat lymphangitis with penicillin. Consider the need for a blood culture; manage the primary infection. Apply warmth and elevate the extremity.

Bibliography ■

Blumer JL et al: Changing therapy for skin and soft tissue infections in children: Have we come full circle? *Pediatr Infect Dis J* 1987; 6:117.

Echeverria P, Vaughn MC: "Tropical pyomyositis": A diagnostic problem in temperature climates. *Am J Dis Child* 1975; 129:856.

Fleisher G, Ludwig S, Campos J: Cellulitis: Bacterial etiology, clinical features and laboratory findings. *J Pediatr* 1980; 97:591.

Ginsburg CM: Management of selected skin and soft tissue infection. *Pediatr Infect Dis J* 1986; 5:735.

Sirihaven S, McCracken GH: Primary suppurative myositis in children. *Am J Dis Child* 1979; 133:263.

Wilson ME, Haltalin KC: Acute necrotizing fasciitis in childhood. *Am J Dis Child* 1973; 125:591.

119 Osteomyelitis

Jay H. Tureen

Osteomyelitis is a pyogenic infection of one or more bony components, including cortical or cancellous bone, the medullary cavity, and the periosteal envelope. It occurs in about one in 5000 children before age 13, is about twice as common in boys, and shows a predilection for long bones, although any bone may be involved. Infection may arise by hematogenous seeding of the bone, by spread from a contiguous focus, or by direct inoculation due to trauma or surgery.

Etiology and Pathophysiology ■

Osteomyelitis most commonly results from microorganisms that lodge in the metaphyseal region of long bones during episodes of bacteremia. This area has increased susceptibility to infection for several reasons. First, it is an area where blood flow tends to be sluggish, due to sharp turns in bone arterioles as they approach the metaphyseal plate and ramify into sinusoids. Second, this region has few local defense mechanisms owing to the absence of fixed macrophages or other scavenger cells. Finally, it is prone to trauma, which appears to predispose to infection.

About 90% of cases of acute, hematogenous osteomyelitis are caused by *Staphylococcus aureus,* with about 5% caused by beta-hemolytic streptococci and the remainder due to other organisms, including pneumococci, *Haemophilus influenzae,* salmonella species, and gram-negative enteric organisms. Neonates have an increased incidence of disease due to Group B beta-hemolytic streptococcus and gram-negative enteric organisms. Individuals with sickling hemoglobinopathies often have infection due to salmonella, and patients with puncture wounds of the foot often develop infection with *Pseudomonas aeruginosa.*

Clinical Findings ■

Systemic complaints include fever, chills, malaise, and toxicity. Local symptoms include loss of function in the involved area, point tenderness, swelling, warmth, decreased range of motion, redness, drainage, and focal induration.

Ancillary Data ■

Diagnosis rests on clinical suspicion with confirmatory radionuclide and radiographic studies. Blood culture or bone aspiration determines etiology. In the emergency setting, only a presumptive bacteriologic diagnosis is possible, with later laboratory confirmation after hospital admission.

ED evaluation for osteomyelitis includes:

1. Blood cultures
2. Plain film radiographs, which reveal varying time-dependent findings:
   a. Soft-tissue swelling (0–3 days)
   b. Obliteration of fat planes (3–7 days)
   c. Periosteal elevation (10–14 days)
   d. Radiolucency (>14 days)
3. Complete blood count with differential (elevated in about one third of cases)
4. Erythrocyte sedimentation rate (ESR) may be normal early, but usually elevated later. ESR is also a useful means of gauging response to therapy.
5. Tc[99] diphosphonate radionuclide scan (rarely performed in the emergency setting)
6. Bone aspiration may be useful for diagnosis upon admission to hospital, or if cultures are negative at 72 hours and response to therapy is poor; also has a role in therapy.

Treatment ■

The mainstay of effective therapy of osteomyelitis is antibiotics that are active against the usual pathogens and that achieve effective concentrations in bone. In general, identification and sensitivity of the pathogen is not available when the disease is suspected.

548

TABLE 119–1. *Empiric Antimicrobial Regimens for Osteomyelitis*

Clinical Setting	Suspected Pathogens	Empiric Antibiotics
Neonates	Group B streptococcus, gram-negative rods	Ampicillin (200 mg/kg/day) **plus** gentamicin (7.5 mg/kg/day)
Toddlers	*Staphylococcus aureus, Haemophilus influenzae*	Nafcillin (100 mg/kg/day) **plus** cefotaxime (100 mg/kg/day)
Older child	*S. aureus* or streptococci	Nafcillin (100 mg/kg/day)
Sickle-cell patient	Salmonella sp. or *S. aureus*	Nafcillin (100 mg/kg/day) **plus** cefotaxime (100 mg/kg/day)

Therefore, administer antibiotics empirically after obtaining cultures. If Gram's stains or results of blood cultures are available, narrow therapy appropriately. Empiric antimicrobial regimens for osteomyelitis are presented in Table 119-1.

Continue empiric therapy until the etiologic diagnosis is determined by culture, at which time therapy can be selective. Surgical drainage has an important role in therapy if clinical response to antibiotics does not occur in the first 3 or 4 days of therapy, or if an abscess is suspected.

Continue antibiotic therapy for 4 to 6 weeks, with the latter portion on an outpatient basis in most cases.

Complications ■

Eighty-five to ninety percent of patients with acute osteomyelitis are completely cured with no residua. Some patients will develop joint deformity, if there is a coexistent septic arthritis or if the blood supply to the growth center is affected. A minority of patients will develop chronic osteomyelitis, which is a lifelong condition in many instances. Factors that predispose to serious complications are age less than 6 months, delay in diagnosis, and involvement of the femur within the hip joint.

Disposition ■

Admit all patients with suspected or known osteomyelitis to the hospital for definitive studies and initiation of therapy.

Bibliography ■

Brook I: Anaerobic osteomyelitis in children. *Pediatr Infect Dis J* 1986; 5:550.

Dich PQ, Nelson JD, Haltalin KC: Osteomyelitis in infants and children: A review of 163 cases. *Am J Dis Child* 1975; 129:1273.

Jackson MA, Nelson JD: Etiology and management of acute suppurative bone and joint infections in pediatric patients. *J Pediatr Orthop* 1982; 2:313.

Jacobs RF, Adelman L, Sack CM: Management of *Pseudomonas* osteochondritis complicating puncture wounds of the foot. *Pediatrics* 1982; 69:432.

Fischer GW, Potich GA, Sullivan DE: Diskitis: A prospective diagnostic analysis. *Pediatrics* 1978; 62:543.

Nade S: Acute hematogenous osteomyelitis in infancy and childhood. *J Bone Joint Surg* 1983; 65:109.

Nelson JD, Bucholz RW, Kusmiesz H: Benefits and risks of sequential parenteral-oral therapy for suppurative bone and joint infections. *J Pediatr Orthop* 1982; 2:255.

Waldvogel FA, Medoff G, Swartz MN: Osteomyelitis: A review of clinical features, therapeutic considerations, and unusual aspects. *N Engl J Med* 1970; 282:198.

Waldvogel FA, Fasey H: Osteomyelitis: The past decade. *N Engl J Med* 1980; 303:360.

120 Septic Arthritis

Jay H. Tureen

Septic arthritis is an acute infectious disorder involving a joint space and synovial membranes. It may be accompanied by systemic complaints of fever and chills and is almost always associated with local symptoms of pain, swelling, erythema, and reduced range of motion of the affected joint. It is an emergency, since failure to diagnose and treat the condition promptly may result in permanent damage to the joint and permanent loss of function.

Etiology and Pathophysiology ■

Joint infection usually occurs through hematogenous seeding, but it may also result from spread from a contiguous focus (osteomyelitis, cellulitis) or by penetrating injury. Etiologic agents show age specificity: *Haemophilus influenzae, Streptococcus pneumoniae,* and *Staphylococcus aureus* are most common in the patient less than 6 years of age and *S. pneumoniae, Neisseria meningitidis,* and *S. aureus* are common in the school-age child. *Neisseria gonorrhoeae* may cause infection in multiple joints in the sexually active patient as part of the arthritis-dermatitis syndrome (see Chapter 121).

There are special clinical situations involving uncommon pathogens. These include the patient with sickling hemoglobinopathy who is predisposed to Salmonella infection, the patient with intravenous drug use who may be infected with *Candida albicans* or *Pseudomonas aeruginosa,* and neonates who may have infection with Group B streptococcus.

Clinical Findings ■

Suspect acute joint infection in any child presenting with fever, malaise, limitation of motion due to pain, unexplained limp, and clinical signs of joint inflammation. These include tenderness, swelling or effusion, erythema, warmth, and diminished range of motion.

Ask about antecedent illness that may be a source of bacteremia, superficial infection of adjacent structures, skin rash or history of sexual activity in the older child, and history of intravenous drug use.

The differential diagnosis includes immunologic disorders (juvenile rheumatoid arthritis, systemic lupus erythematosus, acute rheumatic fever, serum sickness), trauma, or reactive arthritis that may occur as a postinfectious event (toxic synovitis of the hip, rubella or rubella immunization, varicella, salmonella). See Chapter 44 for discussion of these entities.

Ancillary Data ■

Establish a definitive diagnosis of septic arthritis by needle aspiration of the joint, with cytologic and chemical examination of joint fluid, and Gram's stain and culture. Diagnostic yield is approximately 60% and can be increased to about 80% by blood culture. Joint fluid findings in septic arthritis are compared with the other conditions in Table 120-1.

Other laboratory investigations include:

1. Joint fluid obtained in sterile fashion and sent for:
   a. Cell count and differential
   b. Protein, glucose, mucin clot
   c. Gram's stain and culture
2. Complete blood count with differential
3. Erythrocyte sedimentation rate
4. Blood culture
5. Radiographic studies (optional) may yield some information and generally show soft-tissue swelling or effusion (early), or joint space narrowing (late)
6. Radionuclide studies show diffuse uptake, indicative of increased blood flow, but are not specific for infection.

Treatment ■

Antimicrobial therapy is directed against the likely pathogens based on the age of the patient, Gram's

550

TABLE 120–1. *Joint Fluid Findings in Selected Conditions*

Condition	WBC (%PMN)	Appearance	Mucin	GM Stn/Cult.
Normal	<200 (<25)	Clear	Tight	Negative
Septic	>25,000 (>90)	Turbid	Friable	Positive
Immunologic	5000–50,000 (40–75)	Turbid	Friable	Negative
Trauma	<2500 (<25)	Clear or bloody	Tight	Negative
Reactive	<2500 (<25)	Clear	Tight	Negative

TABLE 120–2. *Empiric Therapy of Septic Arthritis*

Age	Suspected Pathogen	Therapy
0–2 mo	Group B streptococcus, gram-negative rods	Ampicillin (100 mg/kg/day) **plus** gentamicin (7.5 mg/kg/day) *or* cefotaxime (100 mg/kg/day)
2 mo–4 yr	*H. influenzae, S. aureus*	Nafcillin (100 mg/kg/day) **plus** cefotaxime (100 mg/kg/day)
>4 yr	*S. aureus*	Nafcillin (100 mg/kg/day)
Hb SS	Salmonella, *S. aureus*	Nafcillin plus cefotaxime

stain, and any significant historical factors. Table 120-2 presents guidelines for therapy. In certain circumstances, surgical drainage must also be performed (hip joint involvement, infection with gram-negative bacilli).

Complications ■

The most common serious complication of septic arthritis is permanent destruction of the articular surfaces, with resultant joint deformity or loss of function. An additional complication is that septic arthritis can serve as a focus for further hematogenous spread of infection to other organs.

Disposition ■

Hospitalize all patients with suspected septic arthritis for parenteral antibiotic therapy. In most cases, the total duration of therapy is 2 to 3 weeks, although the latter portion of this may be on an outpatient basis.

Bibliography ■

Barton LL, Dunkle LM, Habib FH: Septic arthritis in childhood: A 13-year review. *Am J Dis Child* 1987; 141:898.

Garcia-Kutzbach A, Masi AT: Acute infectious agent arthritis (IAA): A detailed comparison of proved gonococcal and other blood-borne bacterial arthritis. *J Rheumatol* 1974; 1:93.

Goldenberg DL, Cohen AS: Acute infectious arthritis: A review of patients with nongonococcal joint infections (with emphasis on therapy and prognosis). *Am J Med* 1976; 60:369.

Lunseth PA, Heiple KG: Prognosis in septic arthritis of the hip in children. *Clin Orthop* 1979; 139:81.

Nelson JD: The bacterial etiology and antibiotic management of septic arthritis in infants and children. *Pediatrics* 1972; 50:437.

Rotbart HA, Glode MP: *Haemophilus influenzae* type b septic arthritis in children: Report of 23 cases. *Pediatrics* 1985; 75:254.

Tetzlaff TR, McCracken GH, Nelson JD: Oral antibiotic therapy for skeletal infections. *J Pediatr* 1978; 92:485.

121 Sexually Transmitted Diseases

Moses Grossman

Of the many diseases transmitted by sexual contact, the most common are gonorrhea, syphilis, herpes type II infection, chlamydial or Ureaplasma (non-gonococcal) urethritis, scabies, lice, chancroid, and lymphogranuloma venereum.

Children of any age may acquire these diseases; the diagnosis should not be ruled out by virtue of age alone. The diagnosis carries greater emotional, legal, and at times criminal impact in the pediatric age group than for adults. The diagnosis should never be made on clinical grounds alone: laboratory confirmation is essential.

Whenever a preadolescent child acquires a sexually transmitted disease, suspect molestation or abuse and report the case to local authorities as required by law (see Chapters 129 and 132). Many state laws allow children 12 years or older to give consent for treatment of sexually transmitted disease. Informing the parents is desirable but is not required by law; in fact, informing parents often requires the youngster's consent.

The diagnosis of one sexually transmitted disease should lead to a search for others. For instance, if a diagnosis of gonorrhea is made, always perform a serologic test for syphilis.

Identify and treat sexual partners.

Gonorrhea ■

The gonococcus is a gram-negative diplococcus best cultured on chocolate agar or special selective (Thayer-Martin) media. Usually the organisms are easily demonstrable on smear; however, they cannot be distinguished from other members of the Neisseria species, and for that reason cultural confirmation is essential. There is no reliable method of serologic diagnosis.

The disease is transmitted by direct contact between mucous membrane surfaces. In the vast majority of cases, the contact is of a sexual nature; other very intimate contacts can also result in infection.

Both men and women are often asymptomatic carriers; this contributes to the enormous prevalence of this disease.

CLINICAL FINDINGS

The clinical spectrum is broad. See Table 121-1.

DIAGNOSIS

In all but polyarthritis and salpingitis, the diagnosis rests on cultural identification of the gonococcus. In these two particular clinical manifestations, the organism may not be recovered in all cases, and a conclusion is based on clinical evidence.

TREATMENT

The great majority of *N. gonorrhoeae* isolates are susceptible to penicillin and amoxicillin. One to two percent of isolates are resistant, either on the basis of production of penicillinase (PPNG strains) or chromosomally mediated resistance (CMRNG). Ceftriaxone, cefotaxime, or spectinomycin are antimicrobials of choice for treating known or suspected resistant strains. The choice of initial therapy depends on local experience as obtained from the local public-health officer.

The drugs of choice for gonococcal infection with a known or suspected penicillin-resistant strain are ceftriaxone or cefotaxime. For children and adolescents allergic to penicillin, use spectinomycin (40 mg/kg; maximum dose 2 g IM). Current treatment recommendations are summarized in Table 121-2.

Pelvic inflammatory disease is discussed in Chapter 107, epididymitis in Chapter 45.

DISPOSITION

Hospitalization with intravenous antimicrobials is indicated for neonatal gonococcal disease, disseminated gonococcemia, the arthritis-dermatitis syndrome, meningitis, and endocarditis. Outpatient therapy as outlined is appropriate for most other presentations. Follow-up and treatment of sexual partners are mandatory.

Syphilis ■

Syphilis is caused by *Treponema pallidum,* a thin, delicate, actively mobile spirochete. There are many clinical presentations of the disease, including congenital as well as acquired infections in the primary, secondary, and tertiary stages. Each of the stages has multiple manifestations. Locating and treating sexual contacts who may have a silent infection is very important.

CLINICAL FINDINGS

The clinical manifestations most likely to present in the ED are the primary- and secondary-stage lesions.

Primary Stage

Classically, the first sign is a chancre, a painless, inflamed, often ulcerated lesion; it may be hidden under the foreskin. All genital lesions are suspicious. The chancre may be atypical. Extragenital lesions are common.

Secondary Stage

The secondary stage presents with a rash that may be macular, papular, follicular, or pustular. Motheaten alopecia, condylomata lata (anogenital), and mucous patches may be present, accompanied by generalized adenopathy and splenomegaly.

DIAGNOSIS

Diagnosis is based on laboratory confirmation of clinical suspicion.

Dark-field examination should be performed on primary or secondary lesions. Moist lesions on the skin or mucous membranes or an aspirate of a regional node should contain demonstrable spirochetes. An alternate method of examination is by immunofluorescence.

Two serologic tests for syphilis are available. The nontreponemal-antigen test in widest use is the Venereal Disease Research Laboratories (VDRL) test.

TABLE 121-1. *Clinical Spectrum of Gonococcal Infections*

Urethritis
Vulvovaginitis
Endocervical
Epididymitis
Rectal
Pharyngeal
Opthalmis
Desseminated
Meningitis
Endocarditis
Pelvic inflammatory disease

This test generally becomes positive 4 to 6 weeks after infection or 1 to 3 weeks after a primary lesion. It is almost always positive during the secondary stage. Unfortunately, false-positive serologic reactions are found in association with many illnesses, including infectious mononucleosis, collagen diseases, drug addiction, and others.

Of the treponemal-antigen tests, the fluorescent antibody absorption test (FTA-ABS) is in widest use at present. Its principal value is in determining whether a positive nontreponemal test indicates the presence of syphilis or is indeed a false positive. The FTA-ABS has very few false-positive reactions. It is almost always positive during the primary and secondary stages of the disease and often remains positive after treatment. Another treponemal antigen test very similar to the FTA-ABS test is the microhemagglutination test for *T. pallidum* (MHA-TP).

The nontreponemal and the FTA-ABS tests need to be interpreted in light of the total clinical picture.

TREATMENT

Penicillin is the antimicrobial drug of choice. Erythromycin is a poor second choice, to be used only if the patient is definitely allergic to penicillin. Treatment for primary or secondary syphilis in the adult is benzathine penicillin G, 2.4 million units (1.2 million units in each buttock) or aqueous procaine penicillin G, 600,000 units daily for 8 days, for a total of 4.8 million units. For patients allergic to penicillin, give oral erythromycin, 2 g daily for 15 days.

Treat adolescents exactly as adults. In younger children, modify the dose depending on weight and age.

Report syphilis to the health department, which will locate, screen, and treat sexual partners.

Secondary syphilis is quite contagious by nonsexual contact. Wear gloves and use caution in examining

TABLE 121-2. *Treatment of Gonococcal Infection in Childhood*

	Penicillin-Sensitive Isolate	Alternative Regimens*
Neonates†		
Ophthalmia neonatorum‡	Pen G 100,000 U/kg/d in divided doses q6h IV × 7d	CFT 50–75 mg/kg/d in divided doses q8 or q12h IV × 7d *or* CTR 125 mg IM × 1
Sepsis, arthritis, abscess	Pen G 100,000 U/kg/d in divided doses q6h IV for ≥ 7d	CFT 100–150 mg/kg/d in divided doses q8 or q12h IV × 10–14d
Meningitis	Pen G 300,000 U/kg/d in divided doses q6h IV for ≥ 10d	CFT 150–200 mg/kg/d in divided doses q6 to q8h IV × 10–14d
Older Children§		
Urethritis, vaginitis, cervicitis, proctitis,‖ pharyngitis,‖	Amoxicillin 50 mg/kg p.o. × 1 (max 3 g) + probenecid 25 mg/kg p.o. × 1 (max 1 g)	CTR 125 mg IM × 1 (250 mg if > 100 lb) *or* Spectinomycin 40 mg/kg IM × 1 (max 2 g)
Conjunctivitis‡	Pen G 75,000–100,000 mg/kg/d (max 10^7 U) in divided doses q6h IV for ≥ 7d	CTR 250–1000 mg IM q.d. × 5d
Sepsis, arthritis	Pen G 150,000–200,000 (max 10^7 U) in divided doses q4h IV × 7d	CTR 50–100 mg/kg/d (max 2 g) in divided doses q8 to q12h IV × 7d *or* CFT 50–100 mg/kg/d (max 2 g) in divided doses q6 to q8h IV × 7d *or* Tet 40 mg/kg/d in divided doses q6h p.o. × 7d*
Meningitis	Pen G 250,000 U/kg/d in divided doses q6h IV × 10–14d	CTR 100 mg/kg/d (max 2 g) in divided doses q8 to q12h IV for ≥ 10d *or* CFT 200 mg/kg/d in divided doses q6h IV for ≥ 10d *or* Chloro 100 mg/kg/d in divided doses q6h IV for ≥ 10d
PID	See Chapter 45	

Abbreviations: Pen G, aqueous penicillin G; CFT, cefotaxime; CTR, ceftriaxone; Tet, tetracycline; Chloro, chloramphenicol; U, units.
* Sensitivity unknown, penicillin allergy, or >1% prevalence of PPNG and/or chromosomally mediated resistance.
† Parents should be cultured and treated.
‡ Accompany with frequent saline eye washes.
§ Children weighing >100 lb (45 kg) should receive the maximum (adult) dose.
‖ Ceftriaxone is drug of choice.
* Tetracycline should not be used in children <8 years old.
(Reproduced with permission from L. E. R. Patterson Gonococcal Infections in Oski F Principles and Practice of Pediatrics J. B. Lippincott Co. Philadelphia 1990.)

these patients. Adequate penicillin therapy usually ends infectivity within 24 hours.

Have patients return at 3, 6, and 12 months for repeated serologic testing.

Examine the cerebrospinal fluid in all patients with congenital syphilis, suspected neurosyphilis, and acquired untreated syphilis of more than a year's duration.

Other Sexually Transmitted Diseases ■

NONGONOCOCCAL URETHRITIS

This clinical entity is usually caused by *Chlamydia trachomatis* or *Ureaplasma urealyticum*. The presentation is one of urethral discharge, either negative for gonococci initially or persisting after treatment for gonococcal infection. Treat with either tetracycline (500 mg PO four times a day for 10 days) or erythromycin (500 mg PO four times a day for 10 days). Examine and treat sexual partners.

VULVOVAGINITIS

See Chapter 107.

SALPINGITIS (PELVIC INFLAMMATORY DISEASE)

See Chapter 107.

CHANCROID

Chancroid (*Haemophilus ducreyi* infection) is an acute, localized, sexually transmitted disease. It is characterized in the male by the initial appearance of a painful soft ulcer with a necrotic base. Subsequently, large, matted, usually unilateral nodes develop, often accompanied by chills and fever. A chancroid skin test may become positive, sometimes for life. Diagnosis depends on cultural isolation of the causative organism. Treat with erythromycin (0.5 g PO four times a day for 10 days); trimethoprim-sulfamethoxazole is equally effective. Treat sexual partners.

LYMPHOGRANULOMA VENEREUM

LGV is an acute, sexually transmitted disease caused by *C. trachomatis,* type L_1-L_3. After a minor, often unnoticed ulcerative or vesicular lesion on the genitalia, massive inguinal lymph nodes appear. They often break down, drain, and heal with scar formation. Rectovaginal fistulas and fissures occur. Systemic symptoms may occur, including fever, arthralgia, skin rash, and conjunctivitis. The diagnosis depends on a combination of clinical findings, a positive complement fixation test, and possibly a positive skin (Frei) test. Tetracycline or erythromycin orally in a full dose for 10 to 20 days is effective early in the disease,

accompanied by local measures to drain, compress, or aspirate the buboes.

ANOGENITAL WARTS (CONDYLOMATA ACUMINATA)

These wartlike papillomas in and around the rectum and vagina are caused by a sexually transmitted human papilloma virus. They must be distinguished from *Condylomata lata,* which are caused by syphilis (serology and dark-field examination). Treatment is difficult because they tend to recur, but consists of either surgical removal or application of 10% to 20% podophyllin in tincture of benzoin or application of liquid nitrogen.

GENITAL HERPES SIMPLEX

An extremely common sexually transmitted infection, genital herpes simplex is manifested by multiple painful blisters around the genitalia, a vaginal discharge, and painful small lymph nodes. A diagnosis is readily made clinically and confirmed by the laboratory (culturing herpes virus or demonstrating its presence by immunofluorescence or the typical histologic appearance). Oral acyclovir (200 mg five times a day for 5–10 days) given within 6 days of onset of the *primary* infection will shorten the duration of that attack. Acyclovir has no role in the acute management of recurrent infection, but a daily dose will prevent recurrences as long as the drug is being administered.

Several other sexually transmitted diseases are discussed elsewhere: see Chapter 125 for HIV infection and Chapter 104 for scabies.

Bibliography ∎

Centers for Disease Control: Antibiotic-resistant strains of *Neisseria gonorrhoeae. MMWR* 1987; 36(supp):15–185.

Centers for Disease Control. Sexually transmitted diseases: Treatment guidelines. *MMWR* 1989; 38(No. S-8):1–43.

Holmes KK, et al: *Sexually Transmitted Diseases.* New York: McGraw-Hill, 1984.

122 Urinary Tract Infection

Moses Grossman

Urinary tract infection (UTI), one of the most common infections of childhood, is the presence of an abnormal number of microorganisms in the urinary tract (bacteriuria) accompanied by an inflammatory response.

Etiology and Pathogenesis ■

The most common microbial pathogen, *Escherichia coli*, accounts for 75% to 80% of UTIs. Other gram-negative organisms are found less frequently.

The most common condition predisposing to UTI is urinary stasis. In young infants this is commonly caused by a congenital anomaly. UTI is much more common in girls; when found in a boy, it suggests a high likelihood of a congenital anomaly. Regard a UTI in a young child as an opportunity to discover and correct an anatomic anomaly before serious kidney damage is incurred.

Bladder infection results in the production of a vesicoureteral reflux that allows the infection to spread to the upper urinary tract and kidney. There is no reliable laboratory method to distinguish between upper and lower UTIs; use clinical guidelines. Infections that clinically seem to be limited to the lower tract only are associated with a 25% incidence of renal scarring, indicating a high incidence of occult upper tract involvement. Thus, cystitis also requires urgent treatment.

Clinical Findings ■

There are three clinical presentations of UTI: afebrile with frequency and urgency and perhaps abdominal pain; febrile with abdominal pain associated with frequency and urgency; and highly febrile with no localizing finding.

In the history, ask about previous UTIs. A complete physical examination is essential because the urinary findings may be the manifestation of systemic disease. Physical findings are used to distinguish upper tract

disease from cystitis. High fever, chills, costovertebral angle (CVA) tenderness, or kidney tenderness in an infant suggest pyelonephritis. Lower abdominal tenderness alone is more consistent with cystitis.

Ancillary Data ■

URINE COLLECTION METHODS

The key to the diagnosis of UTI is the demonstration of bacteria in the urine, but bacteriuria can be accurately interpreted only if the urine has been collected properly. Three collection methods are available: clean-catch urine, bladder puncture, and catheterization. The clean-catch method is the least invasive and the hardest to interpret. If the catch is really clean and the urine is cultured promptly (or refrigerated), 100,000 colonies/ml is considered to be indicative of UTI. Bladder puncture (see Chapter 139 for procedure) is the most reliable method, since urine obtained in this way should be sterile; 15,000 colonies/ml represents bacteriuria. Bladder catheterization using a #5 feeding tube is another good way to obtain a clean specimen.

EXAMINING THE URINE

1. *Microscopic examination* with or without Gram's stain immediately confirms the presence of bacteria. One hundred bacteria per high-power field in spun urine correlates with 100,000 colonies/ml and is indicative of infection.
2. *Culture.* It is useful to culture the urine so that bacteria can be quantitated, identified, and analyzed for antimicrobial sensitivity.
3. *Pyuria.* The presence of more than five white blood cells (WBC) per high-power field is considered pyuria. Normally, many WBCs and clumps of WBCs are seen in UTI, but it is possible to have a UTI without white cells; on the other hand, pyuria may be due to other causes.
4. *Chemical analysis.* Determination of glucose and

TABLE 122–1. *Oral Antimicrobials for the Treatment of UTI*

Antimicrobial Agent	Dose	Doses per 24 hr
Sulfisoxazole	150 mg/kg/d	4
Amoxicillin	30 mg/kg/d	3–4
Cephalexin (Keflex)	25–50 mg/kg/d	4
Cephradine (Velocet)	25–50 mg/kg/d	4
Trimethoprim-sulfamethoxazole	6 mg TMP, 30 mg SMX/kg/d	2

nitrites in the urine (by dipstick) provides a good screening method for the presence of bacteria.

5. *Blood culture.* With children who clinically appear to have pyelonephritis, particularly young infants, obtain a blood culture as well as a urine culture.

Diagnosis ■

Diagnosis is not always straightforward. The presence of classical clinical findings, bacteremia and pus in the urine, is easy to interpret, but the clinical findings may be poorly differentiated; the urine culture may reveal a mixture of organisms or bacteria unusual for UTI (*e.g., Staphylococcus epididymis*). The initial diagnosis is clinical, based mostly on urinary findings but interpreted in the light of how the urine was collected. Follow-up culture results may be confirmatory but may also be useless or confusing. Since the opportunity to make a correct diagnosis is lost once treatment is initiated, examine a second clean-catch specimen or perform a bladder tap in any ambiguous cases.

Treatment ■

Give a suitable antimicrobial agent. In an essentially afebrile patient with cystitis, a single oral antimicrobial agent chosen with convenience and cost in mind will suffice. Table 122-1 presents a choice of such agents. Sulfisoxazole or amoxicillin are best for a first lower tract infection. Recurrent infection may suggest more resistant organisms, and one of the other three antimicrobials listed in the table may be more suitable.

If pyelonephritis is suspected or if the patient is under 6 months of age or very febrile, hospitalize the child and initiate ampicillin and gentamicin parenterally.

Disposition ■

Hospitalize children with pyelonephritis, infants, and highly febrile children. Others can continue therapy as ambulatory patients.

Secure careful follow-up. If symptoms continue after antibiotics are started, the child must be seen in 48 hours to ensure that the urine is sterilized. Normal oral therapy is for 7 days; see the child 3 to 5 days after stopping therapy to be certain that the bacteriuria is controlled.

Refer all boys after the first infection and girls with the second infection for anatomic studies of the urinary collecting system to rule out obstruction. Normally, these studies consist of an ultrasound and a vesicoureteral reflex study.

Recommend a year-long program to check for bacteriuria, either by teaching the family the dipstick nitrite test for home use on an overnight urine sample or by arranging for parents to drop off urine at the laboratory or physician's office every few months.

Bibliography ■

Bauchner H, Phillip B, Dashefsky B: Prevalence of bacteriuria in febrile children. *Pediatr Infect Dis J* 1987; 6: 239–242.

McCracken GM Jr: Diagnosis and management of acute urinary tract infection in infants and children. *Pediatr Infect Dis J* 1987; 6:107–112.

Ogra PL, Faden HS: Urinary tract infection in childhood: An update. *J Pediatr* 1985; 106:1023–1029.

Turck M: Urinary tract infections. *Hosp Pract* 1980; 15:49–58.

123 Other Infections

Moses Grossman

Fever and other signs and symptoms of infection are the most common reasons in childhood for an unscheduled office visit or a trip to the emergency department. The approach to fever in the young child is outlined in Chapter 24. Specific infections affecting various organ systems are described throughout this book (*e.g.*, Chapter 42, earaches; Chapter 46, sore throat; Chapter 37, red eye; Table 104-2 summarizes infections with skin manifestations). This chapter will provide brief synopses of some other important infections of childhood.

Botulism ■

ETIOLOGY

Neurotoxin of *Clostridium botulinum*.

INCUBATION PERIOD

Food botulism: 12 to 26 hours. Other forms: not applicable

CLINICAL FINDINGS

There are three clinical forms. *Infant botulism* is seen in infants younger than 6 months and is characterized by hypotonia (floppy baby), weak cry, constipation, and weakness. *Foodborne botulism* and *wound botulism* are characterized by diplopia, blurred vision, dry mouth, dysphagia, dysphoria, dysarthria followed by general weakness and hypotonia.

DIAGNOSIS

C. botulinum organisms or toxin in feces, toxin in serum, toxin in suspected food. An electromyogram is helpful.

TREATMENT

Hospitalize all patients with known or suspected botulism.

For foodborne and wound botulism, give antitoxin (see Chapter 138). Trivalent equine antitoxin can be obtained from the local or state health department; if unavailable, call the Centers for Disease Control at (404) 329-3755 during business hours and (404) 329-2888 nights and weekends.

For infant botulism, give supportive therapy.

Chicken Pox (Varicella) ■

ETIOLOGY

Varicella-zoster virus.

INCUBATION PERIOD

14 to 16 days; outer limit of 11 to 20 days.

CLINICAL FINDINGS

Fever, generalized pruritic vesicular rash. Virus persists and may produce herpes zoster later in life.

DIAGNOSIS

Clinical. Scraping of lesion can be examined with Tzanck stain; immunofluorescence.

COMMUNICABILITY

Varicella is contagious 1 to 2 days before and 5 days after onset of rash.

COMPLICATIONS

Pneumonia, otitis media. The disease is serious in immunocompromised individuals (see Chapter 124).

PREVENTION

Varicella zoster immune globulin (VZIG) for exposed immunocompromised susceptibles within 72 hours of exposure.

TREATMENT

Acyclovir for immunocompromised individuals (30 mg/kg/day divided into three doses).

Diphtheria ■

ETIOLOGY

Toxigenic strains of *Corynebacterium diphtheriae*.

INCUBATION PERIOD

Two to five days.

CLINICAL FINDINGS

Formation of pseudomembrane over the nasopharynx, uvula, and tonsils that may extend into larynx and cause upper airway obstruction.

DIAGNOSIS

Clinical suspicion initially. Definitive diagnosis by culture (requires special media) and ultimately demonstration of toxin production in cultured organisms.

DIFFERENTIAL DIAGNOSIS

Infectious mononucleosis, streptococcal infection.

COMPLICATIONS

Myocarditis, peripheral neuritis.

TREATMENT

Diphtheria antitoxin (equine) is the principal mode of therapy and arrests further progress of the disease. Give 40,000 to 60,000 units intravenously after appropriate tests for sensitivity. Hospitalize the child with strict isolation precautions. Begin erythromycin therapy to eradicate the organism and prevent further spread. Arrange for suitable care of exposed susceptible individuals.

Kawasaki Disease ■

ETIOLOGY

Unknown; in autoimmune category.

CLINICAL MANIFESTATIONS

Acute illness predominantly of young children. Fever; bulbar conjunctivitis; oral findings (bright-red, dry lips with cracking and edema); enlarged cervical lymph nodes; swelling and induration of hands and feet with red palms and soles and subsequent desquamation of tips of fingers; polymorphous evanescent rash of varying character; thrombocytosis; many other findings in different organ systems.

DIAGNOSIS

Strictly clinical. Major findings must be present. Early diagnosis is important to institute appropriate therapy.

COMPLICATIONS

Carditis, coronary artery aneurysms that may lead to myocardial infarction.

TREATMENT

Aspirin in high doses and intravenous gamma globulin. Obtain consultation, including cardiac consultation.

DISPOSITION

Hospitalize children in the acute stage for intravenous immunoglobulin therapy.

Malaria ■

ETIOLOGY

Four species: *Plasmodium vivax, falciparum, ovale*, and *malariae*.

INCUBATION PERIOD

Incubation period after the mosquito bite is 6 to 16 days. *P. falciparum* can persist 1 to 2 years, *P. vivax* and *P. ovale* up to 4 years, *P. malariae* much longer.

EPIDEMIOLOGY

Essentially all of the malaria cases seen in the United States are acquired abroad. Transmitted by a bite of the anopheles mosquito, malaria is widely distributed throughout the tropics and subtropics.

CLINICAL FINDINGS

Classically, fever, chills, and headache. Chronic malaria: anemia, splenomegaly. *P. falciparum* can cause very severe infection, so-called "cerebral malaria." Encephalopathy, renal and hepatic failure, and death may ensue.

DIAGNOSIS

Stained smear of blood (thick and thin smear) will demonstrate the presence of the parasite. Speciation requires a good stain and experience.

TREATMENT

P. falciparum infection requires emergent treatment. Hospitalize the child. Children with *P. vivax* infection can be treated as ambulatory patients and followed carefully. Mainstay of therapy is chloroquine phosphate, 10 mg base/kg PO (up to 600 mg, the adult dose) followed by 5 mg base/kg 6 hours later; then 5 mg base/kg/day for two days.

Severely ill children with *P. falciparum* infection known or suspected to be chloroquine-resistant require treatment with quinine or quinidine. Obtain appropriate infectious disease consultation; if necessary, consult malaria branch of Centers for Disease Control: daytime (404) 488-4046, nights and weekends (404) 639-2888.

Pertussis ■

ETIOLOGY

Bordetella pertussis.

INCUBATION PERIOD

Seven to ten days.

CLINICAL FINDINGS

Two weeks of catarrhal stage followed by two weeks of paroxysmal cough with or without whooping or vomiting, followed by several weeks of decreasing cough. Lymphocytosis.

DIAGNOSIS

Clinical. Culture of nasopharyngeal swab on special media (Bordet-Gengov). Immunofluorescence is not very reliable.

COMMUNICABILITY

Very communicable, particularly during catarrhal stage.

COMPLICATIONS

Apneic spells especially in young infants; seizures.

TREATMENT

Erythromycin 30 mg/kg/day divided q.i.d. Hospitalize infants younger than 6 months for monitoring. Protect exposed members of household (vaccine, booster dose and erythromycin).

Tetanus ■

ETIOLOGY

Clostridium tetani produces a potent endotoxin responsible for all clinical manifestation.

INCUBATION PERIOD

Three to 21 days (average 8 days).

EPIDEMIOLOGY

Occurs worldwide; organism is widely distributed. Individuals who sustain dirty puncture wounds are at risk. Incidence low in United States because of widespread immunization. Tetanus is not transmissible from person to person.

CLINICAL FINDINGS

Gradual onset progressing to very severe muscle spasms aggravated by external stimuli.

DIAGNOSIS

Clinical. History of wound not always present.

TREATMENT

Hospitalize the patient. Supportive care is of the utmost importance. Give tetanus immune globulin (human) 500 to 3000 units intramuscularly; infiltrate a portion locally around the wound. Give intravenous penicillin. Obtain infectious disease consultation.

PREVENTION

The mainstay of prevention is the primary immunization of all children with tetanus toxoid and booster every 10 years. Table 62-2 deals with tetanus prophylaxis in the course of wound management.

Tuberculosis ■

ETIOLOGY

Mycobacterium tuberculosis (acid-fast organism)

INCUBATION PERIOD

Two to 10 weeks from infection to a positive tuberculin test.

EPIDEMIOLOGY

Very prevalent worldwide. The vast majority of individuals have inactive disease indicated only by the presence of a positive tuberculin test (*reactors*). Those who have become tuberculin-positive within the past year are known as *converters*. The distinction is important, because converters are at significantly greater risk of developing active disease in the near future. Reaction could reactivate their disease with significant deterioration in their cell-mediated immunity (*e.g.*, after developing a malignancy or an HIV infection).

CLINICAL FINDINGS

Reactor. Asymptomatic child whose intradermal tuberculin test (Mantoux) performed with concentration of 5 tuberculin units (TU) shows more than 10 mm of induration.

Converter. Reactor whose tuberculin test became positive within the past 12 months.

Primary tuberculosis: Enlargement of pulmonary hilar nodes. Many children are asymptomatic, but may have a low-grade fever or cough produced by bronchial compression by the nodes. The sedimentation rate is elevated.

Pulmonary tuberculosis: Parenchymal lung involvement produces more of a clinical illness with cough, weight loss, fever, and debility.

DIAGNOSIS

Clinical. Demonstration of acid-fast organism or diagnostic histology of lesion. Chest films may be diagnostic.

COMPLICATIONS

Disseminated tuberculosis: tuberculous meningitis, miliary tuberculosis, visceral involvement other than lungs.

TREATMENT

Treat converters and reactors (after negative chest film) with 9 months of INH therapy, 10 mg/kg once daily up to a total dose of 300 mg. Treat active tuberculosis with two or three antituberculous drugs as clinically indicated. Finding the source of the infection is important to protect others.

124 The Immunocompromised Host

Chandra G. Gordon

The immune system protects the body against alien substances or organisms by means of cellular and humoral components that are activated by foreign antigens. There are three major cellular components (B cells, T cells, and phagocytes) and a variety of humoral components, including antibodies, the complement system, c-reactive protein, inorganic ions, and mediators of the immune response such as interleukins.

A healthy child with an intact immune system may have seven or eight infections each year that are brief in duration and without sequelae. But an immuno-compromised child is susceptible to infections with rare or opportunistic pathogens and to more frequent and more severe infections with common pathogens. This latter infection profile is sufficiently different from that of the immunocompetent child to warrant separate consideration.

An immunodeficient state may result from either acquired or congenital factors. Depending on the specific immune component(s) affected, the nature of and response to infection will vary (Table 124-1).

Etiology and Pathophysiology ■

ACQUIRED CAUSES

Common etiologies of acquired immunocompromise are malignancy, chemical immunosuppression, as-plenia, certain anatomic defects, chronic illness, and certain infections, the most notable of which is AIDS.

Malignancy

Children with lymphoproliferative disorders have a higher rate of infection than do children with solid tumors. This phenomenon is due both to the nature of the malignancy and the aggressive antineoplastic therapy given to patients with leukemia and lymphoma.

All components of the immune system can be affected in malignancy. B cells and T cells are affected by corticosteroids and cytotoxic drugs. T cells are affected in Hodgkin's disease. Phagocytes may be decreased in number and activity in leukemia and lymphoma, when bone marrow is infiltrated by tumor, by cytotoxic agents used in chemotherapy, and by radiation therapy.

The most common presenting symptom of infection in the child with cancer is fever. Agranulocytic patients have fever due to infection four to five times more often than do those who have an adequate neutrophil count. When the granulocyte count is adequate, the infectious agent varies with the type of underlying malignancy. For example, the child with acute lymphocytic leukemia on maintenance chemotherapy tends to develop infections characteristic of T cell dysfunction (*e.g., Pneumocystis carinii* pneumonia), while the patient with acute nonlymphocytic leukemia undergoing induction chemotherapy develops infections related to neutropenia. Once the child becomes granulocytopenic (absolute granulocyte count <500 cells/μL), the infecting organisms to which they are susceptible are the same, regardless of the underlying malignancy.

When the granulocytopenic patient becomes newly febrile, the vast majority of infecting organisms are bacteria. *Streptococcus viridans, Staphylococcus epidermidis, Staphylococcus aureus, Escherichia coli, Klebsiella,* and *Pseudomonas* are common pathogens. Uncommon bacterial agents that are often implicated are *Corynebacterium* species, clostridia, *Bacillus* species, *Enterobacter* species, *Citrobacter* species, nonaeruginosa pseudomonas, *Aeromonas hydrophilia,* and *Acinetobacter.*

Fungal organisms (commonly *Candida* species, *Aspergillus, Mucor, Rhizopus,* and *Torulopsis*) often infect patients with chronic granulocytopenia. Finally,

TABLE 124–1. *Clinical Infections in Immunodeficient States*

Immune Component Affected	Clinical Presentation	Causative Organisms

B cells	Recurrent infections:
	    Dermatitis
	    Otitis media
	    Pneumonia
	    Meningitis
	Chronic infections:
	    Otitis media
	Failure to respond to standard therapy
	Diarrhea
	Failure to thrive
	Eczema
	Arthritis
		Bacterial:
		    Encapsulated organisms:
		        Streptococcus pneumoniae
		        Haemophilus influenzae
		        Neisseria meningitidis
		    Staphylococcus aureus
		    Pseudomonas
		Viral:
		    rotavirus
		Protozoal:
		    Giardia lamblia

T cells	Intractable infections:
	    Thrush
	    Candidal diaper rash
	    Esophagitis
	    Intestinal (diarrhea)
	    Pneumonia
	Failure to thrive
	Prolonged viral infections
	Illness following live virus vaccine
		Bacterial:
		    Intracellular organisms:
		        M. tuberculosis
		        Listeria monocytogenes
		        Nocardia asteroides
		Viral:
		    Cytomegalovirus
		    Varicella zoster
		    Epstein-Barr virus
		    Herpes simplex
		Protozoal:
		    Pneumocystis carinii
		    Toxoplasma
		    Cryptosporidium
		Fungal:
		    Candida
		    Cryptococcus

Phagocytes	Recurrent infections:
	    Dermatitis
	    Lymphadenitis
	    Pneumonitis
	    Osteomyelitis
	    Stomatitis
	    Conjunctivitis
	Abscess formation
	    Cutaneous
	    Hepatic
	    Perianal
		Bacterial:
		    Staphylococcus aureus
		    Serratia marcescens
		    Pseudomonas
		    Klebsiella pneumoniae
		    E. coli
		Fungal:
		    Aspergillis
		    Candida
		    Torulopsis

Complement	Pneumonia
	Meningitis
		Bacterial:
		    Streptococcus pneumoniae
		    Neisseria meningitidis
		    Klebsiella pneumoniae

polymicrobial sepsis occurs often in neutropenic cancer patients.

Chemical Immunosuppression

Corticosteroids and cytotoxic agents cause a multifaceted derangement of immune function. Steroids may inhibit lymphocyte function, deplete lymphatic tissue, depress local inflammatory response, inhibit chemotaxis, interfere with granulocyte function, and rarely cause neutropenia. Cytotoxic agents depress B cell, T cell, and phagocyte function.

Infections are responsible for significant morbidity and mortality in patients receiving immunosuppres-

TABLE 124–2. *Congenital Causes of Immunodeficiency: Suggested Mechanism and Clinical Picture*

Defect	Genetics/Mechanism	Common Infections/ Associated Features	Common Organisms
B Cell Defect (See Table 124-1)			
Transient hypogammaglobulinemia of early childhood	Insufficient synthesis of gamma-globulin until age 20–40 mo	Sinopulmonary: otitis media, meningitis; diarrhea	*S. pneumoniae; H. influenzae; N. meningitidis; S. aureus; G. lamblia*
X-linked agammaglobulinemia	X-linked B-cell defect with absence of antibody and plasma cells	Similar to above	Similar to above
Selective IgA deficiency	Autosomal; dominant or recessive/ decreased serum or secretory IgA	Sinopulmonary infections associated with allergy and autoimmune disease	
T Cell Defect (See Table 124-1)			
Thymic aplasia (DiGeorge syndrome)	Failure of 3rd and 4th branchial pouch; thymus and parathyroid gland are dysplastic T cells deficient and sometimes defective	Associated with hypocalcemia, diaphragmatic hernia, cardiac and brain anomalies	(See Table 124-1) Intracellular bacteria: *M. tuberculosis, Listeria, Nocardia;* Viruses: Cytomegalovirus, measles virus; Protozoans: *P. carinii;* fungi
Combined Cellular Deficiency			
Severe combined immunodeficiency syndrome	Autosomal recessive or X-linked; B-cell and T-cell function is impaired; associated adenosine deaminase or nucleoside phosphorylase deficiency; possible metabolic defect	Pneumonia, thrush, diarrhea, failure to thrive (see Table 124-1)	Organisms common in B-cell and T-cell deficiencies (see Table 124-1)
Wiskott-Aldrich syndrome	X-linked B-cell and T-cell defect	Associated eczema and thrombocytopenia	Bacteria—polysaccharide encapsulated organisms: *S. pneumoniae, H. influenzae, N. meningitidis;* viruses; Protozoans: *P. carinii*
Ataxia-telangiectasia	Autosomal recessive; B-cell and T-cell defect	Sinopulmonary infection causing bronchiectasis associated with cerebellar ataxia in 2nd year of life; telangiectasias, dysarthria, and choreoathetosis occur by the 5th year of life	Saprophytic organisms
Granulocyte Dysfunction			
Chronic granulomatous disease (CGD)	Most commonly X-linked; absent leukocyte glutathione peroxidase; disorder of phagocyte oxidative metabolism with inability to generate hydrogen peroxide—phagocytes ingest but cannot kill certain bacteria; decreased nitroblue tetrazolium dye reduction	Pneumonitis, lymphadenitis, dermatitis, hepatic abscess, osteomyelitis, diarrhea, conjunctivitis, perianal abscess, stomatitis; obstruction of GI and GU systems due to granuloma formation	*S. aureus, Aspergillis, Pseudomonas;* also *Serratia, Nocardia, Clostridium*
Job's syndrome	Molecular basis is not known; elevated serum IgE, defects of T-suppressor cells, poor delayed hypersensitivity, chemotactic defect of neutrophils	Recurrent "cold" abscess formation of skin, subcutaneous tissue, lymph nodes; little surrounding inflammatory response; liver abscess,	*S. aureus, H. influenzae;* also *S. pneumoniae* and enteric gram-negative rods; *Candida*

TABLE 124–2. Congenital Causes of Immunodeficiency: Suggested Mechanism and Clinical Picture (*continued*)

Defect	Genetics/Mechanism	Common Infections/ Associated Features	Common Organisms
		pneumonia, lung abscess, otitis media, chronic nasal discharge, eczematoid rashes, mucocutaneous candidiasis	
Myeloperoxidase deficiency	Complete absence of myeloperoxidase	Recurrent candidal infections	*Candida*
Leukocyte glucose-6-phosphate dehydrogenase deficiency	Leukocytes deficient in NADH and NADPH	Spectrum similar to CGD	Spectrum similar to CGD
Chediak-Higashi syndrome	Autosomal recessive; delayed neutrophil chemotaxis, delayed delivery of lysosomal contents, neutropenia	Recurrent pyogenic infections associated with partial occulocutaneous albinism	Common pyogenic organisms
Congenital neutropenia	Many varieties; may occur with aplastic anemia, agammaglobulinemia, or pancreatic insufficiency; cyclic variety with depression of granulocytes at 3-week intervals	Pyogenic infections	Common pyogenic organisms; occasionally *S. epidermidis, Herrellea, Serratia, Pseudomonas*
Complement Deficiency C3 deficiency	C3 is absent	Severe and recurrent pneumonia and meningitis	*S. pneumoniae, N. meningitidis, Klebsiella*
C8 and C9 deficiency	Terminal portions of C8 and C9 are absent	Recurrent infections with *Neisseria*	*Neisseria*

sive therapy for the management of malignancy (see discussion above), collagen vascular disease, and nephrotic syndrome, and for organ transplantation. *Escherichia coli, Klebsiella, Pseudomonas, Serratia,* and *Proteus* are commonly seen in these patients. *Staphylococcus* and *Streptococcus* are less common but still important agents of disease. Viruses that are implicated include cytomegalovirus, varicella zoster, herpes simplex, Epstein-Barr virus, hepatitis virus, and measles virus. *Candida, Aspergillus,* and other fungal agents are commonly seen in patients with chemically induced immunodeficiency.

Asplenia

Asplenia is seen in cases of surgical splenectomy. Asplenia can also be congenital or the result of sickle-cell disease (splenic atrophy; see Chapter 108). Because the spleen represents a major portion of the reticuloendothelial system, its loss results in diminished phagocytosis and opsonization of antibody.

Streptococcus pneumoniae is the most common cause of infection in the asplenic child. *Neisseria*

meningitidis, Haemophilus influenzae type B, and *Escherichia coli* are also often involved. *Staphylococcus aureus, Klebsiella, Pseudomonas,* and *Salmonella* are less common pathogens.

Selected Anatomic Defects

The skin and mucous membranes are the first line of defense against infection. This barrier is disrupted when a cerebrospinal fluid shunt or central venous catheter is surgically placed. These foreign bodies may in addition serve as a nidus for infection. Infections in patients with a cerebrospinal shunt are commonly caused by *Staphylococcus epidermidis, Staphylococcus aureus,* diphtheroids, and gramnegative bacilli.

In the patient with a central venous catheter, polymicrobial sepsis is frequent. Such multiple infections may involve *Staphylococcus epidermidis, Staphylococcus aureus, Streptococcus, Klebsiella, Escherichia coli, Enterobacter, Pseudomonas, Acenitobacter, Haemophilus influenzae, Candida, Malassezia furfur,* and other organisms.

Chronic Illness

1. *Protein-calorie malnutrition* is associated with decreased T cell function, defective phagocytosis, and decreased serum complement. These children present with pneumonia, urinary tract infections, and diarrhea. They are predisposed to gram-negative bacterial infections, infections with measles virus and herpes simplex, and parasitic infestation.
2. *Cystic fibrosis* predisposes children to *Staphylococcus aureus* lung infections in the first year of life; thereafter, mucoid *Pseudomonas aeruginosa* is most prevalent.
3. *Diabetes mellitus* has been associated with ineffective phagocytosis and opsonization. These patients often present with pyelonephritis and perinephritic abscesses due to *Staphylococcus aureus, Staphylococcus epidermidis, Escherichia coli, Proteus,* clostridia, and actinomycetes. Fungal infections with *Candida, Mucor,* and *Torulopsis* are more common in these children.
4. *Sickle-cell disease:* see above discussion of asplenia and Chapter 108.
5. *Infectious causes of immunodeficiency:* see Chapter 125.

CONGENITAL CAUSES

Congenital causes of immunodeficiency are rare (one per 100,000 children) and are outlined in Table 124-2. The nature of the infection depends on the specific immune component affected (Tables 124-1 and 124-2).

Diagnosis and Treatment ■

The following principles can be applied to the diagnosis and treatment of infections in the immunocompromised child, regardless of the specific immune system defect.

CLINICAL DATA

Obtain a careful history. Reviewing a child's prior infections can help identify a previously undiagnosed immunodeficient state. If the child has a known immunologic defect, elicit details of the child's specific disease process. It is important to identify organisms responsible for prior infections because the patterns of infection in these patients often repeat. Review recent culture results.

Perform a careful, complete physical examination, paying special attention to sites of recent procedures or injury and the systems primarily involved in the child's specific condition. The signs and symptoms of infection are muted in many immunocompromised patients.

ANCILLARY DATA

Obtain appropriate laboratory and other studies. These tests may include a chest x-ray, complete blood count, urinalysis and urine culture, blood cultures from different sites (including central venous catheters), and obtaining tissue and fluid from sites that suggest infection (which may require performing a

TABLE 124–3. *Antibacterial Therapy in Selected Immunodeficient States*

Etiology of Immunologic Defect	Clinical Setting	Initial Antimicrobial Regimen
Malignancy	Granulocytopenic patient with fever	Vancomycin and aminoglycoside and ticarcillin or ceftazidime
Asplenia	Serious infection with high fever, chills, severe headache, drowsiness, stiff neck, or coma	Parenteral high dose of 3rd-generation cephalosporin
	Minor infection with low-grade fever, sore throat, cough, headache, or vomiting	Oral penicillin or ampicillin therapy
Cerebral spinal fluid shunt infection		Vancomycin and aminoglycoside or 3rd-generation cephalosporin
Central venous catheter infection		Vancomycin and aminoglycoside and ticarcillin or ceftazidime; amphotericin B if fungus is suspected
T-cell deficiency	*Pneumocystis carinii* pneumonia (see Chapter 125)	Trimethoprim-sulfamethoxazole

TABLE 124–4. *Additional Treatment Modalities*

Disease Process	Acute Intervention	Delayed Intervention
Abscess formation (*e.g.,* Job's syndrome); perirectal cellulitis and necrotizing enterocolitis (malignancy)	Surgery	
E. coli sepsis; immunoglobulin deficiency; combined immunodeficiency	IV immunoglobulin	
Neutropenia	Granulocyte transfusion	
Varicella zoster; herpes virus	Acyclovir	
Severe combined immunodeficiency syndrome; Wiskott-Aldrich syndrome		Bone-marrow transplant
Chronic granulomatous disease	Granulocyte transfusion	Bone-marrow transplant

lumbar puncture, bronchial lavage, or biopsy). Notify the laboratory that the patient is immunocompromised. No organism isolated in the laboratory can be discounted as a contaminant without careful correlation with the clinical picture.

TREATMENT

Institute antimicrobial therapy immediately if an infectious agent is suspected. Infection can disseminate quickly in these children, with significant morbidity and mortality. Use antimicrobials that are broad in spectrum, synergistic, and bactericidal. As a guide for initial treatment, consider the organisms most often responsible for infection in the disease process (see Table 124-3).

Tailor the antimicrobial therapy according to the Gram's stain and culture results when they are available. If possible, select the antimicrobial(s) with the narrowest spectrum to avoid toxicity and the risk of superinfection. Polymicrobial and sequential infections are common in these patients, and the duration

TABLE 124–5. *Preventive Measures for Selected Immunodeficiency States*

Mechanism of Intervention	Specific Intervention	Disease Entity in Which Benefit Has Been Demonstrated
Enhancement of host defenses	Pneumococcal vaccine	Hodgkin's disease; asplenia; sickle-cell disease; complement deficiency
	Meningococcal vaccine	Asplenia; complement deficiency; Hodgkin's disease
	Haemophilus influenzae vaccine	Asplenia; sickle-cell disease
Reduction of colonization	Isolation; hand washing	Granulocytopenia
Suppression of potentially pathogenic organisms	Trimethoprim-sulfamethoxazole	Malignancy; chemical immunosuppression; transplantation; chronic granulomatous disease; severe combined immunodeficiency
	Acyclovir	Transplantation
	Penicillin	Sickle-cell disease to age 5 years; asplenia (controversial)
Education	Early intervention	Generally applicable
	Avoid live virus vaccine	T-cell deficiency, in particular
	Avoid exposure to varicella	T-cell deficiency

of therapy will often be longer than that required in immunocompetent hosts. In certain disease processes, additional treatment modalities may be indicated (Table 124-4).

Disposition ■

Institute immediate parenteral antimicrobial therapy and hospitalize any immunocompromised patient who shows evidence of a severe infection (*i.e.*, high fever, chills, severe headache, stiff neck, or a change in level of consciousness). Most of these patients have a physician who is familiar with the details of their condition; notify the treating physician to ensure continuity of care and appropriate follow-up.

Preventive Measures ■

Prophylaxis plays an important role in reducing the morbidity and mortality of infection in some of the immunodeficient conditions (Table 124-5).

Bibliography ■

Albano EA, Pizzo PA: Infectious complications in childhood acute leukemias. *Pediatr Clin North Am* 1988; 35:873–901.

Decker MD, Edwards KM: Central venous catheter infections. *Pediatr Clin North Am* 1988; 35:579–612.

Feigin RD, Matson DO: The compromised host. In: *Textbook of Pediatric Infectious Diseases,* 2nd ed. Philadelphia: WB Saunders, 1987, pp 1008–1043.

Frommell GT, Todd JK: Polymicrobial bacteremia in pediatric patients. *Am J Dis Child* 1984; 138:266–269.

Hughes WT: Infection of the immunosuppressed host. In AM Rudolph, JIE Hoffman (eds): *Pediatrics,* 18th ed. Los Altos: Appleton & Lange, 1987, pp 473–475.

Kinney TR, Ware R: Advances in the management of sickle cell disease. *Pediatr Consult* 1988; 7:1–7.

Pachman LM, Lynch PA, Silver RK, et al: Primary immunodeficiency disease in children: An update. *Curr Prob Pediatr* 1989; 16:1–64.

Wara DW, Ammann AJ: Immunologic disorders. In: AM Rudolph, JIE Hoffman (eds): *Pediatrics,* 18th ed. Los Altos: Appleton & Lange, 1987, pp 387–410.

125 HIV Infection

Peggy S. Weintrub

Acquired immunodeficiency syndrome (AIDS) is a growing problem in the pediatric population. Many HIV-infected children are asymptomatic, have only mild symptoms, or have AIDS-related complex (ARC).

About 80% of infected children acquire the virus perinatally from an infected mother. Blood transfusions (between 1978 and 1985) and factor concentrates are responsible for most of the remaining cases. In a small percentage of pediatric cases, the mode of transmission is sexual, drug related, or unknown because an adequate history is not available. In instances of perinatal transmission, the most common risk factors or behaviors in the mother are intravenous drug use or heterosexual contact with a bisexual or drug-using partner; drug use in either parent accounts for more than 70% of perinatal transmission. Perinatal AIDS occurs more commonly in blacks (about 60% of cases) and Hispanics (25%).

Etiology and Pathophysiology ■

Human immunodeficiency virus (HIV) is the causative agent of AIDS. Laboratory investigations of these children have shown a variety of defects, which vary depending on the stage of the child's infection (*i.e.,* asymptomatic, ARC, or AIDS). Both B- and T-cell abnormalities have been described and may correlate with the spectrum of clinical manifestations.

Some HIV-infected children have an absolute lymphopenia ($\leq 1200/\mu L$); others, despite clinical evidence of severe T-cell dysfunction, have normal numbers of lymphocytes, lymphocyte subclasses and normal nonspecific mitogen responses. Opportunistic infections can occur in children who have normal laboratory values.

Evidence of B-cell dysfunction, manifested by recurrent bacterial infections, is very common in infected children. Although these children often have hypergammaglobulinemia, they do not make adequate amounts of specific antibody. Therefore, an HIV-infected child may have normal or elevated quantitative immunoglobulin levels, yet fail to make an adequate primary or secondary response to encapsulated organisms. This leads to an increase in the number and severity of what are usually considered common infections in childhood.

Clinical Findings ■

Children with HIV infection present to the ED with a wide spectrum of initial presentations and associated complications. Many who live in chaotic social environments use the ED as their primary source of medical care. Table 125-1 indicates the most common presentations of HIV infection in children.

The typical case of pediatric HIV infection is a child born to a mother at risk who develops recurrent bacterial infections, thrush, failure to thrive, lymphadenopathy, and hepatosplenomegaly in the first few years of life. However, both those who acquire HIV perinatally and those who acquire infection by transfusion may not present with symptoms until several years of age.

BACTERIAL INFECTIONS

The types of infections are similar to those in patients with hypogammaglobulinemia. Infections with the encapsulated organisms, *Haemophilus influenzae* type B, *Streptococcus pneumoniae,* and enteric gram-negative rods are common and can cause chronic or recurrent otitis media, pneumonia, lymphadenitis, bacteremia, mastoiditis, and meningitis. Malignant external otitis, a disease usually seen in older patients, also occurs. Other common conditions include dermatitis, particularly eczema; in those patients *Staphylococcus aureus* is also an important pathogen. Salmonella infections can be quite severe and may cause prolonged gastroenteritis or bacteremia; frequent relapses may occur.

TABLE 125–1. *Common Clinical Manifestations of Pediatric HIV Infections*

Recurrent Bacterial Infections
  S. pneumoniae
  H. influenzae
  S. aureus
  Enteric gram-negative rods

Pneumonitis
   LIP
   PCP
  Oral thrush
  Diarrhea
  Lymphadenopathy
  Hepatosplenomegaly
  Failure to thrive
  Developmental delay
  Encephalopathy
  Parotitis
  Thrombocytopenia
  Severe herpesvirus infections
  Chronic herpes simplex (disseminated varicella zoster)

RESPIRATORY INFECTIONS

Pulmonary infection is a common and serious manifestation of HIV infection. The most commonly diagnosed infection is *Pneumocystis carinii* pneumonia (PCP), which can present acutely with respiratory distress or with a history of progressive cough and respiratory symptoms over days to weeks. Clinically, it may be difficult to distinguish PCP from more typical causes of childhood pneumonia. The chest x-ray typically shows a diffuse interstitial pneumonitis, although almost every pattern of infiltrate has been seen with PCP.

A second common pneumonitis is lymphoid interstitial pneumonitis (LIP); the cause is unknown. Children with LIP often have a longstanding history of pulmonary symptoms, particularly cough. They are usually not febrile or acutely dyspneic, and rarely have significant auscultatory findings. A concomitant infection can cause a child with pre-existing LIP to present acutely. LIP is most often seen in children with other lymphoproliferative manifestations of HIV such as lymphadenopathy and parotitis; these patients may have signs of chronic pulmonary disease such as clubbing. The chest x-ray shows a diffuse interstitial infiltrate similar to that seen with PCP, but in some longstanding cases there may be a diffuse nodular pattern with widening of the superior mediastinum and hilum. LIP is currently a diagnosis of exclusion.

In addition to PCP and LIP, other routine and opportunistic infections must be considered in an HIV-infected child with respiratory distress. Bacterial pathogens are frequent. Another common pathogen is respiratory syncytial virus (RSV), an extremely common viral infection in young infants and children, which can cause giant cell pneumonia in the compromised host. Cytomegalovirus can be cultured from the lung in these patients, although it is not always clear that it is the primary pathogen. Other opportunistic pulmonary infections are also in the differential diagnosis, including atypical mycobacteria and fungi.

CENTRAL NERVOUS SYSTEM DISORDERS

CNS disorders are a prominent part of the clinical spectrum of HIV infection in children. Encephalopathy, either static or progressive, is often noted. Manifestations often include acquired microcephaly, progressive motor dysfunction, loss of developmental milestones, ataxia, and extrapyramidal rigidity. Isolated seizures are unusual but may occur with a concomitant febrile illness. Focal neurologic signs are uncommon in pediatric AIDS and should suggest possible CNS lymphoma. Opportunistic infections, particularly cryptococcal meningitis, may be present in the child with CNS symptoms. However, in most series of children dying with HIV encephalopathy, opportunistic infection of the CNS is rare, and most signs and symptoms are secondary to HIV infection of the nervous system.

GASTROINTESTINAL ILLNESS

GI illnesses, especially diarrhea, are a major problem for HIV-infected patients. Salmonella can be a persistent problem, particularly in patients with blood or mucus in the stool. Severe or prolonged diarrhea in pediatric AIDS patients also occurs with parasitic enteric pathogens, most notably *Giardia lamblia,* and cryptosporidium. In some instances, even after extensive evaluation, no specific etiology can be found to account for the diarrhea.

OTHER ENTITIES

Many of the usual childhood infections are seen in HIV-infected patients, but they may present in a more severe form. Oral candidiasis (thrush) is extremely common, particularly in infancy. HIV-infected patients often have extensive thrush, in the absence of previous antibiotic therapy. Infection may extend to the esophagus or the larynx and is resistant to the usual forms of therapy. Viral diseases such as herpes simplex, varicella, and measles can be quite aggressive in HIV-infected children. Herpes simplex may cause prolonged or recurrent ulcerations and varicella may disseminate to cause pneumonia, encephalitis, or hepatitis. Measles can also cause a severe pneumonia; the first measles deaths in the United States in several years have recently occurred in HIV-infected children.

A unique feature in pediatric HIV infection is the development of parotitis. This can be chronic, with slow, progressive, painless growth, or it can be acute, associated with rapid enlargement, fever, and pain. The etiology is unknown.

A number of other entities described in pediatric HIV infection are also important to recognize. These include a nonspecific hepatitis, cardiomyopathy, and the nephrotic syndrome.

Hematologic syndromes are also well described; thrombocytopenia is the most common, but anemia, secondary to hemolysis, and neutropenia can be seen.

Clinical Evaluation and Ancillary Data ■

Use an aggressive diagnostic approach, because many of the acute illnesses are treatable. For example, a child with HIV infection who presents with fever is quite likely to have a bacterial infection; obtain a complete blood count (CBC), blood culture, urinalysis, and chest x-ray if there is no obvious source of fever on examination. Other imaging studies such as sinus films may be indicated. If the child has a history of neutropenia or is receiving azidothymidine (AZT), the absolute neutrophil count may be depressed, which would influence therapeutic decisions.

The new onset of pulmonary symptoms requires a thorough evaluation. Although many of these patients may not have an easily treated form of pulmonary disease, early therapy is important. Because it is difficult to clinically differentiate the common forms of pneumonia in pediatric AIDS patients, hospitalization is often required. In such patients, the initial diagnostic tests include chest x-ray, CBC, blood culture, and, in the appropriate epidemiologic setting, nasopharyngeal swabs for immunofluorescence or culture.

Weight loss and diarrhea may be acute or chronic and are often quite severe. In addition to routine bacterial culture, obtain stool for ova and parasites. Assess the patient's state of hydration clinically and measure serum electrolytes, blood urea nitrogen, and creatinine, since enormous fluid losses and profound electrolyte imbalances are sometimes present.

CNS symptoms and physical signs will determine whether lumbar puncture or scanning is appropriate. If a spinal tap is performed, obtain more fluid than necessary to diagnose bacterial meningitis, because additional tests are often indicated, such as a culture for acid-fast organisms, viral culture, and cryptococcal antigen. If focal neurologic signs are present, arrange for a CT scan to evaluate for lymphoma or toxoplasmosis.

Treatment and Disposition ■

The treatment plan and the decision to hospitalize the patient must be made in conjunction with the family; many families want aggressive diagnostic and therapeutic plans, while others may prefer to keep medical intervention limited, with the goal of making the patient comfortable.

Consider hospitalizing HIV-infected patients with fever without a focus of infection, recent onset of pulmonary or CNS manifestations, or severe failure to thrive or diarrheal disease.

Patients who are not acutely ill and do not require hospitalization may require antibiotic therapy. If a focal infection is identified, such a sinusitis or otitis media, and there is no evidence of bacteremia, the patient can ordinarily be managed as an outpatient. However, a longer duration of therapy is required; for example, treat sinusitis for a minimum of 3 weeks.

In cases of possible bacteremia, the antimicrobials must be effective against the encapsulated organisms and the enteric gram-negative rods.

For any HIV-infected patient who does not require hospitalization, arrange for the necessary follow-up of the acute problem with the primary physician and make appropriate referrals for long-term management. Because of the chronic and complex nature of pediatric HIV infection, non-urgent problems are best handled in the calmer, more familiar outpatient office or clinic, not the ED.

Caveats ■

Many of the HIV-infected patients who present for care in the ED are not identified by the caretaker as seropositive. In a large proportion of pediatric AIDS cases, the child is the index case in the family, and the mother or caretaker may not even be aware that the child is at risk.

Thus, the emergency physician must have an increased index of suspicion. There is no way to identify all infected children in the acute setting, but a history of transfusion, parental drug use, or paternal bisexuality must always raise the possibility of HIV infection. In addition, consider HIV infection in unknown patients from a high-risk geographic area, for children with severe failure to thrive, developmental delay, unusual or recurrent infections, or those with unexplained lymphadenopathy or hepatosplenomegaly on physical examination.

A history in the ED may reveal that an infant is HIV antibody-positive or seropositive, and yet the child may or may not be truly infected. All the current HIV assays use IgG anti-HIV; therefore, antibody that has previously been detected in an infant may represent transplacental passage of maternal antibody. Until better methods are devised to accurately assess which of these infants are HIV-infected, proceed with the evaluation and therapy as if the child were immunodeficient.

Bibliography ■

Bernstein LJ, Krieger BZ, Novick B, et al: Bacterial infection in the acquired immunodeficiency syndrome of children. *Pediatr Infect Dis J* 1985; 4:472.

Ellaurie M, Burns ER, Bernstein LJ, et al: Thrombocytopenia and immunodeficiency virus in children. *Pediatrics* 1988; 82;905.

Epstein LG, Sharer LR, Oleske JM, et al: Neurologic manifestations of human immunodeficiency virus infection in children. *Pediatrics* 1986; 78:678.

Falloon J, Eddy J, Weiner L, Pizzo PA: Human immunodeficiency virus infection in children. *J Pediatr* 1989; 114:1.

Rubinstein A, Morecki R, Silverman B, et al: Pulmonary disease in children with the acquired immune deficiency syndrome and AIDS-related complex. *J Pediatr* 1986; 108:498.

Task Force on Pediatric AIDS: Perinatal human immunodeficiency virus infection. *Pediatrics* 1988; 82:941.

Weintrub PS, Scott GB: Pediatric human immunodeficiency infection. In: Leoung GS, Mills J, eds: *Opportunistic Infection in Patients with the Acquired Immunodeficiency Syndrome.* Marcel Dekker, 1989 (pp 153–168).

XII

Psychosocial Emergencies

126 Sudden Infant Death Syndrome

Carol D. Berkowitz

The sudden and unexpected death of a previously well infant is a tragic occurrence that has been reported since Biblical times. Sudden infant death syndrome (SIDS) or crib or cot death is defined as the sudden death of any infant or young child that is unexpected by history and for which a post-mortem examination fails to demonstrate an adequate cause. Often the emergency physician is most able to assist the victim and the parents and relatives. The physician may be able to resuscitate a potential SIDS victim, but if the attempt fails he or she may be able to allay overwhelming parental guilt and guide the early grief reaction.

Epidemiology ■

About 10,000 infants die annually from SIDS. Overall, the disorder affects two infants per 1000 live births, but there is wide variation among ethnic groups, from 0.51 infants per 1000 among Asian-Americans to 5.93 infants per 1000 among Native Americans.

The disorder is rare during the first month of life, although the reason for this is unknown. Most affected infants are between 1 month and 1 year, and SIDS is the leading cause of death in this age group. The peak incidence occurs between 2 and 3 months of age.

A number of epidemiologic risk factors have been identified, including genetic components; prenatal, maternal, and socioeconomic factors; and antecedent infections (Table 126-1). Information about these components assists the physician in counseling the family about other offspring or future pregnancies.

Etiology and Pathophysiology ■

The precise etiology of SIDS has not been determined. Most of the information about the patho-physiology of SIDS comes from autopsy data on victims and from clinical studies on infants who were successfully resuscitated from an apparent life-threatening event (ALTE; formerly called "near-miss" SIDS). Autopsy data reveal changes in multiple organ systems consistent with longstanding hypoxemia. Pulmonary edema and intrathoracic petechiae are associated with hypoxemia at the time of death.

Apnea and abnormalities of ventilation have been implicated in many cases of SIDS, and disorders producing apnea are part of the differential diagnosis in ALTE. Apnea, defined as the transient absence of ventilation of all or part of the alveolar bed, may be of three types: inspiratory apnea; partial or complete airway obstruction (obstructive apnea); or prolonged expiratory apnea. The latter is associated with the rapid onset of cyanosis, and severe hypoxemia, probably related to ventilation-perfusion inequalities. Expiratory apnea, the most common cause of infantile apnea, appears to be the mechanism of death in a significant number of cases of SIDS. Chapter 18 presents a detailed discussion of infantile apnea.

Cardiac arrhythmias are a terminal event following the ventilatory abnormalities and are *not* a primary cause of SIDS. Prolonged QT interval or Wolff-Parkinson-White are rarely reported in infants presenting with an ALTE.

Gastroesophageal reflux has been noted in some infants with an ALTE, but the association is likely to be coincidental rather than causal. Infantile botulism has been reported to be associated with SIDS in about 5% of cases.

Occasionally, parental actions directly contribute to the death of the child. There are about 2000 cases of death from recognized child abuse annually in the United States. Studies using videotape recordings have documented parental smothering as a key factor in the ALTE of some infants. The presence of other signs of trauma, such as fractures, bruises, or failure to thrive, should raise the index of suspicion about the possibility of abuse in a SIDS or ALTE victim (See Chapter 128).

Clinical Findings ■

Infants who have experienced an ALTE may present to the ED with a wide range of symptoms. Some infants appear completely well, and the only evidence of an ALTE is the parents' history that the child stopped breathing momentarily. Other infants may be carried in the arms of a paramedic who is actively administering cardiopulmonary resuscitation. Both these infants require a careful and complete assessment. Administer vigorous CPR to every infant unless signs of irreversible death are present (see Chapter 6).

Obtain a complete history of the ALTE, including any interventions. In general, infants who display pallor or cyanosis, or who have required CPR or vigorous stimulation, most likely have experienced an ALTE. Other infants, particularly those who are completely well at the time of presentation, may have manifested normal behavior (*e.g.*, periodic breathing or Valsalva's maneuver) that was misinterpreted. A past medical history, paying specific attention to the birth history, family history (particularly of other infant deaths), and the epidemiologic factors associated with SIDS is essential. All infants require a complete physical assessment.

Ancillary Data ■

The appropriate laboratory evaluation includes a complete blood count, serum electrolytes, calcium, magnesium and phosphates, 12-lead electrocardiogram, chest x-ray, and evaluation for sepsis (blood culture and lumbar puncture). Other tests might include an electroencephalogram if it appears the infant had a seizure, or a barium swallow if gastroesophageal reflux is suspected.

Treatment ■

See Figure 126-1. In the ED, initial treatment consists of standard resuscitation (Chapter 6) for the child in arrest, or appropriate advanced life support for selected organ dysfunction. Usually, ALTE is a diagnosis of exclusion and may be difficult to establish in the ED.

Long-term management of an infant who has experienced an ALTE is directed at preventing further episodes that may lead to death. Patients who might benefit from therapy are identified after inpatient workup; such infants are often treated with xanthine derivatives such as theophylline (6 mg/kg/day) or caffeine (5–7.5 mg/kg/day). These medications may

TABLE 126–1. *Identified Risk Factors for SIDS*

Familial or Genetic
  Siblings of SIDS victim
  Twin of SIDS victim

Maternal
  Lower socioeconomic class
  Lack of prenatal care
  Single mother
  Maternal youth
  Maternal substance abuse

Neonatal
  Prematurity
  Respiratory distress syndrome
  Bronchopulmonary dysplasia

Postnatal
  Antecedent infection
  Respiratory syncytial virus
  Pertussis

have a beneficial effect in treating apnea of prematurity because they exert an excitatory effect centrally, but their role in preventing SIDS in a term infant with an ALTE is unproven.

Home monitoring for apnea or bradycardia is almost universally recommended, although there is some controversy on the benefits of such a policy. In 1986, the NIH Consensus Statement recommended home monitoring for term infants with apnea, an ALTE, or abnormal pneumocardiogram, preterm infants with apnea beyond 40 weeks postconception, and siblings in families where two or more previous siblings had died of SIDS. Home monitoring is initiated and supervised by the primary physician, however, never by the ED. All parents must receive appropriate CPR training and must have access to a support team that is available 24 hours a day. Monitoring is generally continued until at least 2 or 3 months pass without any ventilatory problems.

Home monitoring is not a guarantee that an infant will not succumb to SIDS: reports indicate that even with monitoring, 50% of such infants will die.

Disposition ■

See Figure 126-1. In general, admit all infants with a history of an ALTE, or new-onset apnea to the hospital. Evaluate the infant for the presence of ventilatory abnormalities with pneumocardiograms and polysomnography; the latter detects the presence of obstructive apnea. Certain centers may be equipped to obtain more elaborate studies such as ventilatory response to elevated CO_2 or diminished O_2.

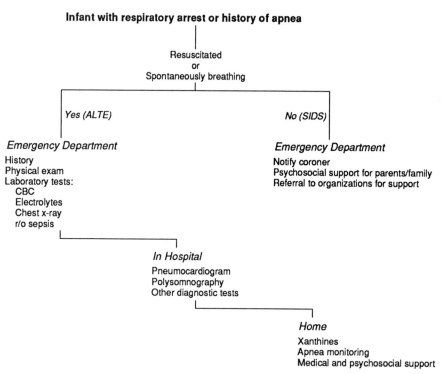

Infant with respiratory arrest or history of apnea

Resuscitated
or
Spontaneously breathing

Yes (ALTE)   *No (SIDS)*

Emergency Department
History
Physical exam
Laboratory tests:
  CBC
  Electrolytes
  Chest x-ray
  r/o sepsis

Emergency Department
Notify coroner
Psychosocial support for parents/family
Referral to organizations for support

In Hospital
Pneumocardiogram
Polysomnography
Other diagnostic tests

Home
Xanthines
Apnea monitoring
Medical and psychosocial support

FIGURE 126–1. Management algorithm: the infant with SIDS or ALTE.

Families of a child with an ALTE require intensive support. They live with the fear that their child may suddenly die and are often unwilling to leave their child in the care of another. Often they are troubled by frequent false alarms on the apnea monitor and sometimes feel compelled to seek medical advice about the significance of these alarms. The emergency physician is expected to differentiate a true from a false alarm. An infant who has required stimulation or resuscitation probably experienced a more serious episode. Refer equipment malfunction to the monitoring company.

One of the greatest challenges facing the physician is counseling the dead infant's family. Often the family is overwhelmed with a sense of guilt that they were in some way responsible for the death. Often, the mother is the last person to see the infant alive: in many cases, she gave the infant a nighttime feeding and, when she checks on him in the morning, she finds him still and lifeless. Invariably there is self-recrimination for not having checked on the baby in the interim. Also take into account the effect of the infant's death on other siblings (see Chapter 127).

In most jurisdictions, SIDS cases must be referred to the coroner's office for an autopsy, but the physician should advise the family of his or her impression that death was secondary to SIDS or, in lay terms, crib death. Complete a death certificate with this diagnosis as the initial impression pending autopsy confirmation. The physician must remain in contact with the family and facilitate their obtaining the results of the post-mortem examination.

Often there is a tendency to encourage a couple to have a replacement child. Sometimes this is more acceptable to the father. Mothers, on the other hand, may need to go through a full period of grieving for the lost infant before they are emotionally able to parent a new offspring. Sometimes they experience difficulty becoming pregnant or suffer a miscarriage. If a couple decides to have a subsequent child, they may fear that the new baby will meet a similar fate; reassure them that SIDS is not a hereditary disease. If one out of 350 infants dies of SIDS, 349 do not.

Several agencies offer support to parents of children who died of SIDS. These agencies have chapters on the national and local levels. Information can be obtained by writing the Council of Guilds for Infant Survival, 510 Fifth Street NW, Washington DC 20001, or the National Foundation for Sudden Infant Death, 101 Broadway, New York, NY 10036. Pamphlets on SIDS are available for distribution by the emergency physician.

Bibliography ■

Bass M, Kravath RE, Glass L: Death-scene investigation in sudden infant death. *N Engl J Med* 1986; 315:100.

Dunne K, Matthews T: Near-miss sudden infant death syndrome: Clinical findings and management. *Pediatrics* 1987; 79:889.

Kahn A, Blum D, Muller MF, et al: Sudden infant death syndrome in a twin: A comparison of sibling histories. *Pediatrics* 1986; 78:146.

Kelly DH, Shannon DC: Sudden infant death syndrome and near sudden infant death syndrome: A review of the literature, 1964–1982. *Pediatr Clin North Am* 1982; 29:1241.

Merritt TA, Bauer WI, Hasselmeyer EG: Sudden infant death syndrome: The role of the emergency room physician. *Clin Pediatr* 1975; 14:1095.

Oren J, Kelly D, Shannon D: Familial occurrence of sudden infant death syndrome and apnea of infancy. *Pediatrics* 1987; 80:355–358.

Peterson DR, Sabotta EE, Dalind JR: Infant mortality among subsequent siblings of infants who died of sudden infant death syndrome. *J Pediatr* 1986; 108:911.

Rosen CL, Frost JD Jr, Glaze DG: Child abuse and recurrent infant apnea. *J Pediatr* 1986; 109:1065.

Shannon DC, Kelly DH: SIDS and near-SIDS, Part 1 and 2. *N Engl J Med* 1982; 306:959, 1022.

Southall DP: Role of apnea in the sudden infant death syndrome: A personal view. *Pediatrics* 1988; 80:73–84.

127 Death of a Child in the Emergency Department

Ronald A. Dieckmann

To cure sometimes, to relieve often, to comfort always. —DR. EDWARD TRUDEAU

The emergency physician sometimes confronts the sudden and unexpected death of an infant or child. The tragedy of childhood death is often devastating to parents, family, and ED staff as well as to the physician. Preparation, organization, and thoughtful communication during resuscitation and after death can facilitate appropriate grief reactions, minimize ED chaos, and ease the physician's anxiety. Through careful, compassionate dialogue with bereaved parents about transplantation, the physician and ED staff may be able to enrich the lives of children with debilitating diseases who await organ and tissue donation.

The physician's reaction sets the stage for the coping process of family and staff. The physician must be sensitive and sympathetic while remaining in control. Often, a short respite from the ED will give the physician an opportunity to calm down, become composed, organize his or her thoughts, and more capably face the bereaved family. Informing parents of the death or impending death of their child is perhaps the most agonizing responsibility in medical practice. A thoughtful plan for essential history-taking, combined with an adaptable, expectant approach to a myriad of grief reactions will facilitate this task. Parents report that their initial encounters and dialogue with ED staff have a long-lasting imprint on their own grief process.

Family Reactions to Death ■

Although family reactions to the death of a child have sociocultural and personal idiosyncracies, predictable patterns exist. In all cases, respect the uniqueness of each family's response, even though it may conflict with the physician's. Often family members can identify their own needs and expectations when the interview is sensitively guided by trained staff. Circumstances of death differ and may influence parental reactions.

UNEXPECTED DEATH

The unexpected death of a child precipitates a profound grief response that is without any psychological preparation (see Chapter 126). The ED is usually poorly suited to assist the parents' grief process because of high patient volume, brief staff encounters, unfamiliarity of the environment, lack of privacy, and dearth of psychosocial support systems. Indeed, the ED is usually frightening and hostile to the distressed parents. In-servicing and proper preparation of ED staff for the sudden-death scenario is imperative so that the death protocol (Table 127-1) can be immediately implemented, and these adverse factors mitigated.

In some cases, resuscitation interventions are perceived as desecration of the child. Parents may not desire heroic measures when the circumstances are hopeless. The physician must initially assess the appropriateness of resuscitation before instituting a process for revival that may be utterly hopeless (see Chapter 6). ED staff must have an extraordinary degree of sensitivity and accommodation when dealing with the bereaved family and should use the communication guidelines outlined in Table 127-2.

NONACCIDENTAL TRAUMA (NAT)

NAT is increasingly common in childhood mortality. Child abuse or neglect, homicide, and suicide may be the basis for the death (see Chapters 128 and 131 for discussion of the physician's role in collecting evidence and notifying legal authorities). When unusual circumstances of death are suspected by the physician:

1. Do not inflame parents. Remain nonjudgmental in obtaining information.

TABLE 127–1. *Death Protocol*

1. Establish primary family liaison for consistent communication. Limit family access to medical information to liaison and attending physician.
2. Place family in private room, with drinks and telephone.
3. Ensure family support services: clergy (minister, priest, rabbi); key family members (other parent, children); psychologist when necessary.
4. Monitor friends and family members to ensure supportive environment for parents.
5. Contact primary physician and enlist his/her assistance.
6. Notify coroner about death. Establish necessity for autopsy before speaking to family about death.
7. After the body is cleaned and the room restored to order, encourage the parents to view the body and touch the child.
8. Explain to family the purpose of lines and tubes before they view the child.
9. Ensure complete chart documentation.
10. Administer rights of baptism to the Roman Catholic child. This can be done by any person of any faith: "I baptize you in the name of the Father, Son, and Holy Ghost. Amen."
11. Consider organ and tissue donation.
12. Give the family names and telephone numbers of the attending physician, coroner, and funeral home.
13. Encourage follow-up with primary physician.

2. Give the family the respect and compassion extended to the parents of the child with accidental trauma or illness. Reactions from parents may be the same, more subdued, or more exaggerated. Fear and recrimination may be prominent.
3. Inform parents of the need to report circumstances to legal authorities and what they should expect from authorities.

OTHER CIRCUMSTANCES

SIDS is the most common cause of death in the child under 1 year. Chapter 126 addresses this condition and the physician's role.

Death of the child with a known fatal disease can be less emotional in the ED setting. Here, parents have often experienced some of the grief process and may already be integrated into psychosocial support networks. On the other hand, despite psychological preparation, the family may react in a highly emotional manner.

In families of children with longstanding, degenerative diseases, parents may request modified resuscitative measures or no resuscitative measures. Physicians need to respect *appropriate* parental requests concerning the nature and extent of resuscitative interventions, usually in concert with the primary treating physicians.

Effect on Siblings ■

Siblings of the dead child require special attention. Their reactions are variable and age-specific. Erickson provides a developmental model for age differences in viewing death:

1. From 6 months to 2 years, there is no concept of death. Instead, children respond with fear of loss of personal attention from parents.
2. From 2 to 4 years, children's view of death is primarily fear of similar separation of themselves from parents.
3. From 4 to 6 years, children may see death as punishment for misdeeds.
4. From 7 years through adolescence, the child regards death as permanent and final, and may experience a sense of culpability or responsibility.

Siblings must be approached candidly, with an age-appropriate expectation of children's responses to death. Fear, guilt, and anger are common among siblings and need open expression. Younger children may not understand euphemisms about death such as "God took him" or "he is sleeping now." These may confuse and instill unnecessary fears in children for their own well-being. Sometimes siblings feel responsible for the death. This requires careful reassurance over time, and physicians can assist parents in expecting and identifying such reactions. Siblings may regress, begin bed-wetting, lose interest in school performance or other activities, or become socially withdrawn or especially fearful of separation.

Acknowledgment of the importance of directed discussions by parents with siblings is an important component of physician communication. Grief responses of over a year are common. Children older than 6 or 7 years can safely attend the funeral, after proper preparation by parents about what to expect.

TABLE 127–2. *Communication Guidelines After Death of a Child*

1. The family feels terrified and helpless when a child is acutely ill or injured. A single staff liaison must be assigned to them at the onset, usually a nurse or social worker. Communication with the family thereafter should come mainly from the single staff contact, in concert with the physician. Consistency and continuity are essential for effective communication.
2. The family liaison should elicit key historical factors from the family. A history of a bleeding disorder, poisoning, or observed aspiration, for example, may assist resuscitation and must be directly communicated to the physician.
3. Allow parents to express fears and concerns about care of their child, as this will decrease anxiety and helplessness. Moreover, sympathetic listening and reassurance that everything possible is being done for the child will minimize medicolegal risk. Legal actions against EDs are strongly associated with parental perceptions that ED staff are distant, impersonal, and uncaring.
4. The physician's first responsibility is to the child. However, when the resuscitation is long, brief physician contact with the family is desirable. When death is pronounced, the physician must devote adequate time with the family discussing the resuscitation process, circumstances of the illness or injury, and post-mortem considerations.
5. Often, *anger* is a first response. This may be directed at another family member, friend, or health-care provider. Sometimes, irrational rage may be directed at the hospital or the physician who is unable to revive the child. Do not respond with defensiveness or hostility. Do not take such assertions personally. Patience and compassion are foremost.
6. Parental *denial* is common and expected. "It can't be. He was fine an hour ago!" Shock and disbelief may be powerful and render the parent unable to accept the death of a previously healthy child. Reactions may vary from screaming, crying, and hyperventilations to silence or overintellectualization. The parent may seek a greatly detailed scientific explanation for the disease or the treatment, unable to face the death itself.
7. Avoid methods of questioning of parents that imply blame. Give parents the benefit of the doubt. Even when there is apparent culpability (*e.g.,* the submersion victim who was left unsupervised), the physician and liaison cannot be judgmental. Listen to the parents; reassure them they were probably not at fault *whenever possible,* and avoid reproach. The ED is not the place for assessing responsibility and fault.
8. *Guilt* may be overwhelming. The "responsible" parent can be suicidal. Parents need to express their own feelings of inadequacy and irresponsibility. Respect parents' rights to sadness, grief, and depression. Do not attempt to talk them out of these feelings. Follow-up physician or support group counseling may be most helpful.
9. Monitor the support systems for each family in the ED. Well-meaning friends or family may disrupt or destroy a controlled grief process with recriminations or misdirected statements to parents. Parents need protection from inappropriate behaviors in the ED.

When possible, integrate the primary physician of the sibling into management of sibling grief processes.

Effect on the ED Staff ■

The death of a child can be frustrating, demoralizing, and sometimes infuriating to the ED staff. Loss of young, healthy life is inevitably associated with feelings of failure and injustice. The physician should expect and contend with these feelings as soon as family communications are attended to. Principles in helping staff cope with death include:

1. Review the care and interventions immediately afterward.
2. Give staff the opportunity to discuss their concerns about the case or the nature and appropriateness of treatment.
3. Allow staff time to get away from the clinical area, whenever possible, to calm down and think.
4. Apply compassion and understanding to staff responses. Listen. Avoid argument. Arrange for follow-up discussion later, when necessary.
5. Prepare staff with in-services on death and grief reactions.

Protocol for Death in the ED ■

A written protocol or checklist may be helpful to staff for ensuring fundamental services to the family. Such a protocol is best developed prospectively; see Table 127-1.

Autopsy ■

The physician must discuss with the family the need for a post-mortem examination (autopsy) and explain the procedure. In the circumstances listed below, the medical examiner (coroner) will usually require an autopsy, but the circumstances for mandatory post-mortem examination have some state-to-state variability. In some cases, after consultation with the emergency physician, the coroner may elect not to require an autopsy.

CIRCUMSTANCES IN WHICH AUTOPSY MAY BE REQUIRED

1. Unnatural, sudden unexpected death (including SIDS)
2. Potential public health hazard (*e.g.*, communicable disease)
3. Suspicion or evidence of trauma or poisoning
4. Suspected abuse or neglect

REASONS FOR ELECTIVE AUTOPSY

The family may choose to have an autopsy based on their own concerns. The possible medical and social value of an elective autopsy includes the following:

1. It may affect living family members, if congenital abnormalities of an inherited nature are discovered.
2. Other children can benefit from information about response to therapy or injury.
3. Autopsy may allay guilt in parents by establishing that the process was not preventable.

Organ and Tissue Donation ■

Transplantation technology has provided an important additional consideration to managing ED death. Currently, transplantation is known to be effective for many organs, including the heart, heart-lung, liver, kidney, and pancreas. Additionally, corneas and connective tissues may be harvested and used in recipients with good success.

Donors must be carefully selected, usually in communication with regional or national transplant organizations. Issues of organ and tissue suitability, brain death determination, maintenance care, consent, and medicolegal concerns are complex and often require guidance by transplantation coordinators.

Approaching the family for donation of organs and tissues is delicate and sometimes highly distressing. Often, discussion is best delayed until later, after death or impending death is communicated to the family and the grief process is initiated. When time permits, a second conversation to broach donation may allow greater acceptance by the family of the child's death, as well as higher cooperation with consent. Families will sometimes initiate such discussions themselves. Indeed, when properly presented by the physician, organ and tissue donation is usually readily accepted by the bereaved family.

Bibliography ■

Berger L: Requesting the autopsy; a pediatric perspective. *Clin Pediatr* 1978; 17:445.

Lorenzen M, Smith L: The role of the physician in the grief reaction. *Clin Pediatr* 1981; 20:466.

Merritt TA, Bauer WI, Hazzelmeyer EC: Sudden infant death syndrome: The role of the emergency room physician. *Clin Pediatr* 1975; 14:1095.

Panides W: Helping parents deal with loss: A psychoanalytic perspective. *Pediatric Soc Work* 1984: 3:53.

Rosen P: Responding to the death of a child. In: Bark R: *The Emergently Ill Child: Dilemmas in Assessment and Management.* Rockville: Aspen, 1987; 391–393.

Soreff SM: Sudden death in the emergency department: A comprehensive approach for families, emergency medical technicians, and emergency department staff. *Crit Care Med* 1979; 7:321.

128 Child Abuse

Moses Grossman

Child abuse is broadly defined as any maltreatment of children or adolescents by their parents or others responsible for their care. Child abuse includes:

1. Physical abuse
2. Sexual abuse, including incest
3. Nutritional neglect
4. Emotional abuse
5. Intentional poisoning
6. Neglect of medical care
7. Lack of appropriate supervision
8. Abandonment
9. Munchausen syndrome by proxy

Child abuse is common: about 1% of children in the United States are reported to be abused or neglected. Some 10% of all injuries seen in EDs are inflicted, rather than accidental in nature. These children are most likely to present to EDs where a prior health record is not available. Child abuse must be ruled out in every pediatric injury so that the child can be protected. The youngest children are at the highest risk of death or permanent disability if the cycle is not interrupted. The ED responsibilities are *recognizing* possible child abuse and *reporting* it as required by law. Prevention is important, but not in the acute setting. Chapter 129 specifically addresses sexual abuse; this chapter deals with the other components of physical abuse.

Recognition ■

The key to recognition is to consider the possibility of inflicted injury (nonaccidental trauma) in every case. Histories are often unreliable; key questions are whether the nature and extent of the injury is compatible with the history, and whether the history from the involved caretakers is consistent. It is difficult to make a certain diagnosis of child abuse in the ED; for that reason, the law requires health personnel to report suspicion of child abuse to protect the child and ensure further investigation. A child even 3 or 4 years old may be able to contribute an account of the injury.

Ninety percent of physical abuse is inflicted by caretakers (parents, other close relatives, and babysitters). While there is no absolute stereotype, abusers often have a history of abuse as a child, low self-esteem, and a certain degree of isolation from family. They often have unrealistic expectations of the child: early toilet training, compliance with parental demands that may be unusual, and an exaggerated need to discipline the child. Injuries often occur as a result of such "discipline." If the family unit has two caretakers (usually parents), one is the active abuser, but the other is a silent participant by not intervening. Delay in seeking medical care is fairly common since the parents are torn between the desire to help the child and the fear that a medical visit may bring intervention from the authorities.

HEAD INJURIES

Injuries to the head are the most serious form of abuse, often resulting in death or permanent injury. Direct blows to the head may cause subdural hematoma and other intracranial injuries. Fractures and skin marks may or may not be found. More than 50% of head injuries in young children are inflicted, and the physician must evaluate the cause of such injuries with careful attention. A particular type of head injury that leaves no marks is the "shaken baby syndrome" in which a young infant is shaken vigorously, usually as a result of the caretaker's frustration with the child's crying. Further crying elicits further shaking, resulting in whiplash-like injuries, tearing of intracranial veins, and hemorrhages. A subdural hematoma or rarely an epidural hematoma may result. Another manifestation of the shaking syndrome is bilateral retinal hemorrhage, often suggesting chronic subdural blood. For that reason, fundoscopic examination is particularly important when child abuse is suspected.

SKIN MANIFESTATIONS

Dermatologic signs of abuse include bruises, welts, lacerations, and ecchymoses of different ages as well as healed scars. The clinician must distinguish the normal bruises on an active toddler's shins from those on the buttocks and lower back, which are almost always the result of punishment. Skin marks may indeed reveal the identity of the instrument of punishment: loop marks of a rope, cigarette burns, belt-buckle marks, and the angle of a wire coat hanger leave telltale scars.

FRACTURES

Inflicted fractures of the shaft of long bones are often spiral fractures incurred by twisting. A classic child abuse fracture is a chip fracture (tearing off the corner of a metaphysis of a long bone along with the epiphysis and periosteum). A bone survey will often reveal fractures of different ages, one of the absolute bits of legal evidence denoting child abuse.

BURNS

Some 10% of inflicted injuries are burns. The physician must distinguish the splash burn, which occurs from pulling over and spilling hot water on the neck and thorax, from the scald burn resulting from dunking the child into very hot water as a form of punishment. Inflicted burns are often over the buttocks only, or extend higher but spare the hands and feet. A burn of the palm may be inflicted as a form of punishment for stealing or other activities.

OTHER INJURIES

Blunt blows over the abdomen may produce life-threatening visceral injuries without external markers, usually spleen or liver laceration. Forcible intrusion of a bottle or other objects into the mouth may produce a torn frenulum, tears around the corner of the mouth, or chipped teeth. Many other injuries have been described, including human bites, puncture wounds, and cigarette burns. Sexual molestation may result in injury to the genitalia or arms.

Clinical Findings ■

Treatment begins with the recognition that child abuse may have caused the child's presenting injuries. Emergency physicians must not overlook or deny this possibility in children of *any* socioeconomic class.

TABLE 128–1. *Characteristics of Bruises*

Initially: reddish blue
1 to 3 days: dark blue to bluish brown
7 to 10 days: greenish yellow
>8 days: yellowish brown
Resolution (2 to 4 weeks): yellow

A very thorough physical examination is in order: disrobe the child fully. Carefully inspect the skin for evidence of trauma (bruises, burns, scars). Of particular importance are multiple bruises at different stages of healing. Table 128-1 presents approximate ages of the bruise by color. The medical record must contain accurate descriptions, preferably with diagrams, of the skin findings.

Evaluate the eyegrounds. Retinal hemorrhage is often a clue to inflicted head injuries, either from direct blows or violent shaking. Evaluate for subdural hematoma, a common and life-threatening finding in child abuse (see Chapter 50); early recognition and treatment is imperative.

Assess for intra-abdominal injury, especially if there is evidence of trauma to the epigastrium.

Ancillary Data ■

When the suspicion of child abuse is high enough to warrant reporting, the following studies are in order:

1. Complete skeletal radiographic survey of long bones and skull to demonstrate fresh and old skeletal trauma. CT head scan may be indicated in the presence of neurologic signs or retinal hemorrhage.
2. A hematologic workup if bleeding is present. Screen the whole process of hemostasis.
   a. Complete blood count, smear
   b. Platelet count, size, and morphology
   c. Prothrombin time
   d. Activated partial thromboplastin time
   e. Bleeding time
3. A developmental evaluation of the child
4. Color photographs of the specific injuries. These can often be obtained through a police photographer after reporting the suspicion of abuse.

Treatment ■

Treatment consists of medical management of the injuries. Pay special attention to the child's emotional needs.

Disposition ■

If the suspicion of abuse persists, hospitalize the child for further medical evaluation. Hospitalization protects the child from further injury, allows for more complete evaluation, and underscores the serious concern on the physician's part.

Suspected child abuse must be reported to local authorities as required by the laws of every state. It is wise to discuss the suspicion and the required report with the family *prior* to making the report, because such an approach builds a good foundation for future work with the family. The physician's tone should be nonaccusatory and nonjudgmental: "There is a suspicion of abuse and now the authorities will look into it." The ED or office staff must agree on who will file the report; in most instances, it is the treating physician.

Disposition of the child will usually be in the hands of social services and the juvenile court. Physicians, however, should not abdicate their interest in the child's welfare; they should participate in the whole process, with emphasis on medical follow-up with the primary physician whenever possible.

If the suspicion of child abuse is sustained, criminal charges may be filed against the suspected abuser. Thus, the physician may have to testify in juvenile court and in criminal court as well. Good documentation of the medical record is *imperative*.

Prevention ■

During the course of an ED visit, it may become apparent that the child who has not yet sustained injuries is at high risk of being abused. Sensitive health personnel can reach this conclusion based on parental attitudes and behavior toward the child in a stressful situation. One particular example is a parent who repeatedly brings the child to the ED without any objective signs of disease or injury. Recognizing the risk and making multidisciplinary efforts to support the caretakers may well serve to prevent future abuse.

Bibliography ■

American Academy of Pediatrics: Medical necessity for the hospitalization of the abused-neglected child. *Pediatrics* 1987; 79:300.

Ellerstein NS, ed: *Child Abuse-Neglect. A Medical Reference.* New York: Wiley, 1981.

Helfer RE: The epidemiology of child abuse and neglect. *Pediatr Ann* 1984; 13:745–51.

Helfer RE, Kempe CH: *Child Abuse-Neglect. The Family and the Community.* Cambridge, Mass.: Ballinger, 1976.

Kempe CM, Helfer RE, eds: *The Battered Child,* 3rd ed. Chicago University Press, 1980.

Silverman FN: Child abuse: The conflict of underdetection and overreporting. *Pediatrics* 1987; 80:441–442.

129 Sexual Abuse

Kevin P. Coulter

Sexual abuse is defined as the involvement of children and adolescents in sexual activities they cannot comprehend because of their developmental level; to which they are unable to give informed consent; or that violate the social taboos of family or society. These activities may physically injure the child and leave detectable patterns of trauma, but often sexual abuse may involve genital touching or fondling that does not cause detectable injury, and may even be physically pleasurable to the child.

Most victims of sexual abuse are female (70%–90%); the mean age of victims is 7 to 8 years. Adolescents are at significant risk for sexual assault because of their increasing independence and sexual naiveté.

Preadolescent victims usually are molested by males (90%) who are known, depended on, or trusted by the victim (*e.g.*, mother's boyfriend, stepfather, neighbor, teacher, coach). Adolescents are more commonly molested by strangers; this tends to be the traditional sexual assault or rape that happens once and often is reported soon after it occurs.

Sexual abuse may involve an adult's exposing his genitals to the victim, displaying sexually explicit pictures, or taking photographs of a child disrobed or engaged in sexual activity with other children. Sexual conduct may involve genital touching or fondling of the child or by the child. Of female victims, 50% will report vaginal penetration or at least genital-to-genital contact. One third of females and one half of male victims report anal penetration. The reported incidence of orogenital contact ranges from 20% to 50%. It is uncommon, particularly with victims of intrafamilial sexual abuse, for signs of physical abuse to be present. Adolescent victims of sexual assault by a stranger have a much higher incidence of concomitant physical abuse. Occasionally, children will be given alcohol or drugs to make them more pliable prior to sexual abuse.

Clinical Findings ■

BEHAVIORAL

Many factors determine how a child responds to sexual abuse. Important factors include the child's developmental age, the victim's sex and relationship to the perpetrator, the nature of the sexual abuse, and, very importantly, the reaction of the victim's family to the initial disclosure of the abuse. Table 129-1 lists the various behaviors that may indicate sexual abuse. Many of these indicators are quite nonspecific and may arise from a variety of stresses on the child (*e.g.*, parental divorce, death of a relative). Young children may have no perception that being touched sexually is wrong and thus may not have shown any signs of stress.

Intrafamilial abuse presents the child with numerous obstacles to disclosure. As the perpetrator is typically a trusted adult, the child may feel allegiance to and dependence on the abuser. Because disclosure invariably causes severe family turmoil whether it is believed or not, children may never reveal the abuse or their disclosure may be tentative, incomplete, and later retracted.

Because these factors can be such effective deterrents to disclosure, physicians must have a high index of suspicion for sexual abuse when examining a child or adolescent who presents with behavioral changes or vague somatic complaints. A physician's ability to diagnose sexual abuse may rest on his or her willingness to consider the diagnosis.

PHYSICAL FINDINGS

Table 129-2 lists physical indicators of sexual abuse. These include various types of genital and nongenital trauma and the presence of sexually transmitted infections. Pregnancy in an adolescent may have re-

TABLE 129–1. **Behavioral Indicators of Sexual Abuse**

Preschool Children
Fear state (*e.g.,* fear of adult males)
Nightmares
Precocious sexual behavior
Enuresis and encopresis
Regression of behavior

School-Aged Children
Precocious sexual behavior
Sexual aggression toward other children
Cross-dressing
School failure, truancy
Running away
Withdrawal, depression

Adolescents
Drugs, promiscuity
Prostitution
Running away
Sexual aggression toward other children
Depression, somatic complaints
School failure

sulted from a sexual assault or an incestuous relationship. To recognize physical signs of sexual abuse, the physician must be familiar with the normal anatomy of pediatric genitalia at the different developmental stages. Figure 129-1 shows the normal anatomy of the prepubertal female genitalia and anus.

The hymen is the thin tissue covering the vagina, present from birth. All females are born with a hymen, which undergoes dramatic changes as the child progresses from birth to sexual maturity. At birth the hymen is thickened and redundant and often has protruding tags. This thickening may persist for 1 to 2 years. After that, the hymen becomes quite thin with a usually smooth free margin outlining the opening into the vagina. In less than 1% of young girls, an imperforate hymen may exist. A hymen may be cribriform, with multiple openings, or septate,

TABLE 129–2. **Physical Indicators of Sexual Abuse**

Sexually transmitted diseases
Vaginitis, urethritis
Vaginal, rectal bleeding
Genital injuries
Pregnancy
Bruising, bites
Oral trauma

with a band of hymenal tissue across the vaginal opening. In most prepubertal females, the hymen will either be annular, completely circling the vaginal opening, or crescentic, leaving the superior portion of the vaginal opening uncovered. Less than 10% of prepubertal females will persist with a redundant hymen with many folds.

With the onset of puberty, the hymen again becomes quite thickened and redundant and takes on a scalloped appearance. Because of the many folds in the mature hymenal tissue, the detection of signs of trauma can be difficult in postpubertal females.

The size of the vaginal opening, bordered by the hymenal tissue, is another key anatomic feature. Generally, infants tend to have a vaginal opening no greater than 5 mm, preschool-aged girls tend not to exceed 7 mm, and school-age girls prior to puberty tend to have vaginal openings no greater than 7 to 9 mm. Do not place too much importance on the size of the vaginal opening: other aspects of the genital anatomy, particularly the hymenal and perihymenal tissues, are more important.

A summary of genital findings in sexually abused children is given in Table 129-3. The nature of the findings depends on the extent of the abuse (*i.e.,* fondling versus vaginal penetration), the number of times the child was abused, and time elapsed from abuse to the examination. Thus, children may show acute or chronic changes or a combination of both. Some of the physical findings are quite nonspecific (*e.g.,* labial erythema), while others are quite specific for sexual abuse (hymenal lacerations). All of these findings, however, are important to look for and accurately document.

Digital penetration often causes anterior hymenal trauma as the pelvis is used as a fulcrum. With penile penetration, posterior hymenal trauma is more common as the penis presses against the fossa navicularis and posterior hymen as it is forced into the vagina. Hymenal lacerations are seen as abrupt breaks in the smooth contour of the hymenal rim, often extending to the vaginal mucosa. With healing, the margins of the lacerations may reapproximate or remain apart as a healed transection. Particularly with repeated vaginal penetration, fibrous scar tissue may develop along the margins of a transection, which may retract the hymenal tissue and further distort its appearance.

With vulvar coitus or vaginal penetration, the fossa navicularis and posterior fourchette are often traumatized. Lacerations and abrasions of this area can occur subsequent to abuse. With repeated abuse, mounds of scar tissue may develop in the fossa navicularis. Occasionally an area of hypovascularity, simulating a scar, is found in the six o'clock position in the fossa navicularis. Do not confuse this with an abusive injury.

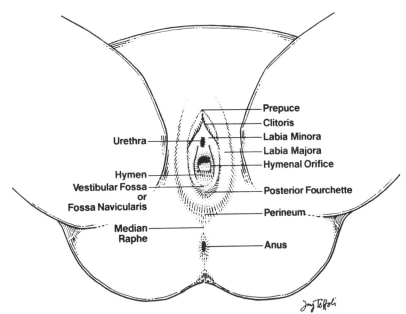

FIGURE 129–1. Normal prepubertal female genitalia.

Accidental genital trauma in girls (*i.e.*, straddle injuries) usually result in injury to the pubic and periclitoral areas. Typical straddle injuries do not cause hymenal lacerations.

Most children examined after anal penetration show no physical findings. Acutely, the perianal tissue may appear swollen, and lacerations, abrasions, erythema, or bruising can occur. Initially, following anal penetration, anal sphincter relaxation may occur and may persist for several hours or up to 2 days, followed by anal spasm. Even with repeated anal penetration, children may have no physical findings. Chronic changes include perianal scars, loss of anal rugae, and skin tags at the site of antecedent fissures. Assessing anal laxity and sphincter tone is very difficult because of a very wide range of normal findings.

Males usually show no evidence of trauma to their genitalia from sexual abuse. Occasionally, if examined soon after molestation, bite marks or bruises may be evident.

Children who are forced to place their mouths on a perpetrator's penis usually have no findings, but with forceful oral copulation, a child may have a laceration of the lip, frenulum, or gingiva. Erythema or abrasions of the palate may also occur, but rarely.

Sexually Transmitted Diseases ∎

Children who are sexually abused are at risk for acquiring a sexually transmitted disease (STD). Finding an STD in a child may be the only indication that the child was molested, but STDs may occur in children by routes other than sexual abuse (*i.e.*, perinatal transmission, nonsexual contact). Be aware of these other mechanisms of infection when suspecting sexual abuse (Table 129-4).

An STD in a female child may present as vaginitis. The differential diagnosis of vaginitis in prepubertal females is extensive, and most of these causes are much more common than sexual abuse (Table 129-5). Even when the vaginal discharge is bloody, sexual abuse is not the most common cause (Table 129-6).

CAVEATS

1. The thin epithelium of the prepubertal vagina is poorly resistant to gonococcal invasion. Thus, gonorrhea in the prepubertal female produces vaginitis as opposed to cervicitis, as in the postpubertal female. Most children with pharyngeal and rectal gonococcal infection are asymptomatic, as are a small portion of children with vaginal infections.

2. Any of the STDs noted in Table 129-3 may infect a child through sexual abuse, but other mechanisms may account for these infections. Of these STDs, *Neisseria gonorrhoeae, Trichomonas vaginalis*, and syphilis are the most specific markers for sexual abuse.

3. Infection of children with STDs by contact with contaminated fomites has never been documented.

4. *Gardnerella vaginalis* has been cultured from re-

TABLE 129–3. *Physical Findings in Child Sexual Abuse*

	Acute	Chronic
Genital Fondling	Erythema, contusions Abrasions of hymen Perihymenal tissue No finding	Usually no finding unless there is digital penetration of the vagina (see below)
Digital-Vaginal Penetration	Abrasions, lacerations of hymen No findings	Healed hymenal transections Hymenal thickening Attenuation of hymen No findings
Vulvar coitus	Erythema, abrasions Bruising of hymenal or perihymenal (particularly posterior fourchette) No findings	Healed hymenal transections Hymenal thickening and attenuation Scarring of posterior fourchette No findings
Penile-Vaginal Penetration	Abrasions, bruising of labia Erythema, abrasions, lacerations of hymen, perihymenal tissue, posterior fourchette	Hymenal scarring Attenuation, thickening of hymen Enlarged hymenal orifice Posterior fourchette scarring
Anal Penetration	Perianal swelling, erythema, abrasions, lacerations, bruises Initially, anal sphincter may be relaxed, then in spasm Frequently no findings	Relaxation of anal sphincter Perianal hypertrophy, scarring Frequently no findings
Penile-Oral Penetration of Child Victim	Usually no findings Rarely, laceration of lip or frenulum Rarely palatal erythema abrasion	Usually no findings

portedly non-sexually active females. Its significance as a marker for sexual abuse remains controversial.

Evaluation ■

Each county or municipality should have a referral center for the evaluation of allegations of sexual abuse of children. Ideally, this center should be staffed by physicians, nurses, and therapists who are expert in the field and who work closely with the police, child protective services, and the judicial system.

The goals of the medical evaluation are to:

1. Treat any medical illnesses or injuries
2. Provide crisis counseling
3. Provide protection for the child if necessary
4. Precisely document injuries and collect evidence for use by the legal system

If a child presents to the ED because of a sexual assault, consider this a medical emergency. A long delay in a crowded waiting room will only add to the trauma and anxiety of the child and family. Whenever possible, assign a nurse or other professional experienced in caring for victims of abuse to be present with the child through the entire evaluation.

Obtain consent prior to the evaluation. Minors 12 years of age or older may give consent to the medical evaluation and treatment of sexual assault, pregnancy, and STDs. Try to contact the parents or guardian of a minor before the examination, unless the examiner believes that person sexually assaulted the minor.

HISTORY

Obtaining the history is the most critical part of the evaluation. Make the setting comfortable for the child; a quiet room with toys and art materials is ideal. Approach the child in a supportive, nonjudgmental manner. Anticipate feelings of guilt, shame, and a sense of loyalty to the abuser on the part of the child. Usually children will experience the evaluation as a therapeutic event if they are given a sense of power over decisions regarding the need for an interview and physical examination.

Do not include the parents for the history, as their presence may be disruptive. Using art materials is a great aid in comforting the child as well as establish-

TABLE 129–4. *Sexually Transmitted Diseases in Children*

Organism	Incubation Period	Clinical Syndrome	Nonabusive Transmission	
			Perinatal Transmission	Nonsexual Contact
Neisseria, gonorrhoeae	3–7 days	Vaginitis (prepubertal females); profuse discharge	Yes, neonatal conjunctivitis	Not documented in children
		Cervicitis, PID (postpubertal females)		
		Pharyngitis, proctitis, urethritis		
		Disseminated disease: rash, arthralgias, tenosynovitis, arthritis		
		Asymptomatic carriage: vagina, cervix, pharynx, rectum		
Chlamydia trachomatis	7–21 days	Vaginitis (prepubertal females)	Yes, may have asymptomatic vaginal, rectal carriage for up to 2 years	Not documented in children
		Cervicitis, endometritis (postpubertal females)		
		Urethritis, proctitis, epidymitis, prostatitis, Reiter's syndrome, perihepatitis		
		Asymptomatic carriage: vagina cervix, rectum		
Herpes simplex virus (HSV) I and II	5–7 days	Painful vesicles on labia, vagina, anus, and rectum (I and II)	Yes	Documented with HSVI: autoinoculation from oral to genital sites
Condyloma acuminata human papilloma virus	2–3 months average ? over 1 year	Mucosa: red, mulberry-type lesions / Skin: verrucous warts common; may be pigmented papules	Yes	Possible
Trichomonas vaginalis	3–28 days	Vaginitis / Asymptomatic carriage in the urethra	Yes, neonate may carry in the vagina for 3–6 weeks after birth	Not documented in children
Syphilis	Primary: 10–90 days	Primary: chancre / Secondary: rash, lymphadenitis, mucous patches, condyloma lata	Yes	Yes

ing the child's knowledge of body parts. By drawing a human figure with genitalia, the examiner can learn what words a child uses for genitalia and then employ those terms in specific questions about sexual abuse.

Phrase questions to the child in a manner that is nonleading and nonthreatening. "Do you know why you were brought here today?" and "Has anything bad been happening to you?" are good general questions to begin with. Eventually, specific questions as to whether sexual touching occurred are necessary. Often children will be able to describe penile erection and ejaculation, what the ejaculate looked and felt like, and what they used to wipe the ejaculate off with. Also ask whether any physical force was used, whether verbal threats were made should the child disclose, or whether money or gifts were given to the child. Young children have a poor concept of time and thus have difficulty answering questions about when or how often something happened.

Some experts advocate the use of anatomically correct dolls in eliciting a history of sexual abuse. These dolls can be useful as an adjunct in helping the child describe what type of sexual acts occurred, but they must not be used as a replacement for a comprehensive history.

Question the patient or the parent about the child's general medical history. Historical points of importance to sexual abuse include:

TABLE 129–5. *Differential Diagnosis of Prepubertal Vaginitis*

Poor hygiene
Chemical irritation
  Soap
  Bubble bath
Trauma
  Tight-fitting underwear or leotards
Infection
  Pinworms
  Group A streptococcus
  Haemophilus influenzae
  Shigella
  Varicella
  Measles
  Sexually transmitted disease

1. Gynecologic information: age at menarche; date of last menstrual period; use of contraception; prior consensual sexual activity; history of vaginal pain, itching, discharge, bleeding; history of rectal pain, discharge, bleeding; history of prior STDs
2. Recent physical injuries
3. Previous history of child abuse
4. Post-assault hygiene that may eliminate evidence from the skin, mouth, vagina, and rectum
5. Recent antibiotic use

The timing of the physical examination depends on several factors. If the sexual assault took place within 72 hours, perform an examination immediately, as seminal fluid and sperm may still be detectable. An immediate examination is also indicated when there is an acute genital or rectal injury, if the child requires protective custody, or if the family is unable to wait because of the emotional crisis surrounding disclosure of the abuse.

Perform a complete medical examination, paying special attention to signs of illness, neglect, and

TABLE 129–6. *Differential Diagnosis of Bloody Vaginal Discharge*

Menses
Tumors
Trauma
  Accidental
  Sexual abuse
Infections
  Shigella
  Group A streptococcus
Urethral prolapse

physical abuse as well as to genital injury. Document signs of physical abuse precisely by drawings or photographs.

The child's comfort is of foremost concern during the examination. Clearly explain to the child the reason for the examination and why the genitals will be examined. Never use forcible restraint. If the child is resistant, defer the examination, as the child may experience a forcible examination as another molestation. If there is suspicion of genital injury that may require emergent treatment, examine a resistant child under general anesthesia.

Different positions can be used to examine a child's genitals (Fig. 129-2). Young girls are usually comfortable in a supine, frog-leg position, on an examination table or on a trusted adult's lap. A knee-chest position will also provide good visualization of the female genitals, but some children become quite anxious in this position. Do an anal examination with the child in a lateral recumbent position or in the knee-chest position.

Adequate lighting and magnification are essential for proper examination of the vagina and anus. This can be achieved quite well with the use of an otoscope. Many referral centers for child abuse use a colposcope, which provides excellent binocular magnification. The colposcope should have a camera attached to provide photographic documentation of genital injuries.

To best visualize the vaginal opening in a young child, retract the labia majora laterally. Downward and lateral traction on the inner thighs or gentle grasping of the labia majora between thumb and forefinger with gentle outward and lateral traction will provide good visualization.

In prepubertal females, an external genital examination is usually sufficient. A speculum exam of the vagina in a prepubertal female is only necessary when there is suspicion of intravaginal trauma that may require treatment (*e.g.*, a laceration); that examination is best done under general anesthesia. With adolescent females, perform a speculum examination following a sexual assault.

Evaluate for STDs as a routine part of a sexual abuse examination. Table 129-7 lists the recommended tests for STDs. Culture children routinely for gonorrhea and chlamydia from the pharynx, vagina, and rectum, as these organisms often cause asymptomatic infection. Culture the vagina, rectum, and urethra using calcium alginate swabs. For the child's comfort, moisten the swab in nonbacteriostatic saline before culturing. Taking swabs of the vagina causes minimal discomfort if hymenal tissue is not touched and if the swabs contact only the posterior floor of the vagina.

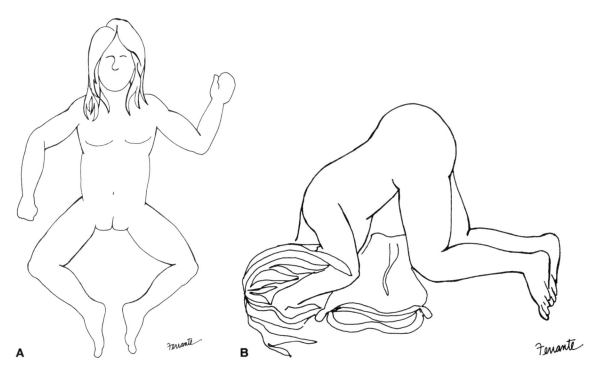

FIGURE 129-2. (*A*) Supine position for genital examination. (*B*) Knee–chest position for genital examination.

Sexually acquired urethritis in male victims of sexual abuse is very unusual. Culturing the urethra of males is indicated only if they have urethral symptoms or give a history of sexual activity, consensual or nonconsensual, that would place them at risk for urethral infection.

Detecting gonorrhea and chlamydia in a child has very serious implications; thus, only cultures should be used as the means of detecting these organisms. Fluorescent antibody or antigen tests are unacceptable for the high degree of certainty required in sexual abuse cases because of the unacceptable level of false positives.

Children who are sexually abused may be at risk for infections with hepatitis B virus (HBV) and human immunodeficiency virus (HIV). Serologic studies for these infections are indicated if the victim or assailant is symptomatic or known to be at high risk for these infections or if the assault occurred in a geographic area with a high prevalence of HBV and HIV.

Retest the victim 12 weeks after the initial evaluation.

Test all adolescent female victims of sexual assault routinely for pregnancy. Urine tests for the detection of beta-subunits HCG can detect pregnancy 10 days after conception.

EVIDENCE COLLECTION

The examiner has a dual role, forensic and medical, in evaluating sexually abused children. Collecting evidence for legal purposes is an important element of the examination. Every examination of an allegedly abused child is an evidentiary exam, as injuries that are documented in the child's records can be used in court. Particularly when examining a child within 72 hours of a sexual assault, when seminal fluid and sperm may still be present on or within a child, the proper collection of evidence is essential. Any phy-

---

TABLE 129-7. *Laboratory Tests in the Diagnosis of Sexually Transmitted Diseases in Sexually Abused Children*

Wet mount and Gram's stain of genital or rectal discharge
Routine genital and rectal cultures for *N. gonorrhoeae* and *C. trachomatis*
Routine pharyngeal culture for *N. gonorrhoeae*
Culture of lesions suspicious for herpes simplex
Serologic studies for hepatitis B and human immunodeficiency virus, if indicated

---

sician who examines sexual abuse victims must be fully knowledgeable of the protocol for evidence collection recommended by the police crime laboratory serving the locale.

Treatment ■

Treat physical injuries as necessary. Evaluate lacerations within the vagina carefully for possible extension into the abdominal cavity. Provide tetanus prophylaxis as indicated.

See Chapter 121 on STDs for treatment recommendations. Offer prophylaxis against gonorrhea and chlamydia to all adolescent victims of sexual assault. Treat prepubertal victims at the time of the examination if the child has a vaginal, rectal, or urethral discharge and the Gram's stain is suggestive of gonorrhea or chlamydia, or if the assailant is known to have gonorrhea or chlamydia. Give prophylaxis for both gonorrhea and chlamydia. Following treatment of documented infections of gonorrhea or chlamydia, arrange re-culture of children for test of cure.

After documentation of a negative urine pregnancy test, offer adolescent females prophylaxis against conception (Ovral, two pills at the time of the examination and two pills 12 hours later). Counsel those females who have been impregnated by a sexual assault about their therapeutic options.

Counseling with therapists experienced in treating victims of sexual abuse is essential following the initial evaluation. Many children will require extensive counseling, particularly those who are victims of long-term incestuous relationships.

Evaluating victims of sexual abuse is very complex and time consuming. Throughout the evaluation, the child's well-being and comfort must be of prime importance. The history, as given in the child's own words, is the most important element of the examination. Many children who give clear and explicit histories of sexual abuse have no physical findings. In almost all of these instances, a normal examination is entirely consistent with the child's history of abuse and should not be used to negate the child's allegations.

Bibliography ■

Berkowitz C: Sexual abuse of children and adolescents. *Adv Pediatr* 1987; 34:275.

Corwin D: Early diagnosis of child sexual abuse. In: Wyatt G, Powell G, eds: *Lasting Effects of Child Sexual Abuse.* London: Sage, 1988.

Emans J: Vulvovaginitis in the child and adolescent. *Pediatr in Rev* 1986; 8:12.

Enos WF: Forensic evaluation of the sexually abused child. *Pediatrics* 1986; 78:385.

Hammerschlag M: Sexually transmitted diseases in sexually abused children. *Adv Pediatr Infect Dis* 1988; 3:1.

Hermann-Giddens ME: Prepubertal female genitalia: Examination for evidence of sexual abuse. *Pediatrics* 1987; 80:203.

Jenny C: Hymens in newborn female infants. *Pediatrics* 1987; 80:399.

Neinstein L, Goldenring J, Carpenter S: Nonsexual transmission of sexually transmitted diseases: An infrequent occurrence. *Pediatrics* 1984; 74:67.

Woodling BA: Sexual abuse and the child. *Emerg Med Serv* 1986; 15:17.

Woodling B, Heger A: The use of the colposcope in the diagnosis of sexual abuse in the pediatric age group. *Child Abuse Negl* 1986; 10:111.

130 Acute Psychiatric Disorders

Stuart A. Bair

Children and adolescents with overt emotional or psychiatric disorders, as well as those who present with altered mental status or disordered behavior, will often be seen first by a pediatrician or emergency physician. Initial goals are twofold: first, rapid, though not necessarily exact, diagnostic evaluation, and secondly, patient control and safety. The specific problems of suicide and altered mental status are discussed in Chapters 131 and 16.

Clinical Findings ■

The primary diagnostic consideration when a patient presents with disturbed thought or behavior is to determine if the problem is due to organic causes, functional mental disorder, or both. Err on the side of excessive organic workup, as misdiagnosis of organic disorders is generally much more dangerous than initially missing a purely psychiatric disorder. History-taking is often very difficult because the patient may not be able to or may not wish to cooperate, and ancillary sources of information may not be available initially. If the family is present, it is usually best to take a history from the parents alone if the child is a preteen and to include the patient if possible if the patient is older. However, the safety and efficacy of each situation must be judged individually.

Psychiatric disorder is not a diagnosis of exclusion: functional disorders have a specific history, signs, and symptoms. *Psychosis* is a general term denoting loss of contact with reality to a significant, though variable, degree. It is not synonymous with schizophrenia. The most common causes of acute functional psychotic disorders in older children and adolescents are listed in Table 130-1. Common causes of organic psychosis are listed in Table 130-2. Findings commonly associated with functional psychiatric disorders are listed in Table 130-3, and those associated with organic psychosis are listed in Table 130-4.

Evaluate clinical findings using a formal mental status format:

1. Appearance, including motor activity
2. Speech: type and rate
3. Mood: how the patient says he feels; affect: how the patient looks to the examiner
4. Thought content: processes as described, as well as suicidal and homicidal ideation
5. Sensorium: orientation, memory, calculations
6. Judgment: tested for simple tasks
7. Insight: degree to which patient perceives that there is a problem and is willing or able to accept help

After the mental status evaluation, assess the overall level of dysfunction using the following parameters:

1. Degree of abnormality: from child's baseline or expected normal
2. Degree of impairment of patient and family: assessment of perceived suffering on the part of the patient
3. Threat to self and others

Treatment ■

Immediate management of all acute mental disorders includes the following steps:

1. Never leave the patient alone. Assign a staff member, not a family member, to the patient at all times.
2. Place the patient in a quiet, low-stimulus environment as far removed from medical emergencies and medical equipment as is reasonably possible.
3. Talk in simple, brief sentences. Reassure the patient that he is in a safe place, that nobody will harm him, and that you are there to help him.
4. If the patient is threatening to harm himself or others, seems to be in danger of running away, or is delirious, consider physical or chemical restraint.
5. If soft restraints are necessary, use them on all four extremities so that the patient cannot untie them himself.
6. Use antipsychotic medication (also known as major tranquilizers or neuroleptics) only in children with

TABLE 130–1. *Common Causes of Acute Functional Psychotic Disorders*

Schizophrenia: first and recurrent episodes
Bipolar affective disorder: manic or depressed, first or recurrent episodes
Major affective disorder: severe or recurrent depressive episodes
Brief reactive psychosis: with identifiable stressor
Acute psychotic episode: without identifiable stressors

It is not crucial to attempt to make a specific diagnosis among the above initially, as they are all treated in a similar fashion emergently.

extreme agitation or when overt psychotic symptoms are present.

ANTIPSYCHOTIC MEDICATION

High-potency medications are preferable for initial management, especially when organicity is still in question, because they have fewer anticholinergic side effects; unfortunately, these medications as a group are more likely to cause extrapyramidal side effects. Common preparations, routes, and dosages are listed in Table 130-5; common side effects are listed in Table 130-6.

The patient population most likely to require antipsychotic medication (*i.e.*, adolescent males) is also at highest risk for dystonic reactions; therefore, consider antiparkinsonian agents prophylactically. These dystonias are usually apparent fairly quickly, but onset may be delayed several hours. Drugs for treatment of dystonia are listed in Table 130-7. Doses may be required every 4 to 6 hours, since the half-life of the antipsychotic agents is quite prolonged.

TABLE 130–2. *Common Causes of Organic Psychotic Disorders*

Drug ingestion and intoxication (street drugs and prescribed medication): sympathomimetics, hallucinogens, PCP, steroids, anticholinergic agents
CNS infection: viral and bacterial
CNS insults or injury: CVA (especially in patients with blood dyscrasias or CHD); vasculitis associated with systemic diseases; occult trauma, especially subdural hematoma
Psychomotor seizures: ictal and interictal
Metabolic disorders: hypoglycemia, electrolyte abnormalities, Wilson's disease, porphyria, hypo- and hyperthyroidism.

TABLE 130–3. *Characteristics of Functional Psychiatric Disorders*

History of long-standing behavior problems
Insidious, increasing symptoms over days to weeks, including day-night reversals, time distortion, strange dietary patterns, bizarre religious preoccupations
Auditory hallucinations, often a running commentary on thoughts and actions
Ideas of reference: the belief that common events or information have special meaning to the patient
Well-organized or complex delusions
Somatic complaints, especially that one's body is being controlled by outside forces
Paranoia, often as part of a larger delusional system
Grandiosity, often associated with mental abilities or lineage
Thought broadcasting or thought insertion: the belief that others can steal unspoken thoughts or put thoughts into one's head against one's will
Loose associations: little or no logical connections between topics
Tangentiality: ideas somewhat connected but increasingly off the topic
Circumstantiality: series of loosely connected ideas, often incorporating immediate surroundings, that eventually come back to the topic
Flight of ideas: scattered, unconnected topics
Klang associations: rhyming words without logical connection
Word salad and neologisms: random or nonsense words that seem to make sense to the patient
Memory: may be intact or psychotically altered
Orientation: lack of concern or delusional
Judgment: no recognition that thoughts or behavior are abnormal

Use a flow sheet listing medications, dosage, route, target symptoms, and efficacy whenever psychoactive medication is given. Use all medications cautiously in cases of suspected encephalopathy or other organic disorder. Nonetheless, if the patient is awaiting specific treatment for a medical disorder, antipsychotics are generally quite safe and do not add excess sedation.

SECONDARY MANAGEMENT

1. Try to get a more detailed history.
2. Get psychiatric consultation, even when organicity is strongly suspected, for help with medication management, family intervention, and disposition.
3. Do not be too eager to make a specific psychiatric diagnosis. Differentiating functional disorders in the acute situation, especially in adolescents, is generally impossible. The correct diagnosis usually is clear only over time.

TABLE 130–4. *Clinical Findings in Organic Psychosis*

Known or suspected ingestion in a previously well child
Diffuse autonomic arousal
Simple delusional ideation
Paranoia, often isolated
Grandiosity, often related to physical prowess
Auditory hallucinations, often unstructured words, phrases, music
Tactile, olfactory, or visual hallucinations
Pressured or inarticulate speech
Disorientation
Impaired memory functions
Inability to do simple calculations
Comprehension that one's thoughts or behavior are not normal

4. Do not attempt family counseling in the acute setting. Etiologic considerations and long-term prognosis both depend on a more firmly established diagnosis. The short-term prognosis may not be clear. It is entirely appropriate to say "I don't know" in these circumstances.

Disposition ■

Even if medication clears symptoms acutely, it is in the best interest of the patient and family to hospitalize, even if briefly, all patients who are acutely psychotic.

Specific Conditions ■

EATING DISORDERS

This group of disorders includes a spectrum of illnesses from self-starvation and associated symptoms

TABLE 130–5. *Antipsychotic Drug Therapy*

Fluphenazine (Prolixin) PO concentrate; do not use decanoate or enanthate
Haloperidol (Haldol) IM or PO (concentrate)
Thiothixene (Navane) IM or PO
Trifluoperazine (Stelazine) PO (concentrate)

Typical initial dose of any of the above, depending on the size and age of the patient, not the severity of the symptoms, is 0.5 to 5 mg IM or 2 to 5 mg P.O. Do not use pills unless liquid is unavailable. This may be repeated hourly as necessary up to a total dose of no more than about 50 mg/24 hr.

TABLE 130–6. *Side Effects of Antipsychotic Drugs*

Dystonia (pseudoparkinsonism): stiffness, rigidity, tremors, thick tongue, or dysarthria
Torticollis: alarming in appearance but rarely dangerous
Laryngospasm and oculoguric crisis: rare but treated the same as other dystonias
Dry mouth
Blurred vision
Motor (especially leg) restlessness
Neuroleptic malignant syndrome (rare)

to binging and purging. The diagnostic criteria for anorexia nervosa and bulimia are listed in Table 130-8 and Table 130-9.

By the time a patient is brought to see a physician with significant weight loss or abnormalities associated with vomiting or laxative abuse, the problem is generally beyond control. In anorexia nervosa, there may be outright psychotic delusions about body habitus. The primary goal of initial treatment is medical stabilization. Although patients with bulimia may be of normal weight, they may still be at significant risk for metabolic derangement. In those who starve themselves, the critical weight at which metabolic homeostasis is in jeopardy is approximately 30 kg. Given that a basic feature of these disorders is the patient's denial or refusal to accept the seriousness of the illness, the patient will often require involuntary psychiatric hospitalization or legal injunction to be hospitalized for medical treatment. *All patients who show any of the major abnormalities listed in Table 103-10 must be hospitalized for their own safety.* Long-term mortality from anorexia nervosa is between 5% and 20%.

Psychiatric consultation may be helpful in the initial phase of treatment to establish a behaviorally oriented weight-gain plan and to begin to work with the families of these patients, who are often very difficult to engage in treatment.

SELF-INJURIOUS AND DANGEROUS BEHAVIOR

Adolescents and occasionally younger children will engage in self-destructive and self-mutilative behav-

TABLE 130–7. *Drugs for Treatment of Dystonia*

Benztropine (Cogentin) 1–2 mg PO or IM
Diphenhydramine (Benadryl) 25–50 mg PO, IM, or slow IV
Trihexyphenidyl (Artane) 5 mg PO

TABLE 130–8. *Diagnostic Criteria for Anorexia Nervosa*

Refusal to maintain body weight over a minimal normal weight for age and height (*e.g.,* weight loss leading to maintenance of body weight 15% below that expected)

Intense fear of gaining weight or becoming fat, even though underweight

Disturbance in the way in which one's body weight, size, or shape is experienced (*e.g.,* the patient claims to "feel fat" even when emaciated, believes that one area of the body is "too fat" even when obviously underweight)

In females, absence of at least three consecutive menstrual cycles when otherwise expected to occur (primary or secondary amenorrhea). A woman is considered to have amenorrhea if her periods occur only following hormone (*e.g.,* estrogen) administration

---

TABLE 130–10. *Indications for Hospitalization in Eating Disorder*

Major Medical Problems
Bradycardia
Prolonged Q-T interval
Dysrhythmias
Orthostatic pulse and blood pressure instability
Hypothermia
Electrolyte abnormalities, especially hypokalemia and hypocalcemia
Superior mesenteric artery syndrome

Minor Problems
Pyuria (not associated with UTI)
Proteinuria
Leukopenia with normal platelet count
Elevated liver function tests

(Adapted from Palla B, and Litt I: *Medical complications of eating disorders in adolescence.* Pediatrics 1988;81:613)

---

iors that are not obviously suicidal. These behaviors include such injuries as nonlethal lacerations, punctures of various parts of the body, scarification, and burning with matches and cigarettes. These patients usually have longstanding and severe psychopathology. Precipitating factors often include a change of routine, even minor, or an episode of personal rejection, real or imagined.

Motivations for these behaviors are diverse and may include command auditory hallucinations, either drug induced or secondary to pre-existing psychiatric disorder; a hidden agenda (*e.g.,* to get drugs); or primitive revenge fantasies ("I'll cut myself and you'll feel the pain").

Attempts to reason with these patients or persistent efforts to determine why they have done it are generally of little value and often only further enrage them. In the absence of overt psychotic signs and symptoms, antipsychotic medications are inappropriate except with extreme agitation or uncontrollable behavior. Often these patients have an ongoing therapist, but this information is rarely volunteered unless specifically asked for. The physician may be

unable to identify the precipitant and probably cannot do much about it. Therefore, *admit these patients for their own protection, involuntarily if necessary, and consider a 24-hour sitter.* Obtain psychiatric consultation as quickly as possible, since these patients often become suddenly and impulsively suicidal and act without warning.

VIOLENCE TOWARD OTHERS

While predicting future violence is difficult, it is possible with psychiatric consultation to determine short-term risk in the face of recent or imminent behavior. Differential diagnosis of acute violent behavior is presented in Table 130-11.

Two factors may have predictive value for subsequent violent behavior in life: firesetting, cruelty to animals, and enuresis; or fighting, temper tantrums, inability to get along with others, school problems, and truancy. While neither is definitive nor diagnostic, their presence or absence is significant.

When there is definite or suspected risk of violence toward family, staff, or other patients, contact hospital

---

TABLE 130–9. *Diagnostic Criteria for Bulimia*

Recurrent episodes of binge eating (rapid consumption of a large amount of food in a discrete period of time)

A feeling of lack of control over eating behavior during the eating binges

Regular self-induced vomiting, use of laxatives or diuretics, strict dieting or fasting, or vigorous exercise to prevent weight gain

A minimum average of two binge-eating episodes a week for at least 3 months

Persistent overconcern with body shape and weight

TABLE 130–11. *Causes of Acute Violent Behavior*

Drug and alcohol intoxication or withdrawal or personality changes associated with chronic substance abuse

Organic psychosis or psychomotor epilepsy: ictal and interictal

Functional psychosis with delusions and paranoia

Early manifestations of intermittent explosive or antisocial personality disorders

security or police immediately, even on a standby basis. In the absence of a treatable medical condition or a psychotic mental disorder, avoid admitting the patient to a pediatric unit, but if necessary obtain a 24-hour sitter. Psychiatric consultation may be helpful to determine whether a given individual is best dealt with by the mental health system or the criminal justice system.

Bibliography ■

Hillard J, et al: A retrospective study of adolescents' visits to a general hospital psychiatric emergency service. *Am J Psychiatry* 1987; 144:432.

Hodas G, Sargent J: In: Fleisher GR, Ludwig S, eds: *Textbook of Pediatric Emergency Care.* Baltimore: Williams & Wilkins, 1983.

Morrison G: Emergency intervention. In: Harrison S, ed: *Basic Handbook of Child Psychiatry.* New York: Basic Books, 1979.

Palla B, Litt I: Medical complication of eating disorder in adolescents. *Pediatrics* 1988; 81:613.

Popper R: Child and adolescent psychopharmacology. In: Michaels R, Cavener J, Brodie H et al, eds: *Psychiatry.* Philadelphia: JB Lippincott, 1988.

Rosenn D: Psychiatric emergencies in childhood and adolescence. In: Bassuk E, Birk A, eds: *Emergency Psychiatry: Concepts, Methods and Practices.* New York: Plenum, 1984.

131 Suicide

Graeme Hanson

A significant number of children and adolescents consider and attempt suicide at some point in their young lives. Physicians treating children and adolescents must be alert to suicidal ideas and actions in these patients and must develop an effective approach to intervention. A suicide attempt is an emergency that elicits complex feelings and reactions on the part of the treating physician.

Epidemiology ■

COMPLETED SUICIDES

Suicide is the third leading cause of death in 15- to 24-year-olds (accidents are the leading cause and homicide second). Eight to 10 percent of children under 12 consider suicide and sometimes act on suicidal wishes, but the number of children under 12 who actually kill themselves is quite small. The rate increases in every successive year beginning at age 13 and peaks around age 23 for the younger population. The highest rate is in white males, followed by black males, then white females and black females.

In completed suicides in the United States, death by firearm is the most common method in adolescents, followed by hanging for males and jumping from a high place for females. Stabbing and drug overdose are also very common. In children under 12, jumping from a high place, hanging, and drug overdose are the most common.

UNSUCCESSFUL SUICIDE ATTEMPTS AND GESTURES

It is this group of patients the physician will be treating. The ratio of suicide attempts to completed suicides is probably between 50:1 to 100:1. In adolescents, females far outnumber males in making suicide attempts. Any act of self-destruction by a young person with a conscious wish to die must be taken very seriously, even though the act may be seen as a gesture and not a serious attempt at suicide. The overall meaning of the act and what it portends for the child's

future may become clear only after extensive assessment and follow-up.

Clinical Findings ■

In all cases, the act results from a combination of factors that have a cumulative effect: individual emotional problems, family difficulties and discord, environmental or social stress, etc. Increasingly, substance abuse has become associated with suicide attempts.

DEPRESSION

Many, but by no means all, children and adolescents who make suicide attempts present with a history and clinical picture of depression. Depression in childhood is characterized by:

1. Dysphoric mood that includes sadness, moodiness, helplessness, crying, and a sense of hopelessness
2. Self-depreciation and a sense of failure; low self-esteem
3. Insomnia and other sleep disorders
4. Social withdrawal
5. Somatic complaints
6. Changes in school attitudes and performance
7. Lethargy and chronic fatigue
8. Increased aggression and aggressive outbursts
9. Eating disorders

In depressed children and adolescents, suicide is often thought about and planned. The attempt is often carried out in a manner that minimizes discovery, and a suicide note is often left. Sometimes the actual attempt is impulsive. In some instances, the child or adolescent may demonstrate an apparent sudden improvement in mood and may appear happier for a short time before the attempt: this dangerous sign usually reflects the patient's relief at having made the decision to kill himself and to be released from his anguish.

ACTING OUT

In the impulsive, acting-out teenager:

1. There is not a consistent history of depression.
2. There is a history of increasing antisocial and aggressive behavior.
3. Often there is a deterioration in school performance and a change in friends.
4. There are increasing struggles with and defiance of parents.

In these cases, the suicidal act is an impulsive one, following an interpersonal confrontation with a parent or parents, a teacher, or a friend. The attempt often takes place in the presence of others. The victim does not leave a note. These attempts can be very dangerous depending on what was available as a suicide method (firearms, combination of pills, etc.).

PSYCHOSIS (See Chapter 130.)

In the child/adolescent with a psychotic condition:

1. There is a history of increasing isolative, inappropriate and bizarre thinking and behavior.
2. The suicide attempt is in response to bizarre thoughts, delusions, or hallucinations (*e.g.,* a voice telling the patient to fly off a bridge).

This situation is quite rare. Because of the patient's overall psychiatric disorder and the bizarreness of the underlying motives for suicide, this situation is most difficult to predict. The patient's psychiatric condition almost invariably warrants psychiatric hospitalization.

Risk Factors and Precipitating Events ■

Specific risk factors include a previous suicide attempt, a history of suicide in a family member or close friend, a combination of chronic depression and somatic difficulties, and increased aggression and hostility.

Common precipitating events are a disciplinary crisis, usually by a parent or sometimes by a teacher; rejection by an important person, such as the break-up of a close relationship; a humiliating experience or failure: a school failure, failure at some event with public exposure, or outright humiliation by another person, especially an important adult (*e.g.,* parent or teacher); or the loss of an important person through death or moving away. Other possible precipitants include incest or sexual molestation, anxiety over possible pregnancy (or sexual activity), fear that illicit drug use or illegal activity will be discovered, or recent publicity about a suicide.

Treatment ■

INITIAL CARE

Treat the emergent medical complications created by the particular method of the attempt. Since drug overdose is the most common method in attempts and since teenagers have access to a wide range of prescribed and nonprescribed drugs, often in fatal combinations, obtain a broad toxicology panel and ask family and friends about drugs to which the victim may have had access. See Chapter 63.

While managing the medical emergency, perform a careful assessment (or consult a trained mental health professional) of the immediate and ongoing suicide risk. If there is any possibility for immediate re-attempt during medical management, take appropriate steps (*e.g.,* a sitter) to ensure the patient's safety.

PSYCHOSOCIAL ASSESSMENT

Once the child is medically stabilized and in a safe environment, complete a more comprehensive assessment of the child's psychosocial problems and what led to the suicide attempt, in order to develop an appropriate treatment plan and disposition. This requires careful, sensitive interviewing of the child and family members. Often friends and teachers can give very useful information. Allow enough time for this assessment. Use support personnel (*e.g.,* a social worker or nurse) to help. Consult a psychiatrist for assistance, if assessment cannot be properly accomplished by the treating physician.

1. Establish an alliance with the patient. Interview the patient alone, away from parents whenever possible. These patients often have troubled relationships with their parents and may have concerns, complaints, and information they do not want their parents to know.
2. Ensure confidentiality regarding the information the patient gives, except for information with life-or-death implications (*e.g.,* further suicide threats). In that instance, the patient needs to know that the physician will take whatever steps are necessary to protect the patient from hurting himself/herself, and the family will need to be involved.
3. Acknowledge that the suicide attempt is taken very seriously and that the patient must have felt desperate to have done something so drastic.
4. Offer to help find ways to resolve the difficulties that led to the suicide attempt, even though the

patient may feel hopeless and helpless. Most children and adolescents who make suicide attempts do so because at the time, they feel their dilemma is unsolvable.

5. Avoid statements that could be interpreted as critical or punitive. Many suicide attempts occur after a negative confrontation with parents or after a disciplinary crisis in which the child feels criticized and humiliated. In addition, some parents, rather than being sympathetic to the child's plight, become angry with him or her for making the suicide attempt.

6. Ask directly about suicidal ideas and preoccupations, previous attempts, current wishes and plans: Are you sorry you didn't succeed? Do you feel like making another attempt? Do you wish you were dead?

FAMILY ASSESSMENT

Interview parents both with the patient and separately, and evaluate:

1. Overall family functioning: level of discord, changes in family composition, family socioeconomic status, any serious health problems in family members

2. Parents' understanding of the suicide attempt: Do they appreciate the seriousness of the situation, do they see it as a manifestation of underlying difficulties in their child, or do they deny that it is a serious problem?

3. Are they sympathetic to their child's plight and interested in helping the child? Or are they primarily accusatory and critical of their child, seeing the child as bad or defiant and causing a range of problems in the family?

4. Are the parents willing to agree to and participate in further psychiatric assessment and treatment for their child and the family?

Disposition ■

There are no reliable and consistent predictors of suicidal behavior, especially in children and adolescents. Whenever possible, develop the disposition plan after the medical crisis is treated, in collaboration with a mental health specialist.

Hospitalize the patient in the pediatric unit if there is any doubt regarding the patient's continued suicidal potential or the family's/environment's ability to support and protect the patient. Immediate hospitalization:

1. Protects the patient from further suicidal acts
2. Removes the patient from precipitating stresses
3. Provides the opportunity to assess the overall situation from different perspectives
4. Provides the opportunity to evaluate changes in the family equilibrium as a result of the attempt
5. Allows time to work out appropriate follow-up arrangements (e.g., inpatient psychiatric hospitalization, outpatient treatment, a change in living arrangements)
6. Emphasizes to both child and parent the seriousness of the suicide attempt and the need for follow-up intervention
7. Allows time to secure the parents' and child's co-operation in the follow-up plan

Consider referral for *psychiatric* hospitalization when:

1. The patient continues to express suicidal ideas and wishes. For seriously suicidal patients, the fact that they failed in the attempt adds to their sense of failure.
2. The attempt was planned and done in a manner to minimize the chances of discovery or rescue.
3. Parental support is minimal or absent, or parents are openly hostile to the patient.
4. There is a history of depression and previous suicide attempts.
5. The method used in the attempt was especially dangerous, and the patient was clearly aware of the lethality of the method (e.g., using a firearm, attempted hanging, massive overdose of dangerous drug).
6. A suicide note was left indicating a commitment to die.

Discharge the patient to family and outpatient follow-up care if:

1. The patient denies continuing suicidal ideation and plans.
2. The suicide attempt was impulsive, not planned, and done in such a way as to guarantee discovery.
3. The patient does not appear to be seriously depressed.
4. The patient agrees to cooperate with the mental health follow-up plan.
5. The parents are supportive of the patient and agree to observe and to support the follow-up plan.
6. A mental health follow-up appointment is arranged before the patient is discharged.

Compliance with follow-up care is greatly enhanced if a specific appointment is made for the patient before leaving the emergency department or hospital. Establish some arrangement to provide support for the parents and family of the seriously suicidal child or adolescent (*e.g.*, a social worker in the pediatric unit, the physician him/herself, or the mental health system).

Bibliography ■

Eisenberg L: Adolescent suicide: Or taking arms against a sea of troubles. *Pediatrics* 1980; 66:315.

Litt IF, Cuskey WR, Rudd S: Emergency room evaluation of the adolescent who attempts suicide. *J Adolesc Health Care* 1983; 9:106.

Marks A: Management of the suicidal adolescent on a non-psychiatric adolescent unit. *J Pediatr* 1979; 95:305.

Pfeffer CR: *The Suicidal Child*. New York: Guilford, 1986.

Shaffer D, Fisher P: The epidemiology of suicide in children and young adolescents. *J Am Acad Child Psych* 1981; 20: 545.

Sudak HS, Ford AB, Rushforth NB, eds: *Suicide in the Young*. Boston: PSG-Wright, 1988.

132 Medicolegal Issues

Aidan R. Gough

The practice of pediatric emergency medicine inevitably involves exposure to legal risks, some of which are inherent in any emergency practice and some of which are particular to, and are exacerbated by, the patient's status as a minor. This chapter will identify the major risk areas and suggest means for reducing or controlling them. Because state laws vary widely and synoptic treatment is difficult, generally accepted legal principles and standards are presented.

The Standard of Care ■

A physician has the duty to "use that degree of care and skill which is expected of a reasonably competent practitioner in the same class to which (s)he belongs, acting in the same or similar circumstances." (*Blair vs. Eblen,* 461 S.W. 2d 370, 376, Ky. 1970). An unexcused or unjustified failure to use that degree of care and skill will expose the practitioner to legal liability. The trend is toward the law's recognition of nationally accepted standards of practice, rather than those rooted in the medical custom of a particular locality.

Medical Negligence ■

Although American laws governing the civil redress of wrongs recognize a number of different kinds of harms, the legal subset of most concern to the healthcare practitioner is that of medical negligence, or medical malpractice law.

To succeed in a suit for medical negligence, a plaintiff must prove four elements:

1. The provider's duty to the patient, which is to meet the standard of care
2. A breach of that duty (that is, a failure to exercise the requisite degree of care and skill)
3. Harm resulting to the patient
4. A causal link between the breach of duty and the harm sustained

The treatment of pediatric emergencies presents significant difficulties. Patients may be very young, and communication directly with the patient may be very difficult. Parents may be upset and frightened or may be very young themselves; their judgment may be impaired through the use of alcohol or other drugs; and they may be poor historians of their child's injury or illness. Communicating with the parents or patient will probably be even more difficult if the encounter takes place in the ED. The atmosphere is often noisy, crowded, and chaotic; waits are likely to be long, particularly with a high volume of patients; registration and other personnel may be impersonal, rude, or overburdened; waiting facilities may be uncomfortable, even dreary; and many parents and patients will not understand why patients who came after them are seen first because of greater acuity. When the patient is finally seen by the physician, the visit may be comparatively brief, and the parents may perceive this as being short-changed. Moreover, the ED physician has probably not seen the child before, so there is no established and continuing relationship of care.

The ED setting places a special burden on the harried clinician to meet the standard of care and to ensure that:

1. Adequate communication is established
2. An appropriate history is taken and examination carried out
3. Suitable rapport is established with the patient and family
4. The examination and treatment are thoroughly documented

Steps taken to ensure these ends are prudent and will help abate anger and fear, which impel litigation.

Statutes of Limitation ■

Every state provides timeframes within which lawsuits must be filed, although the precise periods may vary

602

from state to state. These statutes of limitation present particular problems in pediatric cases because parents may pursue legal actions on behalf of their children (and often, in addition, for vindication of their own rights). Children also have independent rights to pursue legal actions on their own behalf. But because persons below the age of majority cannot sue in their own right, the law provides a period after the attainment of majority (18 years, in most states) within which a patient may sue in his or her own right for treatment rendered when he or she was a minor. This means that clinicians treating children remain vulnerable to claim for much longer periods of time than would be the case if the patient were an adult. That extended susceptibility underscores the importance of thorough documentation.

Child Abuse Reporting ■

Every state requires clinicians and hospitals to report to specified authorities instances of suspected child abuse or neglect, including child sexual abuse (see Chapter 129). Statutes commonly require reporting both by telephone and in writing, and they impose specific duties to report on large numbers of persons: clinicians, pre-hospital care personnel, law-enforcement officers, teachers, counselors, and ministers. Failure to report carries criminal penalties as well as civil liability and may also result in loss of licensure for health-care providers. Liability in these cases is often found in a "second-strike" situation in which a child has sustained harm that arguably could have been averted if an earlier instance or condition had been reported as required. This liability can extend to third persons who have never been seen by the provider, if injury to that person could have been forestalled by a timely report of harm to the original patient. *In virtually all states, persons with a duty to report suspected child abuse or neglect are immune from liability for a mistaken report or if abuse or neglect is not substantiated.*

When a number of persons are involved in a case (paramedics, nurses, physicians, etc.) and each has a duty to report, one telephone call and one written report will usually suffice for all, but it is essential to make the required reports. Too often, it is assumed wrongly that someone else is making the reports. This may be a particular problem in an ED setting when pediatric services are called in to assume care of a child: the ED staff may assume that pediatrics will make the report, and vice versa. As a result, no one reports, and all are in violation of the law.

Consent and Refusal of Care ■

Consent issues present some of the most durable and vexing problems encountered in pediatric emergencies. The law's basic tenet, based on constitutionally protected rights of privacy and personal autonomy, is that an adult patient in possession of her or his faculties has an inviolable right "to determine what shall be done with his own body" (*Schloendorff v. Soc. of N.Y. Hosp.*, 211 N.Y. 125, 129, 105 N.E. 92, 93, 1914). Since children below the age of majority are not adults and lack the legal capacity to make decisions about their care, parents exercise those rights in the child's place and stead.

The right to consent—and the correlative right to decline to consent and to refuse care—is exercised in three different forms, as shown in Table 132-1.

American law requires not only that the patient or a legal surrogate must have consented to examination and the proposed medical intervention, but also requires that such consent must be informed. This essentially means that, in order to be valid, a consent must be grounded upon, and the person consenting must have received, sufficient information about the condition requiring intervention and the risks and

TABLE 132–1. *Types of Consent*

Type of Consent	Definition	Example
Express consent	Manifested permission to treat—verbal, signature, or conduct (presenting for treatment, no objection when able to object)	Minor fully or partially emancipated (married, court order, on active duty with armed forces, presents with STD)
Implied consent	Cannot obtain substituted consent of parent or guardian; minor's condition may endanger life, health, or physical function unless intervention	Minor unconscious; or unknown ingestion; fractured radius and unable to reach parent/guardian
Substituted derivative, or surrogate consent	Parent, guardian, or court has legal right to consent on minor's behalf.	Parent or guardian presents with minor, and child receives care.

benefits of the proposed treatment as opposed to other courses of action, including the alternative of no intervention at all.

Since parents have the legal right to provide substituted consent for the care of their children, it is primarily they (or another legal surrogate, such as a legal guardian) who must be informed, although dictates of prudence and good medical care require that the child receive explanations as well, tailored to his or her ability to comprehend. The duty to inform and to explain rests with the physician and cannot be delegated to other personnel. This is especially important (and too often overlooked in a highly fractionated and specialized teaching center practice) because the scope of consent, and of the information that must be conveyed and assented to, includes not only what is to be done, but the person(s) by whom it will be performed.

The optimal legal standard thus requires that enough information and advice be given to a person fully empowered to consent to permit the latter to make a reasoned decision about the course of care, even if in fact that decision turns out to be unreasonable. However, the exigencies of emergency practice often make the giving of such information impossible, and some states have recognized this by enacting laws limiting the liability of physicians for failure to obtain informed consents in truly emergent cases.

In pediatric emergency care, the problems are often compounded because the actual caretaker of the child may not be a parent, legal guardian, or other legally authorized surrogate. Siblings, grandparents, aunts, uncles, cousins, neighbors, or other friends may have physical care of the child, but they are not legal surrogates unless they are so designated by the parents in writing (and even this is not effective in all states) or by court order. *Make and document all reasonable efforts to reach a parent or other legal representative.*

In short, where the child's condition permits, informed consent should be obtained from the parent or other legally authorized representative. Where the child's condition does not permit this, and lasting harm or impairment may result if prompt and appropriate medical intervention is not accomplished, institute care under the rubric of implied consent. The policies of many hospitals mandate that in such cases, consultation should be obtained from another physician and both physicians should document in the medical record their concurrence that timely intervention is required. Even if this is not spelled out by hospital policy, it is a prudent practice.

If the child's condition is actually or potentially serious, although not immediately urgent, and the parents refuse consent to treatment, contact hospital counsel at once to obtain a court order for treatment.

Every ED should have established policies and procedures detailing these steps. However, if immediate care is required to avert serious harm, notify law-enforcement or child protective services, and provide necessary treatment on the basis of implied consent.

Also seek legal counsel when a child's condition is not urgent but warrants treatment, and a parent or legally authorized surrogate cannot be found within a reasonable time. If there is doubt as to whether delay will harm the child, institute treatment on the basis of implied consent.

In all instances, scrupulously document the circumstances leading to the decision to treat. When a child requires treatment, a parent's or guardian's refusal of care itself may represent child neglect, thus requiring a report to appropriate authorities.

Emancipated and Mature Minors ∎

Although the criteria for inclusion may differ, every state recognizes a class of minors who are legally able to act as adults and contract for and consent to their own medical care, even though they have not yet attained adult age. Those minors are *emancipated*. At common law, emancipation was accomplished by court order, or when a parent formally gave up the right to the child's earnings. Today, the marriage of a minor also works an emancipation, and married minors are able to act as adults with respect to their medical care. Pregnancy also commonly emancipates a minor for the purpose of procuring medical care and other necessities of life, although there is some divergence state-to-state as to whether the minor retains that status after the child is born. Active-duty status in the armed forces emancipates a minor, at least to the extent that the minor has the power to consent to or to refuse medical care.

Additionally, and largely stemming back to the widespread incidence of youthful runaways in the 1960s, many states have laws, often called "mature minor statutes," that recognize other situations in which a minor alone has the power to consent to his or her medical care. These may include situations in which the child is living apart from the parents or when a minor seeks treatment for drug abuse or sexually transmitted diseases. The legal effect of these statutes is to establish a partial or limited emancipation for children who fit the criteria, empowering them to arrange their own health care. Table 132-2 delineates the statutes operative in California, a state with a more complex and elaborate statutory scheme than most. Some exceptions recognized there may not be found in other jurisdictions.

TABLE 132–2. *Parental Consent and Medical Treatment of Minors (under age 18) Under California Law (January 1989)*

Civil Code Section	Parental Consent Not Needed for Care in Non–Life-Threatening Situations
25.5	Seventeen years or older may donate blood without parental consent
25.6	Lawfully married, divorced, or had an annulment
25.7	On active duty with armed forces
25.8	Parent has given written authorization to procure medical care to any adult (over 18) taking care of minor.
25.9	Twelve years or older may get mental health treatment as outpatient if mature enough to participate in treatment and (1) would present danger of serious physical or mental harm to self or others without counseling, or (2) has been alleged victim of incest or child abuse.
34.5	Seeks *prevention or treatment* of pregnancy (does *not* include sterilization or abortion)
34.6	Fifteen years or older, living separate and apart from parent
34.7	Minor is 12 years or older and may have an STD or a reportable disease.
34.8	Twelve years or older is alleged victim of rape.
34.9	Victim of a sexual assault (applies to both boys and girls and has no age limit)
34.10	Twelve years or older and seeks care for drug- or alcohol-related problem.
63(a)	Minor 14 years or older is emancipated by declaration of Superior Court.

Medical Information ■

As a general rule, a person who has the power to consent to medical treatment also has the right to receive medical information about the patient's condition. *If a minor is emancipated or empowered under "mature minors" laws to procure care on his or her own, information about medical intervention should not be released to parents without the patient's written permission.*

Documentation ■

Appropriate, thorough documentation is an essential part of medical care. The legal standard, essentially, is that if something is not charted, it did not exist or it was not done.

First, every patient has the right to an adequate medical record to ensure continuity of care. Second, a comprehensible, thorough medical record is vital for the provider's protection, because that record is the principal (indeed, the only acceptable) evidence of the assessment and treatment of the patient. These injunctions lie with special force in cases of pediatric emergencies, in light of the extended statutes of limitation and the fact that the clinician is most often dealing with substituted consent for treatment given by the parents.

The medical record must:

1. Clearly identify the patient
2. Indicate how, when, and with whom the patient arrived at the ED or other location for care. Any pre-hospital care rendered must be described in accurate detail.
3. Contain a concise but thorough history of the present illness
4. Carefully reflect the results of a complete physical examination, including weight, vital signs repeated as needed, physical findings, and clinical observations
5. Contain the orders for and the results of any diagnostic tests ordered
6. Clearly indicate any diagnostic impressions
7. Fully record procedures undertaken and treatments administered
8. Clearly show the final disposition and the child's condition on discharge
9. Detail any follow-up instructions. Carefully explain these to the parents or other responsible caretaker, and document that explanation. It is helpful to have copies of the after-care instructions in the chart and to have a statement signed by the parents or other responsible party attesting to their understanding of the instructions and their willingness to carry them out.

If the child is not accompanied by a parent or other legally responsible adult, all reasonable attempts must be made to reach the parents, including, in some cases, the use of police or other agencies. These actions must be documented, including times of request and persons spoken to. If telephone consent is obtained, that consent must be recorded and witnessed, and all pertinent data recorded, including the times, persons spoken to, and the identity of the witnesses. If the parents cannot be reached, try to reach other responsible adult family members, even though they do not have the legal power to consent to treatment. Provide intervention on the basis of implied consent in such cases, depending on the urgency of the child's condition. Relatives may be able to help locate parents and can help establish that reasonable attempts were made to contact the parents.

As in other instances of medical documentation, avoid flippant colloquial, jocular, or jargonistic remarks: such comments as "FLK" (for "funny-looking kid") have absolutely no place in a proper medical record. Use only readily understandable and commonly recognized abbreviations approved by the facility and generally customary in medical practice. If correction or emendation is necessary, make it in an approved manner, by singly lining out the erroneous entry so that the original remains readable. The added or corrected entry should be dated, timed, and signed by the person making it.

Transfers of Care ∎

Recent federal and state laws forbid the inappropriate transfers of emergency patients where the deferrals of care are occasioned by financial considerations and are not based on the patient's need for medical treatment and the transferring hospital's abilities to provide the level of care required (42 U.S. Code Ann. §§ 1395 et seq., Supp. 1989). These strictures apply to both children and adults. When transfer is appropriate, there must be consultation with, and agreement to assume care by, a suitable physician at the receiving facility. The transfer must be made by medically appropriate means (e.g., ambulance if required), and the reasons and arrangements for transfer, as well as the agreement of the receiving facility,

must be thoroughly documented. Transfer is a form of treatment, and consent must be obtained from the parent or legal guardian.

Telephonic Advice ∎

The issue of telephonic advice arises frequently in pediatric emergency practice, and the only safe legal counsel is that it should *not* be given. This is especially true when there is not an ongoing physician-patient relationship (as is usual in the ED) and the child or caller is a stranger to the physician. No matter how well-intentioned the caller and the person giving the advice may be, a practitioner cannot adequately assess what he or she cannot examine, and advice without examination is medicolegally perilous.

The only appropriate response to such requests is to advise the caller that the practitioner or facility will be happy to evaluate the child if the child is brought in, but that evaluation cannot be done competently over the telephone.

Sometimes, when the patient or family is known to the physician, it is difficult to withhold telephonic advice. In these cases, records in writing and/or tape recordings are essential if any advice is given. In every case, the practitioner must suggest a standard visit to the ED or office, and the advice must be only for interim care in the setting of minor complaints.

Bibliography ∎

Appelbaum PS, Lidz CW, Meisel A: *Informed Consent & Clinical Practice.* New York: Oxford University Press, 1987.

George JE: *Law & Emergency Care.* St. Louis: CV Mosby, 1980.

Holder AR: *Legal Issues in Pediatrics & Adolescent Medicine,* 2nd ed. New Haven: Yale University Press, 1985.

King JH Jr: *The Law of Medical Malpractice,* 2nd ed. St. Paul: West, 1986.

Selbst SM: Medicolegal aspects. In: Luten R, ed: *Problems in Pediatric Emergency Medicine.* New York: Churchill-Livingstone, 1988.

XIII

Quick
Reference

133 Age-Adjusted Vital Signs

Ronald A. Dieckmann

Careful initial and serial recording of vital signs is paramount in the evaluation, follow-up, and treatment of most children visiting the ED. Table 133-1 lists the expected vital signs for normal children of various ages.

TABLE 133–1. *Age-adjusted Vital Signs*

Age	Mean Wt. in Kg.	Minimum Syst. BP	Normal HR	Normal RR
Premature	2.5	40	120–170	40–60
Term	3.5	50	100–170	40–60
3 mo	6	50	100–170	30–50
6 mo	8	60	100–170	30–50
1 yr	10	65	100–170	30–40
2 yr	13	65	100–160	20–30
4 yr	15	70	80–130	20
6 yr	20	75	70–115	16
8 yr	25	80	70–110	16
10 yr	30	85	60–105	16
12 yr	40	90	60–100	16

134 Growth Curves

Ronald A. Dieckmann

Evaluating pediatric illness usually includes assessing physical growth. Plotting the age-specific growth characteristics of the child on the following curves (Figures 134-1 through 134-8) provides a gross measure of individual physical development against national percentiles. Ninety-four percent of normal children will fall between the 3rd and 97th percentiles, or between −2 standard deviations and +2 standard deviations from the population mean.

However, evaluating growth parameters systematically *over time* in the same child is more accurate, because ethnic and socioeconomic backgrounds exert a powerful influence on a child's percentile growth ratings. Deviations from established patterns of growth are important clues to system insult.

The following growth charts provide curves for the 5th, 10th, 25th, 50th, 75th, 90th, and 95th percentiles for height, weight, head circumference, and physical growth in boys and girls age 0 to 36 months; then height, weight, and physical growth in boys and girls age 2 to 18 years.

(Adapted from Hamill PVV, Drizd TA, Johnson CL, et al: Physical Growth: National Center for Health Statistics percentiles. *Am J Clin Nutr* 1979; 32: 607–629.)

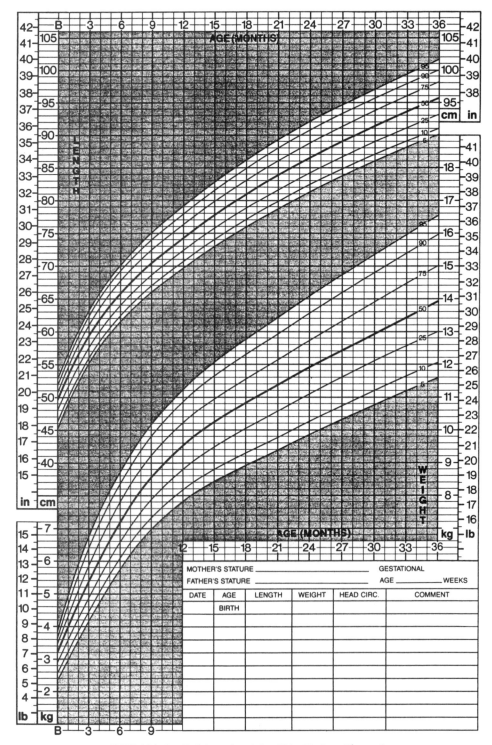

FIGURE 134–1. Height and weight. Girls: Birth to 36 months.

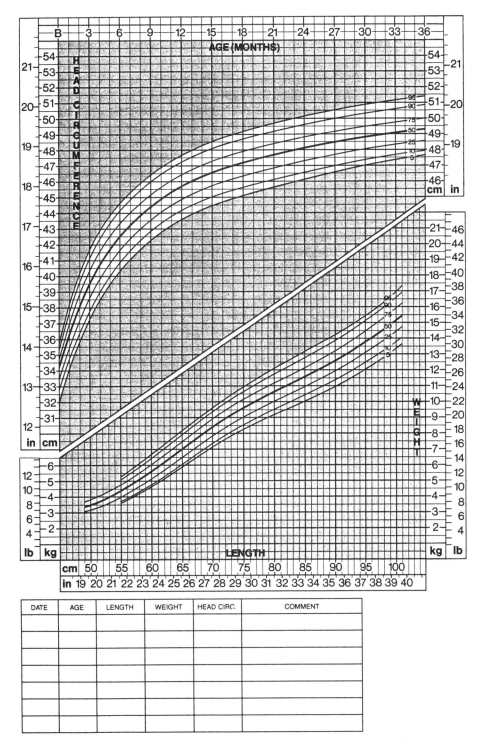

FIGURE 134–2. Head circumference and physical growth. Girls: Birth to 36 months.

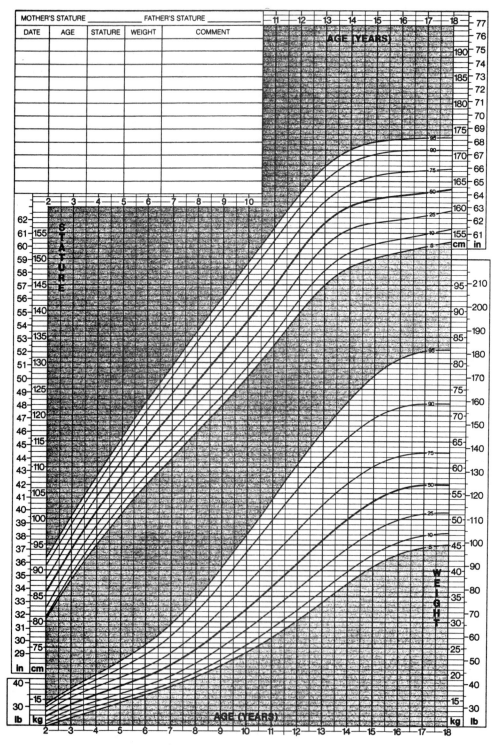

FIGURE 134–3. Height and weight. Girls: 2 to 18 years.

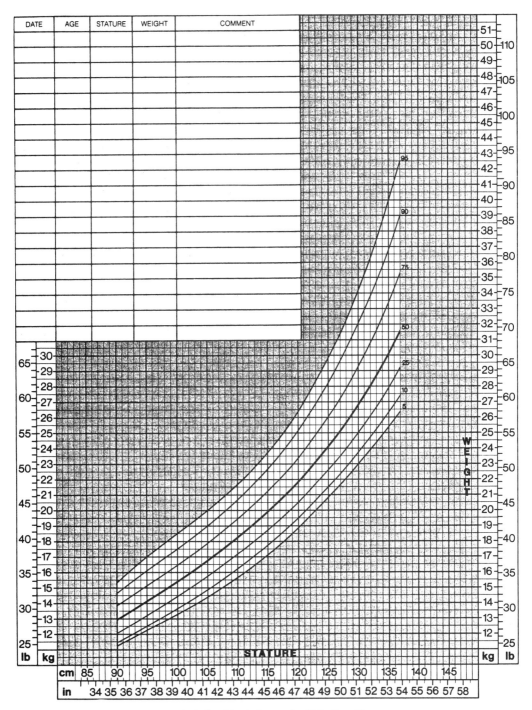

FIGURE 134–4. Physical growth. Girls: 2 to 18 years.

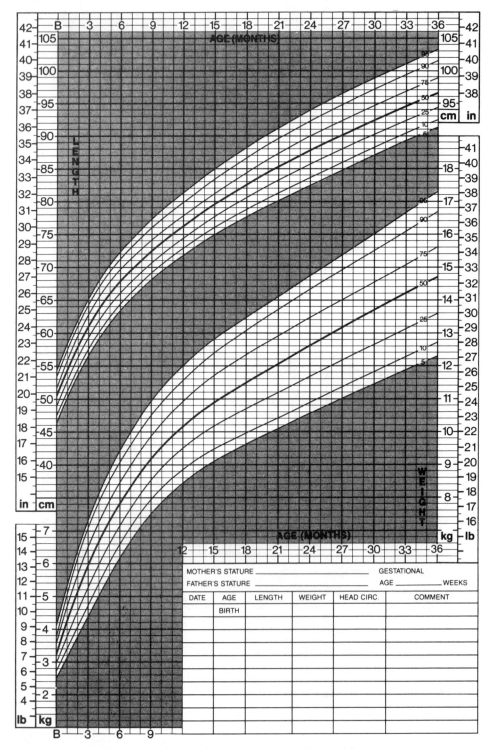

FIGURE 134–5. Height and weight. Boys: Birth to 36 months.

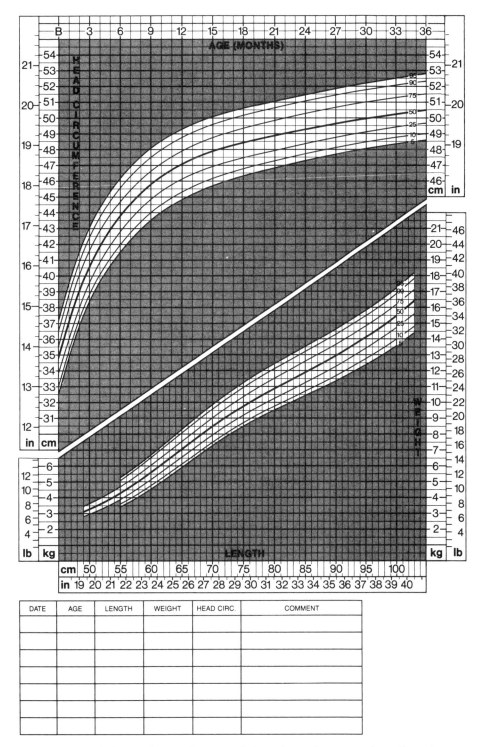

FIGURE 134–6. Head circumference and physical growth. Boys: Birth to 36 months.

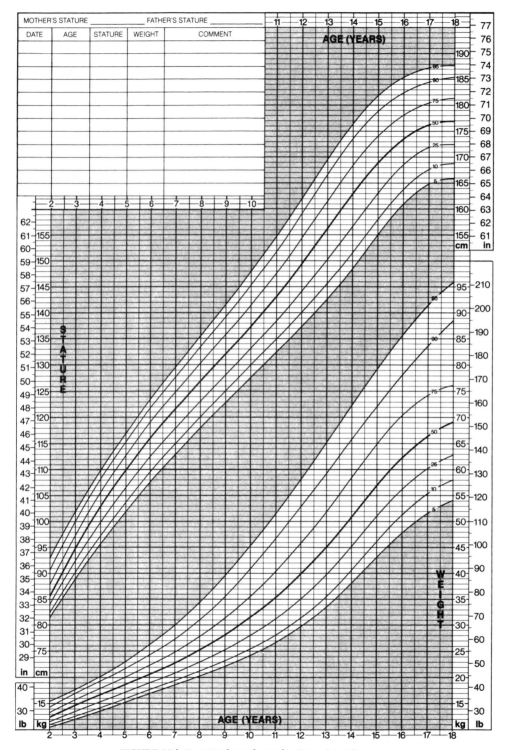

FIGURE 134–7. Height and weight. Boys: 2 to 18 years.

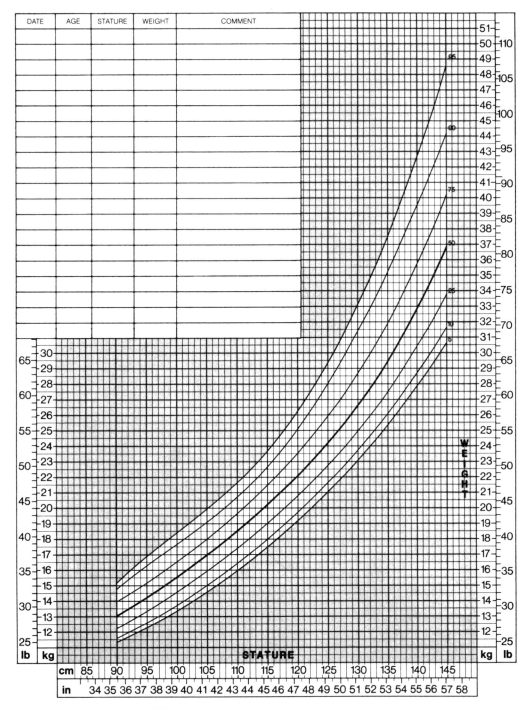

FIGURE 134–8. Physical growth. Boys: 2 to 18 years.

135 Denver Developmental Screening Test

Ronald A. Dieckmann

Assessing a child's developmental status is part of a thorough evaluation of pediatric illness. Appreciating appropriate age-related developmental stage also permits an optimal approach to overall assessment of the sick or injured child (see Chapter 3). The Denver Developmental Screening Test (DDST) is a rapid, accurate method of evaluating developmental status in children 0 to 6 years of age. The DDST has been standardized on a large cross-section of Denver children. The following are simple instructions, followed by the test itself, then the legend.

Test Materials ■

Skein of red wool; box of raisins; rattle with a narrow handle; small clear glass bottle with ⅝" opening; bell; tennis ball; test form; pencil; 8 one-inch cubical, colored (red, blue, yellow, green) blocks.

General Instructions ■

Tell the parent that this is a developmental screening device to obtain an estimate of the child's level of development, and that the child is not expected to perform each of the test items. This test relies on observations of what the child can do and on the report of a parent who knows the child. Use direct observation whenever possible. Since the test requires active participation by the child, make every effort to put the child at ease. The younger child may be tested while sitting on the parent's lap; this should be done in such a way that he or she can comfortably reach the test materials on the table.

Give the test before doing any frightening or painful procedures. It may be started by laying out one or two test materials in front of the child while asking the parent whether the child performs some of the personal-social items. Administer the first few test items well below the child's age level in order to ensure an initial successful experience. To avoid distractions, remove all test materials from the table except those required for the test being given.

Steps in Administering the Test ■

1. Draw a vertical line on the examination sheet through the four sectors (personal-social, fine motor-adaptive, language, and gross motor) to represent the child's chronologic age. Place the date of the examination at the top of the age line. For children who were born prematurely, subtract the number of months of prematurity from the chronologic age.
2. The items to be administered are those through which the child's chronologic age line passes, unless there are obvious deviations. In each sector, establish the area in which the child passes all the items and the point at which he or she fails all the items.
3. If the child refuses to do some of the items requested by the examiner, have the parent administer the item in the prescribed manner.
4. If a child passes an item, write a large letter "P" on the bar. "F" designates a failure, and "R" designates a refusal.
5. Note how the child adjusted to the examination (*i.e.*, cooperation, attention span, self-confidence) and how he or she related to the parent, the examiner, and the test materials.
6. Ask the parent if the child's performance was typical of his or her performance at other times.
7. To retest the child on the same form, use a different color pencil for the scoring and age line.
8. Instructions for administering footnoted items are on the back of the test form.

DIRECTIONS

DATE
NAME
BIRTHDATE
HOSP. NO.

1. Try to get child to smile by smiling, talking or waving to him. Do not touch him.
2. When child is playing with toy, pull it away from him. Pass if he resists.
3. Child does not have to be able to tie shoes or button in the back.
4. Move yarn slowly in an arc from one side to the other, about 6" above child's face. Pass if eyes follow 90° to midline. (Past midline; 180°)
5. Pass if child grasps rattle when it is touched to the backs or tips of fingers.
6. Pass if child continues to look where yarn disappeared or tries to see where it went. Yarn should be dropped quickly from sight from tester's hand without arm movement.
7. Pass if child picks up raisin with any part of thumb and a finger.
8. Pass if child picks up raisin with the ends of thumb and index finger using an over hand approach.

9. Pass any enclosed form. Fail continuous round motions.

10. Which line is longer? (Not bigger.) Turn paper upside down and repeat. (3/3 or 5/6)

11. Pass any crossing lines.

12. Have child copy first. If failed, demonstrate.

When giving items 9, 11 and 12, do not name the forms. Do not demonstrate 9 and 11.

13. When scoring, each pair (2 arms, 2 legs, etc.) counts as one part.
14. Point to picture and have child name it. (No credit is given for sounds only.)

  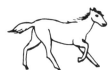

15. Tell child to: Give block to Mommie; put block on table; put block on floor. Pass 2 of 3. (Do not help child by pointing, moving head or eyes.)
16. Ask child: What do you do when you are cold? ..hungry? ..tired? Pass 2 of 3.
17. Tell child to: Put block on table; under table; in front of chair, behind chair. Pass 3 of 4. (Do not help child by pointing, moving head or eyes.)
18. As child: If fire is hot, ice is ?; Mother is a woman, Dad is a ?; a horse is big, a mouse is ?. Pass 2 of 3.
19. Ask child: What is a ball? ..lake? ..desk? ..house? ..banana? ..curtain? ..ceiling? ..hedge? ..pavement? Pass if defined in terms of use, shape, what it is made of or general category (such as banana is fruit, not just yellow). Pass 6 of 9.
20. Ask child: What is a spoon made of? ..a shoe made of? ..a door made of? (No other objects may be substituted.) Pass 3 of 3.
21. When placed on stomach, child lifts chest off table with support of forearms and/or hands.
22. When child is on back, grasp his hands and pull him to sitting. Pass if head does not hang back.
23. Child may use wall or rail only, not person. May not crawl.
24. Child must throw ball overhand 3 feet to within arm's reach of tester.
25. Child must perform standing broad jump over width of test sheet (8½ inches)
26. Tell child to walk forward, ⊂◯⊃⊂◯◯⊃➤ heel within 1 inch of toe. Tester may demonstrate. Child must walk 4 consecutive steps, 2 out of 3 trials.
27. Bounce ball to child who should stand 3 feet away from tester. Child must catch ball with hands, not arms, 2 out of 3 trials.
28. Tell child to walk backward, ◀⊂◯⊃⊂◯◯⊃ toe within 1 inch of heel. Tester may demonstrate. Child must walk 4 consecutive steps, 2 out of 3 trials.

DATE AND BEHAVIORAL OBSERVATIONS (how child feels at time of test, relation to tester, attention span, verbal behavior, self-confidence, etc.):

FIGURE 135–1. Denver Developmental Screening Test. (Reproduced with permission from LADOCA Project and Publishing Foundation, Inc., East 51st Avenue and Lincoln Street, Denver, Colorado)

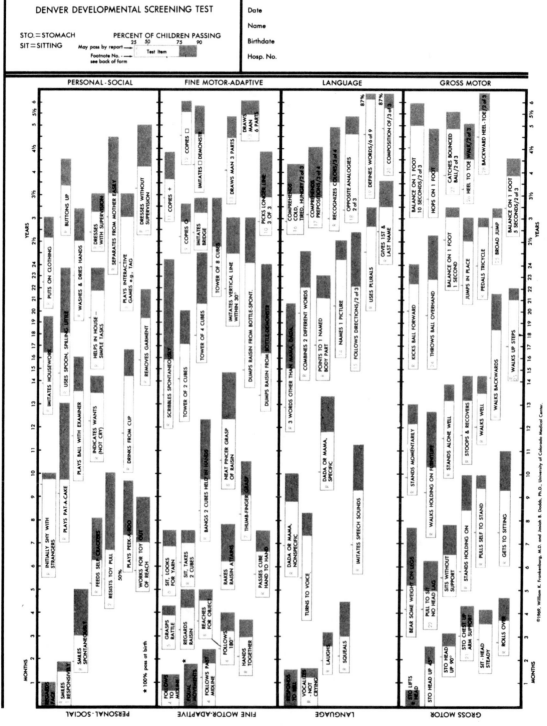

FIGURE 135-1. (Continued)

Interpretation ■

The test items are placed into four categories: personal-social, fine motor-adaptive, language, and gross motor. Each test item is designated by a bar located under the age scale so as to indicate clearly the ages at which 25%, 50%, 75%, and 90% of the standardization population could perform the particular item. The left end of the bar designates the age at which 25% of the standardization population could perform the item, the hatch mark at the top of the bar 50%, the left end of the shaded area 75%, and the right end of the bar 90% (see below).

Failure to perform an item passed by 90% of children of the same age should be considered a delay. Such a failure may be emphasized by coloring the right end of the bar of the failed item. Performances are scored as:

1. *Abnormal* if two or more sectors have two or more delays, or if one sector has two or more delays and one other sector has one delay, and in the same sector the age line does not intersect one item that is passed

2. *Questionable* if any one sector has two or more delays, or if one or more sectors have one delay *and* in the same sectors the age line does not intersect an item that is passed

3. *Untestable* if refusals occur in numbers large enough to cause the test to be questionable or abnormal if the refusals were scored as failures

4. *Normal* if the performance is not abnormal, questionable, or untestable

136 Blood Component Therapy

Pearl T. Toy

Because artificial blood cells are not currently available, blood is still a limited resource. The blood supply, primarily donated by unpaid community volunteers, today is safer than ever, although some risks remain.

The Bleeding Patient ■

In the ED, blood products are used primarily for bleeding patients (see Chapter 19). Prior to transfusions, evaluate bleeding hemostasis and signs and symptoms of hypovolemia (see Chapter 8). Determine abnormal hemostasis by the history and physical examination.

When abnormal bleeding is suspected, a panel of laboratory tests will detect almost all coagulopathies. This panel includes the platelet count, prothrombin time (PT), partial thromboplastin time (PTT), and fibrinogen concentration. Table 136-1 shows levels generally adequate to achieve hemostasis.

Treatment of Hypovolemia ■

Treat acute hypovolemia with crystalloid with or without packed red cells. The use of whole blood is controversial. Never use fresh-frozen plasma as a volume expander.

Crystalloid solutions (normal saline solutions given in amounts approximately three times the volume deficit) will restore blood volume. Colloid solutions provide oncotic pressure but may have side effects, including pulmonary edema (albumin), hypotension (plasma protein fraction), and hemostatic abnormalities (dextran, hydroxyethyl starch).

Packed red cells and crystalloid, rather than whole blood, is the treatment of choice in patients who bleed less than one blood volume. However, in patients who lose more than one blood volume, the safety and efficacy of using packed red cells and crystalloid alone without whole blood or plasma are unknown. If whole blood or modified whole blood is used, prophylactic plasma transfusions are unnecessary.

In emergencies, ABO and Rh-identical (type-specific) blood should be available 5 to 10 minutes after the blood bank receives a patient blood specimen. Universal donor blood (O-negative packed red cells) is limited resource and must be reserved for extreme emergencies. O-positive packed cells are almost always acceptable in dire emergencies but may cause sensitization in women of child-bearing age. Rarely, previously sensitized individuals receiving Rh-positive packed cells experience hypersensitivity reactions.

Autologous salvaged blood can be reinfused within 4 hours from the start of collection. Do not salvage autologous blood that may be contaminated with bacteria from the gastrointestinal tract or with malignant cells.

Patients With Abnormal Hemostasis ■

PLATELET CONCENTRATES

Platelet concentrates are available as a regular or a pheresis unit. A regular unit of platelets is made from a unit of whole blood from one donor. A pheresis unit contains the equivalent of platelets from about six units of whole blood. In the pheresis process, blood is removed from the donor and centrifuged in a pheresis machine. A component such as platelets is removed, and the rest of the blood is returned to the donor. Regular and pheresis platelets are used interchangeably, depending on availability.

Give therapeutic platelet transfusions to patients who are bleeding and who have a platelet count of less than $50,000/\mu L$, if bleeding is not self-limited and cannot be controlled by surgical correction. Bleeding due to an anatomic defect must be corrected by surgery and will not cease with platelet transfusion alone.

TABLE 136–1. *Evaluation of Hemostasis*

Laboratory Test	Generally Adequate Levels
Platelet count	≥50–100,000/μL
Prothrombin/partial thromboplastin time	<1.5 times normal
Fibrinogen	≥100 mg/dL

Do *not* give prophylactic platelet transfusions in massively transfused patients who do not have clinical abnormal bleeding.

The initial dose of platelets is about one unit per 10 kg body weight to raise the platelet count by approximately 50,000/μL. Obtain platelet counts before transfusion and within 1 hour post-transfusion to adjust the dose and to monitor efficacy.

FRESH-FROZEN PLASMA (FFP)

Suspect multiple coagulation factor deficiency in a patient with prolonged PT and PTT, if the prolongations are not due to a single coagulation factor deficiency, heparin, or another inhibitor. Causes of multiple coagulation factor deficiency include liver disease, massive transfusion, disseminated intravascular coagulation (DIC), and plasmapheresis. Consider using FFP in such patients if they have abnormal bleeding and have PT or PTT more than 1.5 times normal and platelet counts above 50,000 to 70,000/μL, if the bleeding cannot be controlled by sutures or cautery.

Give FFP at the time of bleeding or within an hour of the anticipated bleeding. The maximal effect of FFP declines 2 to 4 hours after transfusion; therefore, to assess the efficacy of FFP transfusion, determine PT and PTT immediately before the transfusion and within 2 hours post-transfusion.

CRYOPRECIPITATE AND FACTOR CONCENTRATES

Obtain hematology consultation in patients who have hypofibrinogenemia and need cryoprecipitate, or who have congenital coagulation disorders such as hemophilia and need coagulation factor concentrates.

Immunocompromised Patients ■

Immunocompromised patients may need special blood products such as cytomegalovirus (CMV) an-tibody-negative blood or irradiated blood products. CMV infection transmitted by transfusion is usually asymptomatic except in immunocompromised patients. If such patients (*e.g.*, premature infants, bone-marrow transplant recipients) are CMV antibody-negative, give them CMV antibody-negative donor blood. These and other patients (*e.g.*, some leukemia and lymphoma patients) should also receive irradiated blood products. Irradiation inactivates donor lymphocytes and prevents graft-versus-host disease.

Transfusion Reactions ■

FEVER

The cause of febrile reactions is recipient antibody in previously transfused or pregnant patients against donor white cells, which are present in packed red cells, whole blood platelet concentrates, and granulocyte concentrates. For subsequent transfusions, premedicate the patient with antipyretics. Use leukocyte-poor blood products for patients who have had febrile reactions to two or more units.

HEMOLYTIC REACTION

The most common cause of an acute hemolytic reaction is giving the wrong unit of red cells, and the donor and recipient are ABO incompatible. Patients may be confused because of some similarity (same name, diagnosis, ethnic origin, etc.) Errors occur when patient blood samples are switched during labeling or testing, or when the patient is not correctly identified before blood is administered.

Symptoms and signs of an acute hemolytic reaction are fever and chills, back or chest pain, shock, burning at the intravenous site, anxiety, or hemoglobinuria. If the patient is unconscious, the reaction may not be recognized until hemolysis leads to shock, DIC, and generalized oozing.

Management is outlined below. Give fluids and mannitol 0.5–1 g/kg intravenously over 5 minutes. Treat shock, DIC, and renal failure if they develop.

URTICARIA

Hives after transfusion are due to reactions to unknown allergens in donor blood. These reactions are benign. Give antihistamines and resume the transfusion slowly.

ANAPHYLAXIS

Anaphylaxis occurs in congenital IgA-deficient recipients who are exposed to IgA in donor plasma.

Prevention consists of use of washed, plasma-free blood products. Blood from donors who are IgA-deficient is rarely necessary.

NONCARDIOGENIC PULMONARY EDEMA

Donors who have been pregnant or transfused may have an antibody to leukocytes. Rarely, these antibodies react with recipient leukocytes, which lodge in the pulmonary microcirculation and cause pulmonary edema. Symptoms include fever and shortness of breath during or hours after a transfusion. Management is supportive. No special blood products are necessary for subsequent transfusions. Leukocyte-poor blood products are not helpful because the cause is the antibody in donor plasma. Plasma-free blood products are unnecessary because most plasma does not cause the reaction. To prevent this rare reaction, some blood centers do not use plasma from multiparous women for transfusion to others.

OTHER RARE REACTIONS

1. Venous air embolism causes cyanosis, respiratory failure, and shock. Put the patient in a head-down, feet-up position on the left side.
2. Sepsis from contaminated blood products occurs rarely in platelet concentrates because they are stored at room temperature.
3. Fluid overload occurs when patients cannot tolerate large volumes given over a short period of time. This may occur in infants and small children, in patients receiving large volumes of plasma to correct coagulopathy, and in patients with minimal anemia who receive preoperatively donated autologous blood because it is available.

Management of Transfusion Reactions ■

1. Stop the transfusion.
2. Change the intravenous set and keep it open with saline.
3. Check for clerical errors.
4. Evaluate the patient and initiate treatment if necessary.
5. Fill in a transfusion reaction form.
6. Draw red- and lavender-top blood samples to repeat pretransfusion testing.
7. Collect first urine sample (for hemoglobinuria).
8. Send unit and samples to the laboratory.

TABLE 136–2. *Tests Performed on Blood Donors*

	Test	
Blood Group	Hepatitis	Other
ABO typing	HBsAg	anti-HIV (AIDS)
Rh typing	anti-HBc	VDRL (syphilis)
Antibody screen	ALT	anti-HTLV-I

Infections Transmitted by Transfusion ■

Table 136-2 shows the tests performed on donor blood to maximize safety to the recipient.

Hepatitis was and is the greatest risk. Donors who give a history of or exposure to hepatitis are excluded. Other measures also help to decrease the hepatitis risk (*e.g.*, testing of donor blood for hepatitis, deferral of donors at risk for AIDS, and decrease in hepatitis in the donor population). The current risk of post-transfusion hepatitis is unknown but is estimated to be about 1:100 or less per unit.

The risk of transfusion-associated AIDS was highest in 1982, but has decreased now that high-risk donors are excluded and donor blood is tested for antibody to human immunodeficiency virus (HIV). Again, the risk of transmission of HIV through seronegative units is unknown but is estimated to be 1:40,000 to 1:1,000,000 per unit.

Syphilis may be transmitted by transfusion via nonrefrigerated blood products such as fresh blood and platelet concentrates. Spirochetes are inactivated by refrigeration. Donors with early active syphilis may be seronegative.

CMV transmitted by transfusion rarely causes symptoms. Morbidity occurs in premature infants under 1200 g who are born of seronegative mothers, and in seronegative bone-marrow transplant recipients. Give such patients CMV antibody-negative blood products.

Theoretically, any other infectious agent in donor blood can be transmitted via transfusion. Rare examples include HTLV-I, malaria, trypanosomes, Epstein-Barr virus, and Yersinia enterocolitis.

Bibliography ■

Fresh-frozen plasma. NIH Consensus Conference. *JAMA* 1985; 253:551.

Perioperative red cell transfusion. NIH Consensus Conference. *JAMA* 1988; 260:2700.

Platelet transfusion therapy. NIH Consensus Conference. *JAMA* 1987; 257:1777.

137 Maintenance Fluid Infusion Rates

Ronald A. Dieckmann

The calculation of daily and hourly maintenance fluid rates is based on the child's body weight. The following table shows appropriate infusion rates for normothermic patients with normal sensible and insensible water losses and normal metabolic status. Maintenance infusion rates must be adjusted for temperature alterations (*e.g.*, fever), abnormal losses (*e.g.*, vomiting, diarrhea, burns), and altered metabolic states (*e.g.* hypothermia, hyperthyroidism). Chapter 22 presents a complete discussion of dehydration in childhood.

TABLE 137–1.

Kg	Ml/hour	Volume (ml/24°)
1	4	100
2	8	200
3	12	300
4	16	400
5	20	500
6	24	600
7	28	700
8	32	800
9	36	900
10	42	1000
12	45	1100
14	50	1200
16	54	1300
18	58	1400
20	62	1500
25	66	1600
30	70	1700
35	76	1800
40	80	1900
45	84	2000

138 Immunoprophylaxis

Moses Grossman

Immunization can be either active or passive. *Active immunization* supplies the child with an antigen (vaccine, toxoid, etc.); the child makes his or her own antibodies. The B cells, once primed, will respond to booster doses or clinical or subclinical infection by making more antibody. *Passive immuni-* *zation,* on the other hand, provides the child with preformed antibodies that have a limited life and are not automatically renewed.

Passive immunization provides the patient with *temporary* immunity. It should be used only if active immunization is unavailable or has not been given

TABLE 138–1. *Preparations Available for Passive Immune Prophylaxis*

Disease	Material Available	Dose	Route	Remarks
Measles	Immune globulin (human)	Prevention 0.25 ml/kg (max 15 ml)	IM	Should be followed by active immunization 8 weeks later
Viral hepatitis type A	Immune globulin (human)	0.02 to 0.04 mg/kg	IM	For household and other close contacts
Viral hepatitis type B	Hepatitis B immune globulin	0.06 ml/kg	IM	For accidental inoculation with infected blood or other material
Varicella zoster	Zoster immune globulin	0.5 mg/kg	IM	For prevention of varicella in severely immunosuppressed children
Tetanus				
Prophylaxis	Tetanus immune globulin	250 to 500 units	IM	Use separate site and syringe if tetanus toxoid is also used.
	Tetanus anti-toxin equine or bovine	3,000 to 5,000 units	IM	Use only if human immune globulin is unavailable. Screen and test for animal hypersensitivity.
Treatment	Tetanus immune globulin	500 to 3,000 units	IM	
	Tetanus anti-toxin equine or bovine	50,000 to 100,000 units	IM	
Diphtheria	Diphtheria antitoxin	40,000 to 100,000 units	IV preferable, IM possible	Sensitivity tests must be performed prior to use. This is equine sera.
Rabies	Human rabies immune globulin	20 IU/kg	IM	Supplied in 2 ml (300 IU) and 10 ml (1500 IU) vials.
	Antirabies serum, equine	40 IU/kg	IV or IM	Second best to human globulin. Screen and test for animal serum hypersensitivity.
Botulism	Trivalent anti-toxin (ABE) and type E antitoxin		IM	Call C.D.C. in Atlanta (404) 639-3356 days, (404) 639-2888 eves & weekends

TABLE 138–2. *Vaccines Available in the United States, by Type and Recommended Routes of Administration*

Vaccine	Type	Route
BCG (Bacillus of Calmette and Guérin)	Live bacteria	Intradermal or SC
Cholera	Inactivated bacteria	SC or intradermal*
DTP	Toxoids and inactivated bacteria	IM
D = diphtheria		
T = tetanus		
P = pertussis		
HB (hepatitis B)	Inactive viral antigen	IM
Haemophilus influenzae b		
Polysaccharide (HbPV)	Bacterial polysaccharide	SC or IM†
Conjugate (HbCV)	Polysaccharide conjugated to protein	IM
Influenza	Inactivated virus or viral components	IM
IPV (Inactivated Poliovirus Vaccine)	Inactivated viruses of all 3 serotypes	SC
Measles	Live virus	SC
Meningococcal	Bacterial polysaccharides of serotypes A/C/Y/W-135	SC
MMR	Live viruses	SC
M = measles		
M = mumps		
R = rubella		
Mumps	Live virus	SC
OPV (Oral Poliovirus Vaccine)	Live viruses of all 3 serotypes	PO
Plague	Inactivated bacteria	IM
Pneumococcal	Bacterial polysaccharides of 23 pneumococcal types	IM or SC
Rabies	Inactivated virus	SC or intradermal‡
Rubella	Live virus	SC
Tetanus	Inactivated toxin (toxoid)	IM§
Td or DT‖	Inactivated toxins (toxoids)	IM§
T = Tetanus		
D or d = Diphtheria		
Typhoid	Inactivated bacteria	SC**
Yellow fever	Live virus	SC

* The intradermal dose is lower.
† Route depends on the manufacturer; consult package insert for recommendation for specific product used.
‡ Intradermal dose is lower and used only for preexposure vaccination.
§ Preparations with adjuvants should be given IM.
‖ DT = tetanus and diphtheria toxoids for use in children aged <7 years. Td = tetanus and diphtheria toxoids for use in pesons aged ≥7 years. Td contains the same amount of tetanus toxoid as DTP or DT but a reduced dose of diphtheria toxoid.
** Boosters may be given intradermally unless acetone-killed and dried vaccine is used.

TABLE 138–3. *Recommended Schedule for Active Immunization of Normal Infants and Children**

Recommended Age	Immunization(s)†	Comments
2 mo	DTP, OPV	Can be initiated as early as age 2 wk in areas of high endemicity or during epidemics
4 mo	DTP, OPV	2-mo interval desired for OPV to avoid interference from previous dose
6 mo	DTP	A third dose of OPV is not indicated in the U.S. but is desirable in geographic areas where polio is endemic.
15 mo	Measles, mumps, rubella (MMR)	MMR preferred to individual vaccines; tuberculin testing may be done at the same visit.
18 mo	DTP,‡§ OPV,¶ PRP-D	See footnotes.
4–6 yr	DTP,‖ OPV	At or before school entry
14–16 yr	Td	Repeat every 10 yr throughout life.

* For all products used, consult manufacturer's package insert for instructions for storage, handling, dosage, and administration. Biologics prepared by different manufacturers may vary, and package inserts of the same manufacturer may change from time to time. Therefore, the physician should be aware of the contents of the current package insert.

† DTP = diphtheria and tetanus toxoids with pertussis vaccine; OPV = oral poliovirus vaccine containing attenuated poliovirus types 1, 2, and 3; MMR = live measles, mumps, and rubella viruses in a combined vaccine (see text for discussion of single vaccines versus combination); PRP-D = *Haemophilus* b diphtheria toxoid conjugate vaccine; Td = adult tetanus toxoid (full dose) and diphtheria toxoid (reduced dose) for adult use.

‡ Should be given 6 to 12 months after the third dose.

§ May be given simultaneously with MMR at age 15 months.

¶ May be given simultaneously with MMR at 15 months of age or at any time between 12 and 24 months of age.

‖ Up to the seventh birthday.

(From American Academy of Pediatrics: *Report of the Committee on Infectious Diseases*. 21st ed. Elk Grove, IL: 1988.)

prior to exposure. Active immunization will not provide protection in the acute setting. The duration of passive protection is short (1 to 6 weeks) and often must be accompanied by or followed by active immunization; untoward reactions may occur with animal sera. Human immune serum globulin is always preferable to animal antisera. Usually, there is no real emergency about administering passive immunization; there should be ample time for specialist consultation.

The most common ED passive immunoprophylaxis is with tetanus immunoglobulin, hepatitis immunoglobulin, and human immune globulin. The most common form of active immunoprophylaxis is tetanus toxoid. See Chapter 123 for a discussion of tetanus.

Human immune globulin is derived from the pooled serum of adults prepared by the Cohn alcohol fractionation procedure. It is sterile, does not transmit hepatitis or human immunodeficiency virus, and is a concentrated solution containing 165 mg/ml. Give ordinary immune globulin intramuscularly into deep muscles. A purified form of intravenous gamma globulin is available for children in whom the intravenous route is preferable. Special immune globulins are unavailable for intravenous use at present.

Human globulin is always preferable to animal sera, but some materials are available only as animal sera. In these instances, perform sensitivity tests to the animal material first. Always be prepared for an anaphylactic reaction when performing the sensitivity test or when administering the animal serum (see Chapter 17).

Table 138-1 lists the preparations available for passive immune prophylaxis. Table 138-2 lists the different vaccines available in the United States. Table 138-3 gives the normal immunization schedule for children in the United States.

139 Emergency Procedures

Ronald A. Dieckmann

Arthrocentesis ■

Arthrocentesis is needle aspiration of joint fluid. Usually this technique is used to evaluate joint space infection, but sometimes it is a therapeutic maneuver to relieve joint pressure that causes severe pain.

INDICATIONS

1. Suspected septic joint
2. Joint effusion of unknown etiology
3. Severe pain from joint effusion of known etiology (*e.g.*, trauma)

EQUIPMENT AND SUPPLIES

Prep solution, sterile gloves and drape
Gown and mask
1% lidocaine
25-gauge ⅝" needle and 3-ml syringe
18- or 20-gauge 1.5" needle
10-ml syringe (30 ml for large effusion)
Three-way stopcock
Sterile specimen tubes

POSITION AND PROCEDURE

Knee (Fig. 139-1)

1. Place the child in the supine position, then extend and stabilize the knee by applying distal traction on the leg. Restrain the young child who cannot cooperate.
2. Gown and mask.
3. Carefully prep and drape the area medially or laterally. Choose the side with the most swelling.
4. Anesthetize the entry site with a 25-gauge needle and lidocaine in a 3-ml syringe.
5. Attach the 18-gauge needle to the 10-ml syringe.
6. Advance the needle underneath the midpoint of the patella and above the patellar groove of the femur, at an angle 15 degrees above the horizontal, while applying negative pressure. Flexing the knee

to about 15 or 20 degrees may ease advancement of the needle.
7. Enter the joint space and evacuate all the fluid. Use stopcock and 30-ml syringe for serial collections.
8. Withdraw the needle, cover the site with a sterile dressing, and immobilize the knee.
9. Send fluid for analysis (see Tables 44-3 and 120-1).

Ankle (Fig. 139-2)

1. Place the child in the supine position with the knee fully extended and the foot stabilized in a plantar-flexed position. Restrain the young child who cannot cooperate.
2. Gown and mask.
3. Carefully prep and drape the area medially or laterally. Choose the side with the most swelling. The medial approach is easier.
4. Anesthetize the entry site with a 25-gauge needle and lidocaine in a 3-ml syringe.
5. Attach the 20-gauge needle to the 10-ml syringe.
6. If the swelling is lateral, advance the needle slightly medial and distal to the distal tip of the fibula (lateral malleolus), while applying negative pressure. The entry site is just medial to the extensor digitorum communis tendon, which can be identified by having the child extend the toes.
7. If the swelling is medial, advance the needle anterior and slightly proximal to the distal end of the tibia (medial malleolus), medial to the extensor hallucis longus tendon, while applying negative pressure. The extensor hallucis longus tendon is easily identified by having the child flex and extend the big toe.
8. After evacuating the joint, withdraw the needle, apply a sterile dressing, and immobilize the ankle.

Elbow (Fig. 139-3)

1. Place the child in the prone position with the forearm held midway between supination and prona-

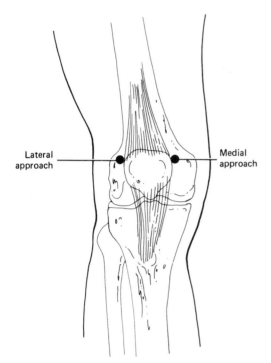

FIGURE 139–1. Entry site for knee arthrocentesis. (From Ho MT, Sanders CE, eds: *Current Emergency Diagnosis and Treatment,* 3rd ed. Los Altos: Lange Medical Publishers, 1990, 834)

tion, and the elbow in a 135-degree extended position. Restrain the young child who cannot cooperate.

2. Mask and gown.
3. Carefully prep and drape the area laterally.
4. Anesthetize the entry site with a 25-gauge needle and lidocaine in a 3-ml syringe.
5. Attach the 20-gauge needle to the 10-ml syringe.
6. Enter the needle at the midpoint of a triangle formed by the lateral epicondyle, olecranon, and radial head. The landmarks may be identified most easily with the elbow extended. Advance the needle at a perpendicular angle while applying negative pressure.
7. After evacuating the joint, withdraw the needle, apply a sterile dressing, and immobilize the elbow.

COMPLICATIONS

1. Bleeding. This complication usually occurs in the child with a bleeding diathesis, especially hemophilia.

2. Joint infection, secondary to improper sterile technique or from aspiration through cellulitis
3. Nerve or blood vessel injury

Needle Cricothyrotomy ■

When tracheal intubation is impossible in a child and surgical cricothyrotomy cannot be immediately performed, needle cricothyrotomy provides a less effective but temporary means of oxygenation and ventilation. *After needle cricothyrotomy, either a definitive surgical airway (cricothyrotomy or tracheostomy) must be established immediately in the emergency department or operating room, or endotracheal or nasotracheal intubation must be accomplished by a skilled physician.*

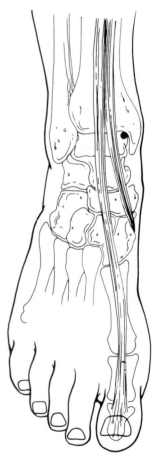

FIGURE 139–2. Entry site for ankle arthrocentesis. (From Ho MT, Sanders CE, eds: *Current Emergency Diagnosis and Treatment,* 3rd ed. Los Altos: Lange Medical Publishers, 1990, 836)

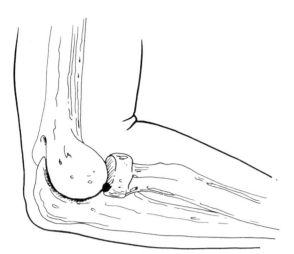

FIGURE 139–3. Entry site for elbow arthrocentesis. (From Ho MT, Sanders CE, eds: *Current Emergency Diagnosis and Treatment,* 3rd ed. Los Altos: Lange Medical Publishers, 1990, 835)

INDICATIONS

1. Airway obstruction, usually in setting of tongue hematoma, uncontrollable nasopharyngeal bleeding, laryngeal edema or vocal-cord paralysis, gross anatomic deformity, congenital abnormalities (atresia, tumor, cyst, vascular malformation), severe subglottic stenosis, epiglottitis with respiratory arrest
2. Failure of orotracheal or nasotracheal intubation in a child requiring assisted ventilation
3. Cervical spine fracture, suspected or proven, in a child who needs an emergency airway and who cannot be safely intubated using in-line axial traction with orotracheal or nasotracheal intubation technique.

EQUIPMENT AND SUPPLIES

Prep solution, sterile gloves, sterile drape
14- or 16-gauge over-the-needle plastic catheter
25-gauge needle and 3-ml syringe
1% lidocaine
10-ml syringe
No. 3 pediatric endotracheal tube adapter
Ventilating system

POSITION

If the child is a trauma victim with altered mental status and head or neck injury, assume cervical spine injury is present and avoid moving the neck. Restrain the child in the supine position with the head held in a neutral position by an assistant using in-line axial traction. If cervical spine injury is not suspected, gently hyperextend the neck by using a towel roll under the shoulder.

PROCEDURE (FIG. 139-4)

1. Prep and drape the anterior neck at the site of the cricothyroid membrane.
2. Stand at the patient's head and locate the entry site in the middle of the cricothyroid membrane, between the thyroid cartilage above and the cricoid cartilage below.
3. If the patient is conscious, anesthetize the entry site with a 25-gauge needle and lidocaine in a 3-ml syringe.
4. Attach the over-the-needle catheter to the 10-ml syringe, then advance the needle through the membrane at a 45-degree angle, while stabilizing the trachea between the thumb and index finger of the opposite hand.
5. Apply negative pressure; entry into the trachea is signaled by a "pop" and free aspiration of air.
6. Advance the catheter into the trachea, while withdrawing the needle and syringe.
7. Attach the No. 3 pediatric adapter to the hub of the catheter and to the ventilating system.
8. Ensure effective ventilation by watching the chest rise and by monitoring pulse oximeter or arterial blood gas measurements.

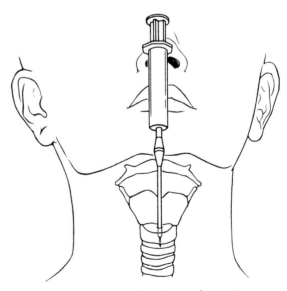

FIGURE 139-4. Needle cricothyrotomy.

9. Tape the apparatus to the neck securely and arrange for immediate operating room or emergency department placement of a definitive airway by surgical technique or by controlled endotracheal or nasotracheal intubation by a skilled physician.

COMPLICATIONS

1. Hemorrhage
2. Posterior tracheal or esophageal perforation
3. Mediastinal or pleural perforation
4. Hypoxia
5. Hypercapnea, especially if complete airway obstruction is present
6. Subcutaneous emphysema

Cricothyrotomy ■

If the equipment and expertise are immediately available for surgical cricothyrotomy, perform this procedure in preference to needle cricothyrotomy.

INDICATIONS

See Needle Cricothyrotomy above.

EQUIPMENT AND SUPPLIES

Prep solution, sterile gloves, sterile drape
No. 11 scalpel
Endotracheal tube or tracheostomy tube
Skin hooks
Curved clamp
Tracheal suction catheter
Ventilating system

POSITION

See Needle Cricothyrotomy above.

PROCEDURE (FIG. 139-5)

1. Prep and drape the anterior neck at the site of the cricothyroid membrane.
2. Gently grasp and stabilize the trachea, then incise the skin and platysma muscle transversely at the location of the cricothyroid membrane.
3. Ensure the skin incision is correctly located directly above the cricothyroid membrane, then continue the incision through the membrane.
4. Twist the scalpel 90 degrees to establish the airway.
5. Use skin hooks or curved clamp to maintain airway patency.
6. Insert the largest possible tracheostomy tube or

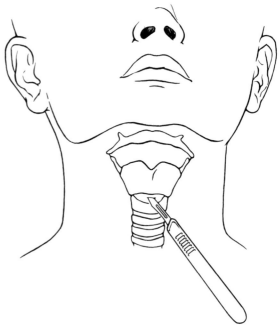

FIGURE 139-5. Cricothyrotomy.

endotracheal tube into the tracheal opening. Cut the tube to proper size after it is properly placed.
7. Secure the apparatus to the neck and connect to the ventilating system.

COMPLICATIONS

See Needle Cricothyrotomy above.

Endotracheal Intubation ■

Endotracheal intubation permits definitive control of the airway and allows optimal oxygenation and ventilation, and also serves as a means for hyperventilation in patients with increased intracranial pressure. In addition, the endotracheal tube provides a conduit for delivery of several important drugs (see Endotracheal Drug Delivery below).

INDICATIONS

1. Cardiac arrest
2. Respiratory arrest
3. Profound shock
4. Severe head trauma with unresponsiveness
5. Loss of protective airway reflexes

TABLE 139–1. *Proper-Sized Pediatric Equipment*

Age	ID of ET Tube (mm)	Laryngoscope Blade	Chest Tube (Fr)	NG/Foley (Fr)
Newborn	2.5–3	0–1	8–12	5
1 mo	3.5	1	12	8
6 mo	3.5	1	16	8
1 yr	4	1	20	8
2–3 yr	4.5	1	24	8
4–5 yr	5–6	2	28	10
6–8 yr	6–6.5	2	32	10
10–12 yr	7	2–3	32	12
14 yr	7.5	3	40	12

EQUIPMENT AND SUPPLIES

Laryngoscope
Appropriate-sized laryngoscope blade (see Table 139-1)
Appropriate-sized endotracheal tube (see Table 139-1)
Stylet
Suction
Pulse oximeter with pediatric adapter

POSITION

The child must be in the supine position. Apply cervical traction and minimize neck movement in patients with head or neck trauma. The larger head of a child under 12 months may require a shoulder towel roll to maintain a neutral spine position. Do not overflex or overextend the neck, as this can occlude the airway: the tracheal orifice is tiny in young children and easily obstructed. Also, hypoxia induced by the intubation procedure develops more rapidly with younger age.

PROCEDURE (FIG. 139-6)

1. Ensure correct positioning and normal airway anatomy. Consider rapid sequence induction if the child is conscious (see Table 48-1).
2. Select a proper-sized endotracheal tube (ETT). Table 139-1 lists tube sizes vis-a-vis age of the child. For children, tube size can be calculated by the following formula:

$$\frac{\text{Age (years)} + 16}{4}$$

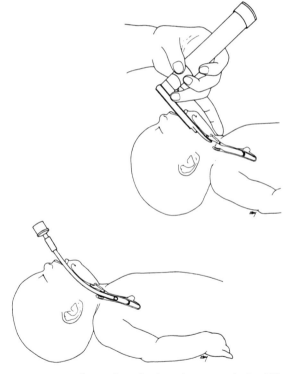

FIGURE 139-6. Endotracheal intubation: With the fifth finger applying cricoid pressure, pass the straight laryngoscope blade behind the tongue and deep to the epiglottis; lift the epiglottis to expose the vocal cords (***above***). Insert the properly-sized, uncuffed endotracheal tube past the glottis, halfway between the vocal cords and carina (***below***). (Reproduced with permission from Motoyama EK, Davis PJ, eds: *Smith's Anesthesia for Infants and Children*, 4th ed. St. Louis: CV Mosby, 1980)

Alternatively, the tube size can be determined by approximating the diameter of the tip of the child's little finger. *Do not use cuffed ETTs in children less than 8 years.*

3. Insert a stylet into the ETT and ensure that the stylet does not extend beyond the ETT tip.
4. Select a proper-sized laryngoscope blade, either straight or curved (see Table 139-1); fit to laryngoscope and test light.
5. If possible, do bag-valve-mask ventilation with 100% oxygen for 1 to 3 minutes before attempting intubation, to fully saturate the hemoglobin. Attach pulse oximeter to monitor oxygen saturation during the procedure.
6. Apply firm cricoid pressure with the fifth finger (Sellick maneuver) or instruct an assistant to do so. Cricoid pressure will occlude the esophagus at the cricoid level, reducing aspiration risk. *Do not release cricoid pressure until ETT placement in the trachea is confirmed.*
7. Use copious suction to clear the airway.
8. Carefully position the laryngoscope in the oropharynx and visualize the vocal cords.
9. Insert the ETT 2 or 3 cm past the vocal cords under direct vision.
10. Remove the stylet and bag-ventilate.
11. Confirm position by auscultation of the epigastrium, then both hemithoraces. Ensure chest rises with bag ventilation. Check oximeter for oxygen saturation.
12. When proper ETT position in the trachea is confirmed, remove cricoid pressure and secure the tube with tape.
13. Limit the intubation attempt to a total of 30 seconds.
14. Keep the child's head in the neutral position to avoid extubation or mainstem-bronchus intubation.

COMPLICATIONS

1. Esophageal intubation
2. Mainstem-bronchus intubation
3. Laryngeal trauma
4. Aspiration
5. Hypoxia
6. Shock

Endotracheal Drug Delivery ∎

When vascular access is not immediately available in an unstable, intubated patient, the endotracheal tube is an effective conduit for delivery of lifesaving drugs. Agents with known efficacy when administered through the endotracheal tube are represented by the mnemonic NAVEL (naloxone, atropine, Valium, epinephrine, lidocaine).

The pharmacokinetics and safety of endotracheal drugs are not well established. Standard intravenous doses of epinephrine, and possibly other drugs, are probably inadequate when given by this method.

INDICATIONS

1. Cardiac arrest
2. Respiratory arrest
3. Status epilepticus
4. Opiate overdose
5. Shock with ventricular dysrhythmia or bradycardia

EQUIPMENT AND SUPPLIES

Measured dose of desired drug
Normal saline
10-ml syringe
5f or 8f infant feeding tube

POSITION

The child must be intubated and well ventilated, with a properly sized and well-secured endotracheal tube.

PROCEDURE

1. Draw the calculated dose into a 10-ml syringe.
2. Dilute with normal saline to 5 ml, *not to exceed 1 ml/kg total volume.*
3. Insert the tip of the feeding tube past the distal tip of the endotracheal tube.
4. Instill the solution directly into the trachea.
5. Clear the feeding tube with an air bolus.
6. Ventilate three to five times to disperse the solution distally into the tracheobronchial tree.

POSSIBLE COMPLICATIONS

1. Post-resuscitation malignant hypertension (epinephrine)
2. Pneumonitis
3. Hypoxia or hypercarbia

Foreign Body Removal ∎

A foreign body (FB) lodged in a body orifice is a common emergency among children under 5 years old. Frequent locations are the ear and the nose. The FB is most likely to be an insect (e.g., a roach), paper, toy part, earring part, or hair bead. Removal must be gentle and rapid to avert complications.

NOSE

Equipment and Supplies

Nasal speculum
Good light source
Headlight
Frazier suction tip and wall suction
Forceps, either straight, alligator, or mosquito
Hook or loop
Topical vasoconstrictor (1% epinephrine or 0.25% phenylephrine)
No. 8 Foley catheter

Position

Restrain the child in a supine position, if uncooperative. Place the older child in a sitting position with a "sniffing" posture.

Procedure

1. Instruct the child to blow the nose vigorously.
2. Apply the vasoconstrictor with a cotton-tipped applicator to the nasal mucosa.
3. Visualize the FB with a speculum and directed light.
4. Try to remove the FB with careful suction.
5. If unsuccessful, use forceps if the FB is small, a loop or hook if it is large.
6. If unsuccessful, insert a lubricated Foley catheter past the FB, inflate with 2 or 3 ml normal saline, then withdraw.

Complications

1. Infection
2. Bleeding (epistaxis)
3. Aspiration of FB

EAR

Equipment and Supplies

Otoscope and speculum
1% lidocaine
Curette
Irrigation system with angiocath or cut-off butterfly tubing and 10-ml syringe
Forceps, either straight, alligator, or mosquito
Frazier suction tip with wall suction

Position

Restrain the uncooperative child in the prone position with the involved ear superior. Alternatively, sit the cooperative child on the parent's lap and have the parent hold the child's head securely.

Procedure

1. Visualize the tympanic membrane and FB with an otoscope.
2. Try to remove the FB with a curette.
3. If unsuccessful, try suction.
4. If unsuccessful, attempt forceps removal through otoscope speculum.
5. If the FB is a live insect, first kill it with 1% lidocaine solution, then remove it by the above methods.
6. If above techniques are unsuccessful and the FB is not vegetable material, use irrigation if the tympanic membrane is intact. Do not use the irrigation technique with vegetable or porous material, to avoid further enlarging the mass.
7. After removal, treat ear canal irritation with topical antibiotic ear drops.

Complications

1. Laceration of canal
2. Otitis externa
3. Tympanic membrane perforation
4. Damage to ossicles

Lumbar Puncture ∎

Lumbar puncture (LP) is the definitive diagnostic procedure for evaluation of infection in the central nervous system (CNS). *Never* perform an LP in a child with evidence of increased intracranial pressure from a mass lesion, prior to computed tomography (CT) imaging of the brain. *Brain herniation and cardiopulmonary arrest may result.*

INDICATIONS

1. Suspected CNS infection
2. Other CNS disorders (*e.g.*, malignancy, subarachnoid hemorrhage), after CT imaging excludes dangerous elevation in intracranial pressure from a mass lesion

EQUIPMENT AND SUPPLIES

Prep solution, sterile gloves, sterile drape
Mask and gown
1% lidocaine
25-gauge needle and 3-ml syringe

22-gauge spinal needle (under 12 months: 1.5"; 12 months to 5 years: 2.5"; 5 years to adult: 3.5")
CSF manometer and three-way stopcock
Sterile collection tubes

POSITION

Two positions are acceptable: lateral decubitus or sitting. The site of entry for either position is the midline of the lumbar spine, at the L3-L4 or L4-L5 interspace. The L4-L5 interspace is easily identified on the horizontal axis between the iliac crests.

If the lateral decubitus position is selected (see Figure 139-7A), ensure that the child is properly restrained by a skilled assistant. Place the patient in a fetal position on the near side of the examining table, with the shoulders and back at a 90-degree angle with the table. If the sitting position is selected (see Figure 139-7B), restrain the child sitting forward (to fully flex the spine), with the knees against the chest. Put the child's hands between the knees.

PROCEDURE (FIG. 139-7)

1. Gown, glove, and mask.
2. Prep and drape the area.
3. With a 25-gauge needle, anesthetize from the skin to the level of the spinous process with lidocaine.
4. Advance the spinal needle under the spinous process at a 90-degree angle.
5. Slowly enter the subarachnoid space. Usually, a "pop" and change in resistance indicates proper needle placement.
6. Attach the three-way stopcock and perform manometry to measure cerebrospinal fluid (CSF) pressure.
7. Collect CSF for standard laboratory analysis, as noted below. Additional measurements of CSF characteristics may be indicated as well. Table 114-3 provides normal and selected abnormal cell counts, glucose, protein, and Gram's stain results in various disease states.
   Tube 1: Gram's stain, India ink stain, culture and sensitivity.
   Tube 2: Glucose and protein
   Tube 3: Cell counts (Do cell counts on tubes 1 and 3 if the CSF is bloody.)
8. Keep the patient in a prone position for several hours after the procedure to minimize post-lumbar puncture headache.

COMPLICATIONS

1. Cardiac arrest
2. Brain stem herniation
3. Infection
4. Bleeding
5. Headache
6. Back pain
7. Transient neuropathy
8. Spinal subdural or epidural hematoma
9. Intraspinal epidermoid tumor (months later)

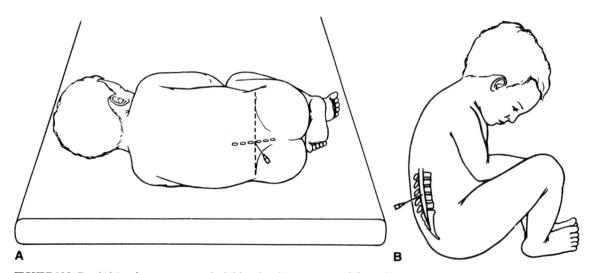

FIGURE 139-7. (**A**) Lumbar puncture with child in decubitus position. (**B**) Lumbar puncture with child in sitting position.

Nasogastric Intubation ◼

Placement of a nasogastric (NG) tube is an important emergency procedure, usually employed for gastric lavage or gastrointestinal (GI) decompression.

INDICATIONS

1. Ingestion of a dangerous poison
2. Need for GI decompression in disorders such as intestinal obstruction, pancreatitis, or abdominal trauma
3. GI hemorrhage
4. Administration of agents unpalatable or unsuitable orally (*e.g.*, activated charcoal, drugs, contrast agents)

EQUIPMENT AND SUPPLIES

Appropriately sized NG tube (see Table 139-1)
Lubricating jelly
Fitted 30-ml syringe with proper connector tip
Suction tube and suction device
Glass of water and straw

POSITION

Place the infant or the uncooperative child in a decubitus position or in a restrained supine position, with the head turned. Place the cooperative child in a sitting position at 60 degrees from the horizontal. *If the patient has altered mental status and loss or impending loss of protective airway reflexes, perform orotracheal intubation prior to nasogastric intubation.*

PROCEDURE (FIG. 139-8)

1. Enlist the assistance of the child and parent.
2. Determine the length of tubing by measuring from ear to umbilicus.
3. Select the largest NG tube that will fit the nasal orifice (usually a 8f in infants and a 10f in children). Lubricate the end with ample jelly. Examine the nose and both nares to select the most patent side for intubation.
4. Have the patient take a sip of water and hold it in the mouth.
5. Advance the tube perpendicularly along the *inferior* nasal passage into the nasopharynx with a steady slow motion. Stiffen the NG tip with cold water if direction cannot be adequately controlled. To prevent intracranial intubation, do not attempt to pass the tube in the presence of severe facial or skull trauma with nasopharyngeal fluid or blood leaks.

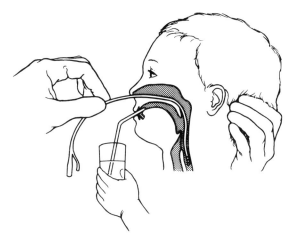

FIGURE 139–8. Nasogastric intubation.

6. Flex the neck and pass the tube into the esophagus as the child swallows.
7. Airway obstruction, cough, or violent gagging indicate tracheal intubation. Withdraw the NG tube immediately.
8. If the NG tube meets no resistance, insert it to the measured length and instill 10 ml air with a syringe, while listening over the epigastrium to confirm position in stomach.
9. Secure the tube with tape to the nose.

COMPLICATIONS

1. Tracheal intubation
2. Epistaxis
3. Nasopharyngeal or hypopharyngeal trauma
4. Aspiration
5. Passage of NG tube intracranially
6. Cribriform plate fracture

Needle Pericardiocentesis ◼

Emergency needle pericardiocentesis is rarely needed but may be lifesaving in the setting of pericardial tamponade and hemodynamic instability.

INDICATIONS

Pericardial tamponade
Bacteriologic diagnosis of purulent pericarditis

EQUIPMENT AND SUPPLIES

Prep solution, sterile gloves, sterile drape
1% lidocaine

25-gauge needle and 3-ml syringe
3.5″ 18-gauge spinal needle
Three-way stopcock
30-ml syringe
Alligator clips
V lead and electrocardiograph (ECG) machine

POSITION

Place the child in a restrained position elevated 30 degrees from the horizontal.

PROCEDURE (FIG. 139-9)

1. Prep and drape the area below the xiphoid process.
2. Attach the metal spinal needle, with stylet removed, to the syringe and stopcock.
3. Attach the V lead from the ECG machine to the hub end of the needle with an alligator clip.
4. Anesthetize the left subxiphoid area.
5. Advance the needle slowly at a 30-degree angle

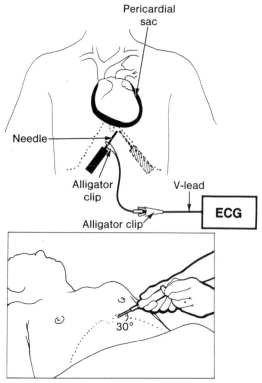

FIGURE 139–9. Needle pericardiocentesis. (From Simon RR, Brenner BE, eds: *Emergency Procedures and Techniques.* Baltimore: Williams & Wilkins, 1987)

from horizontal, directed toward right scapular tip.
6. Apply negative pressure on the syringe and enter the pericardial sac after penetrating the diaphragm.
7. Monitor the ECG, and pull back the needle if injury current (PR or ST segment elevation, depending on atrial or ventricular location) or dysrhythmia is noted on the ECG strip.
8. Aspirate blood or fluid from the pericardial sac and evacuate through stopcock, until dry.
9. Recollection of fluid may necessitate leaving the needle in place, clamped at the point of skin entry.
10. If unsuccessful, change needle direction and aim at left scapular tip.
11. After fluid removal or dry tap, remove the needle quickly and apply a dressing.

COMPLICATIONS

1. Coronary artery laceration
2. Myocardial penetration
3. Pneumothorax
4. Dysrhythmia

Rectal Diazepam Administration ■

Rectal administration of diazepam is a rapid treatment method for status epilepticus. Although the time to onset of action is slightly more than with the IV mode of administration, the ultimate success in stopping seizures is essentially equivalent to IV use, and complications are fewer.

INDICATIONS

1. Active seizures more than 15 minutes
2. Recurrent seizures without return of consciousness for more than 15 minutes

EQUIPMENT AND SUPPLIES

Size 5f pediatric feeding catheter
Lubricant
Measured dose of intravenous diazepam
3-ml syringe

POSITION

Restrain the child in the supine position, with an assistant holding the legs apart in a frog-leg position.

PROCEDURE

1. Ensure that the airway is open. Give 100% oxygen. Use suction to clear oropharyngeal secretions.
2. Draw up the calculated diazepam dose, 0.5 mg/kg, into the syringe.
3. Introduce a lubricated 5f pediatric feeding tube into the rectum, about 5 cm proximal to the anus.
4. Squirt the solution into the rectum and clear the line with 1 ml normal saline.
5. Tape buttocks closed.

COMPLICATIONS

1. Rectal injury
2. Respiratory depression
3. Hypotension

Suprapubic Bladder Aspiration ■

Standard urine collection techniques are ineffective in young children who are not toilet-trained. When accurate urine collection and analysis are necessary for assessment and treatment, suprapubic bladder aspiration is simple and efficacious. In children older than 2 years, perform urethral catheterization instead.

INDICATIONS

1. Diagnosis of sepsis in child under 2 years
2. Diagnosis of urinary infection in child under 2 years
3. Relief of urinary obstruction, when urethral catheterization is impossible or contraindicated (See Urethral Catheterization below.)

EQUIPMENT AND SUPPLIES

Prep solution, sterile drape, sterile gloves
1.5" 22-gauge needle
5-ml syringe
Sterile container

POSITION

Restrain the child in a supine frog-leg position. Wait at least 1 hour after last urination.

PROCEDURE (FIG. 139-10)

1. Percuss the abdomen to help identify bladder level. Prep and drape the area one fingerbreadth above the midline of the pubic bone. Place a sterile collection bag on the child to catch a specimen if spontaneous voiding occurs during the procedure.

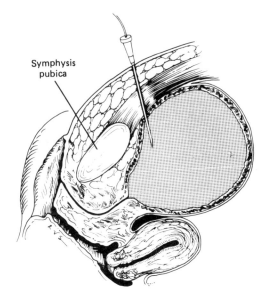

FIGURE 139–10. Suprapubic bladder aspiration. (From Ho MT, Sanders CE, eds: *Current Emergency Diagnosis and Treatment,* 3rd ed. Los Altos: Lange Medical Publishers, 1990, 826)

2. Attach the needle to the syringe and quickly advance the needle 15 degrees off the vertical plane, directed cephalad.
3. Completely advance the needle into the bladder, while putting negative pressure on the syringe.
4. Withdraw the needle slowly while aspirating for urine.
5. If unsuccessful, repeat the attempt at perpendicular, then at 15 degrees off the vertical, pointing caudal.

COMPLICATIONS

1. Infection
2. Bleeding at puncture site or into bladder
3. Bowel perforation

Bladder Catheterization ■

Bladder catheterization is a simple method for accurately monitoring perfusion in children, as well as for diagnostic urine collection and for relief of urinary retention.

INDICATIONS

1. Shock or uncertain perfusion status
2. Post-resuscitation hemodynamic monitoring

3. Urinary retention
4. Need for diagnostic urinalysis or urine culture and sensitivity when other collection methods fail

EQUIPMENT AND SUPPLIES

Prep solution, sterile gloves, sterile drape
Appropriately sized catheter (see Table 139-1)
Sterile lubricant
Normal saline solution
10-ml syringe
Urine collection system

POSITION

See Suprapubic Bladder Aspiration above.

PROCEDURE

Males (Fig. 139-11A)

1. Select a properly sized feeding tube (children under 2 years of age) or Foley catheter (children above 2 years). See Table 139-1 for correct size. If a Foley catheter is selected, test the balloon first.
2. Grasp the penis below the glans and gently extend.
3. Drape, then prep the urethral meatus.
4. Insert the properly sized, well-lubricated catheter, with balloon deflated, into the urethra and advance into the bladder to the point of the Y connection on the catheter. When a feeding tube is used, advance it until urine flow is established or resistance is encountered. *Do not attempt insertion in the presence of prostatic displacement, perineal hematoma, or urethral blood.*
5. Inflate the balloon with normal saline.
6. Withdraw the catheter until the inflated balloon rests snugly against the trigone.
7. Connect the catheter to the collection system and tape it securely to the leg.

Females (Fig. 139-11B)

1. Select a properly sized feeding tube (children under 2–3 years of age) or Foley catheter (children above 2–3 years). See Table 139-1 for correct size. If a Foley catheter is selected, test the balloon first.
2. Drape the perineum. Separate the labia and prep the urethral meatus.
3. Insert a properly sized, well-lubricated catheter with balloon deflated into the urethra and advance into the bladder to the Y connection. If a feeding tube is used, advance it until urine flow is established or until resistance is encountered. *Do not attempt insertion in the presence of perineal hematoma or urethral blood.*

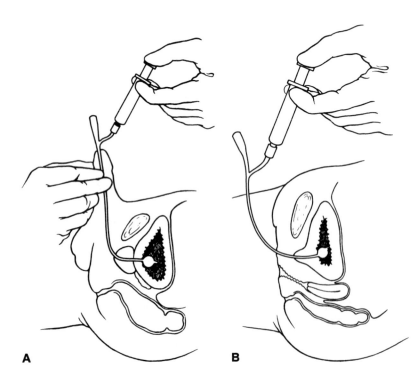

A **B**

FIGURE 139-11. (**A**) Bladder catheterization, male (**B**) Bladder catheterization, female

4. Inflate the balloon with saline.
5. Withdraw the catheter until the balloon rests snugly against the trigone.
6. Connect the catheter to the collection system and tape it securely to the leg.

COMPLICATIONS

1. Urethral injury
2. Bladder injury
3. Vaginal injury
4. Creation of a false passage
5. Bleeding
6. Infection

Needle Thoracostomy ■

This procedure must be used only as a temporizing measure while assembling equipment or obtaining a qualified physician to perform tube thoracostomy.

INDICATION

Pneumothorax with hemodynamic instability

EQUIPMENT AND SUPPLIES

Prep solution, sterile gloves, sterile drape
1% lidocaine
25-ml needle and 3-ml syringe
14-gauge over-the-needle catheter
10-ml syringe
Three-way stopcock

POSITION

Place patient in a restrained position 60 degrees from horizontal, with ipsilateral arm extended over the head.

PROCEDURE (FIG. 139-12)

1. Prep and drape the area at the level of the second intercostal space at the mid-clavicular line.
2. If the patient is conscious, anesthetize the entry site generously.
3. Attach the 14-gauge catheter to the 10-ml syringe and advance it into the pleural space at a 45-degree angle caudal, over the superior edge of rib, while applying negative pressure.
4. Advance the catheter and needle into the pleural space and maintain the 45-degree tangential angle to avoid lung laceration. A change of resistance or "pop" signals entry into the pleural space.
5. Withdraw the needle, attach the stopcock to the

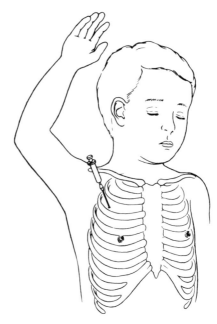

FIGURE 139–12. Needle thoracostomy.

catheter, and perform pleural decompression. Do multiple aspirations and evacuations through the stopcock without removing the catheter.
6. Remove the catheter after tube thoracostomy.

COMPLICATIONS

1. Pneumothorax
2. Hemothorax
3. Lung laceration

Tube Thoracostomy ■

Tube thoracostomy decompresses the pleural space of blood, fluid, or air. This procedure must be performed immediately in the hemodynamically unstable child with the appropriate indication, to avoid irreversible cardiovascular collapse.

INDICATIONS

1. Open pneumothorax (sucking chest wound)
2. Closed pneumothorax
3. Hemothorax

EQUIPMENT AND SUPPLIES

Prep solution, sterile gloves, sterile drape
Mask and gown

1% lidocaine
Two curved clamps
Sterile sponges
10-ml syringe
25-gauge needle
No. 15 scalpel
Siliconized, straight chest tube (see Table 139-1 for size)
Silk suture
Drainage system with adequate suction
Autotransfuser device

POSITION

See Needle Thoracostomy above.

PROCEDURE (FIG. 139-13)

1. Drape the area and prep the entry site at the level of the nipple (fourth or fifth intercostal space), in the mid-axillary line.
2. If the child is conscious, anesthetize generously from the skin to the parietal pleura, including intercostal muscle.
3. Select a large-bore tube from Table 139-1 or use any tube that approximates the size of the child's middle fingertip. A smaller tube may be suitable if only air is being evacuated.
4. Incise a 2- to 3-cm area parallel to the top of the rib, through subcutaneous tissue and fascia.
5. Insert the curved clamp tip through the skin passage, tunnel it superiorly, enter the pleural space, and widen the parietal pleural opening with blunt dissection.
6. Sweep the pleural space with a gloved finger to ensure that the lung is not adherent.
7. Grasp the tip of the chest tube with the curved clamp and insert the tube into the pleural space.
8. Advance the tube posteriorly and superiorly until the tube tip abuts on the mediastinum.
9. Attach the tube to underwater seal at 10 to 20 cm H_2O pressure, and reinforce tube attachments. Inspect the system for air leaks.
10. Suture the tube in place and apply a dressing in sterile fashion. Obtain a chest radiograph.
11. If a large amount of blood is evacuated, capture and return it to the patient with an autotransfuser device.

COMPLICATIONS

1. Hemothorax
2. Infection
3. Lung laceration or contusion
4. Pericardial tamponade
5. Subcutaneous emphysema

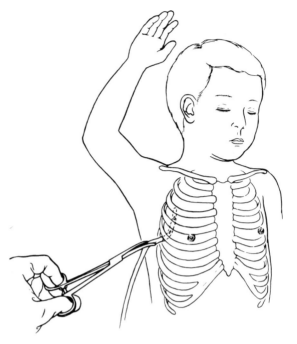

FIGURE 139-13. Tube thoracostomy.

Vascular Access ■

Obtaining vascular access is necessary for diagnostic venipuncture as well as for administration of drugs and fluids. A variety of sites are available; the choice of location depends on urgency, safety, and purpose of the procedure.

PERIPHERAL VENOUS CANNULATION AND VENIPUNCTURE

The most common peripheral venous access sites for venipuncture or cannulation are illustrated in Figure 139-14.

Equipment and Supplies

Prep solution
Alcohol sponge
0.5'' tape and sterile gauze
21-, 23-, or 25-gauge butterfly needle
14-, 16-, 18-, 20-, 22-, or 24-gauge over-the-needle catheter
5- or 10-ml syringe
Intravenous extension tubing, regular infusion set, and intravenous solution
Rubber band or tourniquet
Razor

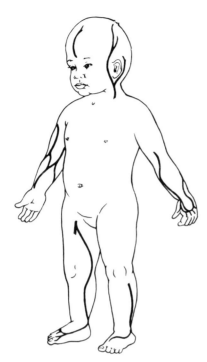

FIGURE 139–14. Peripheral access sites for superficial venous cannulation. (From Kempe CH, Silver HK, O'Brien D, Fulginiti VA, eds: *Current Pediatric Diagnosis and Treatment.* Norwalk: Appleton & Lange, 1987)

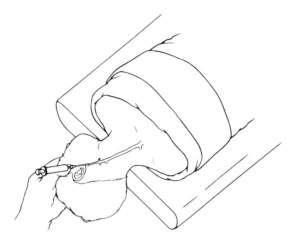

FIGURE 139–15. External jugular vein cannulation.

Position

For venipuncture or percutaneous cannulation of the external jugular vein, restrain the child in a supine position with the head gently turned to the contralateral side and held below the heart level, off the end of the examining table (Fig. 139-15).

For venipuncture or cannulation of the scalp vein in the infant (Fig. 139-16), restrain the child in a supine position and shave the area over the puncture site. Use a rubber band to occlude the vessel proximally.

For venipuncture or cannulation of other peripheral vessels, restrain the child in a supine position if uncooperative, or sit the child on the parent's lap, if older and cooperative. Use either a rubber band or tourniquet to increase venous pressure in the selected vessel.

Procedure

1. Prep the site with alcohol.
2. Apply a tourniquet or rubber band.
3. Select an appropriately sized butterfly needle or over-the-needle catheter.
4. Apply skin traction, then introduce the needle with the bevel up through the skin approximately 0.5 cm distal to the projected site of venous entry.
5. Enter the vessel, attach the syringe, and apply negative pressure to collect blood for laboratory analysis. Release the tourniquet or cut the rubber band.
6. For an indwelling cannula, secure the butterfly needle with gauze and tape in position to maximize flow (Fig. 139-17), then connect to infusion set.
7. *An over-the-needle catheter is superior as an indwelling cannula.* After penetrating the vessel with the needle, slowly advance the catheter with a rotational movement over the needle into the vessel. Then attach it to the infusion set and secure it to the skin.

Complications

1. Bleeding and hematoma formation
2. Infection
3. Thrombophlebitis

DEEP VENOUS CANNULATION

Deep or central venous cannulation is usually reserved for emergency cases requiring fluid or drug delivery with a high level of urgency, or for central venous pressure monitoring. Occasionally, venipuncture is performed at the femoral area for collection of blood for laboratory analysis. *Deep venous catheters do not permit faster fluid infusion rates than short small-gauge peripheral catheters, since their greater length increases resistance to flow.* Be-

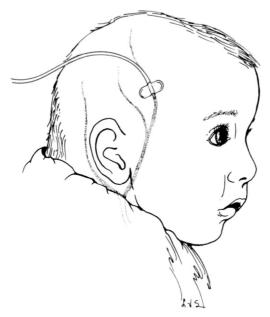

FIGURE 139–16. Scalp vein cannulation in an infant. (From Ho MT, Sanders CE, eds: *Current Emergency Diagnosis and Treatment,* 3rd ed. Los Altos: Lange Medical Publishers, 1990, 789)

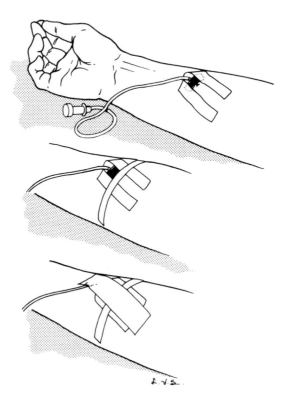

FIGURE 139–17. Technique of securing butterfly needle. (From Ho MT, Sanders CE, eds: *Current Emergency Diagnosis and Treatment,* 3rd ed. Los Altos: Lange Medical Publishers, 1990, 790)

cause emergency deep venous cannulation in children has a high complication rate, other venous access methods are usually preferred. The procedure can be accomplished using percutaneous, open, or Seldinger guide wire techniques.

Indications

1. Emergent need for drug or fluid delivery when no peripheral access is available
2. Central venous pressure monitoring
3. Swan–Ganz pulmonary pressure monitoring
4. Transvenous pacemaker insertion
5. Venipuncture when no peripheral access is available

Equipment and Supplies

Prep solution, sterile gloves, sterile gown, sterile drape
1% lidocaine
25-gauge needle and 3-ml syringe
21- or 23-gauge butterfly needle (for femoral venipuncture)
8'' 18-gauge intracath
Plastic skin guide
No. 11 scalpel
10-ml syringe
Silk sutures
Sterile clamp
Seldinger catheter kit (metal needle, guide wire, infusion catheter)

Position and Procedure

FEMORAL (Fig. 139-18)

1. Restrain the patient in a supine frog-leg position.
2. Prep and drape the femoral area at the mid-inguinal region.
3. Palpate the femoral pulse with the gloved finger, then anesthetize at the entry point 1 cm medial to the pulse, or at the point midway between the anterior-superior iliac spine and the pubic tubercle.

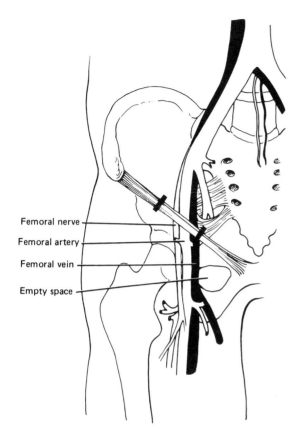

FIGURE 139–18. Anatomic relationships of the femoral vein at the inguinal ligament. (From Ho MT, Sanders CE, eds: *Current Emergency Diagnosis and Treatment,* 3rd ed. Los Altos: Lange Medical Publishers, 1990, 798)

Femoral nerve
Femoral artery
Femoral vein
Empty space

4. For venipuncture or arterial puncture, use a butterfly needle at 60 degrees from the horizontal. Advance the needle toward the umbilicus to enter the vein or artery.
5. After blood collection is complete, withdraw the needle and apply constant pressure on the puncture site for 5 minutes.
6. For percutaneous venous cannulation with a long intracath, attach the metal needle to a syringe and advance the needle at a 45-degree angle to the horizontal into the vein.
7. After blood flow is established, grasp the needle hub with a clamp, disconnect the syringe, occlude the port with a sterile finger, then thread the plastic intracath and stylet into the vessel.
8. After the intracath is fully advanced into the vessel, remove the stylet, attach the cannula to the in-

fusion set-up, and secure the cannula to the skin with the skin guide and a suture.
9. If the Seldinger kit is available, first cannulate the vein with the small needle. Once flow is established, grasp the needle hub with a clamp, disconnect the syringe, and insert the guide wire through the needle. Withdraw the needle over the guide wire while holding the guide wire with sterile fingers at the point of skin entry.
10. Advance the infusion catheter over the guide wire into the vessel with a rotational movement. A skin nick with a scalpel tip will facilitate entry. Then withdraw the guide wire.
11. Attach the Seldinger infusion catheter to the intravenous infusion set-up and tape or suture the catheter at the entry site on the leg.
12. Dress the catheter site in sterile fashion.

Internal Jugular (Fig. 139-19)

1. Restrain the patient in a Trendelenberg position and gently turn the head to the contralateral side.
2. Visualize the course of the vein between the two heads of the sternocleidomastoid muscle and under the clavicle. The carotid artery lies medial to the vein.
3. Prep and drape the patient.
4. Using sterile technique with either the Seldinger approach or the metal intracath needle, enter the anesthetized skin at the apex of the triangle created by the heads of the sternocleidomastoid and the clavicle (anterior approach).
5. Direct the needle at a 45-degree angle off the skin of the neck and aim at the ipsilateral nipple. If unsuccessful, attempt a slightly more lateral direction.
6. Enter the vessel and use the techniques for cannulation described above with Femoral Vein.

Subclavian (Fig. 139-20)

1. Restrain the patient in a Trendelenberg position and hyperextend the back with a towel roll under the mid-thorax. Gently turn the head to the contralateral side.
2. Visualize the course of the vein crossing the first rib and running deep to the medial third of the clavicle.
3. Prep and drape the patient.
4. Using sterile technique with either the Seldinger approach or the metal intracath needle, enter the skin inferior to the clavicle, with a 30-degree angle from the skin, at the juncture of the middle and medial thirds of the clavicle.
5. Advance the needle medially and cephalad toward the finger placed in the sternal notch.

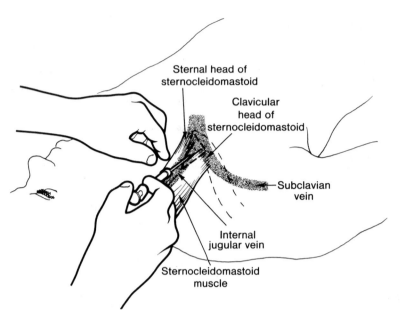

FIGURE 139–19. Cannulation of the internal jugular vein using the anterior approach. (From Simon RR, Brenner BE, eds: *Emergency Procedures and Techniques.* Baltimore: Williams & Wilkins, 1987)

6. Enter the vessel and use the techniques for cannulation described above with Femoral Vein.

Complications

1. Bleeding
2. Infection
3. Air embolism
4. Catheter fragment in circulation or skin
5. Bowel perforation (femoral approach)
6. Hip joint infection (femoral approach)
7. Pneumothorax or hemothorax (internal jugular and subclavian approaches)

SAPHENOUS VEIN CUTDOWN

Open saphenous vein cutdown is useful for emergent drug and fluid administration in the child with no available peripheral venous access. This procedure is technically quite difficult in the child under 2 years. A major advantage is that large-bore catheters with high flow rates can be inserted under direct vision.

Equipment and Supplies

Prep solution, sterile gloves, sterile drape
Mask and gown
1% lidocaine
25-gauge needle and 3-ml syringe
No. 15 scalpel
Two curved clamps
Scissors
Forceps
5f or 8f feeding tube
Vein introducer device
Silk suture

Position

Restrain the child and externally rotate the leg and ankle. Secure the foot in a position to expose the saphenous area at the medial malleolus.

Procedure (Fig. 139-21)

1. Prep and drape the area.
2. Mask and gown. If the child is conscious, generously anesthetize the cutdown site. Select an incision site 1 to 2 cm proximal and 1 to 2 cm anterior to the medial malleolus.
3. Incise 2 to 3 cm through the skin and bluntly dissect the surrounding tissues to isolate the vein.
4. If the vein is not visible, sweep the point of a curved clamp across the surface of the tibia to locate the vessel.
5. Pass two silk sutures under the vessel, ligate the vein distally, and use a clamp to apply traction on the distal suture inferiorly to enhance exposure of the vein.
6. Incise the skin 1 to 2 cm distally and tunnel the feeding tube under the skin to the venotomy site.

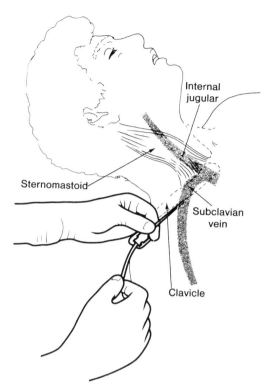

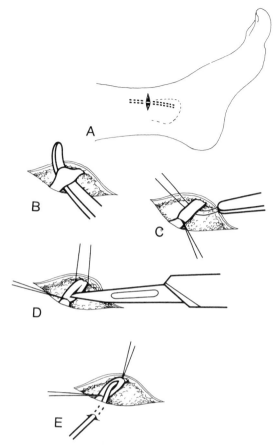

FIGURE 139–20. Cannulation of the subclavian vein by the infraclavicular approach. (From Simon RR, Brenner BE, eds: *Emergency Procedures and Techniques.* Baltimore: Williams & Wilkins, 1987)

7. Loop the proximal suture around the vessel, and with a clamp apply gentle traction on the proximal suture in a superior direction to further expose the vein.
8. Incise the vein on the superficial side, carefully enlarge the venotomy site with the tip of a forceps, and introduce the feeding tube into the vessel under the introducer device.
9. Advance the catheter proximally until either blood returns or rapid flow of intravenous fluid is achieved. Then tie the proximal suture around the vein over the catheter to secure it in place.
10. Connect to infusion set-up.
11. Suture the incision closed over the catheter and tape and dress the cutdown site and tunnel site securely.

Complications

1. Infection
2. Bleeding
3. Thrombophlebitis
4. Scar formation

FIGURE 139–21. Procedure for venous cutdown at saphenous vein in ankle. (*A*) Identify site superior and lateral to medial malleolus. (*B*) Isolate vessel with clamp. (*C*) Ligate vessel distally. (*D*) Perform venotomy with traction on vessel. (*E*) Tunnel catheter (feeding tube) through distal skin site. (From Simon RR, Brenner BE, eds: *Emergency Procedures and Techniques.* Baltimore: Williams & Wilkins, 1987)

UMBILICAL VESSEL CANNULATION

The umbilical vessels provide easy vascular access in the immediate newborn period for emergency delivery of drugs and fluids, hemodynamic monitoring, and blood specimen collection. Either the vein or artery can be used.

Equipment and Supplies

Prep solution, sterile gloves, sterile drape
Mask and gown

No. 15 scalpel
Curved clamps
Scissors
3-0 silk umbilical tie
3.5f (premature babies) or 5f (full-term babies) umbilical catheter
Normal saline (with heparin 1 unit/ml) infusion set-up
10-ml syringe
Three-way stopcock

POSITION AND PROCEDURE (FIG. 139-22)

1. Restrain the child in a supine frog-leg position.
2. Drape and prep the cord and surrounding area from xiphoid to pubis.
3. Place a purse-string umbilical 3-0 silk tie around the base of the umbilicus and trim the cord 2 cm above the skin. Tighten the tie to arrest significant bleeding.
4. Identify the larger, thin umbilical vein and two thick-walled umbilical arteries. Grasp two sides of the umbilicus with curved clamps to fully expose the vessel. Gently enlarge the vessel opening with the forceps.
5. Insert the tip of a umbilical catheter filled with saline into the vessel lumen with the prongs of the forceps and advance the catheter until blood returns.
6. If resistance is encountered, pull back the catheter and gently re-insert it.
7. When the flow is unobstructed, attach the catheter to the three-way stopcock and infusion set-up. Secure the catheter by tightening the silk purse-string suture on the cord. Tape to abdomen.

8. If the catheter is left in place after resuscitation, confirm T6-T9 or L4-L5 position with an abdominal radiograph.

Complications

1. Embolization or thrombosis
2. Infection
3. Bleeding
4. Arterial occlusion
5. Air embolism

INTRAOSSEOUS INFUSION

Intraosseous cannulation is an effective method for delivery of drugs and fluids into the highly vascular intramedullary bone space, in a patient with low venous pressures requiring emergent vascular access. This technique is especially useful in the child under 2 years, and becomes more difficult in children over 5 years. The flow dynamics and pharmacokinetics of intraosseous drugs and fluids appear to be equivalent to peripheral venous administration. Complications are few. A principal advantage of this technique is speed; an intraosseous line can usually be established in 1 to 2 minutes.

Indications

1. Cardiac arrest
2. Respiratory arrest
3. Unstable cardiac dysrhythmias
4. Shock
5. Any life-threatening emergency requiring rapid drug or fluid administration where peripheral access is unavailable

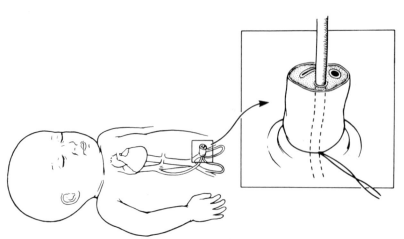

FIGURE 139–22. Umbilical vessel cannulation.

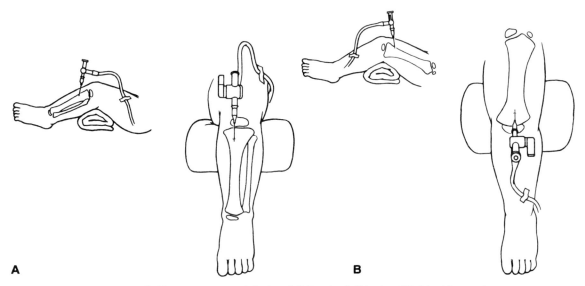

FIGURE 139–23. Intraosseous infusion. (*A*) Proximal tibia site. (*B*) Distal femur site.

Equipment and Supplies

Prep solution, sterile gloves, sterile drape
1% lidocaine
25-gauge needle and 3-ml syringe
16- or 18-gauge intraosseous needle, bone-marrow aspiration needle, or spinal needle
Three-way stopcock
10-ml syringe with normal saline
Infusion set-up
Silk suture

Position

Restrain the child in a supine position. Place a towel roll behind the knee and secure the foot. Select either a tibial or femoral site for entry. The tibial site (Fig. 139A) is easier and is located 2 cm medial to the inferior tip of the patella in the flat portion of the proximal bone. The femoral site (Fig. 139B) is in the midline of the distal femur 2 cm above the superior tip of the patella.

Procedure (Fig. 139-23)

1. Prep and drape the area.
2. If the child is conscious, anesthetize the area from skin to periosteum.
3. Introduce the intraosseous needle directed at 60 degrees off the horizontal, away from the growth plate of the bone. Direct the needle superiorly in the femur and inferiorly in the tibia.
4. Pierce the anterior cortex and enter the intramedullary space with a gentle, steady rotational movement.
5. Remove the stylet and confirm proper placement by instilling 10 ml of normal saline without resistance.
6. Attach the stopcock to the needle hub and to the infusion set-up.
7. Secure the needle to the skin with a suture, and tape the infusion tubing to the skin.

Complications

1. Osteomyelitis
2. Soft-tissue infection
3. Compartment syndrome
4. Bleeding

140 Diagnostic Imaging

Ronald R. Townsend

Recent technological advances have significantly improved the radiologist's ability to help the clinician achieve a rapid, correct diagnosis. Optimal evaluation of a particular problem might involve use of any combination of standard radiographs, fluoroscopic studies, angiography, ultrasound, computed tomography (CT), nuclear medicine, magnetic resonance imaging (MRI), or other studies. These advances have also created the potential for much confusion. The myriad of available radiographic procedures may leave the clinician uncertain as to the best test for a particular patient. This can result in blindly ordering all the studies available, putting patients through unnecessary procedures and increasing health-care expenditures. The following are general guidelines for appropriate imaging that are particularly applicable in the emergency setting:

1. If you are uncertain as to which test is appropriate, discuss the case with the consulting radiologist. Local equipment availability and expertise will influence which procedure is of choice for a given clinical question. For example, for a clinical question of pyloric stenosis, the diagnostic procedure of choice may be a barium fluoroscopic study (upper GI exam) or ultrasound, depending on local expertise.
2. Before ordering a test, ask yourself how the result of the test will alter patient management. If the procedure will not make a difference in patient treatment, it is generally not indicated.
3. Optimize conditions to maximize diagnostic information and minimize patient risk. Do not move a patient with potential spine injury to the radiology department for radiographs that could adequately be obtained in the emergency department. Avoid placing an unstable or potentially unstable patient in an unsupervised environment. Another consideration, particularly for young infants, is the risk of hypothermia when the patient is left uncovered for multiple radiographic procedures. Monitor the infant's temperature and bundle the patient carefully.

4. If several studies are likely to have equal diagnostic yield, ask yourself:
   a. Which study is actually most readily available and rapidly completed on an emergent basis?
   b. Which study offers the least risk or potential risk to the patient? For example, ultrasound has the advantage of no ionizing radiation.
   c. Which does the patient prefer?
   d. What is the cost to the patient and to society in general?
5. Avoid reflex ordering of radiographs. Not everyone with arm pain needs radiographs of the entire arm. If radiography is indicated, a good history and physical examination will limit the radiographic examination to the area of concern, limiting radiation exposure and costs.
6. Use common sense.

In the patient with complex abnormalities (*e.g.*, trauma with injuries to multiple organ systems), multiple imaging studies may be indicated. Make a diagnostic plan before initiating the evaluation, as some studies may preclude others (*e.g.*, abdominal ultrasound or CT is of limited utility after the GI tract is filled with barium). A single study (*e.g.*, abdominal CT) may answer all the questions that otherwise would require multiple studies (barium enema, intravenous urogram, etc.). Such cases particularly demand close communication of radiologist and physician.

Some examinations (particularly CT, MRI, and angiography) may require patient sedation. The need for sedation must be addressed for each patient individually; important considerations include the patient's age, medical condition, and the length and nature of the examination. The best form of sedation varies with the patient's medical condition, the type of examination, the monitoring equipment and personnel available, etc. Discuss these factors with the radiologist when arranging the examination.

General considerations for specific symptoms and signs in different anatomic regions are discussed below. Local factors, including equipment availability,

650

the radiologist's expertise, and the particular circumstances of a given patient's presentation may alter the examination of choice.

Specific Anatomic Areas ■

ABDOMEN

Abdominal Mass

Radiographs to rule out bowel obstruction, calcified mass, soft-tissue mass. Further evaluation depends on patient age and findings on physical examination/laboratory evaluation. Ultrasound is commonly employed, but CT or organ-specific evaluation (*e.g.*, intravenous pyelography) may be performed based on the specific case and local expertise.

Acute Abdomen

Radiographs: to evaluate for bowel obstruction or perforation; abnormal calcifications (especially nephrolithiasis, appendicolith, or radiopaque gallstones); or masses or organomegaly.

Further evaluation depends on findings of physical examination and radiographs (see Chapter 40).

1. *Ultrasound*: especially for a question of cholecystitis, renal obstruction, or ascites, or to evaluate the nature of a palpable mass. In centers with appropriate expertise, graded compression ultrasound may be useful for evaluating appendicitis.
2. *Barium enema*: to further evaluate etiology of bowel obstruction in patients without peritoneal signs on physical examination (*e.g.*, intussusception)
3. *Intravenous urogram*: for possible renal stone
4. *Chest radiographs*: to rule out pneumonia, which may present with abdominal symptoms

GI Bleeding

Initial evaluation may include endoscopic or radiographic methods, depending on factors such as patient's age, likely pathology, severity of bleeding, and local expertise (see Chapter 32).

Barium enema (or rectal air in some medical centers): for suspicion of intussusception. Study may be diagnostic and therapeutic.

Radionuclide studies: can be useful to identify the source of bleeding in some situations (*e.g.*, Meckel's diverticulum)

Angiography: may be indicated with brisk bleeding for both diagnosis and therapy

Hematuria

Intravenous urogram: to rule out renal stone disease/mass. Further evaluation depends on findings and accompanying symptoms/signs (see Chapter 112).

Ingestion

Radiographs: especially with ingestion or a question of ingestion of radiopaque tablets (*e.g.*, iron, calcium, bismuth antacids, phenothiazines, etc.) or other radiopaque material (see Chapter 63)

Renal Failure

Ultrasonography: to rule out obstruction or identify the site of obstruction in the urinary tract, and to evaluate for evidence of renal parenchymal disease (cystic disease, etc.) (see Chapter 111). Further evaluation depends on ultrasound findings and symptoms/signs.

Trauma

Patients with massive blunt abdominal trauma who are hemodynamically unstable or those with penetrating trauma (knife, bullet) to the peritoneal cavity usually undergo attempted life-saving surgery without imaging.

Abdominal/pelvic CT: In more stable patients with significant suspicion of injury (*e.g.*, slowly falling hematocrit, suspicious findings on physical examination), CT has proven highly effective in diagnosis of parenchymal organ injuries and detection of hemoperitoneum. Even in the absence of clinical suspicion of abdominal injury, abdominal CT may be useful to exclude injury in patients with extensive trauma and neurologic impairment or young age such that abdominal symptoms and signs can not be well evaluated (see Chapter 56).

Intravenous urography may be useful for evaluating injury clinically felt to be limited to the kidney, but CT is more sensitive in detecting and more effective at characterizing these and other associated injuries (see Chapter 57).

Radiographs: useful for evaluating associated skeletal injuries and to exclude free air seen with gross bowel perforation or penetrating injury

Radionuclide studies (*e.g.*, liver-spleen scan with a question of hepatic laceration) or *ultrasound* have proven useful in the setting of trauma in some institutions.

CHEST

The initial, and often the only, imaging modality for complaints referable to the chest is the *chest radio-*

graph. Variations in standard radiographic technique or additional study may be indicated in specific situations as discussed below.

Airway Obstruction (see also Neck)

Radiographs: include an expiratory view. In a child too young to cooperate with expiration, consider decubitus views to evaluate for air-trapping in the dependent hemithorax. Evaluate for radiopaque foreign body, mass, unilateral increased lung volume with obstructing foreign body, bilateral increased lung volumes with obstructive pulmonary disease (*e.g.*, asthma) (see Chapter 13).

Assessment of Medical Intervention

Radiographs: for placement of catheters, endotracheal tube, chest tubes, etc.; evaluation for rib fractures or lung contusions after CPR

Asthma Exacerbation

Radiographs: to rule out focal consolidation (pneumonia), bronchial inflammation (thickening), pneumothorax, pneumomediastinum. See Chapter 15 for consideration of when radiographs are indicated.

Congestive Heart Failure

Radiographs: to confirm diagnosis. Evaluate for presence of cardiomegaly, vascular congestion, interstitial or alveolar edema, pleural effusions (see Chapter 9).

Infection

Radiographs: to detect focal consolidation with bacterial pneumonia. Multifocal abnormalities, especially perihilar/peribronchial increased densities, suggest viral inflammation. Utility of chest radiography in patients with fever and no respiratory signs or symptoms is questionable and depends on circumstances (see Chapter 116).

Near-Drowning

Radiographs: evaluate for evidence of diffuse aspiration or edema and superimposed focal consolidation (see Chapter 99).

Pericarditis/Tamponade

Radiographs: to look for increased size of cardiac silhouette, evidence of congestive heart failure (see Chapter 10)
  Echocardiography: to rule out pericardial effusion

Respiratory Distress

Radiographs: to evaluate for edema, focal consolidation, congestive heart failure, airway obstruction, etc.

Smoke Inhalation

Radiographs: to evaluate for diffuse edema, focal atelectasis or consolidation (see Chapter 61)

Trauma

Radiographs: to evaluate for fracture, pneumothorax, hemothorax, lung contusion, mediastinal widening (see Chapter 55)
  Arteriography: with deceleration injuries (motor vehicle accident, fall from a height) and mediastinal widening on chest radiograph; possible traumatic aortic aneurysm may be excluded with arteriography.

EXTREMITIES

Child Abuse

Radiographs: standard views of symptomatic areas and standard evaluation of presenting symptoms and signs (*e.g.*, head CT scan with neurologic findings); skeletal survey (includes chest, abdomen, extremities, skull) to look for evidence of unexplained trauma and epiphyseal or metaphyseal injuries (see Chapter 128)

Foreign Body

Radiographs (soft-tissue technique), xeroradiographs, or *ultrasound* depending on circumstances and local availability/expertise. Ultrasound may effectively localize non-radiopaque objects such as wood fragments.

Gas in Soft Tissues

Radiographs: to look for presence and extent of gas collection accompanying necrotizing infections (see Chapter 118)

Infection

Radiographs: to look for evidence of bone destruction, demineralization, periostitis, soft-tissue mass to rule out osteomyelitis (see Chapter 119). If radiographs are negative, consider radionuclide imaging (bone scan, or combination of bone scan and gallium scan) to differentiate osteomyelitis from overlying soft-tissue infection.

With prominent soft-tissue swelling and suspected soft-tissue abscess, *ultrasound* can be useful to localize fluid collections for diagnostic aspiration/drainage.

Pain

Radiographs: In the joint, evaluate for presence of effusion, bone destruction, or demineralization to suggest infectious or noninfectious arthropathy (see Chapters 44 and 120); in the bone shaft, for evidence of infection, tumor, stress fracture, or associated soft-tissue mass.

Trauma

Radiographs: Use standard views for anatomic area of interest. If radiographic evaluation is indicated by the clinical examination, avoid the temptation to order a single view to limit exposure. Subtle injuries may not be detected in one view. Comparison views of the opposite normal extremity may be necessary, but their use can be minimized with reference to a standard atlas, such as that by Keats and Smith (see Chapter 58).

Angiography may be indicated with displaced/comminuted fractures to evaluate for possible associated vascular injuries.

FACE

Foreign Body

Radiographs, especially to evaluate for a question of intraorbital metallic foreign body (see Chapter 52)

CT may provide more precise localization if needed for surgical planning.

Infection

Radiographs:

1. To evaluate for sinus opacification or air/fluid levels accompanying sinusitis (see Chapter 117)
2. To rule out bone destruction from osteomyelitis

3. Mandibular or maxillary views may be indicated to rule out complications of dental infection, especially osteomyelitis (see Chapter 47).

Trauma

Radiographs: to rule out fracture or sinus opacification associated with occult fracture (see Chapter 51)

CT: to evaluate complex fractures and for surgical planning

HEAD

Coma/Altered Mental Status

CT or *MRI* of brain, depending on circumstances and local availability/expertise. Evaluate for any intracranial abnormality. Radiographic evaluation for systemic causes of altered mental status may be indicated, depending on circumstances (see Chapter 16).

Infection

CT (with contrast) or *MRI* of brain: to evaluate complications of meningitis (subdural/epidural fluid collection, hydrocephalus) or abscess (see Chapter 114)

Seizure (Without Trauma)

CT (contrast enhanced) or *MRI* of brain, depending on circumstances and local availability/expertise. Evaluate for any potential seizure focus (tumor, infection, congenital abnormality, etc.) (see Chapter 26).

Trauma

CT of brain (non-contrast), when history and physical examination (especially with focal neurologic symptoms and/or signs) suggest significant injury. Evaluate for subdural, epidural, or parenchymal hematoma, and associated mass effect. Associated skull fracture or foreign body (in case of penetrating trauma) may be visualized (see Chapter 50).

Skull *radiographs* are rarely indicated due to inability to visualize intracranial structures. Significant intracranial pathology requiring urgent intervention may be present without skull fracture, and skull fracture may be present without significant intracranial injury.

Caution: If cervical spine injury is also a consideration, radiographs of the cervical spine should generally be obtained before the patient is transported to the radiology department for head CT (see Chapter 54).

NECK

Airway Obstruction (Patient Supervised)

Lateral radiograph: for evaluation of possible epiglottitis, retropharyngeal mass, or foreign body (see Chapter 13)

A-P radiograph: for question of croup (subglottic narrowing of airway), mass, foreign body

CT: to further evaluate mass (*e.g.*, define retropharyngeal abscess, allow surgical planning, etc.)

Dysphagia/Odynophagia

Neck radiographs: to rule out epiglottitis, mass, foreign body. If radiographs are nondiagnostic, consider contrast esophagram to rule out esophagitis, foreign body, mass.

Trauma

Radiographs: for spine trauma (see also Spine)

CT: may be useful for evaluation of laryngeal trauma

Angiography: for penetrating injuries, depending on location of injury

PELVIS/GENITALIA

Pain (Gynecologic)

Ultrasound: to evaluate for ovarian torsion, infection (abscess complicating pelvic inflammatory disease), hematometrocolpos, etc (see Chapter 107).

Pain (Scrotal)

Ultrasound (preferably with Doppler) or *radionuclide perfusion study* (depending on local availability/expertise): for clinical question of torsion (see Chapter 45)

Ultrasound: for evaluation of testicular mass, epididymitis, orchitis

Trauma

Radiographs: to evaluate for pelvic fractures, accompanying hematoma

CT: may be necessary to evaluate sacral or acetabular fractures, etc., for treatment planning

Contrast cystogram: to evaluate possible bladder rupture associated with pelvic injury (See Chapter 57.)

Ultrasound: for scrotal trauma with possible testicular injury

SPINE

Acute Myelopathy

Myelogram (subarachnoid injection of water-soluble contrast)/*CT myelogram* or *MRI* of spine: to evaluate for intrinsic cord pathology (tumor, syrinx, hematoma, transverse myelitis) or subdural/epidural mass causing cord compression (see Chapter 54)

Infection

Radiographs: to exclude discitis (irregular vertebral end plates on both sides of a disc) or osteomyelitis

CT at level of radiographic abnormality is useful for better definition and guidance of diagnostic needle aspiration.

Myelogram (usually with CT): in cases with neurologic symptoms to evaluate extent of epidural mass

Trauma

Radiographs: with patient immobilized until unstable injury is excluded. Evaluate alignment, rule out fractures/dislocations. CT may be indicated to further evaluate a radiographic abnormality or question of abnormality.

Bibliography ■

Federle MP, Brant-Zawadzki M: *Computed Tomography in the Evaluation of Trauma,* 2nd ed. Baltimore: Williams & Wilkins, 1986.

Harris JH Jr, Harris WH: *The Radiology of Emergency Medicine,* 2nd ed. Baltimore: Williams & Wilkins, 1981.

Hayden CK, Swischuk LE: *Pediatric Ultrasonography.* Baltimore: Williams & Wilkins, 1987.

Keats TE, Smith TH: *An Atlas of Normal Developmental Roentgen Anatomy.* Chicago: Year Book, 1977.

Kirchner SG, ed: Symposium on pediatric radiology. *Pediatr Clin North Am* 1985; 32:1351.

Kirks DR: *Practical Pediatric Imaging.* Boston: Little, Brown, 1984.

Swischuk LE: *Emergency Radiology of the Acutely Ill or Injured Child,* 2nd ed. Baltimore: Williams & Wilkins, 1986.

141 Pediatric Emergency Equipment and Supplies

Ronald A. Dieckmann

All facilities that may be called upon to see pediatric emergencies must have the necessary equipment and supplies. The location of such equipment and supplies must be known and available to all ED personnel. Often a pediatric emergency cart provides the best location. This chapter lists such necessary equipment and supplies.

Monitoring devices:
1. ECG monitor-defibrillator/cardioverter (0 to 400 watt-seconds), with 4.5-cm and 8-cm paddles and hard-copy recording capability
2. Otoscope/ophthalmoscope/stethoscope
3. Pulse oximeter with pediatric adapter
4. Doppler ultrasound blood-pressure device
5. Arterial and venous pressure monitoring equipment immediately available to ED
6. Rectal temperature probe
7. Blood pressure cuffs (neonatal, infant, child); arm and thigh for adult

Specialized pediatric trays for the following procedures:
1. Thoracotomy, including pediatric rib spreaders and aortic clamp
2. Tube thoracostomy and water seal drainage
3. Cricothyrotomy and tracheostomy
4. Peritoneal lavage
5. Spinal tap
6. Open surgical venous cutdown
7. Deep venous cannulation or Seldinger vascular access technique
8. Umbilical vessel cannulation
9. Minor procedures
10. Plastic surgery procedures

Vascular access equipment:
1. Intravenous fluid warmer
2. Infusion pumps, drip or volumetric with microinfusion capability

Respiratory equipment:
1. Bag-valve-mask resuscitator
2. Suction devices
3. Laryngoscope handle
4. Laryngoscope blades (curved 1, 2, 3; straight 0, 1, 2, 3)
5. Stylets for endotracheal tubes
6. Magill forceps

Fracture management devices:
1. Spine board (child and adult)
2. Femur splint (child and adult)
3. Traction device
4. Rigid neck collars (child and adult)
5. Gardner-Wells tongs
6. Halo device
7. Sandbags
8. K-wire surgical set

Miscellaneous equipment:
1. Infant scale
2. Heating source
3. Cardiac backboard

Supplies:
1. Endotracheal tubes (uncuffed sizes 2.5, 3, 3.5, 4.0, 4.5, 5.0, 5.5, 6.0; cuffed sizes 6.0, 6.5, 7.0, 7.5, 8.0)
2. Tracheostomy tubes (Shiley tube sizes 00, 1, 2, 3, 4, 6)
3. Oral airways (sizes 0, 1, 2, 3, 4, 5)
4. Nasopharyngeal airways (sizes 12, 16, 20, 24, 28, 30 f)
5. Clear masks (standard and non-rebreathing; neonatal, infant, child, adult)
6. Nasal cannulae (child and adult)
7. Needles:
   Butterfly: 21, 23, 25
   Over-the-needle: 14, 16, 18, 20, 22, 24
   Intracaths (8"): small, medium, large
   Intraosseous: 16 and 18

8. Syringes (sizes TB, 3, 5, 10, 20, 30, 60 ml)
9. Needles (regular sizes 16, 18, 21, 22, 23, 25; spinal 18, 20 [1.5, 2.5, 3"])
10. Three-way stopcocks
11. Tourniquets and rubber bands
12. Armboards (infant and child)
13. Urinary catheters (sizes 5, 8, 10, 12)
14. Chest tubes (sizes 8, 12, 16, 20, 24, 28, 32, 40)
15. Intravenous solutions (normal saline and 5% dextrose in water: 100 ml, 250 ml, 500 ml; mannitol 20%: 500 ml)
16. IV administration sets and extension tubing
17. Suction catheters (sizes 6f, 8f, 10f, 14f)
18. Yankauer suction tip
19. Feeding tubes for endotracheal drugs (sizes 3.5, 5, 8f)
20. Nasogastric tubes (sizes 5, 8, 10, 12, 14, 16 f)
21. Lubricating jelly
22. Arm boards (neonatal, infant, child)
23. Bulb syringes (sizes 1, 2, 3 oz)
24. Diapers (sizes small, medium, large)
25. Casting materials
26. Medications (see Chapter 146 for doses and concentrations): acetaminophen, activated charcoal, topical antibiotics, atropine, bretylium, calcium chloride, dexamethasone, diazepam, diazoxide, digoxin, diphenhydramine, dobutamine, dopamine, 50% dextrose in water, epinephrine, furosemide, heparin, insulin, ipecac, isoproterenol, lidocaine, mannitol, metaproterenol, methyl prednisolone, morphine sulfate, naloxone, pancuronium, phenobarbital, phenylephrine, phenytoin, potassium chloride, propranolol, racemic epinephrine, sodium bicarbonate, sodium chloride, succinylcholine, tetracaine-epinephrine-cocaine topical anesthetic, thiopental.

142 Reportable Diseases

Moses Grossman

All states and municipalities require the reporting of communicable disease to the Department of Health. In most instances the reporting can be done by the child's regular physician after laboratory confirmation, but some diseases must be reported on an urgent basis for public protection. Table 142-1 lists diseases reportable in California. This list may vary slightly from state to state but is quite representative.

TABLE 142–1. *Reportable Diseases or Conditions in California*

Acquired Immune Deficiency Syndrome (AIDS)	+ Malaria
+ Amebiasis	+ Measles (rubeola)
* Anthrax	+ Meningitis (specify etiology: viral, bacterial, fungal, parasitic)
* Botulism (infant, foodborne, wound)	+ Meningococcal infections
Brucellosis	+ Meningococcal infections
+ Campylobacteriosis	Mumps
Chancroid	Non-gonococcal urethritis (excluding laboratory confirmed chlamydial infections)
Chlamydial infections	
* Cholera	Pelvic inflammatory disease (PID)
Coccidioidomycosis	Pertussis (whooping cough)
+ Conjunctivitis, acute infectious of the newborn (specify etiology)	* Plague
Cryptosporidiosis	+ Poliomyelitis, paralytic
Cysticercosis	+ Psittacosis
* Dengue	+ Q fever
* Diarrhea of the newborn, outbreaks	* Rabies, human or animal
* Diphtheria	+ Relapsing fever
+ Encephalitis (specify etiology: viral, bacterial, fungal, parasitic)	Reye syndrome
Foodborne illness	Rheumatic fever, acute
Giardiasis	Rocky Mountain spotted fever
Gonococcal infections	Rubella (German measles)
Granuloma inguinale	Salmonellosis (other than typhoid fever)
Haemophilus influenzae, invasive disease	Shigellosis
+ Hepatitis A	+ Streptococcal infections (outbreaks and cases in foodhandlers and dairy workers only)
Hepatitis B, cases and carriers (specify)	
Hepatitis, Delta (D)	+ Syphilis
Hepatitis, Non-A, Non-B	Tetanus
Hepatitis, Unspecified	Toxic shock syndrome
Kawasaki syndrome (mucocutaneous lymph node syndrome)	+ Trichinosis
Legionellosis	Tuberculosis
Leprosy (Hansen's disease)	Tularemia
Leptospirosis	+ Typhoid fever, cases and carriers
+ Listeriosis	Typhus fever
Lyme disease	* Yellow fever
Lymphogranuloma venereum (lymphogranuloma inguinale)	

The urgency of reporting each disease or condition is indicated by the following symbols: (*) To be reported immediately by telephone. (+) To be reported by mailing a report or telephoning within one (1) working day of identification of the case or suspected case. (no star or cross symbol) To be reported within seven (7) calendar days from the time of identification.

143 Patient Instructions

Kevin P. Coulter

Parental Instructions ■

1. Your child has been examined in the emergency department. The physician who examined your child will not become your child's regular doctor. You should schedule an appointment with your child's regular doctor in _____ days.
2. If your child's condition worsens in the next 24 hours, return to the emergency department.
3. Your child's regular doctor will receive a copy of the medical records, test results, and a written description of any x-rays taken on your child.
4. If you do not have a regular doctor for your child, ask the emergency department staff for help in finding one.
5. If you have any questions, call your regular doctor or the emergency department.

Medications ■

1. If you were given a medicine, follow the directions on the label. If the medicine is an antibiotic, take it until it is finished.
2. If you think your child is having an allergic reaction to the medicine, stop it and call your regular doctor or the emergency department.

Fever ■

1. Fever is a normal body response to infection or injury. It is not unusual for children to have high fevers with a mild cold.
2. To take your child's temperature:
   a. Use a rectal thermometer.
   b. Shake it until the mercury falls below 97°F (36°C).
   c. Put Vaseline or K-Y Lubricating Jelly on the tip.
   d. With the child on his/her stomach, hold the buttocks apart and gently put the thermometer one inch into the rectum.
   e. Hold the child still and do not let go of the thermometer while it is in place.
   f. Read the thermometer in 2 minutes.

3. To read the thermometer:
   a. Rotate the thermometer until the wide silver line can be seen.
   b. Read the number at the end of the silver line.
4. To treat a fever:
   a. A rectal temperature up to 100.4°F (38°C) is considered normal.
   b. A mild fever (less than 101°F) does not require treatment.
   c. For temperature over 101°F, give your child acetaminophen. Acetaminophen comes under different names (Tylenol, Tempra, Liquiprin).
   d. Give acetaminophen drops _____ ml every _____ hours. Give acetaminophen liquid __ tsp every _____ hours.
   e. If the fever is over 104°F, give your child a lukewarm bath for 30 minutes. Do not allow your child to become chilled. Towel-dry immediately after bathing.
   f. Dress your child lightly. Do not bundle your child up.
   g. Encourage your child to drink a lot of fluids.
   h. Keep the room temperature normal.
   i. Do not bathe your child in alcohol.
5. Call your doctor if:
   a. Your child is under 3 months old and has *any* degree of fever.
   b. Your child's fever is over 105°F.
   c. The fever lasts over 48 hours.
   d. Your child has unusual movements of face, arms, or legs.
   e. Your child looks sicker than you would expect.

Common Childhood Illnesses ■

COLD

1. Colds are virus infections of the nose and mouth. Your baby may have a runny nose, watery eyes, cough, and fever. You can help your baby by giving him/her plenty of fluids to drink.

2. Your child can breathe easier if you add moisture to the air. You can do this by:
   a. Using a vaporizer or humidifier
   b. Running a hot shower in a closed bathroom and letting your baby breathe the steamy air
   c. Putting salt-water drops in your baby's nose. Mix ¼ teaspoon salt in 4 ounces water. Put two drops in each side of the nose, then suck out the nose with a bulb syringe.
3. Treat fever over 101°F with acetaminophen.
4. Call your doctor if:
   a. The fever lasts longer than 3 days
   b. Your child is unable to take fluids, is vomiting, or has abdominal pain
   c. Your child complains of earache, or pulls at ears
   d. Your child has trouble breathing or is breathing rapidly
   e. Your child is abnormally irritable or sleepy

EAR INFECTION

1. Your child has been prescribed an antibiotic to treat his/her ear infection. Follow the instructions, finishing the antibiotic entirely. Acetaminophen will help relieve the ear pain.
2. Your child should be rechecked in 2 weeks to be sure the infection is cured.
3. Contact your doctor if:
   a. Your child is no better in 48 hours
   b. Your child becomes irritable or listless

CONJUNCTIVITIS

1. Eye drops may be prescribed. Gently wipe the discharge from your child's eye with a washcloth or moistened cotton. Pulling the lower eyelid down, put two drops in each eye four times per day. Alternatively, ointment may be prescribed: squeeze a small amount into each eye four times per day.
2. Conjunctivitis is contagious. Wash your hands after cleaning your child's eyes. Use separate towels and washcloths for your child.
3. Cool-water compresses over the eyelid may be soothing.
4. Contact your doctor if:
   a. Symptoms don't improve in 4 days
   b. Pain develops in the eye itself
   c. Any change in vision develops
   d. The eyelid becomes red, swollen, or tender

SORE THROAT

1. Acetaminophen may help relieve throat pain and fever.
2. Gargle with salt water (¼ tsp. in 4 oz. water).
3. If your child is thought to have strep throat, an antibiotic will be prescribed. He/she can return to school or daycare 48 hours after antibiotics are started.
4. If a throat culture was done, we will contact you in 48 hours with results.
5. Call your doctor if:
   a. Symptoms don't improve in 2 days
   b. Your child begins to drool
   c. Swallowing or breathing becomes difficult

CROUP

1. Acetaminophen will help your child feel better if he/she has a fever.
2. Moistened air will help your child breathe easier. You can accomplish this with a humidifier or vaporizer or by turning on a hot shower in a closed bathroom and having your child breathe the steamy air.
3. Call your doctor if:
   a. Breathing becomes more difficult
   b. Drooling develops or swallowing becomes difficult
   c. Your child becomes very irritable or listless
   d. Moistened air does not improve symptoms
   e. Your child turns blue

CHICKEN POX

1. If your child has a fever, treat it with acetaminophen. *DO NOT USE ASPIRIN.*
2. To treat itchy skin, bathe your child in cool water to which is added ½ cup of baking soda. You can also place calamine lotion on the sores.
3. Trim your child's fingernails short. Scratching the sores may cause them to get infected.
4. Your child is *very* contagious. Keep him/her at home for at least 7 days after the rash begins.
5. Contact your doctor if:
   a. The sores get very red
   b. The temperature is over 103°F
   c. Your child gets a severe headache, is vomiting, or acting very sick or very sleepy
   d. Your child has trouble breathing or develops a bad cough

DIARRHEA AND VOMITING

1. Stop all milk and solid foods. These will irritate the bowel and make the diarrhea worse. Begin the special diet listed below. If you are breastfeeding, continue to do so.
2. Dietary instructions:
   a. First day: clear fluids only. For infants or toddlers: Pedialyte, Lytren, or Gatorade; for older children: Gatorade, soda, clear soup, Popsicles.

b. If your child has diarrhea, give as much fluid as your child wants, but at least 3 to 4 ounces every 3 to 4 hours.

c. If your child is vomiting, give clear fluids ½ ounce every 15 to 20 minutes until vomiting has stopped, then give 3 to 4 ounces every 3 to 4 hours.

d. Second day: mashed bananas, applesauce, crackers, bread, boiled potato. Begin half-strength formula or milk and gradually advance to full strength over the next day.

3. Contact your doctor if:
   a. Fever is higher than 103°F
   b. Blood is in the stool
   c. Abdominal pain develops or worsens
   d. Diarrhea lasts longer than 7 days
   e. Adding foods other than clear liquids makes diarrhea worse
   f. Signs of dehydration appear (when the body has lost too much water): dry mouth, crying without tears, no urine in 12 hours, sunken eyes or sunken soft spot in baby's head

Common Injuries ■

HEAD INJURY

1. Although your doctors feel it is safe for your child to go home, any head injury has a small chance of causing delayed bleeding around the brain and may be dangerous. If any of the following problems arise in the next 7 days, return to the emergency department or contact your own doctor immediately:
   a. Abnormal behavior: strange or changed behavior; drowsy, forgetful
   b. Irritable, violent
   c. Unconsciousness; cannot be awakened
   d. Severe headache
   e. Repeated vomiting
   f. Slurred speech
   g. Blurry or double vision
   h. Weakness of an arm or leg; inability to walk normally
   i. Bleeding or leakage of clear fluid from ears or nose
   j. Seizure
   k. Temperature over 100°F
2. If your child goes to sleep within 8 hours of the injury, you should awaken him/her every 2 hours for the first 12 hours after the injury to make sure that he/she is not in a coma.

3. The following symptoms are normal and to be expected after any head injury:
   a. Mild headache
   b. Mild nausea
   c. Mild dizziness

SPRAIN OR SOFT-TISSUE INJURY

1. Keep the injured part elevated.
2. Apply an ice pack to the injured area for _____ days.
3. Give aspirin/acetaminophen _____ ml/tsp/tab every _____ hours.
4. Use crutches for _____ days.
5. Do not allow the child to walk on the injured part for _____ days.

CAST INSTRUCTIONS

1. A cast takes 24 to 72 hours to dry thoroughly. Contact a physician if any of the following conditions occur:
   a. Swelling or discoloration of toes or fingers
   b. Inability to move toes or fingers
   c. Pain or odor from cast
   d. Numbness or loss of feeling in hand and fingers or foot and toes
   e. Foot or arm slips in cast
2. Return for a cast check in _____ hrs/days.

DRESSING CARE AND WOUND CARE

1. If pain from the wound is severe or persistent, contact your regular doctor or the emergency department.
2. Watch for signs of wound infection (swelling, redness, pain, warm to touch, fever, red streaks from the wound).
3. Do not allow the dressing to get wet.
4. Clean the wound _____ times per day with soap and water.
5. The wound needs to be examined in _____ days by your doctor.
6. It is necessary to change the dressing in _____ days. It may be changed sooner if it becomes dirty or you are concerned about infection.
7. Sutures should be removed in _____ days.

MINOR BURNS

1. A minor burn will heal quickly, usually in 1 to 2 weeks. Ways to help it heal without infection and less scarring are:
   a. Keep the burn area or dressing clean and dry.

b. Do not break any blisters or remove skin unless directed by the doctor.

c. Raise the burned area above the level of the heart to reduce pain and swelling. Prop on pillows at night.

d. Take aspirin/acetaminophen _____ ml/tsp/tab every _____ hours for pain.

2. After healing, the new skin may dry or crack. Apply a lotion or cream such as cocoa butter, Eucerin, or vitamin E for 4 to 8 weeks *after* healing.

3. Avoid exposing the burned area to excessive sunlight for 6 months. Apply a sunscreen to the burned area.

4. Do not use strong soaps or tight clothing on the burned area.

5. Remember to keep your appointment to recheck the burn.

6. Contact the emergency department or your doctor if:

a. The burn becomes red, feels hot, or drains pus

b. Fever is over 101°F

c. The burned area swells or becomes numb or more painful

Infestations ■

SCABIES

1. Scabies are very small insects that live in the top layer of the skin. They cause an itchy rash on the fingers, wrists, armpits, waist, and groin. In infants, they can spread to the face.

2. Scabies can be spread by close personal contact and by having sex.

3. To treat scabies:

a. Shower with soap and water, then apply Kwell lotion from neck to toes. Leave on for 8 hours (overnight), then wash completely off.

b. Repeat this once, in one week.

4. All household members and sex partners should be treated also.

5. Wash your bed linen, pajamas, and clothing in hot, soapy water.

6. Itching can be expected for at least several days after treatment.

7. Clean and trim fingernails to prevent infection.

8. Signs of infection are redness, warmth, pus, and fever.

9. Children under 2 years of age should not be given Kwell. Instead, your doctor has given you 6% sulfur in petrolatum. Put this on your infant nightly for three consecutive nights; wash off in the morning. It has a bad smell and can stain clothing.

LICE

1. Lice are small insects that bite and suck blood, causing a very itchy rash. Different types of lice infest the scalp and groin. They are visible to the naked eye. Pin-sized eggs may be stuck on the hair.

2. To treat head lice and pubic lice:

a. Shampoo hair regularly.

b. Wash Nix Cream Rinse into the hair for 4 to 5 minutes, then rinse out.

c. Wash linens, caps, combs, pillowcases, and clothing in soapy water.

d. Eggs (nits) are killed by treatment but remain on hair until combed with a fine-toothed comb. The presence of eggs does not prevent return to work or school.

3. Groin lice (pubic lice) are transmitted while having sex. Your sex partner will also need treatment.

144 Normal Laboratory Values

Alan Adler

TABLE 144–1. *Hematology*

Age	Hbg (g/dL)	Hct %	MCV (u/m)	MCHC (pg/cell)	Platelets (10^3/mm³)	Comments
1 day	17.1–21.5	55.5–68.4	110.4–128.4	29.2–35	84–478	Premature infants have slightly lower values. Values are from capillary blood.
1 week	15–19.6	48–62	93–131	29.2–35	150–400	Capillary blood values
2 mo	9–24	28–42	93–109	26–34	150–400	Adult platelet counts are achieved at 1 week of age.
6–12 yr	11.5–15.5	35–45	77–95	25–33		
12–18 yr (female)	12–18	36–46	78–102	25–35		
12–18 yr (male)	12–16	37–49	78–98	25–35		

Erythrocyte sedimentation rate (Wintrobe units): Child: 0–13; adult female: 0–20; adult male: 0–9

TABLE 144–2. *Leukocyte Counts and Differentials ($\times 10^3$/mm³)*

Age	Total WBCs	Neutrophils	%	Lymphocytes	%	Mean Monocytes	%	Mean Eosinophils	%	Basophils
Newborn	9–30	6–26	81	2–11	31	1.3	6	0.4	2	0–0.75%
1 week	5–21	1.5–10	45	2–17	41	1.9	9	0.5	4	No change with age
1 mo	5–19.5	1–9	35	2.5–16.5	56	0.7	7	0.3	3	No change with age
1 yr	5–17.5	1.5–8.5	31	4–10.5	61	0.6	5	0.3	3	No change with age
4 yr	5.5–15.5	1.5–8.5	42	2–8	50	0.5	5	0.3	3	No change with age
8 yr	4.5–13.5	1.5–8	53	1.5–6.8	39	0.4	4	0.2	2	No change with age
16 yr	4.5–13	1.8–8	57	1.2–5.2	35	0.4	5	0.2	3	No change with age

TABLE 144–3. *Tests of Coagulation*

	Fibrinogen	Fibrin Degradation Products	Prothrombin Time (PT)	Partial Thromboplastin Time (PTT)
Newborn	125–300 mg/dL	<10 μg/ml	11–15 sec	25–35 sec
Child	200–400 mg/dL	<10 mg/ml	11–15 sec	25–35 sec

TABLE 144–4. *Serum Chemistries (Values for Serum or Plasma)*

Na (mmol/L)	136–148
K (mmol/L)	3.5–5.5
Cl (mmol/L)	95–108
CO_2* (mmol/L)	20–28
Ca^{+2} (mg/dL)†	8.9–10.8
Phosphorus (mg/dL)‡	2.4–8.9
Mg (meg/L)	1.5–2.1
Anion Gap	
(Na + K) − (Cl + CO_2) (mmol/L)	7–19
Plasma Osmolality (mosm/L)	270–285
BUN (mg/dL)§	9–18
Glucose (serum fasting levels) (mg/dL)¶	
Newborn–1 day:	30–60
>1 day:	50–90
Child:	60–100
Creatinine (mg/dL)	
Newborn:	0.3–1
Infant:	0.2–0.4
Child:	0.3–0.7
Adolescent:	0.5–1

* Newborn values are lower.
† Infants have larger normal ranges; values are a function of serum albumin and pH.
‡ Values are age specific.
§ Values rise during childhood.
¶ Plasma values are 5–15% higher.

TABLE 144–5. *Serum Proteins*

Amylase*	5–65 u/L
Alanine transaminase (ALT)†	3–30 u/L
Asparate transaminase (AST)‡	15–40 u/L
Alkaline phosphatase	65–263 u/L
Albumin§	3.7–5.5 g/dL
Total protein¶	6–8 g/dL
Bilirubin	Total: 2 mg/dL
	Direct: <0.2 mg/dL

* Values decrease throughout childhood.
† Infant: 3–55
‡ Infant: 15–60
§ Infant: 2.7–5
¶ Newborn: 4.4–7.6

Reference ranges may vary among laboratories due to differences in methodologies for any given test and due to variability in standardization and reference groups.

In the following tables, reference values are ranges of normals. About 5% of healthy patients will have values outside the reference ranges. All values are in conventional units.

Bibliography ■

Cherlan AC, Hill JC: Percentile estimates for reference values for 14 chemical constituents in sera of children and adolescents. *Am J Clin Pathol* 1978; 69:24–31.

Gottfried EL: *Clinical Laboratories Manual,* 29th ed. San Francisco: University of California, 1989.

Meites S: *Pediatric Clinical Chemistry,* 2nd ed. Washington DC: American Association for Clinical Chemistry, 1981.

Oski FA, Naiman JC: *Hematology of Infancy & Childhood,* 2nd ed. Philadelphia: WB Saunders, 1981.

Wallach J: *Interpretation of Pediatric Tests.* Boston: Little, Brown, 1983.

Wersberg HF: *Water, Electrolyte & Acid Base Balance,* 2nd ed. Baltimore: Williams & Wilkins, 1962.

The clinical laboratory is an integral component of pediatric emergency medicine, but normal and abnormal laboratory values have meaning only in the context of clinical findings. Rarely is it necessary to provide emergency treatment for an abnormal laboratory value in the absence of clinical findings.

TABLE 144–6. *Arterial Blood Gases*

	pH	PO$_2$ (mm Hg)	PCO$_2$ (mm Hg)	HCO$_3$ (mmol/L)	Saturation %
Newborn	7.27–7.44	65–80	27–40	16–23	>95%
Thereafter	7.35–7.44	83–108	35–45	22–26	>95%

TABLE 144–7. *Cerebrospinal Fluid*

	Color	Opening Pressure (mm H$_2$O)	Glucose (mg/dL)	Protein (mg/dL)
Newborn	Clear*	60–110	34–119	40–120
>1 Month	Clear	<200	40–85	15–40

* May be xanthochromic.

TABLE 144–8. *Cerebrospinal Fluid Cell Count*

	Total WBC/mm^3	% Polymorphonuclear Cells
Newborn	0–25	65
>1 Month	0–5	0

TABLE 144–9. *Urine*

Specific gravity	1.003–1.030
pH*	4.6–8
Osmolality	500–1200 mosm/kg H2O
Protein	<100 mg/24 h
Glucose	0
Ketones	0
Urobilinogen	0–4 mg 24/h
RBC	<1–2
WBC	<1–2
Hyaline casts	Occasional

* Depends on diet

TABLE 144–10. *Miscellaneous Laboratory Values*

	Ammonia (NH^3)	Iron (Fe)	Lead (Pb)
Newborn	90–150 µg/dL	40–100 µg/dL	Levels of >30 Mg/dL require further evaluation.
Child	40–80 µg/dL	50–120 µg/dL	

145 Electrocardiographic Normals

Ronald A. Dieckmann

Accurate interpretation of the pediatric electrocardiogram (ECG) requires adjustments for the patient's age. Table 145.1 provides a summary of the major ECG features, based on age ranges from newborn to 15 years.

TABLE 145–1. Electrocardiographic Normals

Age Group	*Heart Rate (BPM)	Frontal Plane QRS Vector (degrees)	PR Interval (sec)	†Q III (mm)‡	†Q V6 (mm)	RV1 (mm)	SV1 (mm)	R/S V1	RV6 (mm)	SV6 (mm)	R/S V6	†SV1 + RV6 (mm)	†R + S V4 (mm)
<1 day	93–154 (123)	+59 to –163 (137)	.08–.16 (.11)	4.5	2	5–26 (14)	0–23 (8)	.1–U (2.2)	0–11 (4)	0–9.5 (3)	.1–U (2.0)	28	52.5
1–2 days	91–159 (123)	+64 to –161 (134)	.08–.14 (.11)	6.5	2.5	5–27 (14)	0–21 (9)	.1–U (2.0)	0–12 (4.5)	0–9.5 (3)	.1–U (2.5)	29	52
3–6 days	91–166 (129)	+77 to –163 (132)	.07–.14 (.10)	5.5	3	3–24 (13)	0–17 (7)	.2–U (2.7)	.5–12 (5)	0–10 (3.5)	.1–U (2.2)	24.5	49
1–3 weeks	107–182 (148)	+65 to +161 (110)	.07–.14 (.10)	6	3	3–21 (11)	0–11 (4)	1.0–U (2.9)	2.5–16.5 (7.5)	0–10 (3.5)	.1–U (3.3)	21	49
1–2 mo	121–179 (149)	+31 to +113 (74)	.07–13 (.10)	7.5	3	3–18 (10)	0–12 (5)	.3–U (2.3)	5–21.5 (11.5)	0–6.5 (3)	.2–U (4.8)	29	53.5
3–5 mo	106–186 (141)	+7 to +104 (60)	.07–15 (.11)	6.5	3	3–20 (10)	0–17 (6)	.1–U (2.3)	6.5–22.5 (13)	0–10 (3)	.2–U (6.2)	32	61.5
6–11 mo	109–169 (134)	+6 to +99 (56)	.07–16 (.11)	8.5	3	1.5–20 (9.5)	.5–18 (4)	.1–3.9 (1.6)	6–22.5 (12.5)	0–7 (2)	.2–U (7.6)	32	53
1–2 yr	89–151 (119)	+7 to +101 (55)	.08–15 (.11)	6	3	2.5–17 (9)	.5–21 (8)	.05–4.3 (1.4)	6–22.5 (13)	0–6.5 (2)	.3–U (9.3)	39	49.5
3–4 yr	73–137 (108)	+6 to +104 (55)	.09–16 (.12)	5	3.5	1–18 (8)	.2–21 (10)	.03–2.8 (.9)	8–24.5 (15)	0–5 (1.5)	.6–U (10.8)	42	53.5
5–7 yr	65–133 (100)	+11 to +143 (65)	.09–16 (.12)	4	4.5	.5–14 (7)	.3–24 (12)	.02–2.0 (.7)	8.5–26.5 (16)	0–4 (1)	.9–U (11.5)	47	54
8–11 yr	62–130 (91)	+9 to +114 (61)	.09–17 (.13)	3	3	0–12 (5.5)	.3–25 (12)	0–1.8 (.5)	9–25.5 (16)	0–4 (1)	1.5–U (14.3)	45.5	53
12–15 yr	60–119 (85)	+11 to +130 (59)	.09–18 (.14)	3	3	0–10 (4)	.3–21 (11)	0–1.7 (.5)	6.5–23 (14)	0–4 (1)	1.4–U (14.7)	41	50

* 2%–98% (mean)
† 98th percentile
‡ mm at normal standardization
U = undefined (S wave may equal zero)
(Reproduced with permission from Garso A: *The Electrocardiogram in Infants and Children: A Systematic Approach.* Philadelphia: Lea & Febiger, 1983)

XIV
Emergency Drugs

146 Emergency Drugs

Olga F. Woo

Most specific drug therapy for children has been derived from empiric use or has been extrapolated from adult dosages. Only recently have pharmacokinetic studies of drugs in children provided more rational applications of dosages and dosing regimens. Physicians must be familiar with drugs used in emergency situations, and drug administration must be carefully monitored to avoid dangerous errors.

There are several basic principles of emergency drug therapy. First, drugs may have several dosing regimens depending on the disease state; for instance, maximal antibiotic dosages are necessary in serious infections, especially when delivery of the drug into the cerebrospinal fluid is crucial. Second, toxic dosages are based on anecdotal case reports of accidental poisonings and iatrogenic errors, yet for many medications precise toxic levels are unknown.

Third, in emergencies, the route of administration and subsequent absorption characteristics of a drug will determine the onset and duration of the pharmacologic effect of a given dose. Intravascular administration delivers the drug directly to the bloodstream for most drugs. However, in an emergency, conventional intravascular administration (usually peripheral venous) may be impossible and therefore alternative routes must be considered (intramuscular, intraosseous, sublingual, endotracheal, or subcutaneous). Intramuscular absorption may be too slow or inadequate because of vasoconstriction, avascular tissue, shock, or adipose tissue injection.

Errors in emergency drug therapy occur for a variety of reasons. Improper labeling, coding, and placement of drugs are often responsible. Aminophylline may be mistaken for ampicillin because the parenteral vials and lettering appear similar. Simple arithmetic mistakes or copying errors may result in dangerous or life-threatening circumstances: for example, when calculating an epinephrine dose, misplacing a decimal point or forgetting a zero in the concentration results in a dosage error of 1000%! Further, in neonates, intravenous administration may be especially difficult because minute volumes are

required and need appropriate serial dilution to produce a volume that can be measured accurately.

Often, a precise choice of infusion fluid is necessary to avoid drug precipitation (*e.g.*, diazepam, phenytoin, calcium salts). A parenteral drug may be formulated with other incipients (*e.g.*, propylene glycol with diazepam) or accompanied by its own diluent (*e.g.*, phenol with glucagon); these additives may themselves be harmful.

Advance preparation and meticulous attention to detail are imperative for the rational emergency use of drugs. The following are general guidelines:

1. Prelabel all emergency drugs and keep them in an organized crash cart or emergency box that is also equipped with appropriate syringes and needles. The cart must be sealed and inspected regularly to ensure that the contents are complete and the drugs have not expired.
2. Use premixed, ready-to-use syringes whenever possible to avoid extemporaneous preparation of crucial drug concentrations during an emergency.
3. Ensure that everyone who directs or assists in emergency procedures is trained in the indications, doses, side effects, contraindications, and pharmacology of emergency medications, as well as appropriate routes of administration and recognition and treatment of overdoses.
4. When an emergency drug is selected, check the label for expiration date, concentration, pediatric or adult preparation, and vehicle for administration.
5. Ensure the appropriate minimum effective dose for age and know the maximum amount of drug for age.
6. Use appropriate administration routes for maximal absorption and rapid onset of action.
7. Use proper rates of intravenous administration (*e.g.*, fast or slow bolus, IV push, IV infusion) to achieve maximal benefit and to avoid untoward effects.
8. Use the correct diluent.

TABLE 146–1. *Emergency Drugs*

Drug	Route	Dosage Neonate	Dosage Pediatric	Dosage Adult	Administration	Comment
Acetaminophen	PO, PR	5–10 mg/kg/ dose	5–10 mg/kg/dose or 80 mg/yr to 5 yr	325–650 mg/ dose	Every 4–6 hours	Not anti-inflammatory. More than 140 mg/kg is toxic dose.
Acetazolamide	IM, PO		15 mg/kg/dose	250–1000 mg	Single dose	Use single dose to lower intra-ocular pressure. Do not use in salicylate poisoning. Use 5–10 mg/kg/day divided in two doses for treatment of high-altitude sickness.
Acetylsalicylic acid (aspirin)	PO	5–10 mg/kg/ dose	10–20 mg/kg/dose or 81 mg/yr to 5 yr	325–650 mg/ dose	Every 4–6 hours	Use with extreme caution in a child <2 yr old. Avoid use when treating chicken pox or flu in children because of possible risk of Reye's syndrome.
ACTH	IV, IM, SQ, Gel IM		0.4–0.5 U/kg/day	20 U/day	3–4 divided doses	
Acyclovir 20 mg/ ml	IV	30 mg/kg/ day	25–50 mg/kg/day	15 mg/kg/ day	Divide q8 hrs. Give slowly over 1–3 hrs.	For herpes simplex and zoster treatment
	PO		200 mg q4 hrs	200 mg q4 hrs	5 times/day	
	Topical 5%		q.s. to cover lesions		Q3 hrs.	
Albuterol 0.5%	Inhaled		0.05–0.15 mg/kg/ dose (0.01–0.03 ml/kg) max 2.5 mg	1–2 inhalations	Every 4–6 hr	A beta-2 agonist
	PO		2–6 yr: 0.1–0.2 mg/kg/D (max 12 mg total)	2–4 mg/dose	3–4 times daily	2 mg q6 hrs on conventional tablets is equivalent to 4 mg q12 hrs with extended-release tablets.
			6–12 yr: 2 mg/ dose (max 24 mg total)	4–8 mg q12 hrs	Extended-release tablets	
Allopurinol	PO		Infants: 10 mg/kg/ day	300 mg/day	1–3 times daily	Reduce dose if using with 6-MP.
			<6 yr: 150 mg/day			
			6–10 yr: 300 mg/ day			
Amantadine HCl	PO		5–8 mg/kg/day (max 200 mg/day)	100 mg b.i.d.	Once or twice daily	Divide q12 hr
Amikacin	IV, IM	<2000 g 0–7 days: 7.5 mg/kg q12 hrs >7 days: 10 mg/kg q8 hrs	15–20 mg/kg/day	15–24 mg/ kg/day	Divided q8–12 hr	Ototoxicity and nephrotoxicity associated with aminoglycoside antibiotics.

(continued)

TABLE 146–1. Emergency Drugs (*continued*)

Drug	Route	Neonate	Pediatric	Adult	Administration	Comment
		>2000 g 0–7 days: 10 mg/kg q12 hrs >7 days: 10 mg/kg q8 hrs				
Aminocaproic acid	IV		Initial: 100 mg/kg/dose	4000–5000 mg	Initial loading dose	Give slowly to achieve serum level of 130 μg/ml.
			Hourly: 30 mg/kg/dose	1000 mg	Hourly infusion	
	PO		100 mg/kg/dose (max 6 g/day)	1000 mg	Every 6 hr	
Aminosalicylic acid	PO		300 mg/kg/day	10–12 gm/day	Divide q8–12 hrs	
Aminophylline	IV	Loading: 5 mg/kg	5 mg/kg	6 mg/kg	Loading dose followed by hourly maintenance infusion dose	Adjust dosages accordingly to achieve serum levels between 5–20 μg/ml. Avoid levels above 10–15 μg/ml in neonates.
		Maintenance: 2 mg/kg q12–24 hr or 0.16 mg/kg/hr	0.8–1.2 mg/kg/hr for 12 hrs then 0.8–1 mg/kg/hr	0.7 mg/kg/hr for 12 hr then 0.5 mg/kg/hr		
Amitriptyline	PO		25–100 mg	50–100 mg	Once daily	Treatment of chronic pain
Amoxicillin	PO		45 mg/kg/day	250–500 mg t.i.d.	Divide q8 hr	
Amoxicillin-Potassium clavulanate (Augmentin*)	PO		40 mg/kg/day (based on amoxicillin)	250–500 mg q8 hrs	Divide q8 hr	
Amphotericin B	IV		0.25–1 mg/kg/day	1–1.5 mg/kg/day	q1–2 days	Infuse dose very slowly over 6 hours.
Ampicillin	IV, IM	<2000 g 0–7 days: 50 mg/kg q12 hr >7 days: 50 mg/kg q8 hr >2000 g 0–7 days: 50 mg/kg q8 hr >7 days: 50 mg/kg q6 hr	100–200 mg/kg/day 200–400 mg/kg/day for meningitis	1–12 g/day	Divide q6 hr	Maintain good urine flow to prevent crystalluria.
	PO		50 mg/kg/day	250–500 mg q.i.d.	Divide q6 hr	

* Trade Name.

TABLE 146-1. Emergency Drugs (*continued*)

Drug	Route	Neonate	Pediatric	Adult	Administration	Comment
			Dosage			
Amyl nitrite	Inhalation	1 ampule	1 ampule	1 ampule		
Aspirin (see Acetylsalicylic acid)						
Atenolol	PO		50–100 mg/dose	Same as pediatric	Once daily	A beta₁-specific blocker
Atropine sulfate 0.1 mg/ml	IV, IM, IO, ET, SQ, PO	0.01–0.03 mg/kg (min 0.1 mg)	0.02–0.05 mg/kg	0.5–1 mg (max 2 mg/dose)	Repeat dose as needed.	High doses (2–10 mg) and large amounts (50–100 mg) total may be required in severe organophosphate poisoning. Physostigmine is an antidote for atropine poisoning
Augmentin* (see Amoxicillin-Potassium clavulanate)						
Azlocillin	IV		300–450 mg/kg/day	1–5 g q6 hr	Divide q4–6 hr	
Azidothymidine (AZT) (Zidovudine)	IV		25–40 mg/kg/day or 180 mg/m²/day or 80 mg initial load then 0.9–1.4 mg/kg/hr		Divide 4–5 doses	
Aztreonam	IV, IM	<2000 g 0–7 day: 30 mg/kg q12 hr >7 day: 30 mg/kg q8 hr >2000 g 0–7 day: 30 mg/kg q8 hr >7 day: 30 mg/kg q8 hr	90–120 mg/kg/day	1–2 g q6–12 hr	Divide q6–8 hr	
Bacampicillin HCl	PO		25–50 mg/kg/day	200–800 mg q8–12 hr	Divide q12 hr	400 mg tablet equivalent to 280 mg ampicillin
BAL (see Dimercaprol)						
Belladonna tincture	PO		0.03–0.1 ml/kg	1–2 ml	t.i.d.	Approximately 0.3 mg atropine/ml.
Benztropine	PO, IM		0.01–0.03 mg/kg	1–2 mg	b.i.d.-q.i.d.	Alternative to diphenhydramine for treatment of drug-induced dystonic reactions
Bretylium tosylate	IV, IM		5 mg/kg (max 30 mg/kg total)	5–10 mg/kg/dose	Rapid bolus	Use after lidocaine fails. Avoid in tricyclic antidepressant overdoses. Maintenance doses given over 10–30 minutes every 6 hours
Bupivacaine (Marcaine*) 0.25%	Topical		1–2 mg/kg (0.5 ml/kg)		Single application	Not yet approved for use in infants and children.

(*continued*)

TABLE 146-1. Emergency Drugs (*continued*)

Drug	Route	Dosage			Administration	Comment
		Neonate	Pediatric	Adult		
Caffeine sodium benzoate	IV, IM, SQ	Load: 10 mg/kg Maintenance: 2.5 mg/kg q24 hrs	6-10 mg/kg/dose	500 mg	Every 4 hr	Avoid in jaundiced neonate because benzoate competes with bilirubin for albumin binding sites.
Calcium chloride 10% 10% = 100 mg/ml (contains 27% calcium = 14.6 mEq Ca^{++}/10 ml)	IV	20 mg/kg	25 mg/kg	1000 mg	Give slowly; repeat q6 hr if needed.	Avoid extravasation. Do not mix with sodium bicarbonate. May cause metabolic acidosis. Watch for bradycardia.
Calcium disodium versenate (see EDTA calcium)						
Calcium gluconate 10%; 10% = 100 mg/ml (contains 9% calcium = 4.5 mEq Ca^{++}/10 ml)	IV	100 mg/kg	100-200 mg/kg	1000-2000 mg	Give slowly.	Preferred to calcium chloride because it does not cause metabolic acidosis. Do not mix with sodium bicarbonate. Watch for bradycardia.
Captopril	PO		Initially 0.5 mg/kg then increase to 1-2 mg/kg (max 6 mg/kg/day)	Initially 25 mg then increase to 50-150 mg/day (max 450 mg/day)	t.i.d.	Take 1 hour before meals.
Carbamazepine	PO		20-30 mg/kg/day	600-1200 mg/day	Divide in 2-4 doses/day.	
Carbenicillin disodium	IV, IM		400-600 mg/kg/day	24-40 g/day	Divide q4-6 hr	
Carbenicillin indanyl sodium	PO		30-50 mg/kg/day	382-764 mg q.i.d.	Divide q6 hr	
Cefaclor	PO		40 mg/kg/day	250 mg q8 hr	Divide q8-12 hr	Alternative treatment for bites resistant to initial treatment
Cefadroxil	PO		30 mg/kg/day	1-2 g/day	Divide q12 hr	
Cefamandole	IV, IM		150 mg/kg/day	1.5-12 g/day	Divide q4-6 hr	Avoid alcohol.
Cefazolin	IV, IM	<2000 g 20 mg/kg q12 hr >2000 g 0-7 day: 20 mg/kg q12 hr >7 day: 20 mg/kg q8 hr	50-100 mg/kg/day	500 mg q8 hr	Divide q8 hr	
Cefixime	PO		8 mg/kg/day	400 mg q24 hr or 200 mg q12 hr	Divide q12-24 hr	
Cefonicid	IV, IM		20-40 mg/kg/day	1 g q24 hr	q24 hr	Not approved for use in children

TABLE 146–1. Emergency Drugs (*continued*)

Drug	Route	Neonate	Pediatric	Adult	Administration	Comment
			Dosage			
Cefoperazone	IV, IM		100–150 mg/kg/day	2–4 g/day	Divide q8–12 hr	Not approved for use in children. Avoid alcohol.
Ceforanide	IV, IM		20–40 mg/kg/day	0.5–1 g q12 hr	Divide q12 hr	
Cefotaxime	IV, IM	0–7 day: 50 mg/kg q12 hr >7 day: 50 mg/kg q8 hr	100–200 mg/kg/day	1–12 g/day	Divide q6–8 hr	200 mg/kg/day for meningitis divided q6 hrs.
Cefotetan	IV, IM		40–80 mg/kg/day	1–2 g q12 hr	Divide q12 hr	Not approved for children
Cefoxitin	IV, IM		80–160 mg/kg/day	1–2 g q6–8 hr	Divide q4–6 hr	
Ceftazidime	IV, IM	<2000 gm 0–7 day: 50 mg/kg q12 hr >2000 gm *or* >7 day: 50 mg/kg q8 hr	100–150 mg/kg/day	1 g q8–12 hr	Divide q8 hr	150 mg/kg/day for meningitis
Ceftizoxime	IV, IM		150–200 mg/kg/day	1–2 g q8–12 hr	Divide q6–8 hr	
Ceftriaxone	IV, IM	<2000 g 50 mg q24 hr >2000 g 0–7 day: 50 mg q24 hr >7 day: 75 mg q24 hr	50–100 mg/kg/day	1–2 g q24 hr	Divide q12–24 hr	100 mg/kg/day divided q12 hr for meningitis and q24 hr for periorbital cellulitis
Cefuroxime	IV, IM		100–150 mg/kg/day 240 mg/kg/day for meningitis	750 mg–1.5 g q8 hr	Divided q8 hr Divided q6 hr	
	PO		30 mg/kg/day		Divided q12 hr	
Cephalexin	PO		50 mg/kg/day	500 mg q6 hr	Divided q6 hr	For initial treatment of bite wounds
Cephalothin	IV, IM	<2000 g 0–7 day: 20 mg/kg q12 hr >7 day: 20 mg/kg q8 hr >2000 g	75–125 mg/kg/day	0.5–1 g q4–6 hr	Divided q4–6 hr	Large doses may cause renal toxicity.

(continued)

TABLE 146–1.   Emergency Drugs (*continued*)

Drug	Route	Neonate	Pediatric	Adult	Administration	Comment
		0–7 day: 20 mg/kg q8 hr				
		>7 day: 20 mg/kg q6 hr				
Cephapirin	IV, IM		40–80 mg/kg/day	0.5–12 g/day	Divided q6 hr	
Cephradine	IV		50–100 mg/kg/day	2–4 g/day	Divided q6 hr	
	PO		50 mg/kg/day	500 mg q6 hr	Divided q6 hr	For treatment of unknown bite wounds
Charcoal, activated	PO	1 g/kg	1–2 g/kg	50–100 g	Single dose	Avoid aspiration; may cause vomiting.
		0.25–0.5 mg/ kg	0.5 mg/kg	20–25 g	Repeat-dose regimen Q2–4 hr	Watch for excessive diarrhea if combined with a cathartic.
Chloral hydrate	PO, PR		50 mg/kg	1000–2000 mg (max 2000 mg/ dose)	Single dose	For diagnostic procedures.
			25–100 mg/kg/ dose (max 1000 mg)		Every 6 hr	Metabolized to an active long-acting metabolite
Chloramphenicol	IV, PO	<2000 g	50–75 mg/kg/day, 75–100 mg/kg/day for meningitis	50 mg/kg/ day	Divided q6 hr	Serum levels >25 μg/ml can cause gray-baby syndrome in neonates. Rare complication is aplastic anemia.
		25 mg q24 hr				
		>2000 g				
		0–7 day: 25 mg q24 hr				
		>7 day: 25 mg q12 hr				
Chloroquine HCl	IM		5 mg base/kg	160–200 mg base	1–2 doses	
	then					
phosphate	PO		10 mg base/kg	300 mg base	Every 24 hr	
Chlorothiazide	IV, PO	5–10 mg/kg	10–50 mg/kg	250–500 mg	Every 12–24 hr	Thiazide diuretics have flat dose-response; thus, increased doses do not produce comparable effects.
Chlorpheniramine maleate	SC, PO		0.1 mg/kg/dose	4–8 mg	t.i.d.-q.i.d.	Sustained-release tablets also available
Chlorpromazine	PO, IV IM	0.5–0.7 mg/ kg	0.2–1 mg/kg (max 2 mg/kg/dose)	25–50 mg	Every 6 hr	Used in neonatal withdrawal syndrome. Give very slowly IV. Higher doses are used for psychiatric problems.
Cimetidine HCl	PO, IV, IM	4 mg/kg q12 hr has been used.	20–40 mg/kg/day or 1 mg/kg/hr IV infusion	250–500 mg	Every 4–6 hr	Doses greater than 15–40 mg/ kg/day may cause toxicity.
Clindamycin HCl or phosphate	IV, IM	<2000 g	25–40 mg/kg/day	600–1200 mg/day	Divided q6–8 hr	
		0–7 day: 5 mg/kg q12 hr				

TABLE 146–1. Emergency Drugs (*continued*)

Drug	Route	Neonate	Pediatric	Adult	Administration	Comment
		>7 day: 5 mg/kg q8 hr				
		>2000 g				
		0–7 day: 5 mg/kg q8 hr				
		>7 day: 5 mg/kg q6 hr				
	PO		20–30 mg/kg/day	150–450 q6 hr	Divided q6 hr	
Clonazepam	PO		0.01–0.2 mg/kg/day	1.5–20 mg/day	Divide into 2–3 doses per day.	
Clonidine	PO	0.5 μg/kg q6 hr	3–5 μg/kg q6–12 hr	0.05–0.2 mg	b.i.d.-q.i.d.	Used for opiate withdrawal syndrome. Watch for bradycardia.
Cloxacillin	PO		50–100 mg/kg/day	500 mg q6 hr	Divided q6 hr	
Codeine phosphate	PO, IM, SQ		0.2–1 mg/kg/dose	15–60 mg	Every 4–6 hr	Lower doses for antitussive, higher doses for analgesic effects
Cortisone acetate	IM		0.2–0.35 mg/kg/dose	30–40 mg	Single dose	Physiologic dose
			1.2–5 mg/kg/day	150–300 mg	Every 12–24 hr	Pharmacologic dose
	PO		0.7 mg/kg/day	30–40 mg	Every 8 hr	Physiologic dose
			2.5–10 mg/kg/day	150–300 mg	Every 6–8 hr	Pharmacologic dose
Dantrolene sodium	IV		1 to 10 mg/kg	1 to 10 mg/kg		For treatment of malignant hyperthermia
Dapsone	PO		1–2 mg/kg/day	100 mg	Once daily	
DDAVP	IV		0.3 μg/kg	0.3 μg/kg	Slowly over 30 min	For hemophilia A or Type I von Willebrand's disease
	SQ, intranasal		2.5–40 μg/dose	5–40 μg/dose	Single dose or divided 2–3 times a day	Higher doses for diabetes insipidus and enuresis
Deferoxamine	IV		10–15 mg/kg/hr (max 30–45 mg/kg/hr)	1–2 g	Infuse slowly.	Rapid administration may cause hypotension.
	IM		25 mg/kg/dose (max 500 mg/dose)	1–2 g	Every 8–12 hr	May cause hypotension with larger dose
Desoxycorticosterone acetate (DOCA)	IM		1–5 mg/dose	1–10 mg	Single dose	For adrenal crisis
Dexamethasone	PO, IV, IM	0.3 mg/kg/day	0.1–0.2 mg/kg/day	0.75–9 mg/day	Divide 2–4 times daily	Not suitable for alternate-day therapy
Dextromethorphan	PO		0.45 mg/kg/day (max 15 mg/dose)	10–15 mg/dose	q.i.d.	Mixed narcotic and anticholinergic effects with overdoses

(*continued*)

TABLE 146-1. Emergency Drugs (*continued*)

Drug	Route	Neonate	Pediatric	Adult	Administration	Comment
Diazepam	IV, IM, IO, ET	0.1–0.2 mg/kg (max 5 mg/dose)	0.1–0.3 mg/kg (max 15 mg)	5–10 mg (max 15 mg)	Slow IV push	Do not mix with any other drugs or dilute with any IV solutions. Children may exhibit paradoxical hyperexcitability.
	PR		0.5 mg/kg			
	PO		0.2–0.5 mg/kg/dose (max 10 mg)	2.5–10 mg	Every 6–8 hr	
Diazoxide	IV	2 mg/kg (max 5 mg/kg)	2–6 mg/kg	300 mg	Single dose rapid; repeat every 10 min if needed	May produce hyperglycemia
	PO	10–15 mg/kg/day	10–15 mg/kg/day	200 mg/day	Divide q8–12 hr	Oral for treatment of neonatal hypoglycemia
Dicloxacillin	PO		50 mg/kg/day	500 mg q6 hr	Divide q6 hr	For treatment of unknown bite wounds
			50–100 mg/kg/day		Divide q6 hr	For treatment of cat bites
Digoxin	IV, IM	Premature: 30 µg/kg	Full term–2 yr: 45 µg/kg	1–1.5 mg	Digitalizing dose	Divide into 3 portions given every 8 hr
			Over 2 yr: 30 µg/kg			
	PO	10 µg/kg/day	Full term–2 yr: 15 µg/kg/day	0.125–0.5 mg	Maintenance daily dose. Divide in 2 doses for pediatric and once daily for adult patients.	Begin dose 24 hours after last digitalized dose given.
			Over 2 yr: 10 µg/kg/day			
Digibind	IV	Formula to calculate dose: Dose (in number of vials) $$= \frac{\text{Serum Digoxin Concentration (ng/ml)} \times \text{Wt. (kg)}}{100}$$			Administer over 30 minutes through a 22 micron filter.	Each vial of Digibind will bind 0.6 mg of digoxin. Serum digoxin levels will be falsely elevated after Digibind administration.
Dihydroergotamine	IV, IM		0.75 mg	1 mg	Repeat at 1 hr. interval.	Max. 3 mg IM; Max. 2 mg IV. Max 6 mg/week.
Dimenhydrinate	PO		1–1.5 mg/kg/dose	50 mg	Every 6 hr	
Dimercaprol (BAL)	IM			3–5 mg/kg/dose	3–5 mg/kg/dose	Every 4–12 hr. Administer 4 hours before giving EDTA calcium if both chelating agents are used.
D-Penicillamine (see Penicillamine)						
Diphenhydramine	PO, IV IM		1–2 mg/kg/dose	50–100 mg	Every 6 hr	Local anesthetic properties when applied topically
Dobutamine	IV	1–10 µg/kg/min	2.5–10 µg/kg/min	2.5–10 µg/kg/min	Continuous infusion	Watch for tachycardia.
Dopamine	IV	5–20 µg/kg/min	5–15 µg/kg/min (max 50 µg/kg/min)	5–50 µg/kg/min	Continuous infusion	Prepare 1 ampule (200 mg) in 250 ml D_5W or normal saline.

TABLE 146–1. Emergency Drugs (*continued*)

Drug	Route	Neonate	Pediatric	Adult	Administration	Comment
Doxycycline	PO		2–4 mg/kg/day (>7 yrs)	100–200 mg	Every 12–24 hr	Photosensitivity reactions and dizziness common
Edrophonium chloride	IV	1 mg/dose	0.2 mg/kg/dose	2–10 mg	Give very slowly.	Give $^1/_5$ dose initially to evaluate tolerance to effect, then give remainder.
Edetate (EDTA) calcium disodium (calcium disodium versenate)	IV		35–50 mg/kg	1–2 g	Infuse over 2 hr then q12 hr	Do not confuse with *edetate disodium*.
Ephedrine sulfate	IM, SC		0.2–0.3 mg/kg	12.5–25 mg	Every 4–6 hr	
	PO		0.5–0.75 mg/kg	25–50 mg	Every 4–6 hr	
Epinephrine HCl (1:10,000) (0.1 mg/ml)	IV, ET, IO	10–30 µg/kg	10–20 µg/kg	0.1–1 mg	Slow IV. Repeat every 5 min if needed.	Avoid rapid injection. Higher doses (100–300 µg/kg) may be needed. Double doses for ET route. Acidosis decreases efficacy.
	Infusion	0.05–1.5 µg/kg/min	0.1–0.2 µg/kg/min	1–4 µg/min		
(1:1000) (1 mg/ml)	IM, SC		10 µg/kg	0.3–0.5 mg	Repeat every 10–30 min.	
Epinephrine suspension (Susphrine*) (1:200; 5 mg/ml)	SQ, IM		0.005 ml/kg (max 0.15 ml) *or* 0.01–0.03 mg/kg (max 0.5 mg)	0.15–0.3 ml	Every 4–6 hr	Avoid decimal error to prevent administration of 10 times the desired dose.
Epinephrine racemic (1% or 2.25%)	Inhalant		0.05 ml/kg/dose		Repeat once after 1 minute then every 3–4 hr	
Erythromycin	PO	<2000 g 0–7 day: 10 mg/kg q12 hr >7 day: 10 mg/kg q8 hr >2000 g 0–7 day: 10 mg/kg q12 hr >7 day: 30–40 mg/kg/day divided q8 hr	40 mg/kg/day	500 mg q6 hr	Divided q6 hr	Gastrointestinal upset common. May inhibit theophylline metabolism if used together and decreased theophylline doses needed.
Esmolol	IV		25–50 µg/kg/min	25–50 µg/kg/min	Continuous infusion	Duration of action is brief

(*continued*)

* Trade Name.

TABLE 146-1. Emergency Drugs (*continued*)

Drug	Route	Neonate	Pediatric	Adult	Administration	Comment
			Dosage			
Estradiol valerate	IM		10 mg		Weekly for 3 weeks	Combined with medroxyprogesterone for uterine bleeding
Estrogen	IV		20 μg q4–6 hr for 24 hr			
Ethanol 100% (v/v)	IV		Load: 1 ml/kg (1 g/kg)		For treatment of methanol and ethylene glycol poisoning. Goal is to achieve and maintain blood level of 100 mg/dL. Dilute to 5% to administer IV, avoid phlebitis.	
			Maintenance: 0.16 ml/kg/hr			
	PO, NG		Same as IV		Dilute to 20–30% for PO, NG administration.	
Ethacrynic acid	IV		0.5–1 mg/kg/dose	25–50 mg	Every 12–48 hr	Avoid using concurrently with aminoglycoside antibiotics.
	PO		25 mg/dose for older children	25–50 mg	Every 24–48 hr	
Ethosuximide	PO		20–40 mg/kg/day	750–2000 mg	Divide b.i.d.	
Fentanyl	IV, IM		2–20 μg/kg (max 150 μg/kg)	50–100 μg (max 150 μg/kg)	Single dose	Watch for hallucinatory reactions. Larger doses used for general anesthesia
Furosemide	IV, IM PO	1–2 mg/kg/dose	1–3 mg/kg/dose (max 6 mg/kg PO)	40–80 mg/dose		Once daily for prematures. Every 12–24 hr for neonates. For infants > 6 months, may give every 6 hr
Gentamicin	IV, IM	0–7 day: 2.5 mg/kg q12 hr	3–7.5 mg/kg/day	3 mg/kg/day	Divided q8 hr	Larger doses (7–10 mg/kg/day) for patients with cystic fibrosis
		>7 day: 2.5 mg/kg q8 hr				
Glucagon	IV, IM, SC		0.1–0.2 mg/kg	1–10 mg	Single dose	Higher doses cause nausea and vomiting, used in beta-blocker overdose. Do not use and mix with the phenol diluent.
	Infusion		1 mg/hr (max 10 mg)	1 mg/hr	Continuous	
Griseofulvin	PO		15 mg/kg/day	0.5–1 g	Every 24 hr	May give 2 or 3 times a day with difficult infections.
Guanidine HCl	PO		2.5–5 mg/kg/dose (max 35 mg/kg/day)	15–50 mg/kg/day	Divide in 4–5 doses	Use for botulism.
Heparin aqueous	IV	10–24 U/kg/hr	50 U/kg/dose, then 100 U/kg every 4 hr	10,000 U then 2000–4000 U every 4 hr	Bolus, then maintenance infusion	Antidote is protamine sulfate, 1 mg for each 100 U (mg) heparin given in the previous 2 hr
	SQ		25–50 U/kg/dose	5,000–10,000 U	b.i.d.	
Hydralazine	IV, IM	0.1–0.5 mg/kg	0.1–0.5 mg/kg (max 2 mg/kg q6 hr)	20–40 mg	Every 3–6 hr	Reduce dose to <0.15 mg/kg when combined with other antihypertensive agents.
	PO		0.75 mg/kg/day (max 7.5 mg/kg/day)		Divide q.i.d.	

TABLE 146–1. Emergency Drugs (*continued*)

Drug	Route	Neonate	Pediatric	Adult	Administration	Comment
			Dosage			
Hydrochlorothia-zide	PO		1–2 mg/kg (max 2.7 mg/kg)	50–100 mg	Every 12–24 hr	See Chlorothiazide.
Hydrocortisone phosphate, sodium succinate	IV		2.5–10 mg/kg/dose	250–500 mg	Every 6 hr	Use higher dose for cerebral edema.
Hydromorphone HCl	PO		6–12 yrs. 0.5 mg	1 mg	t.i.d.–q.i.d.	Anti-tussive dose
Hydroxyzine HCl	IM		0.5–1 mg/kg/dose	50–100 mg	Single dose	IV route is not an approved use, but has been used under special circumstances.
	PO		0.25–0.5 mg/kg (max 4 mg/kg/day)	25–50 mg	q.i.d.	
Isoniazid	PO, IM		10–20 mg/kg/day (max 300 mg/day)	300 mg	Divide q12–24 hr	
Insulin NPH	SQ		0.1–1 U/kg	20–50 U	Every 12–24 hr	Peaks 8–12 hr. Can be mixed with regular insulin
Insulin protamine zinc	SQ		0.1–1 U/kg	10–50 U	Every 12–24 hr	Peaks 14–20 hr. Usually mixed with regular insulin
Insulin regular	IV, SC		0.1–1 U/Kg	5–50 U	Every 8 hr or low-dose infusion	Peaks in 2.5–5 hr
Insulin lente	SQ		0.1–1 U/dose	20–50 U	Every 12–24 hr	Peaks in 8–12 hr
Regular						
Semi	SQ		0.1–1 U/dose	20–50 U	Every 8–24 hr	Peaks in 5–7 hr
Ultra	SQ		0.1–1 U/dose	20–50 U	Every 24 hr	Peaks in 14–18 hr. All three can be mixed with regular insulin or with each other.
Ipratropium bro-mide	Inhalation		1–2 metered dose	2 metered doses	q.i.d.	Do not exceed 12 inhalations in 24 hrs.
Ipecac syrup	PO		<1 yr 10 ml/dose >1 yr 15 ml/dose	30 ml/dose	Repeat once in 15–20 min	Never use fluid extract, which is 14 times more potent and can lead to cardiotoxicity.
Isoetharine 0.5%–1%	Inhalation		0.25–0.5 ml/dose	0.5–1 ml/dose	1–7 inhalations; repeat q4 hr as needed.	Adult dosages have been tolerated in children without adverse effects.
Isoproterenol HCl (1:5000) (0.2 mg/ml)	IV	0.05–1 µg/kg/min	0.1–1 µg/kg/min	2–20 µg/min	Continuous infusion	Start with low dose and increase every 5–10 minutes to desired effect. Large doses (10 times) may be required in massive beta-blocker poisoning.
Kanamycin	IV, IM	<2000 g 0–7 day: 7.5 mg/kg q12 hr	15–30 mg/kg/day	15 mg/kg/day	Divided q8 hr. Give over 20–60 minutes if IV.	Reduce dose in renal impairment.

(*continued*)

TABLE 146–1. Emergency Drugs (*continued*)

Drug	Route	Dosage Neonate	Dosage Pediatric	Dosage Adult	Administration	Comment
		>7 day: 20 mg/kg/ divide q8 hr				
		>2000 g				
		0–7 day: 10 mg/kg q12 hr				
		>7 day: 10 mg/kg q8 hr				
Kayexalate* (see Polystyrene sodium sulfonate)						
Labetalol	IV		0.3 mg/kg	10–20 mg	Over 2 min	Possesses both alpha$_1$ and non-specific beta blockade.
Levarterenol bitartrate (Levophed*) (norepinephrine)	IV		2 μg/min	2–4 μg/min	Continuous infusion	Preferred vasopressor in phenothiazine poisoning.
Lidocaine (1% = 10 mg/ml) (2% = 20 mg/ml)	IV, ET Load	1 mg/kg/ dose (max 3 mg/kg)	1 mg/kg/dose	50–100 mg	Single bolus. Repeat q8 min if needed for 3 doses.	Observe for seizures with overdose; thus, avoid levels over 5 μg/ml.
	IV Maintenance	10–50 μg/ kg/min	20–50 μg/kg/min	30–50 μg/ min (max 5 mg/kg/min)	Maintenance infusion	
	SQ		4 mg/kg		Repeat as needed.	For wound repair. Avoid absorption of >5 mg/kg total amount used.
Lidocaine 2% viscous	Topical		1–10 ml	1–10 ml	Apply as needed.	Avoid large open mucous membranes.
Lincomycin	PO		30–60 mg/kg/day		Divided q8 hr	
Lorazepam	IV,		0.01–0.02 mg/kg (max 0.04 mg/kg)	1–2 mg	Every 8 hr	Avoid intra-arterial injection, because it may cause arteriospasm.
	IM		0.02–0.04 mg/kg (max 0.05 mg/kg)	2–4 mg	Every 8 hr	
Magnesium citrate	PO		3–5 ml/kg/dose	200–300 ml	Single dose	Use caution in renal impairment.
Magnesium sulfate	IV 1%		20–100 mg/kg	1000–2000 mg	Slow infusion, 150 mg/min	Use 1% solution for hypertension.
	IM 50%	0.2 ml/kg	100 mg/kg	1000 mg	Every 5–6 hr	Use 50% solution when giving IM.
	PO		250 mg/kg/dose	15 g	Every 4 hr as needed.	Observe for diarrhea and hypermagnesemia with repeated doses.
Mannitol	IV		200 mg/kg/dose	200 mg	Single dose over 3–5 minutes	Anuria or oliguria test dose
	IV		500–2000 mg/kg/ dose	100 g	Over 2–6 hr	For edema, ascites, oliguria
	IV 20%		500–3000 mg/kg/ dose	100–200 g	Over 30–60 min	For cerebral or ocular edema. Use 20% solution. Achieve serum osmolarity between 320–330.

* Trade Name.

TABLE 146-1. Emergency Drugs (*continued*)

Drug	Route	Neonate	Pediatric	Adult	Administration	Comment
Mebendazole	PO		100 mg	100 mg	Single dose for pinworms	Give q12 hr for 3 days for other nematodes.
Medroxyprogester-one	PO		Adolescents: 5–10 mg	5–10 mg	Once daily for 5–10 days	Combine with estradiol for uterine bleeding
	IM		50 mg		Once a week for 3 weeks	
Meperidine	IV, IM SQ	0.5 mg/kg/dose q6 hr	1–2 mg/kg/dose (max 100 mg)	50–100 mg	Every 3–4 hr except for neonates	Cumulative repeated doses may result in adverse CNS reactions.
	PO		2–3 mg/kg/dose	100–200 mg	Every 3–4 hr	Poor oral absorption
Mephentermine sulfate (Wyamine*)	IV, IM		0.4 mg/kg/dose	0.5 mg/kg/dose (average dose is 30–45 mg)	Single dose	Generally used to treat hypotension during anesthesia
Metaproterenol	5% inhalant		0.1–0.5 mg/kg (0.002–0.01 ml/kg) (max 15 mg)	2–3 metered inhalations, max 12/day	Every 4–6 hr	Watch for tachycardia.
	PO		<6 yr, 1.3–2.6 mg/kg/day 6–9 yr, 10 mg/dose >9 yr, 20 mg/dose	20 mg/dose	3–4 times daily	
Metaraminol bitartrate	IV		0.3–2 mg/kg/dose	15–500 mg	Infusion dose	Titrate to desired blood pressure.
	IM, SQ		0.1 mg/kg/dose	2–10 mg	Single dose	
Methicillin	IV, IM	<2000 g 0–7 day: 50 mg/kg q12 hr >7 day: 50 mg/kg q8 hr >2000 g 0–7 day: 50 mg/kg q8 hr >7 day: 50 mg/kg q6 hr	150–200 mg/kg/day	1 g q4 hr	Divided q6 hr	For meningitis treatment
Methoxamine HCl (Vasoxyl*)	IV		0.1 mg/kg/dose	3–5 mg	Single dose given slowly	Generally used for hypotension and supraventricular tachycardia during anesthesia
	IM		0.25 mg/kg/dose	10–15 mg	Single dose	
Methyldopa	IV	5–10 mg/kg/dose	10–40 mg/kg/day	250–500 mg/dose	Every 6–8 hr	Observe for drop in blood pressure after 1–2 hr
	PO		10–65 mg/kg/day	250–500 mg/dose	b.i.d.	

(*continued*)

TABLE 146–1. Emergency Drugs (*continued*)

Drug	Route	Neonate	Pediatric	Adult	Administration	Comment
Methylene blue	IV 1%	1–2 mg/kg/ dose (0.1– 0.2 ml/kg/ dose)	1–2 mg/kg/dose (0.1–0.2 ml/kg/ dose)	1–2 mg/kg/ dose (0.1–0.2 ml/kg/dose)	Single dose over 5 min	Use 1% solution (10 mg/ml). Repeat in 20–30 minutes if needed.
Methylpredniso-lone	IV, IM		0.5–8 mg/kg/day	10–40 mg/ dose (up to 100–400 mg)	Every 6 hr	Larger doses used for cerebral edema
	PO		1–2 mg/kg/day			
Metoclopramide	IV, IM	0.5 mg/kg/ day	<6 yr, 0.1 mg/kg >6 yr, 2.5–5 mg/ dose	1–2 mg/kg	Single dose	Used for prophylaxis of chemo-therapy-induced emesis. Overdosage in neonates and in-fants may cause methemoglobin-emia.
	PO		>6 yr, 2.5–5 mg/ dose	10–20 mg/ dose	b.i.d.-q.i.d.	Observe for dystonic reactions.
Metolazone	IV		0.02 mg/kg/dose	5–20 mg (max 100 mg)	Every 12–24 hr	Long-acting diuretic
	PO		0.2–0.4 mg/kg/ dose	5–20 mg (max 100 mg)	Every 12–24 hr	
Metoprolol	PO		Adolescents: Same as adult doses	50–200 mg/ dose (max 450 mg/day)	Twice a day	A specific beta$_1$-blocker
Metronidazole	PO	<2000 g 7.5 mg/kg q12 hr >2000 g 0–7 day: 7.5 mg/kg q12 hr >7 day: 15 mg/kg q12 hr	35–50 mg/day	250 mg or 2 g	T.i.d. for 5–10 days, or single dose	For trichomonas or amebiasis Avoid ingestion of ethanol.
Mezlocillin	IV, IM	0–7 day: 75 mg/kg q12 hr >7 day: 75 mg/kg q8 hr	200–300 mg/kg/ day	200–450 mg/ kg/day	Divide q4–6 hr	
Midazolam HCl (Versed*)	IV		0.035–0.1 mg/kg	1–2.5 mg/ dose	Repeat every 2–3 min if needed.	Duration of action is 30–60 min
	IM		0.08–0.1 mg/kg	5 mg/dose		
Morphine sulfate	IV, IM SQ	0.1 mg/kg/ dose	0.1–0.2 mg/kg/ dose	10–15 mg	Every 4 hr	Higher dose used for Fallot's te-tralogy–induced cyanosis. Anti-dote is naloxone.
Moxalactam	IV, IM		200 mg/kg/day	2–6 g/day	Divided q6 hr	For treatment of meningitis

* Trade Name.

TABLE 146–1. Emergency Drugs (*continued*)

Drug	Route	Neonate	Pediatric	Adult	Administration	Comment
					Dosage	
N-acetylcysteine	PO, NG		140–200 mg/kg	140–200 mg/kg	Loading dose	Dilute 1:4 to give PO. Use higher dose if activated charcoal has been given.
			70 mg/kg q4 hr	70 mg/kg q4 hr	Maintenance dose for 17 doses maximum.	
Nadolol	PO		Adolescents: same as adult dose	80–240 mg (max 640 mg/day)	Once daily	A nonspecific beta-blocker
Nafcillin sodium	IV, IM	<2000 g 0–7 day: 25 mg/kg q12 hr >7 day: 25 mg/kg q8 hr >2000 g 0–7 day: 50 mg/kg/ divide q8 hr >7 day: 75 mg/kg/ divide q6 hr	150 mg/kg/day	1 g q4 hr	Divided q6 hr	
Naloxone (Narcan*)	IV, ET, SL	0.1 mg/kg/dose	0.1 mg/kg til 5 yr or 20 kg then 2 mg/dose	0.4–2 mg/dose	Repeat every 2–3 min as needed.	May need doses 10 times higher in large opiate overdoses. Avoid IM route because of poor absorption.
Neomycin	PO		50–100 mg/kg/day	4–12 g/day	Divide q6 hr	Adjunct therapy for hepatic coma
Neostigmine methylsulfate	IV, IM SQ	0.05–0.1 mg	0.04 mg/kg/dose	0.5–2 mg/dose	Single dose	Test dose for myasthenia gravis
Netilmicin	IV, IM	0–7 day: 2.5 mg/kg q12 hr >7 day: 2.5 mg/kg q8 hr	3–7.5 mg/kg/day	3–7.5 mg/kg/day	Divided q8 hr	
Nifedipine	PO, SL		0.25–0.5 mg/kg	10–20 mg	Single dose. Repeat in 20–30 min if no effect.	For hypertensive emergency. Chew capsule or puncture capsule to administer the liquid from the gel capsule.
Nitroprusside sodium	IV	0.5–10 μg/kg/min	0.5–10.0 μg/kg/min	35–560 μg/min	Continuous infusion	Use infusion pump and add no other drugs to the solution. Metabolized to cyanide; thus, monitor thiocyanate levels (<12 mg/dL). More than the total amount of 3 mg/kg may cause metabolic acidosis.
Nystatin	PO	100,000 U/dose	1–2 million U/day	1–2 million U/day	Every 6–8 hr	Apply to monilia lesions with a cotton tip

(*continued*)

TABLE 146-1. Emergency Drugs (*continued*)

Drug	Route	Neonate	Pediatric	Adult	Administration	Comment
Oxacillin	IV, IM	<2000 g 0–7 day: 25 mg/kg q12 hr >7 day: 100 mg/kg/ divide q8 hr >2000 g 0–7 day: 25 mg/kg q8 hr >7 day: 150 mg/kg/ divide q6 hr	150–200 mg/kg/ day	1 g q4 hr	Divided q6 hr	
Pancuronium bromide	IV	0.02 mg/kg	0.04–0.1 mg/kg	0.1 mg/kg	Single dose. Repeat every 30–60 minutes as needed.	Used to facilitate mechanical respiration
Paraldehyde	PR		0.3 ml/kg/dose	0.3 ml/kg/ dose	Repeat q6 hr if needed.	Dilute in 1–2 parts olive oil or cottonseed oil. Not compatible with most plastics; use glass.
	IV		0.1 mg/kg	5 ml	Infuse slowly.	Use IV route only in emergencies; may cause pulmonary hemorrhages and metabolic acidosis. Dilute with at least 20 volume 0.9% sodium chloride for injection.
Paregoric tincture	PO	2 drops/kg/ dose	2–10 drops/kg/ dose	5–10 ml	Every 3–4 hr	Morphine concentration is 0.4 mg/ml.
Penicillin G Potassium or sodium	IV	<2000 g 0–7 day: 50,000 U/kg q12 hr >7 day: 50,000 U/kg q8 hr >2000 g 0–7 day: 50,000 U/kg q8 hr >7 day: 50,000 U/kg q6 hr	200–400,000 U/ kg/day	1,000,000–3,000,000 units q2–6 hr	Divide q4 hr	For treatment of meningitis
Penicillin benzathine	IM	50,000 units	<60 lbs, 600,000 U >60 lbs, 1,200,000 U	600,000–1,200,000 units	Single dose	
Penicillin procaine	IM	50,000 units	25–50,000 units/ kg/day	1,000,000 units	Single dose	

TABLE 146–1. Emergency Drugs (*continued*)

Drug	Route	Neonate	Pediatric	Adult	Administration	Comment
			Dosage			
Penicillin V	PO		50–100 mg/kg/day	500 mg q6 hr		For treatment of cat bites
Pentamidine	IM		4 mg/kg/day	4 mg/kg/day	Every 24 hr	Infuse over 60 min.
Pentazocine	IV		0.25–0.5 mg/kg	30 mg	Every 3–4 hr	Watch for adverse CNS reactions.
	IM, SQ		0.5–1 mg/kg	30–60 mg	Every 3–4 hr	Drug has both partial agonist and antagonist opiate effects.
	PO		1–2 mg/kg	50–100 mg (max 600 mg/day)	Every 3–4 hr	
Pentobarbital	IV		Load: 15 mg/kg then 0.5–2 mg/kg/hr	5 mg/kg, then 1–2 mg/kg/hr	Bolus then continuous infusion.	To induce pentobarb coma. Observe for hypotension. Solution is highly alkaline; extravasation should be prevented.
Phenobarbital	IV, IO	Load: 15–20 mg/kg	15–20 mg/kg	1000–2000 mg	Give slowly over 20–30 min.	For anti-seizure treatment.
	IV or PO	Maintenance: 3–5 mg/kg/day	3–5 mg/kg/day	100–300 mg/day	Start 12 hr after loading dose.	For sedation, use 1–3 mg/kg/day.
Phenoxybenzamine	PO		1–5 mg/kg (max 10 mg/kg)	10 mg	Every 12 hr.	For treatment of pheochromocytoma.
Phentolamine mesylate (Regitine*)	IV		0.02–0.1 mg/kg	1–5 mg	Single dose	Pheochromocytoma test dose; use lower dose first. Lower dose also used for hypertensive emergencies.
Phenylephrine	IV Load	0.01 mg/kg/dose	0.05–0.1 mg/kg/dose	0.1–0.5 mg	Single dose then	Watch for bradycardia.
	Infusion	0.3–0.5 μg/kg/min	20–60 μg/min	20–60 μg/min	continuous infusion	
Phenytoin	IV, IO then PO	Load: 20 mg/kg	20 mg/kg	1000–1500 mg	Loading dose then	For anti-seizure treatment. Infuse slowly over 20–30 mins. to avoid hypotension, bradycardia, and dysrrhythmias. Poor oral absorption in infants <1 yr; higher dosages may be needed.
		5–15 mg/day	4–8 mg/kg/day	300–600 mg/day	oral maintenance	
	IV		2–5 mg/kg/dose	100–300 mg/dose	Repeat up to 20 mg/kg.	For anti-arrhythmic treatment
Physostigmine salicylate	IV, IM		0.03–0.5 mg/kg	1–2 mg	Single dose. Repeat once in 15–30 min.	Rapidly degraded in 1–2 hr. Do not use in tricyclic and related drug overdoses because it may cause bradycardia, hypotension.
Pindolol	PO		Adolescents: Same as adult dose	10–20 mg (max 60 mg/day)	2–3 times daily	Nonspecific beta-blocker.
Piperacillin	IV		200–300 mg/kg/day	4–24 g/day	Divided q4–6 hr	Not approved for use in children
Piperazine citrate	PO		75 mg/kg/day (max 3.5 g/day)	3.5 g/day	Every 24 hr	For 2 days for ascaris treatment
			65 mg/kg/day (max 2.5 g/day)	2.5 g/day	Every 24 hr	For 7 days for pinworm treatment

(*continued*)

* Trade Name.

TABLE 146–1. Emergency Drugs (*continued*)

Drug	Route	Neonate	Pediatric	Adult	Administration	Comment
Polystyrene sodium sulfonate (Kayexalate*)	PO	1 g/kg/dose	1 g/kg/dose	50 g	Single dose	Each g exchanges 1 mEq K$^+$. Used in suspension with sorbitol.
	PR	1.5–2 g/kg/dose	1.5–2 g/kg/dose	50–100 g	Single dose	Rectal administration requires 30–45 min retention time.
Pralidoxime (2-PAM) (Protopam*)	IV		25–50 mg/kg/dose	1–2 g/dose	Repeat every 4–12 hr as needed.	Used with atropine in serious organophosphate poisoning. Can be given as a continuous IV infusion (500 mg/hr)
Prazosin	PO		25 µg/kg/dose (max. 250 µg/kg/day)	1 mg/dose (max. 20–40 mg total/day)	2–3 times daily	
Prednisone	PO	1–2 mg/kg/day	1–2 mg/kg/day	40–120 mg/day	Once-a-day dose or 3–4 divided doses	Can be used for alternate-day regimens
Primidone	PO		10–25 mg/kg/day	750–1500 mg/day	Divide b.i.d.-q.i.d.	Metabolized to phenobarbital
Probenecid	PO		10–25 mg/kg	1 g	Single dose	Used in co-treatment of gonorrhea
Procainamide	IV		1 mg/kg q5 min (max 10–15 mg/kg) then	50–100 mg Repeat q10–30 min to 500 mg	Slowly over 5 mins.	Metabolized to active metabolite N-acetyl-procainamide (NAPA). Use caution in renal impairment.
	IV infusion or		20–50 µg/kg/min	1–6 mg/min		
	PO		5–15 mg/kg q4–6 hr	0.5–1 g q4–6 hr		
Prochlorperazine (Compazine*)	IV, IM		0.13 mg/kg (max 5 mg)	2.5–10 mg	3–4 doses/day	Watch for delayed-onset dystonic reactions.
	PO, PR		0.4 mg/kg (max 10 mg)	10–25 mg	2–4 doses/day	
Promethazine	IM, PO PR		0.25–1 mg/kg (max 2 mg/kg)	25–50 mg	3–4 doses/day	Larger doses may cause dystonic reactions and CNS stimulation.
Propranolol	IV	0.01–0.15 mg/kg	0.01–0.25 mg/kg (max 1 mg/dose)	1–10 mg	Slow IV (1 mg/min). Repeat in 5 min if needed, up to 0.1 mg/kg, then q4–8 hr	A nonspecific betablocker of moderate duration
	PO	1 mg/kg	0.5–2 mg/kg	10–40 mg	Every 6 hr	Up to 320 mg total dose has been used.
Prostaglandin E1 (PGE1)	IV, IA	0.05–0.1 µg/kg/min (max 0.5 µg/kg/min)	0.002–0.5 µg/kg/min		Continuous infusion	Maintenance dose is usually half the initial dose. IV route is preferred to intra-arterial infusion. Prepared solution is stable for 24 hrs.
Pseudoephedrine	PO		4–5 mg/kg/day	30–60 mg	Every 4–6 hr	Dextro isomer with half the activity of ephedrine

* Trade Name.

TABLE 146–1. Emergency Drugs (*continued*)

Drug	Route	Neonate	Pediatric	Adult	Administration	Comment
Pyridoxine	IV, IM		5–10 g	5–10 g	Single dose	For isoniazid overdose, give 1 g of pyridoxine per g of isoniazid ingested.
	PO, IV		25 mg/kg	25 mg/kg	Single dose	For monomethylhydrazine-type mushroom poisoning.
Quinidine gluconate	IV, IM		2 mg/kg/dose	200 mg	Single test dose	Procainamide is preferred for parenteral use.
sulfate	PO		30 mg/kg/day	200–400 mg	4–5 doses a day	Quinidine is preferred for oral use.
Ranitidine	IV	0.2 mg/kg/hr	0.1 mg/kg/hr or 2–6 mg/kg/day (max 50 mg)	50–100 mg/dose	Every 6 hr	Not approved for use in pediatric patients. Doses stated are based on case reports from the manufacturer.
Reserpine	IM		0.02–0.07 mg/kg/day (max 2.5 mg/day)	0.25–1 mg	1–2 doses/day	May cause nasal stuffiness. Onset of action is delayed up to 12 hr.
	PO		0.02–0.03 mg/kg/day	0.25–0.5 mg	1–2 doses/day	
Rifampin	PO		8–10 mg/kg/dose	300 mg	b.i.d. for 2–4 days	Used for prophylaxis of *Haemophilus influenzae* and meningococcal disease
			10–20 mg/kg/dose	300–600 mg	Single dose	Combined therapy for treatment of tuberculosis. All body secretions turn orange.
Scopolamine HBr	IM, SQ PO		0.006 mg/kg	0.4 mg	Single dose	
Secobarbital	IV, IM SQ		1–2 mg/kg	100–200 mg	Single dose	Use one-half dose as sedative dose
	PO		3–6 mg/kg/dose	100–200 mg		
Sodium bicarbonate	IV	1–2 mEq/kg	1–2 mEq/kg	50 mEq	Single dose. Repeat q5–10 min if needed.	Do not mix with calcium salts, epinephrine, or dopamine. Avoid overcorrection of metabolic acidosis.
	2% lavage		1 ampule (44.6 mEq/50 ml)	in 150 ml of water		Lavage solution used in iron poisoning
Sodium iodide	IV		25 mg/kg/dose	1000 mg	Single dose; repeat if needed.	
Sodium nitrite 3%	IV		10 mg/kg/dose (0.3 ml/kg/dose)	6–8 ml	Single dose given slowly	For cyanide poisoning
Sodium sulfate	PO		300 mg/kg/dose	15 g	Single dose	Used for barium poisoning.
Sodium thiosulfate 25%	IV		250 mg/kg/dose (1 ml/kg/dose)	12.5 g (50 ml)	Single dose	For cyanide poisoning. Use 25% solution. Monitor blood pressure.
Spectinomycin	IM		30–40 mg/kg	2–4 g	Single deep IM injection	Not approved for use in children

(*continued*)

TABLE 146–1. Emergency Drugs (*continued*)

Drug	Route	Neonate	Pediatric	Adult	Administration	Comment
			Dosage			
Streptomycin sulfate	IM		20–50 mg/kg/dose	1–2 g	1–2 doses/day	Reduce dose in renal impairment.
Succinylcholine	IV		1–2 mg/kg	0.3–1.1 mg/kg	Single dose; repeat if needed.	Avoid use in organophosphate and carbamate poisoning. Use caution in patients with preexisting hyperkalemia, or beware of inducing hyperkalemia.
Sulfadiazine	IV, SQ		100 mg/kg/day		Divide q6–8 hr	
	PO		120–150 mg/kg/day	2–4 g/day	Divide q4–6 hr	
Sulfisoxazole	PO		120–150 mg/kg/day	1 g	Every 4–6 hr	Avoid giving to neonates and pregnant women. May cause hyperbilirubinemia
TAC 0.5% tetracaine 1:200 epinephrine 11.8% cocaine	Topical		4–10 ml		Single application for maximum of 10 minutes.	Must avoid mucous membrane absorption, which may cause seizures.
Terbutaline	SQ		0.25 mg/dose	0.25 mg/dose	Single dose	Repeat in 15–30 min to max 0.5 mg q4 hr
	0.1% inhalant		0.1–0.2 mg/kg (1–2 ml/kg) (max 1–2 mg)	400 μg/dose	Single dose; repeat q4–6 hr	Wait 1 minute between inhalations.
	PO		2.5–5 mg (max 7.5 mg/day)	2.5–5 mg (max 15 mg/day)	t.i.d.	
Tetracycline	PO		25–50 mg/kg/day	250 mg q6 hr	Divided q6 hr	Avoid use in children <7 yrs because of teeth discoloration.
	IV		20–30 mg/kg/day	250–500 mg q12 hr	Divided q8–12 hr	Do not exceed 4 g/day, especially in pregnant females.
	IM		15–25 mg/kg/day	300 mg/day or 250 mg q24 hr	Divided q8–12 hr	
Theophylline	PO	Load: 4–5 mg/kg	5–6 mg/kg	200–400 mg/dose	Single dose	Aminophylline is 85% theophylline with ethylenediamine for parenteral use.
		Maintenance: 1–2 mg/kg/dose	12–30 mg/kg/day	200–400 mg/dose	Neonates: Every 12–24 hr	Neonates metabolize theophylline slowly.
					Children and adults: every 6 hr	Some children metabolize theophylline rapidly, and large daily doses (up to 60 mg/kg/day) or frequent dosing may be necessary.
Thiamylal (Surital*)	IV		4 mg/kg			
Thiopental (Pentothal*)	IV		4–6 mg/kg			

* Trade Name.

TABLE 146–1. Emergency Drugs (*continued*)

Drug	Route	Dosage Neonate	Dosage Pediatric	Dosage Adult	Administration	Comment
Ticarcillin	IV	<2000 g 0–7 day: 75 mg/kg q12 hr >7 day: 75 mg/kg q8 hr >2000 g 0–7 day: 75 mg/kg q8 hr >7 day: 75 mg/kg q6 hr	200–300 mg/kg/day	200–300 mg/kg/day	Divide q4–6 hr	Not approved for use in children.
Tobramycin	IV, IM	0–7 day: 2 mg/kg q12 hr >7 day: 2 mg/kg q8 hr	3–6 mg/kg/day	3–8 mg/kg/day	Divide q8 hr	Larger doses (7–10 mg/kg/day) for patients with cystic fibrosis.
Tolazoline	IV		2 mg/kg/ then 1–2 mg/kg/hr	1–2 mg/kg then 1–2 mg/kg/hr	Single bolus	
Trimethadione	PO		Load: 25–50 mg/kg/day Maintenance: 40 mg/kg/day	900 mg/day 300–600 mg/dose	Every 6–8 hr	
Trimethaphan camsylate	IV		50–150 μg/kg/min	0.5–6 mg/min	Slow IV infusion	Very potent ganglionic blocker
Trimethoprim	PO		4 mg/kg/day		Every 12 hr	
Trimethoprim/sulfamethoxazole (TMP/SMX) (Bactrim*, Septra*)	PO IV		8–12 mg TMP–30–60 mg SMX/kg/day 20 mg TMP–100 mg SMX/kg/day		Every 12 hr Every 6 hr	 For *Pneumocystis carinii*
Valproic acid (Valproate)	PO		15–60 mg/kg/day	100–3000 mg	Single or divided doses	
Vancomycin	IV	<2000 g 0–7 day: 10 mg/kg q12 hr >7 day: 10 mg/kg q8 hr >2000 g 0–7 day: 15 mg/kg q12 hr >7 day: 40 mg/kg/ divided q8 hr	40–60 mg/kg/day	1 g q12 hr or 500 mg q6 hr	Divided q6 hr	"Red man syndrome" rash if infused too rapidly (less than 30 min); thus, infuse over 60 min.

(*continued*)

TABLE 146–1. Emergency Drugs (*continued*)

Drug	Route	Dosage: Neonate	Dosage: Pediatric	Dosage: Adult	Dosage: Administration	Comment
Vasopressin	IM		0.2–2 ml/dose	1–2 ml	Single dose	Warm and shake well to dissolve completely before using. Suspension is in peanut oil; thus, use caution in allergic individuals.
	Tannate in oil: 5 U/ml			Repeat once or q2–3 days as needed		
	SQ Aqueous 20 U/ml		1–3 ml/day	1–3 ml/day	Every 8 hr	
	IV		<5 yr: 0.10–0.2 U/min	0.1–0.4 U/min	Continuous infusion	
			5–12 yr: 0.1–0.3 U/min			
Verapamil	IV	Contra-indicated under 6 mo	<1 yr: 0.1–0.2 mg/kg (max 5–10 mg)	5–10 mg/dose	Bolus over 2 min.	Do not give with disopyramide. Lower dose when used with digoxin.
			1–15 yr: 0.1–0.3 mg/kg		Repeat every 30 min once or twice.	
Vitamin B_6 (see Pyridoxine)						
Vitamin C	PO		100–500 mg/day	100–500 mg/day	Single or divided doses	Used in hereditary methemoglobinemia
Vitamin K (phytonadione)	IV	1–2 mg	5–10 mg	10 mg	Single dose	Rapid IV can cause hypotension.
	IM, SQ	0.5–1 mg	1–2 mg		Single dose	For prophylaxis
		1–5 mg	5–10 mg	10 mg	Single dose	For treatment of vitamin K deficiency
						Total doses >25 mg in neonates may cause hyperbilirubinemia.
	PO	2 mg	5–10 mg	10 mg	Single dose	For treatment of vitamin K deficiency

TABLE 146–2. ***Therapeutic Drug Monitoring***

Drug	Therapeutic Range (ug/ml)	Toxic Levels (ug/ml)	Comments
Acetaminophen	5–20	>140 at 4 hrs post ingestion	Use Rumack-Matthew nomogram.
Amikacin	Peak 20–30	>35	Monitor renal function.
	Trough 5–10		
Amitriptyline	50–300 ng/ml	>500 ng/ml	Combined with metabolite, nortriptyline, for a total level
Azidothymidine (AZT, zidovudine)	>1 uM	Undetermined	
Barbiturates (see individual drugs)			
Barbital	5–8	>30	
Butabarbital	10–14	>30	

TABLE 146-2. Therapeutic Drug Monitoring (*continued*)

Drug	Therapeutic Range (ug/ml)	Toxic Levels (ug/ml)	Comments
Caffeine	3–15	>50	
Carbamazepine	4–8	>15	
Chloramphenicol	Peak 10–25	>25	Gray-baby syndrome associated with levels >25 μg/ml
	Trough 5–10		
Cyanide	<0.5	>1	
Diazepam	100–1000 ng/ml	>5000 ng/ml	
Digitoxin	9–30 ng/ml	>45 ng/ml	Obtain blood sample 6–12 hrs after dose.
Digoxin	0.5–2 ng/ml	>2.2 ng/ml	Obtain blood sample 6–12 hr after dose. Toxicity can occur in the therapeutic range.
Ethanol		>50–100 mg/dL	Observe for hypoglycemia in children.
Etchlorvynol		>20	
Ethosuximide	40–100	>150	
Ethylene glycol		>20 mg/dL	
Gentamicin	Peak 6–10	>12	Monitor renal function.
	Trough 1–2		
Glutethimide	5–10	>20	
Iron	50–150 ug/dl	>350–500 ug/dl	
Isopropanol		40–80 mg/dl	
Kanamycin	Peak 25–35	>40	Monitor renal function.
	Trough 4–8	>10–15	
Lidocaine	1.5–6	>8	
Lithium	0.5–1.2 mEq/L	>2 mEq/L	Differentiate between an acute vs. chronic toxic level.
Meprobamate	6–12	>60	
Methemoglobin	<4%	>10%	
Methanol		>20 mg/dL	
Netilmicin	Peak 6–10	>12	Monitor renal function.
	Trough <2	>2	
NAPA (N-acetylprocainamide)—see Procainamide			
Pentobarbital	20–50		For barb coma
Phenobarbital	10–40	>50–60	
Phenytoin	10–20	>40	
Primidone	5–12	>15	
Procainamide	4–8	>10	Active metabolite is NAPA; thus maintain sum of 10–30 ug/ml.
NAPA	2–8		
Quinidine	3–5	>8	
Salicylate	50–350	>400	Differentiate between an acute vs. chronic poisoning. Beware: former units were mg/dL.
Secobarbital	1–5	>10	

(*continued*)

TABLE 146–2. Therapeutic Drug Monitoring (*continued*)

Drug	Therapeutic Range (ug/ml)	Toxic Levels (ug/ml)	Comments
Theophylline	5–20	>20	Differentiate between an acute vs. chronic poisoning
	5–13	>15	For premature apnea
Thiocyanate	5–10	>50–100	Optimally keep below 12 ug/ml.
Tobramycin	Peak 6–10	>10–15	Monitor renal function.
	Trough 1–2	2–4	
Valproic acid	50–100	>100	
Vancomycin	Peak 30–50	>80–100	Monitor renal function.
	Trough 5–10		

9. Avoid drug incompatibilities when giving more than one solution concurrently.
10. Use proper infusion pumps to ensure careful titration. Label infusions with red labels and do not add other medications.
11. Standardize a drug report form or "Code Blue" report. This form must include names and doses of drugs (with concentrations or volumes, when appropriate), start and stop times, and, if possible, response to therapy.
12. Ensure that emergency drugs are properly charted by a knowledgeable person. Designate this person in advance.

Table 146-1 provides detailed information about generic drug dosages, routes of administration, and dosing intervals for emergency medications available for use in neonates, children, and adults. Table 146-2 lists therapeutic and toxic levels of common medications used in pediatric practice.

Index

P

JB Lippincott Titles of Related Interest

Jeffrey L. Brown, MD: *Pediatric Telephone Medicine:*
Principles, Triage and Advice
Ann L. Harwood-Nuss, MD: *Clinical Practice of Emergency Medicine*
Jacob A. Lohr, MD: *Pediatric Outpatient Procedures*
Hugh L. Moffet, MD: *Pediatric Infectious Diseases, 3rd edition*
Frank A. Oski, MD: *Principles and Practice of Pediatrics*